REFERENCE COPY

615.4 ENC

AGNG

LIBRARY
ROYAL
PHARMACEUTICAL SOCIETY
12 OCT 1994
1, LAMBETH HIGH STREET
LONDON SE1 7JN

RPSGB LIBRARY
211114

ENCYCLOPEDIA OF PHARMACEUTICAL TECHNOLOGY

VOLUME 11

ENCYCLOPEDIA OF PHARMACEUTICAL TECHNOLOGY

Editors

JAMES SWARBRICK
Vice President
Research and Development
AAI, Inc.
Wilmington, North Carolina

JAMES C. BOYLAN
Director
Pharmaceutical Technology
Hospital Products Division
Abbott Laboratories
Abbott Park, Illinois

VOLUME 11

NUCLEAR MEDICINE AND PHARMACY TO PERMEATION ENHANCEMENT THROUGH SKIN

MARCEL DEKKER, INC. NEW YORK ● BASEL ● HONG KONG

Library of Congress Cataloging in Publication Data
Main entry under title:

Encyclopedia of Pharmaceutical Technology.
editors: James Swarbrick, James C. Boylan.

Includes index.
1. Pharmaceutical technology—Dictionaries. I. Swarbrick, James.
II. Boylan, James C.
[DNLM: 1. Chemistry, Pharmaceutical-encyclopedias. 2. Drugs—encyclopedias. 3. Technology, Pharmaceutical-encyclopedias. QV 13 E565].
RS192.E53 1988 615'.1'0321-dc19

COPYRIGHT © 1995 BY MARCEL DEKKER, INC. ALL RIGHTS RESERVED.

Neither this book nor any part may be reproduced or transmitted in any form or by any means, electronic or mechanical, including photocopying, microfilming, and recording, or by any information storage and retrieval system, without permission in writing from the publisher.

MARCEL DEKKER, INC.
270 Madison Avenue, New York, New York 10016

LIBRARY OF CONGRESS CATALOG CARD NUMBER: 88-25664
ISBN: 0-8247-2810-6

Current printing (last digit):
10 9 8 7 6 5 4 3 2 1

PRINTED IN THE UNITED STATES OF AMERICA

CONTENTS OF VOLUME 11

CONTRIBUTORS TO VOLUME 11

Michael J. Akers, Ph.D. Senior Research Scientist, Lilly Research Laboratories, Indianapolis, Indiana: *Parenterals: Small Volume*

Carolyn H. Asbury, Ph.D. Director, Health and Human Services Program, The Pew Charitable Trusts, Philadelphia, Pennsylvania: *Orphan Drugs*

Ajay K. Banga, Ph.D. Assistant Professor, Department of Pharmacal Science, School of Pharmacy, Auburn University, Auburn, Alabama: *Peptide and Protein Drug Delivery*

Brian W. Barry Professor of Pharmaceutical Technology, The School of Pharmacy, University of Bradford, Bradford, United Kingdom: *Permeation Enhancement through Skin*

James Blanchard, Ph.D. Professor of Pharmaceutical Sciences, College of Pharmacy, The University of Arizona, Tucson, Arizona: *Ocular Drug Formulation and Delivery*

Richard E. Brownlee, Jr., M.D. Assistant Professor, Department of Otolaryngology, University of Florida, Gainesville, Florida: *Otic Preparations*

Pieter de Haan, Ph.D. Department of Pharmaceutics, Organon International, Oss, The Netherlands: *Optimization Techniques in Formulation and Processing*

Suketu D. Desai, Ph.D. Senior Scientist, Drug Delivery, R&D, Alcon Laboratories, Inc., Fort Worth, Texas: *Ocular Drug Formulation and Delivery*

Durk A. Doornbos, Ph.D. Professor, University Centre for Pharmacy, and Groningen Institute for Drug Studies, University of Groningen, Groningen, The Netherlands: *Optimization Techniques in Formulation and Processing*

Thomas J. Franz, M.D. Professor, Department of Dermatology, University of Arkansas for Medical Sciences, Little Rock, Arkansas: *Percutaneous Absorption*

Isaac Ghebre-Sellassie, Ph.D. Associate Professor Fellow, Product Development, Parke-Davis Pharmaceutical Research, Warner-Lambert Company, Morris Plains, New Jersey: *Pelletization Techniques*

Michael J. Groves, Ph.D. Professor of Pharmaceutics and Director, The Institute for Tuberculosis Research, College of Pharmacy, University of Illinois at Chicago, Chicago, Illinois: *Particulate Matter in Parenteral Products*

Brian H. Kaye, Ph.D. Professor of Physics, Department of Physics and Astronomy, Laurentian University, Sudbury, Ontario, Canada: *Particle-Size Characterization*

Axel Knoch, Ph.D. Godecke AG, Freiburg, Germany: *Pelletization Techniques*

Richard J. Kowalsky, Pharm. D. Associate Professor of Pharmacy and Radiology, Director, Nuclear Pharmacy, UNC Hospitals, The University of North Carolina at Chapel Hill, Chapel Hill, North Carolina: *Nuclear Medicine and Pharmacy*

Paul A. Lehman, M.S. Professor, Department of Dermatology, University of Arkansas for Medical Sciences, Little Rock, Arkansas: *Percutaneous Absorption*

Eric J. Lien, Ph.D. Professor, Biomedical Chemistry and Pharmaceutics, Department of Pharmaceutical Sciences, School of Pharmacy, University of South California, Los Angeles, California: *Partition Coefficients*

Alan F. Parr, Ph.D. Research Leader, Glaxo, Inc., Research Triangle Park, North Carolina: *Nuclear Medicine and Pharmacy*

Rosalie Sagraves, Pharm. D. Professor and Associate Head, Section of Pharmacy Practice, College of Pharmacy, Health Sciences Center, The University of Oklahoma: *Pediatric Dosing and Dosage Forms*

William H. Slattery III, M.D. Associate, House Ear Clinic; Research Coordinator, House Ear Institute, Los Angeles, California: *Otic Preparations*

Stuart R. Suter, Ph.D. Vice President and Patent Counsel, SmithKline Beecham, Philadelphia, Pennsylvania: *Patents in the Pharmaceutical Industry*

Salvatore J. Turco, Pharm. D. Professor of Pharmacy, Temple University School of Pharmacy, Philadelphia, Pennsylvania: *Parenterals: Large Volume*

Lorraine L. Wearley, Ph.D. Director of Product Development, Advanced Care Products, Ortho Pharmaceutical Corp., North Brunswick, New Jersey: *Peptide and Protein Drug Delivery*

Adrian C. Williams, Ph.D. Lecturer in Pharmaceutical Technology, The School of Pharmacy, University of Bradford, Bradford, United Kingdom: *Permeation Enhancement through Skin*

CONTENTS OF OTHER VOLUMES

CONTENTS OF VOLUME 1

ROYAL PHARMACEUTICAL SOCIETY LIBRARY
1, LAMBETH HIGH STREET, LONDON SE1 7JN

CONTENTS OF VOLUME 2

CONTENTS OF VOLUME 3

CONTENTS OF VOLUME 4

CONTENTS OF VOLUME 5

CONTENTS OF VOLUME 6

CONTENTS OF VOLUME 7

CONTENTS OF VOLUME 8

CONTENTS OF VOLUME 9

CONTENTS OF VOLUME 10

ENCYCLOPEDIA OF PHARMACEUTICAL TECHNOLOGY

VOLUME 11

Nuclear Medicine and Pharmacy

Introduction

The application of radiation in medicine began soon after the discovery of x-rays by Roentgen in 1895, when he produced the first x-ray image of his wife's hand. Becquerel discovered radioactivity in uranium salts in 1896, Marie and Pierre Curie discovered polonium and radium in 1898, and isotopes were identified in natural radioactive substances by Soddy in 1910. In 1934 the era of artificial isotopes was initiated when the French radiochemists, J. F. Joliot and his wife Irene Curie-Joliot, discovered induced radioactivity after bombarding a piece of aluminum foil with alpha particles. They produced the first artificial radioisotope, phosphorus-30. In the same year, Lawrence produced artificial radionuclides by bombardment of stable elements with accelerated particles in a cyclotron, which he first conceived and built at the University of California at Berkeley. One of these radionuclides, sodium-24, the first artificial radioisotope used in therapy, was used unsuccessfully to treat leukemia in humans. The discovery of nuclear fission by Hahn and Strassmann in Germany in 1939 led to the eventual development of the first self-sustaining nuclear chain reaction in a uranium graphite "pile" at the University of Chicago under the direction of Fermi. Although nuclear reactors were first developed to produce plutonium, the main product used in atomic bombs, numerous artifical radionuclides or by-products were also obtained. After World War II, these radionuclides were sold for peacetime use. It was during this time that many radiotracer substances, labeled with radioisotopes such as hydrogen-3, carbon-14, phosphorus-32, chromium-51, iodine-131, and mercury-203, were developed and used to study biological processes in plants, animals, and humans. It was also the time when nuclear medicine established its roots. Over the years more sophisticated radiotracers and imaging equipment have been developed to the point that today all the major organ systems in the body can be imaged.

Nuclear medicine not only has evolved into a discipline unto itself, but the radiotracer methodology that it employs has been adopted by other medical disciplines, such as cardiology and pulmonary medicine, as analytical tools in research and clinical practice. In the pharmaceutical industry nuclear medicine techniques are used in the development of new drugs. Indeed, the ability to label dosage forms with gamma-emitting nuclides has permitted researchers to perform in vivo evaluation of dosage forms with the help of nuclear imaging techniques. Nuclear medicine and pharmacy have one common aim, that is, drug targeting in the body. Nuclear medicine uses drug molecules as carriers of radionuclides to target radioactivity to organs for diagnostic evaluation and radiotherapy, while a primary goal of pharmaceutical development in pharmacy is to target drug molecules to receptor body sites for therapeutic effect. Although it is not uncommon for pharmacy researchers to use radiation in the evaluation of a drug's pharmacokinetics and pharmacodynamics, it is also not uncommon for nuclear medicine practitioners to use pharmacologic agents to augment nuclear medicine studies. This article considers these aspects of nuclear medicine and pharmacy.

Radiation in Medicine

Radiation is used in medicine as a diagnostic and therapeutic tool. Several diagnostic radiology modalities use electromagnetic radiation to ''peer'' inside the body. Conventional radiography and x-ray computorized tomography (CT) employ x-rays to produce images of internal body structures. Diagnostic ultrasound uses high frequency sound waves to create sonograms of internal structures, whereas magnetic resonance imaging (MRI) uses magnetic fields and radiofrequency radiation to generate images. In the future, magnetic resonance spectroscopy may also be useful for measuring biochemical changes in vivo. Anatomic information is the principal contribution of these diagnostic imaging modalities.

Nuclear medicine can also provide anatomic information, but its principal purpose is the acquisition of functional information through the measurement of in vivo changes of radiopharmaceutical distribution caused by disease. For example, diagnostic ultrasound can demonstrate the presence of gallstones in the cystic duct of a patient with gallbladder disease, but it cannot determine if these stones obstruct bile flow. However, by means of a radiopharmaceutical that is excreted into the bile, a nuclear hepatobiliary scan can determine whether or not the stones actually obstruct bile flow into the gallbladder and intestinal tract. Thus, a complementary role is sometimes played between imaging modalities. Another example is pulmonary embolism where a blood clot obstructs arterial blood flow in the lung. The obstruction can be detected immediately after it occurs with a perfusion lung scan. In this situation, the nuclear medicine examination can provide early information about the patient's condition, facilitating medical treatment. The embolism could also be identified by an angiogram, a more complicated procedure where an x-ray contrast agent is injected into the pulmonary circulation during an x-ray exam. Although an angiogram can identify the exact location of an embolus, the procedure involves a higher risk and is not necessary in all cases. The lung scan serves as a safe, simple screening procedure and often provides all the information needed to provide good patient care.

Ionizing radiation is also used therapeutically to destroy diseased tissue, such as cancer. Most radiation therapy treatments are conducted by specialists in radiation oncology who use high intensity gamma radiation to treat tumors. The radiation source may be a machine containing a high activity radionuclide such as cobalt-60 (teletherapy) or the source may be contained in a removable applicator which is implanted in the body close to the tumor (brachytherapy). In nuclear medicine, therapy is accomplished with radiopharmaceuticals which direct the radionuclide to the organ being treated.

Radiopharmaceuticals

A radiopharmaceutical is a chemical substance that contains a radioactive atom (radionuclide) within its structure and which is suitable for human use in the diagnosis and treatment of disease. Radiopharmaceuticals are formulated in various physicochemical forms to deliver the radioactive atoms to particular parts of the body. Once localized, a diagnostic radiopharmaceutical emits gamma radiation which escapes from the body, permitting external detection and measurement. A scintillation camera detects the gamma radiation and creates an image of the radioactivity distribution in the organ. In this way, the nuclear medicine physician can evaluate the function and morphology of various organs in the body.

The amount of radioactivity administered to a patient in a nuclear medicine procedure is termed the dosage and is usually measured in units of millicuries (mCi or 10^{-3} Ci). The Curie (Ci), which is equal to 3.7×10^{10} disintegrations (atoms decaying) per second, is the traditional measure of radioactivity currently used in the United States. The international unit (IU) of radioactivity is the Becquerel (Bq) which is equal to one disintegration per second (1 mCi = 37 MBq). The amount of radiation absorbed by tissue in the body in which a radioactive substance resides is termed the radiation dose, traditionally measured in units of rads. One rad (radiation absorbed dose) is equal to 100 ergs of energy absorbed per gram of tissue. The IU of absorbed dose, the Gray (Gy), is equal to one joule of energy absorbed dose per kilogram of tissue (1 Gy = 100 rads). A goal in diagnostic nuclear medicine is to administer the optimum dosage of radioactivity needed with the minimum radiation absorbed to the patient. The clinical usefulness of a radiopharmaceutical is determined, in part, by the radionuclide's physical properties, that is, its radiation, energy, and half-life. In general, the lowest radiation dose and the best diagnostic images are obtained if the radionuclide has a short half-life and emits only gamma radiation of moderate energy. The energy must be high enough to escape the body with minimal scatter and low enough to be efficiently stopped by the gamma camera detector. Technetium, Tc-99m, is a good example, having a six-hour half-life and gamma emission of 140 keV.

Radionuclides for therapy, on the other hand, should emit particulate radiation (beta particles), which deposit their radiation within the organ. Phosphorus P-32 emits only beta radiation. Some radionuclides emit beta and gamma radiation simultaneously and therefore possess both therapeutic and diagnostic usefulness; iodine, I-131, is a prime example.

Aside from its nuclear properties, a radionuclide is dependent on its chemical form for localization in specific organs. Thus I-131, as the iodide anion localizes in the thyroid gland, but covalently bonded to orthoiodohippuric acid is excreted by the kidney, and bonded to an antibody seeks out the tumor that expresses the complementary antigen. Therefore, several different chemical forms may be labeled with the same radionuclide. Technetium, Tc-99m, is another example. In addition to its desirable nuclear properties, its unique chemistry makes it suitable to the production of several different radiopharmaceuticals. Another advantage of Tc-99m is its ready availability in hospitals from a generator system. On a daily basis, Tc-99m is eluted with saline from a molybdenum, Mo-99–Tc-99m generator. The sterile solution of sodium pertechnetate obtained may be used as is or to prepare other Tc-99m-labeled radiopharmaceuticals. Because of these advantages, Tc-99m is the radionuclide used in most nuclear medicine studies. Other examples are listed in Table 1. A wide variety of chemical forms comprise the list of radiotracers used in nuclear medicine, ranging from elemental gases and simple ions to labeled molecules, small particles, and blood cells.

Radioactivity and the attendant risk of biologic damage due to absorbed radiation distinguishes radiopharmaceuticals from traditional drugs. What is less apparent, however, is that radioactive drugs present little, if any, toxicologic risk because of the extremely small amount of chemical substance administered. For example, the largest dosage of radionuclide administered in nuclear medicine (200 mCi of I-131) is equivalent to 1.6 μg of iodine and represents only 0.5% of the average daily intake of iodine from dietary

TABLE 1 Radionuclides in Nuclear Medicine

Radionuclide	Decay Mode[a]	Half-life	Photon Energy (keV)
Carbon-11	Beta+	20.3 min	511
Nitrogen-13	Beta+	10.0 min	511
Oxygen-15	Beta+	2.0 min	511
Fluorine-18	Beta+	109.8 min	511
Phosphorus-32	Beta−	14.3 days	none
Chromium-51	EC	27.7 days	320
Cobalt-57	EC	271.8 days	122,136
Gallium-67	EC	78.3 h	93,185,300
Molybdenum-99	Beta−	65.9 h	740,784
Technetium-99m	IT	6.0 h	140
Indium-111	EC	2.8 days	172,247
Iodine-123	EC	13.1 h	159
Iodine-125	EC	59.9 days	27,35
Iodine-131	Beta−	8.0 days	364,637
Xenon-133	Beta−	5.3 days	81
Thallium-201	EC	73.1 h	69,71,80

[a]EC = electron capture; IT = isomeric transition; Beta+ = positron; Beta− = negatron.

sources. Nevertheless, radiopharmaceuticals are legend drugs in all respects, as defined by the Food and Drug Administration (FDA).

Nuclear Pharmacy

Technetium-99m was discovered in 1937 but not put into clinical use in nuclear medicine until 1964. Prior to that time few pharmacists were involved in nuclear medicine, but the rapid demand for Tc-99m-labeled radiopharmaceuticals and the necessity for their daily preparation created a demand for the pharmacist's expertise in formulation. Thus, an increasing number of pharmacists became trained in the radiation sciences to meet the demand for nuclear pharmacists. During the 1960s and early 1970s most nuclear pharmacists were employed by nuclear medicine departments in hospitals and medical schools. As nuclear medicine services expanded across the country, nuclear pharmacies became established mostly in metropolitan areas. These pharmacies contract with several hospitals in a citywide area, and in some instances statewide area, to provide radiopharmaceuticals on a prescription basis to their nuclear medicine departments. Over the years a few large corporations were formed by merging several smaller nuclear pharmacies. Today most nuclear pharmacists are employed by these large corporations. However, several smaller independent nuclear pharmacies still operate nationwide.

The daily routine in a nuclear pharmacy involves elution of the Tc-99m generator, preparing Tc-99m-labeled radiopharmaceuticals for the day's studies, performing quality control tests on these agents and on radiation-measuring instruments, and checking-in prepared radiopharmaceuticals received from commercial manufacturers. Since most radiopharmaceuticals are parenteral products, aseptic methods must be followed in their preparation and use. Before administration, a prescription order, initiated by a nuclear medicine physician, is reviewed by the pharmacist. Radioactive decay calculations are made and the dose is prepared and radioassayed to ensure the correct amount of radioactivity. The information is recorded and the dose is labeled and appropriately shielded before release for patient use.

The nuclear pharmacist also provides advice to physicians and technologists regarding the clinical use of radiopharmaceuticals, their properties, and stability. A pharmacist's professional opinion is often sought when a scan demonstrates unexpected biodistribution which could be related to a radiopharmaceutical that has degraded or has been improperly formulated, or to patient factors such as disease state or drug interactions. A wide range of questions related to radiopharmaceutical use may be posed to the nuclear pharmacist regarding, for example, the radiation dose to a fetus in utero; pediatric dosage; routes of administration; adverse reactions; drug use in interventional studies; specific physicochemical, pharmaceutical, or kinetic properties of radiopharmaceuticals; and investigational use. The nuclear pharmacist's knowledge of drugs, medical devices, and state and federal regulations make him or her a valuable member of the nuclear medicine health care team.

Procedures

Nuclear medicine studies are used to determine whether a disease is present or to evaluate the progress of disease following therapy and to arrest certain types of illness through the localized in vivo destruction of diseased tissue with radiation.

The types of procedures routinely performed in nuclear medicine with radiopharmaceuticals are imaging procedures, in vivo functional studies, and therapeutic procedures.

Imaging

Imaging procedures provide diagnostic information about organs of body systems based upon the distribution pattern of radioactivity in the body; they are either dynamic or static. Dynamic studies provide functional information through measurement of the rates of accumulation and removal of the radiopharmaceutical by the organ. Static studies provide morphologic information regarding organ size and shape, position, or presence of space-occupying lesions, such as cysts or tumors, and their relative function.

The pattern of radiopharmaceutical distribution observed in a nuclear medicine scan depends on the particular organ being studied and varies with the disease. In some studies, the normal organ concentrates the radiopharmaceutical and appears "hot," whereas the diseased area excludes radioactivity and appears "cold." The Tc-99m sulfur colloid liver scan is an example where a tumor or cyst appears "cold" due to destruction of the phagocytic cells that normally engulf the radioactive colloidal particles. In another type of study, the normal organ excludes the radiopharmaceutical and appears "cold," while the diseased area concentrates activity and appears "hot." An example is the traditional brain scan with Tc-99m gluceptate or Tc-99m pertechnetate, where a brain tumor, for example, disrupts the blood-brain barrier, allowing blood-borne radioactivity to accumulate in the tumor but not in normal brain tissue. In still other studies, the normal organ may concentrate the radiopharmaceutical, but diseased tissue concentrates it to a greater

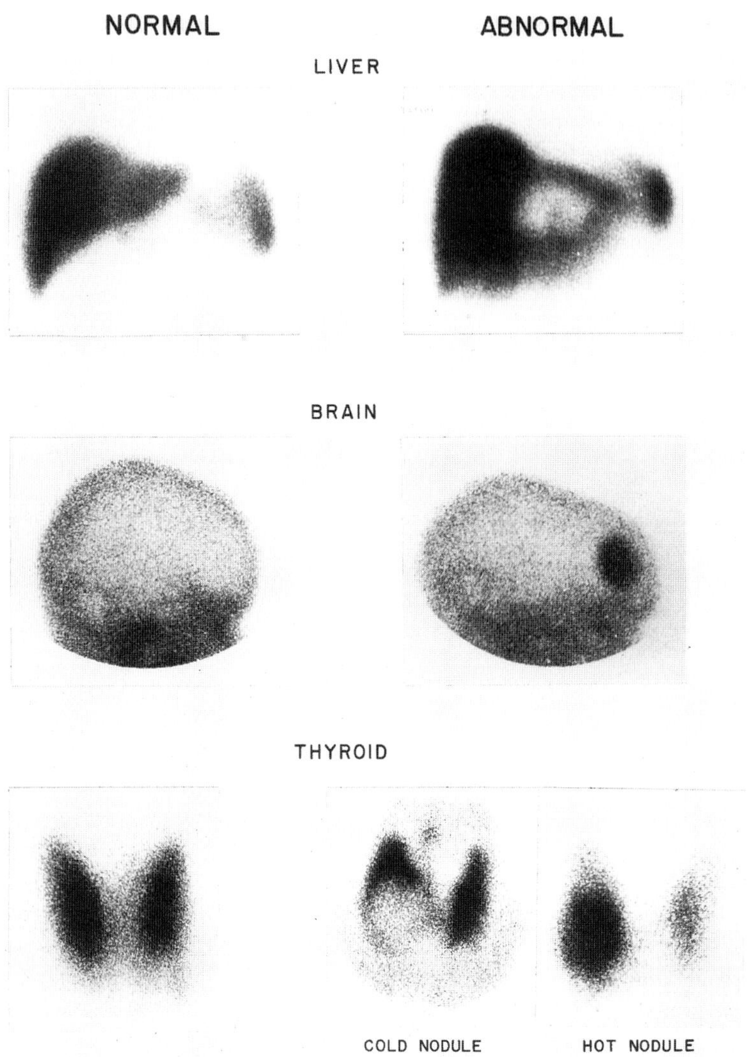

FIG. 1. Typical normal and abnormal static images obtained with a conventional planar imaging gamma camera: anterior view of the liver, lateral view of the brain, and anterior view of the thyroid gland.

extent due to increased function or to a lesser extent to decreased function. An example is thyroid imaging with radioiodide, demonstrating the presence of hyperfunctioning (hot) or hypofunctioning (cold) nodules. Examples of such scans are shown in Fig. 1.

In Vivo Studies

In vivo function studies measure the function of a particular organ or body system. Usually the absorption, dilution, concentration, or excretion of radioactivity is measured and compared to standard values. These studies do not require imaging, but a radiopharmaceutical is administered and analyzed by counting radioactivity directly emitted from organs within the body or from blood or urine samples. An example is the assessment of thyroid function by counting the radioactivity of I-131 taken up by the gland following an oral dose of sodium iodide I-131. Other examples are the measurement of plasma volume with I-125-labeled human serum albumin and red-cell volume with Cr-51-labeled erythrocytes based on the principle of isotope dilution analysis.

Therapeutic Procedures

Therapeutic procedures with radiopharmaceuticals are limited primarily to the treatment of hyperthyroidism and thyroid cancer with sodium iodide I-131. Occasionally, polycythemia vera is treated with sodium phosphate P-32, and peritoneal effusions are treated by instilling insoluble chromic phosphate P-32 into the peritoneal cavity. What distinguishes radiation therapy with radiopharmaceuticals from conventional radiation therapy with implantable and removable sources (brachytherapy) or with radiation therapy machines (e.g., Co-60 teletherapy) is that the radiation source (radiopharmaceutical) undergoes a metabolic change in the body and is not easily removed once administered.

Radiation Detection

In the early years of nuclear medicine, detection of radiation in the body was made by mapping distribution with Geiger counters. This crude method eventually yielded to gamma scintillation counters equipped with sodium iodide crystal detectors of 7.6- or 12.7-cm diameters. These detectors were housed in rectilinear scanners which could map radiation distribution in the body by scanning over an organ in a back-and-forth, top-to-bottom manner, building up an image line by line. The result was a scan of radiopharmaceutical distribution in the organ. In the late 1950s the gamma scintillation camera was developed which, because of its stationary sodium iodide detector (30.5 cm in diameter), could image an entire organ. Two-dimensional or planar images were the standard format, similar to those shown in Fig. 1. Modern-day scintillation cameras employ even larger detectors and are capable of generating three-dimensional images through the use of computor-enhanced reconstruction algorithms. This method is called single-photon emission computed tomography or SPECT because it detects and analyzes radionuclides which emit a single photon per decay. With this camera the detector moves at a controlled rate around the patient in up to a 360° arc, detecting gamma radiation emanating from the organ of interest. The information is stored in a computor which is capable of constructing 6-mm slice images through the organ in transverse (top-to-bottom), sagittal (side-to-side), and coronal (front-to-back) planes (Fig. 2). In this way the physician can obtain a three-dimensional view of radiotracer distribution in the organ. The SPECT method is especially useful where radioactivity in overlying structures may obscure imaging of the organ.

Another modern imaging modality is positron emission tomography or PET. The PET camera has the capability of displaying images in a three-dimensional manner similar to SPECT, but the method of radiation detection is somewhat different. The patient is injected with a positron-emitting radiopharmaceutical capable of producing two 511-keV gamma photons simultaneously at a 180° angle from each other. The patient is moved at

ROYAL PHARMACEUTICAL SOCIETY LIBRARY
1, LAMBETH HIGH STREET, LONDON SE1 7JN

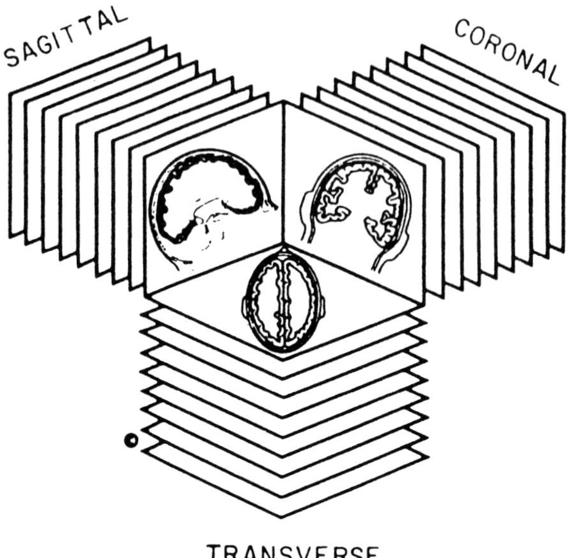

FIG. 2. The three-dimensional imaging technique of a SPECT gamma camera, capable of constructing slice images through an organ in transverse, sagittal, and coronal planes.

a controlled rate through a circular gantry containing an array of sodium iodide detectors. Only those photons detected simultaneously along a straight line path by opposing detectors are counted and stored in the computor. The coordinates of the photon interaction in each detector are recorded and used by the data processor to establish a point of origin in the organ. This process is the basis for generating three-dimensional images and for making quantitative measurements of radiotracer distribution in the organ. Tracer quantitation can be also accomplished with SPECT, but it is easier with PET. Other advantages of PET are higher resolution images and the capability of using physiologic tracers labeled with C-11, N-13, O-15, or F-18. The first three are radioisotopes of the fundamental building blocks of biological systems. Thus, they can label naturally occuring biochemicals or drugs which can be used as radiotracers to evaluate human physiologic processes. (See Burns et al. under Bibliography for more discussion on this topic.)

Targeting Radionuclides in the Body

The main objective in radiopharmaceutical design is to incorporate a radionuclide into a physicochemical form that delivers the radioactive atoms to a target organ. A secondary objective is to minimize uptake into ancillary organs and tissues which would reduce the target-to-background ratio and increase the radiation burden to the patient. Ideally, all of the administered radiotracer would localize in the target organ, remain there for the required imaging time, and then be rapidly excreted from the body. The ideal situation is seldom, if ever achieved. An understanding of target-organ physiology and radionuclide chemistry is important to radiopharmaceutical design.

Radiopharmaceuticals can be labeled isotopically or nonisotopically. Isotopic labeling is the replacement of a stable atom in a compound with its radioisotope. It results in a radiotracer that is physiologically identical to the parent compound. Although this approach is ideal, it is limited by the choice of radionuclides available. For example, radioisotopes of C, H, O, N, S, and P, the elements which make up biological molecules, do not possess ideal imaging properties. Thus, H-3, C-14, P-32, and S-35 are pure beta emitters and therefore cannot be imaged with the gamma camera. The positron emitters C-11, N-13, and O-15 are useful radioisotopic labels but their short half-lives (20, 10, and 2 min) require on-site cyclotron production and applications are limited. Despite the complexity and expense of PET radiopharmaceuticals, however, PET imaging centers are increasingly being established throughout the world.

There are a few isotopically labeled radiopharmaceuticals that are not positron emitters. These are I-123- and I-131- labeled sodium iodide for thyroid studies, Co-57 cyanocobalamin as a marker for vitamin B-12 absorption, Fe-59 ferrous citrate for measuring iron kinetics, and P-32 sodium phosphate for treating polycythemia vera.

The limited number of isotopic labels available often requires nonisotopic or ''foreign'' labeling, that is, introducing a radionuclide not previously present into a molecule. Although this is not the ideal method of labeling, many useful radiopharmaceuticals have been developed by this method. In the past, the empirical approach was taken, that is, a radionuclide with favorable imaging properties was selected, transformed into different chemical entities, and biodistribution studies performed in animals and humans to identify any useful properties. Most radiopharmaceuticals used in nuclear medicine were developed this way, the principal ones being labeled with Tc-99m. Once a greater understanding of technetium's chemistry was gained, radiopharmaceuticals with specific biological properties were developed that included technetium as a ''core'' atom, that is required for the desired targeting in the body. Noteworthy are the technetium-labeled hepatobiliary agents and agents for imaging brain and heart perfusion.

Approximately 80% of nuclear medicine studies employ a technetium-labeled radiopharmaceutical. This demonstrates the importance of technetium's desirable nuclear properties for imaging. Fortunately, technetium also possesses a diverse chemistry, allowing many compounds to be labeled to it. Technetium is positioned in the periodic table along with manganese and rhenium, but its chemistry is more similar to that of rhenium. As a transition metal in group VIIB, technetium has seven electrons beyond the nobel gas configuration and readily loses these electrons to yield the 7^+ oxidation state of pertechnetate, TcO_4^-. Although this is the most stable state in aqueous solution, oxidation states from 1^- to 7^+ have been reported. Tc-99m sodium pertechnetate is readily available on a daily basis from a Mo-99–Tc-99m generator in a nuclear medicine lab. As pertechnetate, technetium does not bind to other chemical species. Being an oxidizing agent, however, it can be reduced to a positively charged species that complexes to a variety of ligands. The type of ligand determines the localization of technetium in the body.

Technetium can be reduced by suitable reducing agents, most notably stannous ion. This powerful reducing agent is capable of producing quantitative yields of technetium-labeled compounds. For the most part, technetium compounds are prepared by addition of Tc-99m sodium pertechnetate to a vial of nonradioactive chemicals, commonly known as a kit. Typically it contains a sterile, lyophilized mixture of the desired ligand, stannous ion, and the necessary adjuvants for labeling and stability. Heating and incubation steps may be involved in the labeling process, and the final product is chromatographed to as-

TABLE 2 Technetium-99m Radiopharmaceuticals

Radiopharmaceutical	Generic Name	Target Organ
Pertechnetate	—	Thyroid, actively trapped
Diethylenetriamine pentaacetic acid (DTPA)	Pentetate	Kidney, glom. filtration
Glucoheptonate (GH)	Gluceptate	Kidney, glom. filtration, cortical binding
Dimercaptosuccinic acid (DMSA)	Succimer	Kidney, cortical binding
Mercaptoacetyl triglycine (MAG_3)	Mertiatide	Kidney, glom. filtration, tubular secretion
Sulfur colloid	—	Liver, phagocytosis via Kupffer cells
Diisopropylacetanilido-iminodiacetic acid (DISIDA)	Disofenin	Liver, active transport via hepatocytes
Trimethylbromoacetanilido-iminodiacetic acid	Mebrofenin	Liver, active transport via hepatocytes
Methylene disphosphonate (MDP)	Medronate	Bone, chemisorption
Hydroxymethylene diphosphonate (HDP)	Oxidronate	Bone, chemisorption
Macroaggretated human serum albumin (MAA)	—	Lung, capillary blockade
Hexamethylpropyleneamine oxime (HM-PAO)	Exametazime	Brain, passive diffusion
Hexakis-2-methoxyisobutyl isonitrile	Sestamibi	Heart, passive diffusion
Chloro[tris(cyclohexane-dionedioxime)methylboronic acid	Teboroxime	Heart, passive diffusion

sess labeling yield. A list of Tc-99m-labeled radiopharmaceuticals is given in Table 2. The following discussion will highlight the development and uses of the major radiopharmaceuticals in nuclear medicine today.

Brain

Radiopharmaceuticals for the evaluation of the central nervous system can be divided into two catagories: brain-imaging agents and cisternography agents.

Brain-imaging radiopharmaceuticals can be divided into four groups. The first group includes hydrophilic compounds that undergo nonspecific mechanisms of localization. The earliest brain-imaging agents fall into this group. They are excluded from entering the normal brain by an intact blood-brain-barrier (BBB). Under pathologic conditions, however, the barrier is disrupted, and radiotracer concentrates in the lesion for positive identification. In such studies, lesions appear as hot spots against a cold background.

Tc-99m pertechnetate and Tc-99m gluceptate (Table 2) are capable of evaluating blood flow to the brain, for example, in confirming brain death (absent flow), and identifying tumors, abscesses, and subdural hematomas.

The second group of brain-imaging agents are lipophilic compounds that readily enter the normal brain by passive diffusion through an intact BBB. These agents are most useful in measuring changes in regional cerebral blood flow caused by disease. The ideal brain-perfusion agent should exhibit the following characteristics:

1. Extraction that is linearly proportional to flow over a wide range of blood flow,
2. BBB permeability (lipid solubility),
3. High initial brain uptake,
4. Retention time long enough for imaging,
5. A fixed regional distribution (no change from its original location),
6. A high brain-to-blood ratio, and
7. Little or no in vivo metabolism that would alter the agent's regional distribution.

Example radiopharmaceuticals in this group are Tc-99m exametazime and I-123 iofetamine [1–3]. Both these agents are lipophilic and have high first-pass extraction into the brain. Tc-99m exametazime (d,l-hexamethylpropyleneamine oxime) is prepared with the help of a Tc-99m kit which must be used within 30 min of preparation because the desired complex is unstable, reverting to a hydrophilic species that does not enter the brain. I-123 iofetamine (iodoamphetamine) is a commercial product which must be purchased daily because of the short half-life of I-123 (13 h); it is produced in a cyclotron. These agents are useful for diagnosing diseases with altered blood distribution such as stroke, dementia, and seizure disorders. For example, in complex partial seizures which have a temporal focus, blood flow increases at the seizure focus during the ictal stage and decreases during the interictal stage, providing a means of localizing the seizure focus with brain-perfusion tracers.

The third group of brain agents are the glucose analogs used to measure brain glucose metabolism. The principal agent in this group is F-18 2-fluoro-2-deoxyglucose or FDG [4]. The importance of this agent is that it exhibits brain kinetics similar to glucose, but differs in that it becomes trapped in the brain long enough for imaging to be accomplished. The trapping is due to the buildup of deoxyglucose-6-phosphate which cannot be metabolized by the hexosephosphate isomerase enzyme. Radiolabeled glucose cannot be used for imaging because it is rapidly metabolized and washed out of the brain as carbon dioxide and water. Because it is physiologically similar to glucose, FDG is useful for evaluating tissue viability, that is, active metabolism of glucose. For example, in a brain tumor treated with radiation therapy, tumor regrowth, evidenced by increased blood flow and glucose metabolism (FDG uptake), can be differentiated from radiation-induced tumor necrosis, evidenced by increased blood flow but absent metabolism (no FDG uptake). Additional uses of FDG PET include the mapping of neuronal activity in regions of the brain following visual, auditory, and somatosensory stimulation. For example, visual stimulation experiments in subjects injected with FDG demonstrate that visual perception involves secondary association areas of the brain as well as primary sensory areas of the cortex.

The fourth group of brain agents are the receptor-imaging agents. Labeled with the positron emitter carbon-11, quantification of dopamine receptors can be made with C-11 *N*-methylspiperone [5] and of opiate receptors with C-11 carfentanil. In the future, PET receptor probes such as these will make it possible to monitor specific effects of drugs on the brain.

Cisternography agents are used to evaluate the cerebrospinal fluid (CSF) space, in particular to diagnose obstruction to CSF flow and identify CSF leaks. A radiopharmaceutical is injected into the lumbar subarachnoid space and imaged with a gamma camera as it diffuses toward the head. Normal egress of radiotracer is via the arachnoid granulations into the superior sagittal sinus. A molecular weight above 200 Daltons is required to keep the radiopharmaceutical from diffusing through the meninges. Two radionuclide chelates of diethylenetriamine pentaacetic acid (DTPA) are used: indium In-111 DTPA ($T_{1/2}$ 2.8 days) for long-term studies such as the evaluation of hydrocephalus [6] and Tc-99m DTPA ($T_{1/2}$ 6 h) for short-term studies such as the identification of CSF leaks (rhinorrhea and otorrhea) caused by meningitis or physical trauma [7]. In-111 is cyclotron produced, and In-111 DTPA is available commercially. Tc-99m DTPA is produced in the hospital from a kit.

Thyroid

The principal radiopharmaceuticals employed for studying the thyroid gland are I-131 or I-123 sodium iodide and Tc-99m sodium pertechnetate. The pertechnetate ion, similar to the thiocyanate, is actively trapped in the thyroid gland by the anion-concentrating mechanism of the epithelial cells, similar to iodide, but it is not organified into thyroid hormone. Pertechnetate is eventually washed out of the gland, but its residence time is long enough to image the thyroid gland in the neck. It is not used to assess thyroid function but to visualize functional anatomy (e.g., thyroid nodules). Its advantages are high-resolution images and low-radiation dose to the patient. Radioiodide, as I-131 and I-123, is used diagnostically to image thyroid tissue in the neck, to identify metastatic lesions in the body from thyroid cancer, and to assess thyroid function during the radioactive iodine uptake test. Iodine-131, because of its beta radiation, is used in the radiation therapy of hyperthyroidism and thyroid cancer. The amount of I-131 administered for therapy is on the order of 1000 to 20,000 times larger than the usual diagnostic dose for assessing thyroid function.

Heart

The goals of cardiac imaging are broad, encompassing the assessment of myocardial perfusion, cardiac chamber function, infarction, and metabolism. Approximately 50% of all nuclear medicine studies involve the assessment of heart disease. A variety of radiopharmaceuticals are available to meet the goals of cardiac imaging.

Cardiac imaging has played a key role in the diagnostic workup of patients with coronary artery disease. The precise measurement of regional myocardial perfusion in humans has clinical applicability for identifying ischemia, defining the extent and severity of disease, assessing myocardial viability, establishing the need for medical and surgical intervention, and monitoring the effects of treatment. The diagnosis of obstructive coronary artery disease is made by measuring coronary perfusion in the heart with radiotracers that exhibit high first-pass extraction by the myocardium in proportion to blood flow. High extraction permits accurate flow measurements at all flow rates and the delineation of perfusion abnormalities. The principal agents used in SPECT imaging are Tl-201 thallous chloride, Tc-99m sestamibi, and Tc-99m teboroxime [8,9]. The perfusion tracers used in PET are Rb-82 rubidium chloride ($T_{1/2}$ 75 s), O-15 water ($T_{1/2}$ 2 min), and N-13 ammonia ($T_{1/2}$ 10 min). Tl-201 and Rb-82, being potassium analogs, localize in the myocardium by active transport via the sodium-potassium ATPase membrane-bound pump. These agents have a similar (Rb-82) or higher (Tl-201) myocardial uptake than potassium and a longer retention time for imaging. Additionally, their nuclear properties are better suited for imaging than those of potassium radionuclides. The remaining agents are extracted by passive diffusion but their retention times and mechanisms vary. Oxygen O-15 water is an inert freely diffusible tracer whose uptake, as a function of blood flow, is less likely to be affected by tissue metabolic changes. N-13 ammonia is a nonionic tracer that crosses the sarcolemmal membrane and is converted to ammonium ion which is trapped by the glutamate–glutamine reaction. Its cardiac half-time is 1–2 h. Tc-99m teboroxime is a neutral lipophilic complex of the general class of compounds known as boronic acid adducts of technetium dioxime. It rapidly diffuses into and out of the myocardium, requiring rapid imaging methods. It also exhibits high uptake in the liver which may interfere with heart imaging. Tc-99m sestamibi is a monovalent cationic, lipophilic complex comprised of one atom of Tc-99m in the 1^+ oxidation state and six molecules of 2-methoxyisobutylisonitrile. It is taken up and bound in the myocardium with a half-time of about 6 h which permits a more convenient time frame for imaging with this agent. Tc-99m teboroxime and sestamibi are relatively new agents and their clinical utility is not as well established as that of Tl-201 chloride.

Clinically, perfusion agents are used to distinguish infarcted or dead myocardium from poorly perfused myocardium and ischemic but viable myocardium which can be restored to health by medical and/or surgical intervention, such as via coronary bypass graft or angioplasty. The assessment is made by imaging the patient under conditions of normal coronary blood flow and at elavated blood flow when regions of diseased myocardium are more likely to exhibit proportionately less increase in flow than normal myocardium. This is because coronary flow reserve of coronary vessels in diseased myocardium is compromised due to stenosis. The routine agent used for this purpose is Tl-201 chloride [10]. Typically, the study is done in two parts. In the first part (the stress study) the patient is stressed, by treadmill exercise or with a pharmacologic agent such as adenosine, to increase coronary blood flow three to four times normal and 2–3 mCi of Tl-201 chloride is then injected intravenously. The heart distribution of Tl-201 activity is imaged within 12–40 min of injection to allow sufficient time for uptake into the heart and for study completion before significant washout. Under these circumstances, normally perfused myocardium takes up the radiotracer well (appears "hot"), whereas poorly perfused (ischemic) or nonperfused (infarcted) myocardium shows decreased or no radiotracer uptake, that is, it appears as a deficiency or defect ("cold" area) in the myocardial image. After a period of rest, usually 4 to 24 h after the stress study, the second part, or redistribution study, is performed. At this time the patient is reimaged to assess myocardial redistribution of the Tl-201 activity administered during the stress study. During the rest phase, Tl-201 ion redistributes in the myocardium, washing out of normal myocardium, but less well from areas of compromised flow during the stress. Thus, the redistribution image of the heart demonstrates "filling-in" of activity in ischemic areas, but no "filling-in" of infarcted areas; hence, the differential diagnosis of ischemia versus infarction. The "filling-in" phenomenon is indicative of viable myocardium and an indirect assessment of viability. The advantage of PET in cardiac studies is that myocardial perfusion, measured with Rb-82, O-15, or N-13, can be compared with an independent PET viability assessment using FDG. With SPECT, viability assessment must be made from perfusion data alone, since no SPECT metabolism agent is available. However, if carefully done, the Tl-201 SPECT study is capable of providing accurate assessments of myocardial viability [11].

Cardiac chamber assessment, usually that of the left ventricle, is made with a radiopharmaceutical that is confined to the blood pool, such as Tc-99m-labeled red blood cells [12]. The patient is injected with stannous pyrophosphate which "tins" the red blood cells. Technetium-99m pertechnetate is then injected, enters the circulating red cells, becomes reduced by the intracellular tin, and binds to hemoglobin. The binding is very stable. Alternatively, red cells can be labeled in vitro by a similar procedure. With the help of this agent, a dynamic motion study of the behavior of the ventricular blood pool during an R–R electrocardiographic (ECG) interval can be made. The study is displayed in cine mode, with a composite R-R interval (one representative heart beat) replayed repeatedly. With the aid of a computer, necessary for acquisition and processing, wall motion abnormalities can be observed, seen as regions of akinesis caused by ischemic or infarcted muscle. Additionally, ventricular ejection fraction, a measure of left ventricular performance, can be calculated from the differences in blood activity present at end systole and end diastole. End-systolic and end-diastolic ventricular volumes can also be measured. These studies are done with the patient at rest or following exercise to define the heart's response to increased workload. They can also be used to assess the therapeutic effects of cardiac drugs and procedures.

Radiopharmaceuticals with an affinity for infarcted myocardium have been used to diagnose myocardial infarction. When heart muscle becomes infarcted, membrane damage occurs which allows a shift of extracellular substances, such as calcium and proteins, into myocytes. This process begins within 12–24 h of infarction. Calcium deposition occurs during irreversible tissue injury and results in the formation of various calcium phosphate complexes, such as amorphous calcium phosphate (ACP) and insoluble calcium hydroxyapatite (HA) crystals. These crystals act as sites of uptake, via chemisorption, for Tc-99m bone-seeking radiopharmaceuticals. The agent used most widely is Tc-99m pyrophosphate [13]. Residual blood flow is required for delivery of the radiopharmaceutical to the infarct, and highest uptake occurs within 24–72 h following the infarct event. Increased uptake of activity into infarcted myocardium has dubbed these agents "hot spot" markers.

The loss of sarcolemmal integrity with cell death exposes myosin, an intracellular contractile protein present in high concentrations. A potentially more specific agent for localizing myocardial infarcts is indium In-111 antimyosin antibody [14]. This agent is actually an Fab monoclonal antibody fragment bound to a DTPA linker molecule which chelates the In-111. This antibody binds with irreversibly damaged myocardial cells with maximal uptake occurring in regions of lowest blood flow, or most necrosis. In-111 antimyosin antibody is still in clinical trials but offers hope of a more infarct-specific agent.

Several agents have been used for measuring cardiac metabolism with PET [9]. The most widely used agent is F-18 2-fluoro-2-deoxyglucose (FDG) a marker of anaerobic glycolysis which is useful in differentiating between viable and scarred myocardium. It is useful in clinical decisions regarding the revascularization of coronary arteries. Carbon-11 palmitate is a marker of oxidative fatty acid metabolism via the mitochondrial tricarboxylic acid (TCA) cycle, and C-11 acetate is a marker of oxidative metabolism via the TCA cycle and is used for measuring effects of hypoxia.

Lung

Pulmonary embolism is the most common acute pulmonary disease seen in the hospital and results in approximately 200,000 deaths per year in the United States. A principal advantage of the nuclear medicine lung scan is that it has the capability of detecting an embolus immediately after it occurs. It is also a relatively safe procedure. In nuclear medicine, the diagnosis of pulmonary embolism entails both lung perfusion agents and lung ventilation agents. Typically, the perfusion agents are radiolabeled particles of heat-denatured human serum albumin macroaggregates (MAA) with a particle size range of 10–90 μm. Albumin microspheres in the 10–35 μm size range have also been used. Following intravenous injection, more than 90% of Tc-99m MAA is extracted by pulmonary arterioles and capillaries first pass through the lungs. The mechanism of localization is by physical entrapment of particles that are larger than the blood vessel lumen. The smallest capillaries are 6–10 μm. Distribution of particles in the lung is a function of regional blood flow. Thus, in a normal lung radiolabeled particles are distributed uniformly throughout the lung tissue, and it appears "hot." Where blood flow is occluded because of an embolus, particles are prevented from passage beyond these points. This is seen as a perfusion deficit or "cold spot" distal to the point of obstruction. Large emboli block larger-sized vessels and produce larger-sized deficits.

Particle flow can also be restricted if capillaries are constricted due to ventilatory problems, such as might occur in asthma or chronic obstructive pulmonary disease (COPD). Perfusion deficits due to these diseases can be ruled out by performing a ventilation lung scan with a radioactive gas, such as Xe-133, or using a radioaerosol, such as nebulized Tc-99m DTPA. In a normal ventilation scan using Xe-133, the radioactive gas moves readily in and out of the lungs. In ventilatory disease, gas flows poorly into obstructed airways compared to normal areas. This is seen as a wash-in deficit. During rebreathing, however, the gas eventually diffuses into obstructed areas. During washout, these areas temporarily retain or trap radioactive gas compared to normal areas which wash out quickly. In general, a normal ventilation scan with an abnormal perfusion scan (mismatch) indicates high probability of blood flow obstruction due to pulmonary embolism. An abnormal ventilation scan, seen as gas trapping with an abnormal perfusion scan (match) indicates higher probability for COPD [15].

The Tc-99m MAA is prepared by adding Tc-99m pertechnetate (typically 30–50 mCi) to a lyophilized kit of stannous MAA. A typical kit contains 5 million particles. Labeling efficiency is greater than 95% and the label is stable for 6 h or longer. The usual adult dose is 3 mCi containing 300,000 to 500,000 particles. This number of particles is quite safe to inject in subjects with normal lungs where less than 1% of capillary segments are occluded and pulmonary circulation is not affected significantly. Patients with pulmonary hypertension, however, receive a smaller number of particles (60,000 to 100,000) because their lung blood flow is compromised [16–18]. Particles trapped in the lung are eventually degraded by mechanical forces to smaller-sized particles which pass into the systemic circulation and become phagocytosed and metabolized by the reticuloendothelial cells, principally in the liver.

Xenon-133 gas is available commercially in unit-dose vials of 10 and 20 mCi. It is administered to the patient via a closed breathing circuit. Xenon's air-to-water partition coefficient is approximately 10:1, and little xenon is absorbed into the body during a typical 5–10 min ventilation study. If a radioaerosol is used, it is prepared by adding Tc-99m DTPA to a nebulizer apparatus attached to a closed breathing circuit; 0.5 to 1 mCi of the aerosol particles are deposited in the lungs during the study. Systemically Tc-99m DTPA is readily excreted by glomerular filtration.

Liver, Gallbladder, and Spleen

The liver, spleen, and bone marrow form a major part of the reticuloendothelial system (RES) in humans. The venous sinuses of these organs are lined with reticular cells that function to remove foreign particles from the blood. The liver sinusoids are vessels that transport blood from the portal vein to the central vein in the liver lobule. The sinusoidal cells contain pores and intercellular spaces where small particles and soluble substances can leave the blood to enter the space of Disse. Here, particles are trapped in collagen fibrils and are phagocytosed by Kupffer cells. Soluble substances can wash back out of this space or be actively transported into the hepatocyte through one of the four independent carrier-mediated membrane transport pathways. These pathways can accomodate organic anions, organic cations, neutral compounds, or conjugated bile salts [19]. Substances within the hepatocyte can then be secreted with the bile into the biliary ducts and gallbladder and eventually into the intestinal tract. These pathways form the basis for targeting radionuclides to the liver and its biliary system.

There are two main groups of radiotracers targeting the liver: radiocolloids, which become entrapped in the liver for a prolonged period of time, permitting the evaluation of liver morphology, and hepatobiliary agents, that are actively cleared from the blood by the hepatocytes and excreted into the bile, permitting an evaluation of hepatobiliary obstruction and function.

The standard radiocolloid used to evaluate the liver, is a Tc-99m–sulfur colloid. This product is prepared by heating a mixture of Tc-99m pertechnetate in acidified thiosulfate in the presence of gelatin. Tc-99m technetium heptasulfide, Tc_2S_7, coprecipitates with colloidal sulfur particles in the 0.1–1.0-μm size range [20]; approximately 70% are below 0.4 μm. The product is buffered to pH 5–6 before use. A Tc-99m-labeled albumin colloid is also available for liver scanning. Following intravenous injection in normal subjects, the particles are removed from the blood stream within 15 min, with 85% localized in the liver, 4–8% in the spleen, and the remainder in the bone marrow. Under normal circumstances, only liver and spleen activity are seen on the image. Distribution may change with disease, however. For example, in severe cirrhosis, significantly decreased liver uptake is seen, with increased uptake in an enlarged spleen, and bone marrow activity is evident. Due to tissue displacement, cysts, tumors and metastatic lesions in the liver appear as ''cold'' spots in an otherwise normal ''hot'' liver. Most liver–spleen scans are requested as part of a workup for metastatic disease in patients with known tumors. Other indications include abscesses, trauma, and alcoholic cirrhosis.

The first effective agent for evaluating the hepatobiliary tree was I-131 rose bengal, developed in 1955. Although it was not ideal, it remained in use for nearly 20 years until an effective Tc-99m agent could be developed. The principal agents used today are derivatives of N-substituted iminodiacetic acid [19] (Table 3). These agents are known as bifunctional chelates because they are comprised of a drug portion (N-substituted group) that can be modified chemically to alter biodistribution, and a metal binding portion (iminodiacetic acid) which chelates Tc-99m. These agents are prepared by the addition of Tc-99m pertechnetate to a kit containing the appropriate ligand. Tc-99m serves as a

TABLE 3 Iminodiacetic Acid (IDA) Analogues

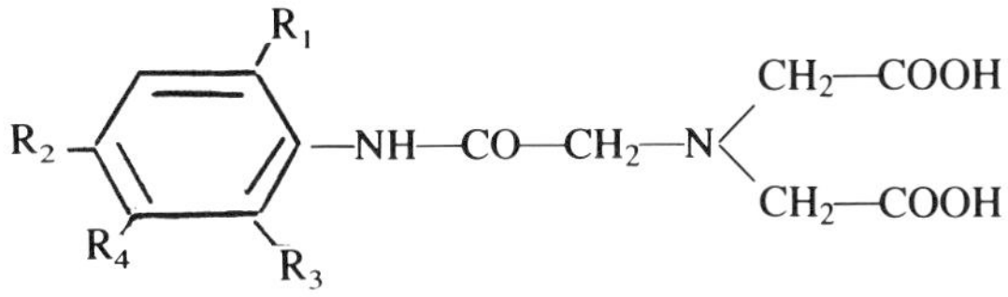

Analogue	Acronym	Generic Name	R-1	R-2	R-3	R-4
2,6-Dimethyl-acetanilido-IDA	HIDA	Lidofenin	CH_3	H	CH_3	H
2,6-Diisopropyl-acetanilido-IDA	DISIDA	Disofenin	$CH(CH_3)_2$	H	$CH(CH_3)_2$	H
2,4,6-Trimethyl-3-bromo-acetanilido-IDA	BrIDA	Mebrofenin	CH_3	CH_3	CH_3	Br

bridging atom between two molecules of the ligand and is required for hepatobiliary excretion. The anionic, lipophilic Tc-99m biscomplex (Fig. 3) is actively transported on the hepatocyte membrane, where it competes for bilirubin excretion. Disofenin and mebrofenin are more efficiently excreted in the presence of high bilirubinemia than the original compound, lidofenin. These agents are rapidly excreted into the bile following intravenous injection. Within 20–30 min, gallbladder and intestinal activity is often seen in normal subjects [21] (Fig. 4). The primary usefulness of these agents is to demonstrate patency of the cystic duct to the gallbladder and of the common bile duct to the intestine. Timing is important because nonvisualization of the gallbladder during the first hour of imaging generally means acute cholecystitis (nonpatency of cystic duct), whereas visualization of the gallbladder between 1 and 4 h usually means chronic cholecystitis [22]. These agents are sensitive indicators of impaired liver function, which is observed as slow clearance from the nearby cardiac blood pool or delayed excretion into the intestine. Nonvisualization of intestinal activity on delayed images indicates obstruction which could be caused by a gallstone or other disease (Fig. 5).

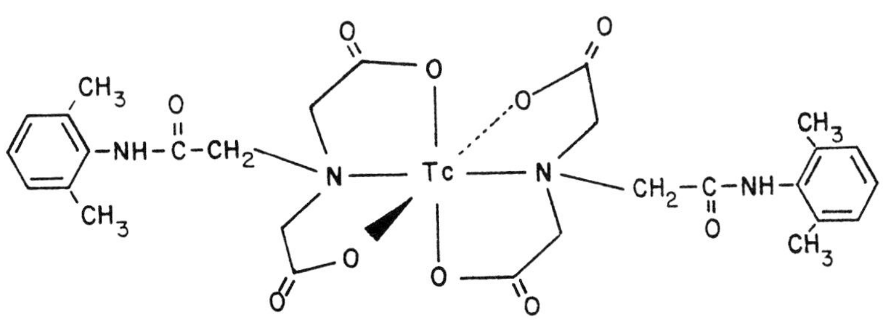

FIG. 3. Dimeric structure of $Tc(HIDA)_2$.

The spleen can be imaged with radiocolloids, which are localized by splenic phagocytes, or denatured radiolabeled red blood cells. Tc-99m sulfur colloid is frequently used because of convenience and simplicity but suffers from a lack of splenic specificity. Heat-

ROYAL PHARMACEUTICAL SOCIETY LIBRARY
1, LAMBETH HIGH STREET, LONDON SE1 7JN

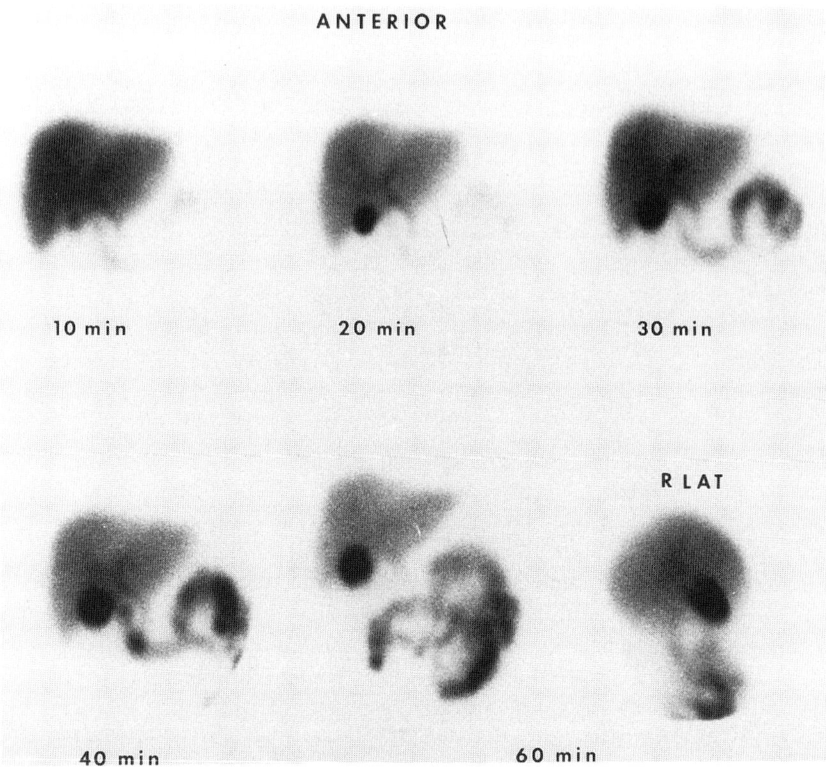

FIG. 4. Normal hepatobiliary study. After intravenous injection of 5 mCi of Tc-99m disofenin, there is a prompt clearance of tracer by the hepatobiliary system. At 10 min, there is evidence of activity in the gallbladder and small intestine that becomes more prominent later (R LAT = right lateral).

denatured red blood cells provide a more spleen-specific agent since this organ is the graveyard for effete red blood cells. The rationale is that heated red cells lose their biconcave disk shape and become fragile spherocytes. Because of this they lyse in the spleen while they squeeze through the splenic sinuses and their radioactive contents are phagocytosed by the RES cells. The red cells are labeled with Tc-99m and heated to 49 ± 1°C for 15 min [23]. Insufficient heating produces insufficient denaturation, resulting in reduced spleen uptake; overheating produces very fragile cells which lyse readily, causing primarily liver uptake. Spleen-specific imaging is usually performed to delineate the spleen from nearby structures and determine its true size and contour, determine the presence and location of accessory spleens in patients who have had a splenectomy, or delineate trauma, infarction, or tumor.

Kidney and Genitourinary System

The kidney functions to conserve fluid and essential electrolytes and excrete waste products from the blood. The processes involved are glomerular filtration and tubular secretion and reabsorption. Several radiotracers have been developed to exploit these renal processes in order to evaluate kidney function and morphology. Radiopharmaceuticals for renal studies can be grouped into two main categories:

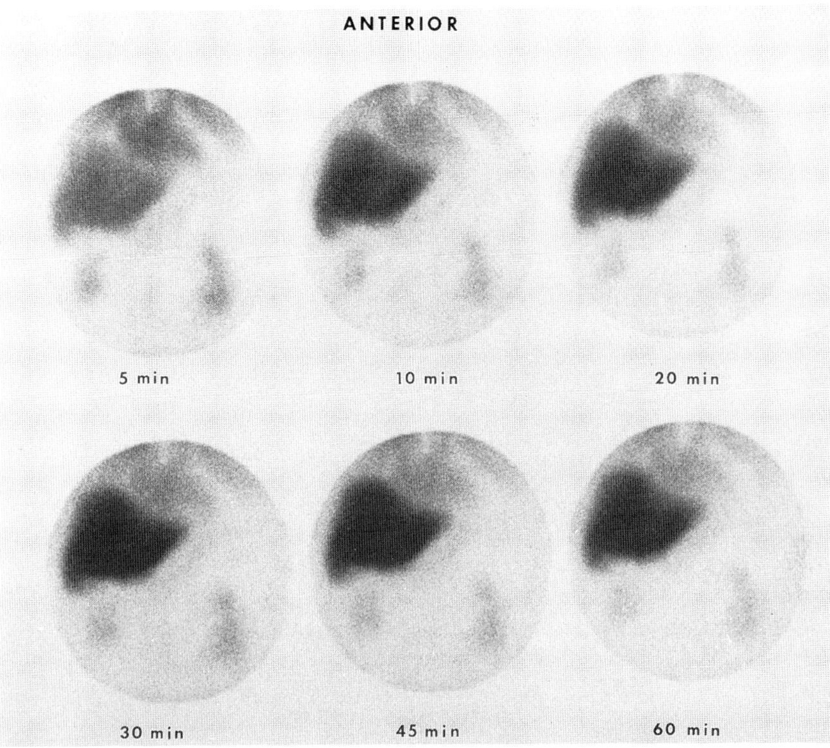

FIG. 5. Abnormal hepatobiliary study following intravenous injection of Tc-99m disofenin; complete obstruction to bile flow is caused by a gallstone lodged in the common bile duct. Liver activity is evident, but tracer clearance from the plasma is slow. Secondary excretion of tracer via the kidneys is evident, which is typically seen in obstruction.

- Agents for renal clearance, which may be further subdivided into agents for assessing glomerular filtration rate and agents for measuring tubular function and renal plasma flow, and
- Agents for renal imaging that bind to the renal cortical cells

If a radiotracer has an extraction ratio of 1.0, it is completely removed in a single pass through the kidney. If none of the tracer appears in the urine, it is completely bound by the kidney. A radiopharmaceutical with this property would be the ideal renal imaging agent for evaluating kidney morphology. On the other hand, if all of the tracer appears in the urine (via glomerular filtration and tubular secretion) and none is bound by the kidney, its clearance is equal to the renal plasma flow. Such a radiopharmaceutical would be the ideal agent for measuring renal function. If a tracer's extraction ratio is 0.2, that is, 20% of renal plasma flow, but none of it is reabsorbed, secreted, or bound by the kidney, the agent would be ideal for measuring glomerular filtration rate (GFR).

Several complexes of Tc-99m have been developed to study the kidney. Tc-99m pentetate (DTPA), a complex of diethylenetriamine pentaacetic acid is a small, hydrophilic chelate (MW < 500), which exhibits low protein binding ($< 5\%$) and is not secreted, reabsorbed, or bound in the kidney [24,25]. It is essentially a GFR agent.

Technetium-99m gluceptate (GH), a complex of glucoheptonic acid, demonstrates renal kinetics similar to DTPA early after injection (good visualization of pelvicalyceal collecting system) but differs from DTPA in that about 15% is bound to the kidney [26,27]. It exhibits about 50% plasma protein binding. Its renal mechanism is believed to be glomerular filtration of the protein-free fraction and tubular secretion because its kidney uptake is inhibited by probenecid and para-aminohippuric acid (PAH) [28].

Technetium-99m succimer (DMSA), a complex of 2,3 dimercaptosuccinic acid, is more highly protein bound (~75%) and undergoes less glomerular filtration than GH or DTPA [26]. Approximately 50% is bound in the kidney cortex. Competition experiments demonstrate that Tc-99m DMSA renal uptake is inhibited by captopril, an agent that lowers filtration pressure, indicating a partial mechanism of glomerular filtration, but it is not inhibited by probenecid, indicating that it is not secreted, at least not by the same enzyme system as probenecid. The data suggest that the filtered fraction is reabsorbed and becomes bound to intracellular proteins of the proximal tubular cells [26,29,30].

Iodine-131 orthoiodohippurate (OIH) was developed in the early 1960s to measure renal plasma flow, because para-aminohippurate (PAH) could not be labeled with a gamma-emitting radionuclide. It undergoes glomerular filtration and tubular secretion, similar to PAH, but its renal extraction is only 80–90% that of PAH [31]. Thus, OIH measures effective renal plasma flow.

The undesirable imaging properties of I-131 stimulated the search for an agent similar to OIH but with a Tc-99m label. Success was finally achieved with the development of Tc-99m mertiatide or (MAG_3), a complex of Tc-99m with mercaptoacetyltriglycine [32]. Although its plasma clearance is approximately 50% that of OIH, its urinary excretion rate is essentially the same as that of OIH. This has been attributed to its higher protein binding and smaller volume of distribution, causing it to have a higher intravascular concentration than OIH. The similar clearance kinetics of these agents has caused them to be used interchangeably for measuring renal function and it is likely that MAG_3 will supplant OIH in the future.

Other procedures are available for assessing renal function, but nuclear medicine procedures are usually simpler and less invasive, and can measure individual functions [33]. Perfusion studies allow observation of gross and differential blood flow to the kidneys. A series of 5- to 10-s images is taken for 1 to 2 min following iv injection of a radiopharmaceutical. Blood flow is best evaluated with a Tc-99m agent because of its high photon flux. For example, blood flow and renal function is usually assessed immediately following kidney transplantation. Blood flow can be assessed with Tc-99m DTPA and tubular function with OIH, but with the availability of MAG_3, both parameters can be evaluated with this one agent.

Renal scans are performed to examine kidney morphology, such as renal size and any space-occupying lesions and gross differences in functioning renal mass between right and left kidneys, and to examine cortical and collecting system function; Tc-99m DMSA and Tc-99m GH are usually employed for this purpose. For example, the differential blood flow to the kidneys can be estimated by counting the DMSA activity accumulated in each kidney.

Renograms are dynamic functional studies that examine the time course of radiotracer clearance by the kidney, namely, the time-to-peak and washout half-time of activity from the kidney. The renogram is very useful for following transplant rejection and recovery after therapy with immunosuppressive drugs or radiation; OIH or MAG_3 are mostly used. A variation on this procedure is the diuretic renogram. It is useful for differentiating between functional and mechanical obstruction of the collecting system. Tc-99m DTPA is usually employed, and a rapidly acting diuretic, such as furosemide, is given halfway through the study. With functional obstruction, activity is held up in the kidney, usually due to a dilated renal collecting system. In this case, the diuretic agent causes a drammatic flush out of pooled activity because of the increased urine flow, whereas with mechanical obstruction, such as that caused by ureteral stenosis or a stone, activity washout does not occur because of mechanical blockade.

Quantitative estimates of glomerular filtration rate, using Tc-99m DTPA and effective renal plasma flow, using I-131 OIH or Tc-99m MAG_3 are possible with well developed procedures which have demonstrated close correlation with inulin and PAH clearance methods. A quantitative measure of residual bladder urine can be made from counts of the accumulated bladder activity pre- and postvoid and by measuring the voided urine volume. Finally, reflux of urine into the ureters can be observed and quantitated by filling the bladder through a catheter with 1 mCi (37 MBq) of Tc-99m pertechnetate and sterile saline. By observing the bladder area during micturition, ureteral reflux can be seen when bladder pressure is highest.

Bone

The composition of bone mineral is mainly calcium, phosphate, and hydroxyl ions. The principal inorganic salts found in bone are amorphous calcium phosphate (ACP) and hydroxyapatite (HA). The former is believed to be the precursor to HA which is the predominant crystalline form found in mature bone. Many radionuclides have been used to study bone, but few of the earlier ones had physical properties desirable for skeletal imaging [34]. Neither calcium nor phosphorus isotopes have useful gamma emitters, and strontium isotopes demonstrated slow biological clearance. F-18 fluoride demonstrated high bone uptake (exchanges with hydroxyl ion) and rapid blood clearance, but its gamma energy was too high and its 1.8 h half-life required daily shipments. The development of a Tc-99m complex with sodium tripolyphosphate in 1971 revolutionized bone imaging because it allowed the use of Tc-99m. However, the discovery that a pyrophosphate impurity was actually responsible for bone uptake led to the use of Tc-99m pyrophosphate for bone imaging. The desire for an agent that exhibited more rapid blood clearance following injection eventually led to the development of a series of Tc-99m complexes with diphosphonic acids. These agents provided more rapid blood clearance than pyrophosphate following intravenous injection (because of less plasma protein and red cell binding) and a bone uptake of about 50% of the injected dose [35]. Tc-99m medronate (MDP), a complex with methylene diphosphonic acid, and Tc-99m oxidronate (HDP), a complex with hydroxymethylene diphosphonic acid, are the current agents of choice for bone imaging [36].

As with other Tc-99m complexes, these agents are prepared with the help of lyophilized kits. Being relatively weak complexes, they are easily oxidized by atmospheric and dissolved oxygen and free-radical species induced by radiolysis. The kits, therefore, are often stabilized with ascorbic or gentisic acid as antioxidants.

There are several clinical indications for bone imaging including metastatic disease, osteomyelitis, avascular necrosis, trauma, metabolic disorders, and arthritic disease. However, the most common indication is the workup for metastatic disease, particularly from breast and prostate cancer. The bone scan replaced the x-ray skeletal survey because it is 95% sensitive for detecting metastatic disease to bone and because lesions could be detected an average of six months earlier than by x-ray examination. The reason for this is the fact that the bone scan demonstrates osseous remodeling, which must precede and is the cause of structural changes seen on the x-ray image. A typical study involves intravenous injection of 20 mCi of Tc-99m agent and imaging within 3 h (Fig. 6). These anionic Tc-99m complexes are believed to localize in bone by chemisorption to calcium ions. Binding is higher to ACP than to HA because ACP contains newly forming hydroxyapatite crystallites that have a crystal growing face configuration of calcium ions best suited for binding to the oxygen atoms of the diphosphonate ligand. Since bone lesions contain a higher concentration of ACP than HA, due to the osseous remodeling process, they appear as focal areas of increased activity uptake compared to normal bone (Fig. 7b). The bone scan is a safe, noninvasive procedure that is useful for staging cancer and following the effects of a clinical treatment course.

Other Studies

Abscess Localization

A fever of unknown origin (FUO) is often due to an occult abscess. The site may be localized with the help of gallium Ga-67 citrate and In-111 leukocytes.

The patient is imaged from 1 to 5 days after iv injection of 5 mCi of Ga-67 citrate. SPECT imaging helps to separate abscess sites of activity accumulation from bowel activity which is a major route of Ga-67 excretion. In-111 leukocytes are more specific than Ga-67 but require preparation [34]. Briefly, the white cells are separated by gravity from 50 mL of whole blood from the patient. The separated white cells are incubated with In-111 oxine for 25 min during which time the neutral, lipophilic complex of In-111 oxine enters the cells and dissociates, and the In-111 binds to intracellular protein [37]. The labeled cells are reinjected (maximum of 500 μCi) into the patient and imaging is done between 4 and 24 h or longer to identify the abscess. The Ga-67 is believed to label circulating leukocytes which then target the abscess and bind to those cells already at the inflammatory site; In-111 leukocytes target the abscess directly.

Gastrointestinal (GI) Bleeding-Site Localization

Successful management of acute GI bleeding may depend upon accurate localization of the bleeding site. Because of the complexity of using angiographic contrast procedures, radionuclide procedures were developed. Both Tc-99m sulfur colloid and Tc-99m labeled red blood cells (RBCs) are used [38,39]. The rationale is that these labeled particles or cells extravasate into the bleeding site, identifying its location. The problem is, however, that most bleeding is intermittent and timing of radiopharmaceutical administration is critical. Because it is removed quickly from the vascular space by the RES, Tc-99m sulfur colloid is less likely to localize in an intermittent bleeding site. It is best used for active bleeding. Its rapid blood clearance, however, is an advantage because blood background is reduced and the site is more easily identified, except if it is near the liver or spleen. For intermittent bleeding sites, Tc-99m RBCs are a better choice since they remain in the circulation for a longer time and are "available" when bleeding does occur.

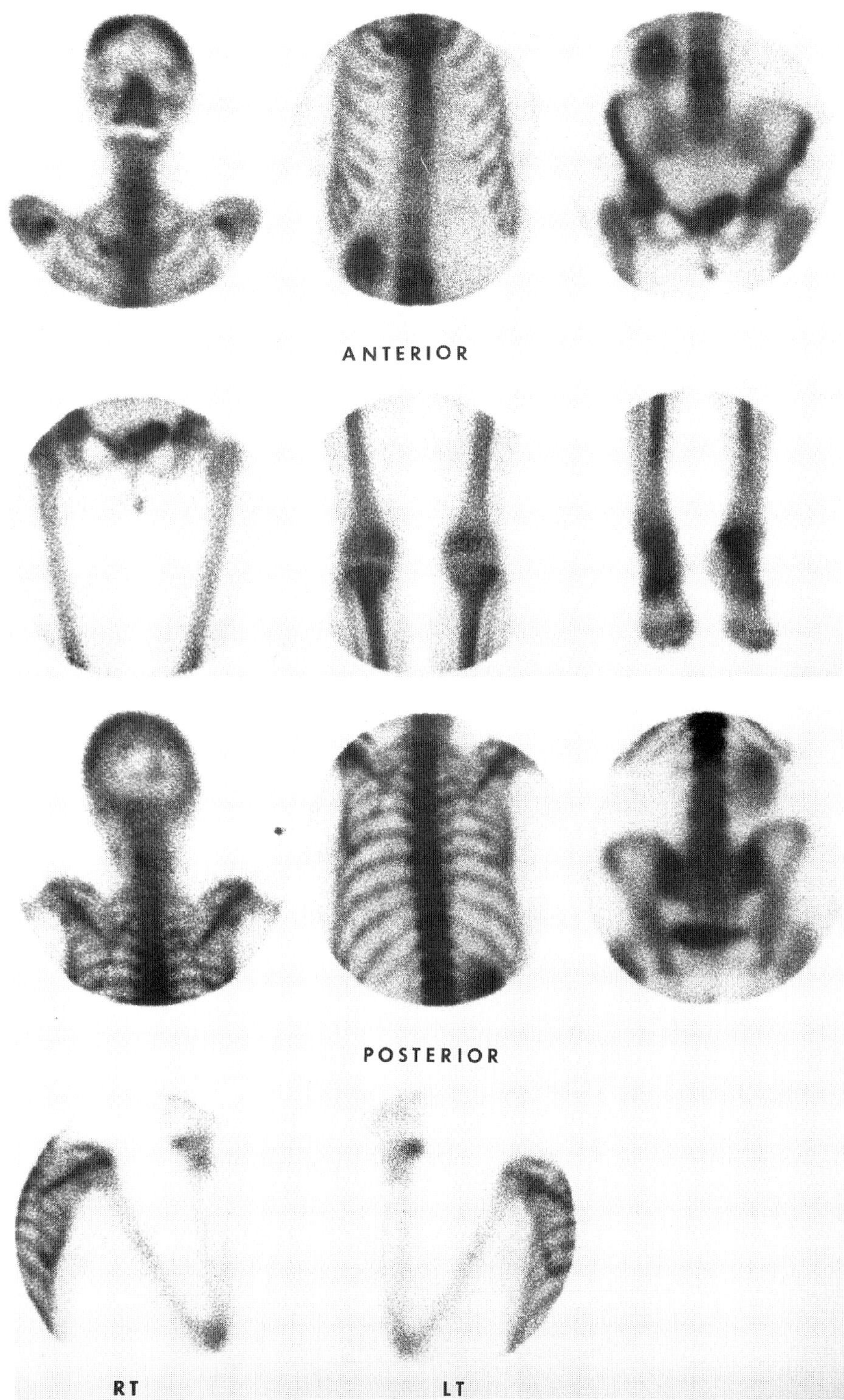

FIG. 6. Normal anterior and posterior bone scan in an adult obtained 3 h after intravenous injection of 15 mCi of Tc-99m medronate. Normal excretion of tracer by the kidneys demonstrates absence of the left kidney in this patient.

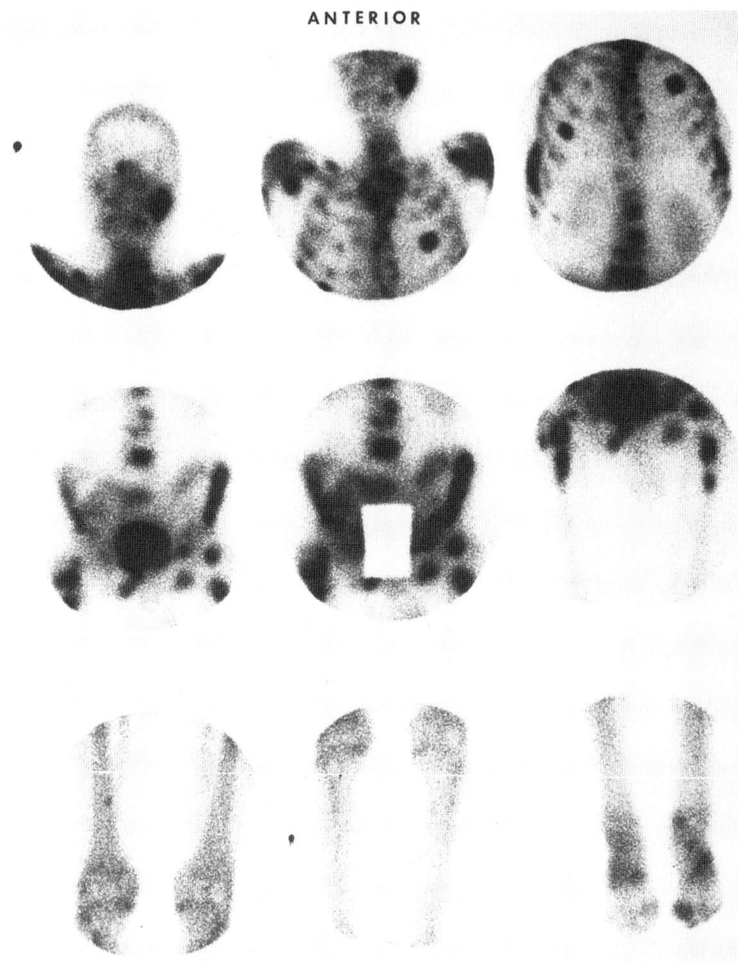

FIG. 7A. Abnormal anterior (A) and posterior (B) bone scan in an 82-year-old man with metastatic prostate carcinoma. Multiple focal areas of increased uptake of Tc-99m medronate are seen in the axial skeleton and the extremities (LLAT = left lateral).

Their disadvantage is that blood background is much higher, making the bleeding site more difficult to identify. The Tc-99m RBCs can be prepared in 30 min using a labeling kit and 3 mL of the patient's own blood.

Gastric-Emptying Studies

The rate of gastric emptying of liquids and solids from the stomach can be measured easily with radiotracers. The study involves ingestion of an appropriate radiotracer "meal" and counting the stomach activity over time. A plot of activity over time is used to measure the rate of gastric emptying. Critical points are to administer a standard-size meal and to use liquid markers that are not absorbed from the stomach and solid markers that do not dissociate from the solid meal ingested [40]. A satisfactory liquid marker is Tc-99m sulfur colloid, which is stable in gastric juice and can be given with juice or

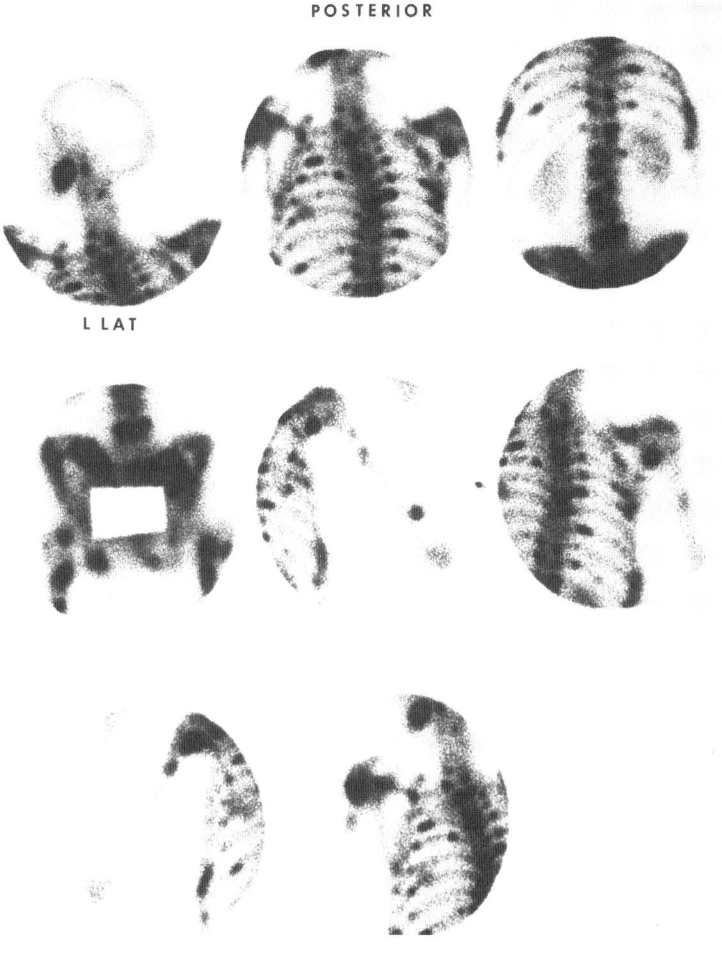

FIG. 7B.

other suitable liquid. A useful solid marker is Tc-99m sulfur colloid mixed into scrambled eggs. Another is Tc-99m labeled to Chelex-100 cation exchange resin suspended in a package of instant oatmeal. If liquid and solid emptying are to be measured simultaneously, two different radionuclides must be used. A useful combination is 100 μCi of In-111 DTPA as the liquid marker and 600 μCi of Tc-99m sulfur colloid in scrambled eggs. Typically, anterior and posterior abdominal counts are collected and the geometric mean (anterior count × posterior count)$^{1/2}$ is used to correct for attenuation caused by variations in tissue depth. Decay correction and down-scatter of In-111 in the Tc-99m window must be made. The normal mean half-times for a 300-g meal based on geometric-mean data analysis are 38 min for a liquid meal and 77 min for a solid meal.

Meckel's Diverticulum

Meckel's diverticulum is the most frequent congenital malformation of the GI tract in humans which occurs most commonly in children [41]. It is a 3-5 cm long sac in the ileum containing all the layers of the bowel wall, but approximately 50% contain gastric tissue. The peptic acid secretion may cause it to rupture, resulting in rectal bleeding which is the most common symptom. It is localized following injection of Tc-99m sodium pertechnetate, because it concentrates in the mucous cells of the gastric mucosa. Typically 50 μCi/kg is injected iv and imaging is done at 5-to-10-min intervals. The diverticulum usually appears coincident with activity uptake into the stomach, about 10–30 min after dosing.

Dacryocystography

The patency of nasolacrimal drainage can be evaluated by placing a drop (100 μCi) of Tc-99m sodium pertechnetate onto the conjunctiva near the lateral canthus and imaging the transit time of radioactivity into the nasolacrimal sac. A transit time longer than 1.5 min indicates obstruction and provides a sensitive means for its detection. The normal eye is done first to provide a control.

Lymph Node Imaging

Lymphoscintigraphy, the evaluation of the lymph nodes and the lymphatic channels, can be done following injection of radiocolloids into the interstitial space [42]. Cannulation of lymph vessels is not necessary, but uptake from the interstitial space into the lymphatics depends on the size of the colloid particles; a size less than 100 nm is required. The agent most widely used is Tc-99m antimony sulfide colloid of particle size 3–30 nm. The most important clinical application has been in the evaluation of internal mammary lymphatics by sequential imaging, following an injection of 500 μCi into the subcostal insterstitial space. A more recent application of radionuclide targeting to lymphatics is immunolymphoscintigraphy [43]. This involves insterstitial injection of radiolabeled monoclonal antibody which targets the lymphatics and is useful in staging malignant disease to these structures.

Adrenal-Gland Imaging

The ability to image the adrenal medulla was made possible by the development of I-131-labeled metaiodobenzylguanidine (MIBG) [44]. This was based, in part, on previous work to develop antihypertensive agents that would selectively block the sympathetic nervous system. The benzyl portion of bretylium tosylate and the guanidine moiety of guanethidine sulfate were combined and eventually iodinated to produce MIBG. It is used to localize pheochromocytomas in the adrenal glands and in extrarenal tissue.

Effusion Therapy

The palliative treatment of peritoneal effusions caused by ovarian or endometrial cancer can be accomplished with P-32 chromic phosphate in the form of an insoluble suspension of approximately 1 μm-sized particles which are instilled into the peritoneal space. The colloidal particles are engulfed by floating macrophages and eventually by fixed tissue macrophages lining the wall of the serous cavity. The intense beta radiation causes fibrosis of the mesothelium and small blood vessels, which reduces fluid production. It is important that the insoluble chromic phosphate salt be used. Erroneous use of the soluble sodium phosphate salt would cause absorption into the systemic circulation and transport to the bone marrow where the P-32 beta radiation could cause bone marrow suppression.

Monoclonal Antibodies

Site-specific localization of radiotracers that target tumors with high affinity and avidity is a diagnostic goal in nuclear medicine. The specificity of the antibody–antigen reaction has been exploited to achieve that goal. The spleens of animals and humans produce B lymphocytes that can develop into antibody-producing plasma cells after exposure to foreign substances. A foreign substance may contain several different antigens, and each antigen may contain several different determinants (epitopes). Each epitope can stimulate one or more B lymphocytes whose plasma cells produce a specific antibody to the specific epitope. After immunization with a foreign substance, the host recipient produces a diverse number of antibodies (polyclonal antibodies). If, however, one could select a single lymphocyte and culture it in vitro, the single cell's progeny, or clone, would produce antibody specific for a single epitope, a monoclonal antibody. In 1975 Kohler and Milstein developed a method of producing monoclonal antibodies in vitro by fusing splenic lymphocytes from immunized mice with mouse myeloma cells [45], resulting in clones of hybrid cells called hybridomas. Because antigenically stimulated lymphocytes do not survive alone in cell culture and myeloma cells cannot be induced to secrete antigen-specific antibodies, the advantage of hybridomas is that the cells exhibit both the lymphocyte's capability of specific-antibody production and the immortal character of the myeloma cells.

Hybridomas usually produce IgG immunoglobulin. Immunoglobulin molecules are Y-shaped structures comprised of two long (heavy or H) chains and two short (light or L) chains of amino acids linked by disulfide bridges (Fig. 8). Two variable regions (Fab) can bind to specific antigenic sites, and the constant region (Fc) interacts with the host immune system. Enzymatic digestion with pepsin removes part of the constant region to produce an $F(ab')_2$ fragment, whereas papain splits the molecule into an Fc fragment and two Fab fragments.

Whole antibodies as well as antibody fragments have been radiolabeled with various radionuclides [46]. Mild iodination of tyrosine moieties with I-123 and I-131 is a common method. Another technique is to link the antibody with DTPA forming an antibody–DTPA conjugate which can be labeled with a radionuclide metal. The most critical factor in radiolabeling is maintaining immunoreactivity of the labeled antibody. A desired goal for a usable antibody is to retain at least 70% immunoreactivity.

Ideally, a labeled antibody would seek out and bind specifically to the tumor tissue and be cleared rapidly from the blood to provide high target-to-background ratios for imaging. Despite the theoretical specificity of the antigen–antibody reaction, a number of problems make this diagnostic approach to tumor detection less than desirable [47]. Specific localization of labeled antibody in tumor tissue is compromised by several factors, and typically only about 0.1% of the injected activity localizes in the tumor compared with 5–10% organ localization for routine nuclear medicine studies. For example, simple dilutional factors are important. A 1-g tumor implanted in a laboratory mouse has a

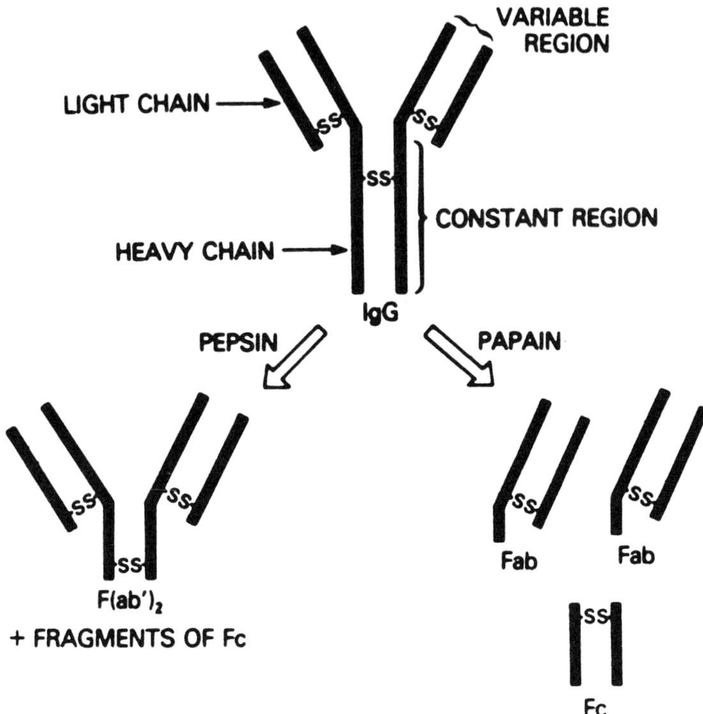

FIG. 8. Immunoglobulin G molecules consist of two heavy and two light protein chains held together by disulfide bonds. Two variable regions can bind to specific antigenic sites, and the constant region interacts with the host immune system. Enzymatic digestion with pepsin removes part of constant region to produce an $F(ab')_2$ fragment, whereas papain splits the molecule into an Fc fragment and two Fab fragments.

greater chance of reacting with tracer antibody than a 1-g tumor in a 70-kg person. Whole (intact) antibody exhibits longer circulation times and increases tumor uptake of activity, but tumor-to-background ratios are low. Ratios are higher with antibody fragments with faster blood clearances, but the absolute quantity of activity localized in tumors is lower than with whole antibody. Thus, intact antibodies appear to be better suited for therapy, whereas fragments perform better in diagnostic applications where higher target-to-nontarget ratios can be achieved earlier after injection.

Nonspecific binding of antibody in nontarget tissue reduces the tumor-to-background ratio and unnecessarily irradiates normal tissue. Antibody administration techniques have been developed to mitigate this problem. One method is to administer a second antibody, entrapped in liposomes, against the primary antibody 24 h after the primary antibody is given to clear it from the circulation, but high liver uptake of the liposomes is a complication. Another approach is to use a bifunctional antibody with one Fab end specific for tumor and the other Fab end specific for a hapten. The unlabeled antibody is administered and allowed to accumulate in tumors and clear from the circulation and normal tissue. Subsequently, a radiolabeled hapten is administered which washes rapidly out of normal tissue but targets the Fab-hapten-specific end in the tumor. This results in higher tumor-to-background ratios and reduced radiation burden to normal tissues.

Tumor localization of antibody is also dependent on the administered dose. In general, larger doses of antibody prolong serum half-life, reduce nonspecific visceral uptake, and increase tumor uptake. This has led to enhanced ability to detect lesions. The assumed mechanism is an increased saturation of antibody binding in the liver and other nonspecific sites with increasing administered dose, leading to decreased blood clearance and greater availability of antibody-to-target antigen.

Although significant advances have been made to improve tumor specificity of radiolabeled monoclonal antibodies, a tumor-specific antibody per se probably does not exist, and even with the purest of antibodies, the range of tumor concentration of the antibody is still suboptimal for imaging and therapy. It appears that biologic response modifiers may be required to develop the clinically successful applications of antibodies, such as recombinant interferon, to enhance antigen expression on the surface of malignant cells.

Several radionuclides have been used to label antibodies; the most important for diagnostic use are I-123, Tc-99m, and In-111 [48]. Radioiodination is accomplished by conversion of iodide to the positively charged electrophilic species which covalently labels tyrosine moieties in the protein. The process is often not quantitative, requiring separation of unlabeled nuclide. Iodine-131 is useful for diagnosis and therapy; I-123 is an ideal diagnostic but its 13-h half-life and cyclotron production make it inconvenient and expensive to use. Clinically, radioiodinated antibodies tend to undergo in vivo deiodination with loss of activity from the antibody and irradiation of nontarget tissue, especially the thyroid gland. Administration of a stable iodide, such as SSKI, is required to protect the thyroid.

The stability of the radiolabel has been improved by the bifunctional chelate method in antibody labeling [49]. A chelating agent, such as EDTA or DTPA, is linked to the antibody via a linker molecule, such as benzyl isothiocyanate or benzylbromoacetamide, which is covalently bound to the antibody via a lysine amino group. The chelating group serves to bind radionuclide metals such as In-111. Potential problems with indium labeling include trace metal contamination and hydrolysis control near neutral pH. However, these problems can be readily overcome and labeling yields are generally quantitative, requiring no further purification. With this method, antibody manufacturers can produce a lyophilized kit of the purified antibody conjugate. At the time of use, In-111 is added to the kit whereupon it firmly binds to the antibody via the chelating group. The 2.8 day indium-111 half-life is desirable when tumor uptake is slow and imaging procedures require several days to complete. Significant uptake occurs in the liver and kidney which may obscure tumor localization in these regions.

Considering availability, cost, and imaging properties, Tc-99m is the ideal nuclide label for antibodies. Its major drawbacks are difficulties in the labeling chemistry of antibodies and its short half-life (6 h), which presents problems where optimal imaging is at more than 18 h following dosing. Technetium-99m is bound to antibody either directly via free sulfhydryl groups made available by prereduction with stannous ion or indirectly via bifunctional chelates [50].

Since most monoclonal antibodies are murine-derived, there is the possibility of human subjects developing human antimouse antibodies (HAMA) [47]. This is particularly a problem where multiple doses of antibody are given over time, such as in radioimmunotherapy. The principal source of immune sensitization to mouse monoclonal antibodies appears to be the constant region of the antibody. An approach to mitigate this problem has been the use of antibody fragments, $F(ab')_2$ or Fab (Fig. 8), but their disadvantages are lower tumor uptake and high renal accretion which may present toxicity problems to the kidneys. Recombinant-DNA techniques make it possible to combine the V region of useful mouse monoclonal antibodies with the C regions of human monoclonal antibodies in order to generate chimeric molecules with less immunogenicity. The same technology can also be used to create molecules in which all or parts of the Fc region are replaced by toxins, chemotherapeutic agents, enzymes, or other molecules intended for targeted drug delivery. (See Cannon et al., under Bibliography for more discussion of this topic.) Regional administration increases antibody contact with cancer cells and avoids the problems of systemic administration. In this regard, intraperitoneal injection and interstitial (lymphatic) administration are being investigated [46].

Many radiolabeled monoclonal antibodies have been developed for nuclear medicine studies, but only a few have had a significant impact on the diagnosis and treatment of disease. There is still the need to improve hybridoma technology and to learn how to modify and use monoclonal antibodies to achieve higher target affinity. Several antibodies have entered clinical trials, but only one has been approved by the FDA Center for Biologics Evaluation and Research for routine application. The greatest progress appears to have been made in identifying colorectal cancer, melanoma, neuroblastoma, lymphoma, breast and ovarian cancer, and prostatic cancer.

Interventional Agents

Probably the closest interaction of nuclear medicine and pharmacy is in the use of pharmacologic agents to augment nuclear medicine studies. Several drugs are used to pharmacologically alter radiopharmaceutical distribution in various organs to facilitate diagnosis.

Cardiac Intervention

The routine assessment of myocardial viability in patients with coronary artery disease is made by observing the myocardial distribution of a perfusion tracer, such as Tl-201 chloride, at normal coronary blood flow (rest) and at elevated blood flow (stress). In general, regions of myocardium demonstrating deficient tracer uptake at rest and at stress indicate infarction, whereas deficient uptake at stress only with normal uptake at rest indicate the presence of viable myocardium whose blood flow under stress is reduced due to coronary stenosis. Coronary blood flow can be increased through exercise (treadmill or bicycle ergometer) or following administration of dobutamine or the coronary vasodilators adenosine and dipyridamole [51]. The required maximal increase in coronary blood flow is often difficult to achieve clinically following exercise because patients suspected of having heart disease can rarely reach the intense exercise level required. The reasons may be physical or emotional or due to beta-blocking medication which prevents patients from adequately exercising their hearts. In these situations, a coronary vasodilator provides the required increase in blood flow to conduct the study.

Hepatobiliary Intervention

Several agents have been used successfully to augment hepatobiliary studies in nuclear medicine [52].

Cholecystokinin

Hepatobiliary studies are performed routinely to evaluate obstruction to bile flow via the cystic duct into the gallbladder. Lack of gallbladder uptake of tracer (Tc-99m disofenin or Tc-99m mebrofenin) is an indication of acute cholecystitis. False positive scans, that is, lack of gallbladder uptake when the cystic duct is patent, can occur in certain situations, such as after fasting longer than 48 h, during intravenous hyperalimentation, and anorexia. In these cases, when the gallbladder is filled and intraluminal pressure is high, it is necessary to empty the gallbladder with the help of cholecystokinin (CCK) or sincalide, the C-terminal octapeptide of CCK. The usual dose is 0.02 μg/kg iv over 3 min. It causes contraction of the gallbladder and relaxation of the sphincter of Oddi prior to administration of the radiopharmaceutical. After contraction, the gallbladder relaxes, creating an optimal state for the accumulation of Tc-99m tracer if the cystic duct is patent.

Cholecystokinin is also used to determine gallbladder ejection fraction in patients with partially obstructed, chronically inflamed, or functionally impaired gallbladders. These patients respond differently to exogenous CCK than individuals with normal gallbladder function; they have a diminished, maximal gallbladder ejection response ($< 35\%$) to CCK. The ejection fraction is determined from the difference in gallbladder counts before and after CCK administration after a prescribed time, usually 20 min.

Morphine Sulfate

Differentiating between acute cholecystitis (lack of gallbladder visualization due to a nonpatent cystic duct) from chronic cholecystitis (delayed gallbaldder visualization due to a sludge-filled gallbladder) can be augmented by morphine sulfate intervention. Nonvisualization of the gallbladder 60 min following injection of radiotracer is indicative of acute cholecystitis. However, imaging must be delayed to rule out chronic cholecystitis. Delayed gallbladder visualization in patients with chronic cholecystitis may take several hours. Administration of 0.04 mg/kg of morphine sulfate in 10 mL of saline over 3 min causes constriction of the sphincter of Oddi and an increased intraluminal common bile duct pressure. The increased pressure is high enough to overcome the increased resistence to bile flow within a functionally obstructed sludge-filled gallbladder and diverts radiotracer into the cystic duct if it is patent. This procedure can easily shorten the study from 4 to 1.5 h.

Phenobarbital

Phenobarbital can be used to differentiate neonatal hepatitis from biliary atresia. Phenobarbital is a potent hepatic enzyme inducer, increasing bilirubin conjugation and excretion and enhancing the uptake and excretion of bile via the membrane-bound hepatic transport system for organic anions, the same system used by Tc-99m hepatobiliary tracers. In essence, neonatal hepatitis is characterized by the inability to conjugate bilirubin due to damaged hepatocytes, whereas biliary atresia is characterized by obstruction to bile flow resulting from sclerosis or absence of bile ducts. It is important to make the distinction between these two liver conditions because patient management depends on it. Biliary atresia requires corrective surgery within the first 60 days of life, whereas hepatitis requires medical management.

Phenobarbital is administered at a dosage of 5 mg/kg orally in two doses for five consecutive days before intravenous administration of Tc-99m hepatobiliary agent. The effect of phenobarbital on liver function enhances tracer excretion. If tracer is excreted into the bowel, biliary atresia is ruled out since the ducts are obviously patent. If not, the distinction between biliary atresia and severe hepatocellular disease, which restricts liver extraction of tracer, must be made by other diagnostic tests.

Renal Intervention

The main areas for pharmacologic intervention in renal studies are in obstructive uropathy and renovascular hypertension [53].

Furosemide

A delayed washout of radiotracer from the kidney may be caused by mechanical obstruction to urine flow or a dilated collecting system without obstruction. A distinction between these two conditions can be facilitated by the use of furosemide, a rapid-acting diuretic. The study, called a diuretic renogram, is conducted by administration of a radiopharmaceutical, such as Tc-99m DTPA or Tc-99m MAG_3, which is cleared into the urine, followed after 15–30 min by an intravenous injection of furosemide. The usual adult dosage is 0.3–0.5 mg/kg (20–40 mg); infants and children should receive 1 mg/kg up to 20 mg in a single dose. Under normal conditions, without furosemide, the radiotracer reaches peak renal concentration in 3–5 min and washes out with a half-time of 12–15 min, producing a normal renogram curve (Fig. 9). If the collecting system is dilated, however, pooling of tracer and an increased transit time occurs, giving the appearance of renal obstruction. However, the administration of furosemide produces an increase in urine flow. If no obstruction is present, the increased urine flow causes the tracer to be washed rapidly out of the kidney. If obstruction is present, no washout occurs.

Captopril

Angiotensin converting enzyme (ACE) inhibitors, such as captopril, can be used in conjunction with renal scintigraphy to evaluate renovascular hypertension. A single dose of captopril, 25 mg, is given orally 1 h before injection of radiotracer (Tc-99m DTPA). In the diseased kidney, the uptake of tracer is dramatically reduced as evidenced by a flat renogram curve.The renogram of the normal kidney is unaffected. When renovascular hypertension is present, angiotensin II is produced which constricts the efferent arteriole on the affected kidney in order to maintain a high filtration pressure. Captopril inhibits the production of angiotensin II, causing dilatation of the efferent arteriole on the affected kidney. The resultant drop in filtration pressure in the affected kidney leads to reduced glomerular clearance of Tc-99m DTPA tracer, creating a flat renogram curve. The normal kidney is unaffected by captopril.

Radionuclides in Drug Development

Within the pharmaceutical industry both beta- and gamma-emitting isotopes have been used. The radioactive isotopes listed in Table 4 have been used to evaluate the metabolic

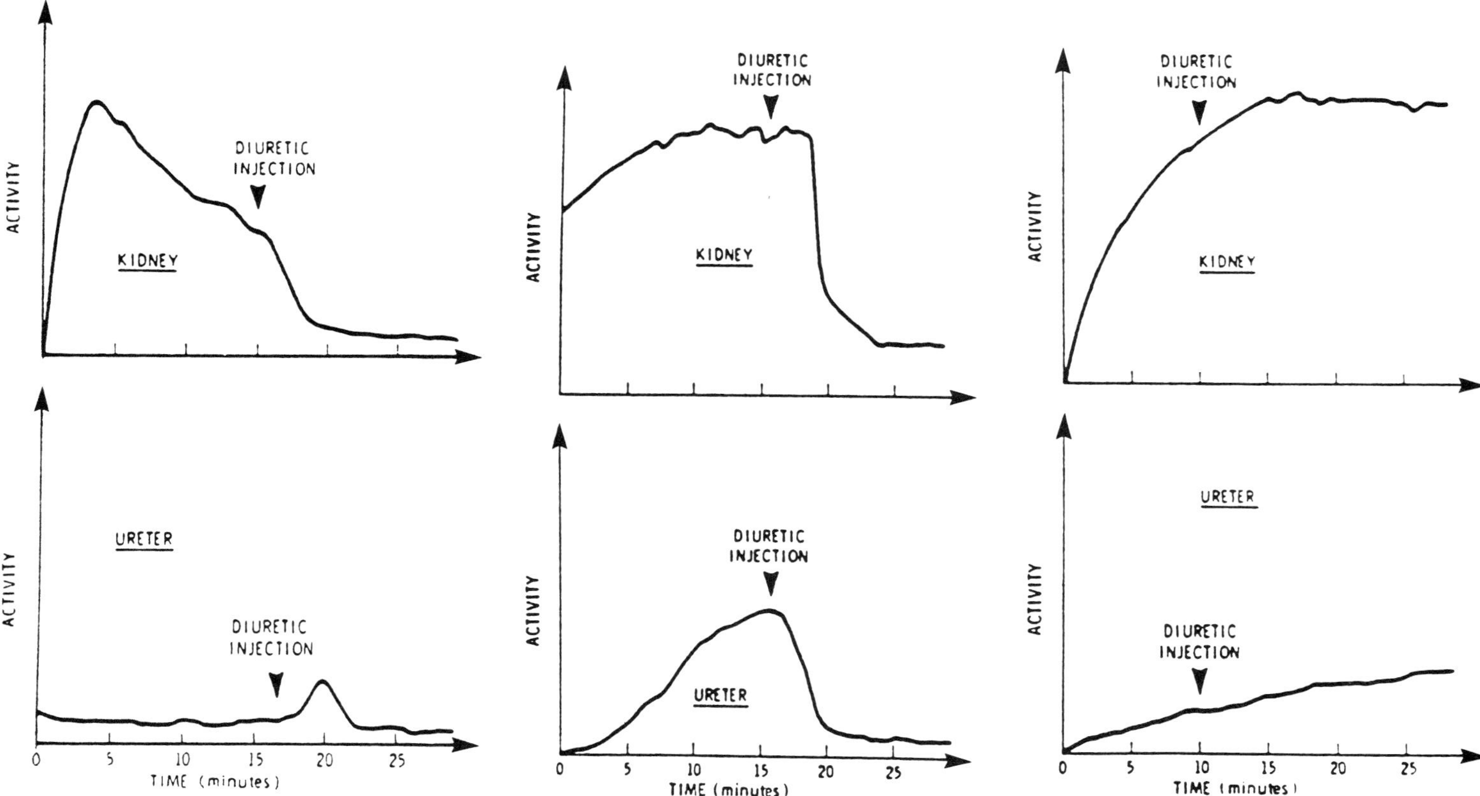

FIG. 9. Representative furosemide renograms showing time–activity curve patterns in a normal patient (A), and in patients with dilated nonobstruction (B) and obstruction (C) of the urinary collecting systems. (From Thrall, J. H., Koff, S. A., and Keyes, J. W., Jr., Diuretic radionuclide renography and scintigraphy in the differential diagnosis of hydroureteronephrosis, *Semin. Nucl. Med.*, 11(20):89–104 (1981), with permission.)

fate of drugs (absorption, distribution, metabolism, and excretion, ADME), DNA sequencing, and receptor localization and binding. Because they lack gamma emission, use of these isotopes limits the investigator to in vitro methods of detection and measurement, such as liquid scintillation counting. The radioactive isotopes listed in Table 5 emit gamma rays and thus have been used for in vivo receptor localization studies and evaluation of various pharmaceutical dosage forms. In addition to these novel applications of short-lived isotopes, pharmaceutical scientists have also used radiopharmaceuticals to evaluate the effect of drugs on various physiological factors such as cardiac output. The subsequent discussion covers the application of short-lived radioactive isotopes in the drug development process. Specifically, it gives a historical view of this area of research and includes labeling methods, applications, and future trends.

TABLE 4 Radioactive Isotopes Used Within the Pharmaceutical Industry for the In Vitro and In Vivo Evaluation of Drugs

Isotope	Decay Mode[a]	Half-Life	Application
Carbon-14	Beta–	5730 years	Metabolism studies
Iodine-129	Beta–	1.59×10^7 years	Peptide–protein studies[b]
Phosphorus-32	Beta–	14.3 days	Peptide–protein studies[b]
Sulfur-35	Beta–	87.2 days	Peptide–protein studies[b]
Tritium-3	Beta–	12.33 years	Metabolism studies

[a]Negatron.
[b]Includes receptor localization and binding studies.

TABLE 5 Radioactive Isotopes Used Within the Pharmaceutical Industry for the In Vivo Evaluation of Dosage Forms and Drugs

Isotope	Decay Mode[b]	Half-Life	Photon Energy (keV)
Barium-139	Beta–	83.8 min	166
Carbon-11[a]	Beta+	20.3 min	511
Erbium-171	Beta–	7.5 h	112, 124, 296, 308
Fluorine-18[a]	Beta+	109.8 min	511
Indium-111	EC	2.8 days	172, 247
Indium-113m	IT	99.8 min	393
Iodine-123	EC	13.1 h	159
Iodine-131	Beta–	8.0 days	364, 637
Oxygen-15[a]	Beta+	2.0 min	511
Samarium-153	Beta–	46.7 h	103
Technetium-99m	IT	6.0 h	140

[a]Cyclotron produced.
[b]EC = electron transfer; IT = isomeric transition; Beta+ = positron; Beta– = negatron.

History and Techniques

The in vitro evaluation of orally administered dosage forms, such as tablet and capsule preparations, has been evaluated on the basis of hardness, disintegration, and dissolution studies and other parameters since the early 1900s. Poor correlation is often observed between these in vitro parameters and the in vivo plasma concentration. This poor correlation has been associated with unequal absorption of the drug throughout the GI tract, variability in gastric emptying, disease states, and a multiple of other factors. Because of this poor correlation between in vitro and in vivo data, alternative techniques have been developed to monitor the in vivo behavior (i.e., disintegration) of dosage forms. These include:

- Use of radiopaque materials (roentgenography),
- String technique,
- Endoscope technique,
- pH detection (radiotelemetry), and
- External scintigraphy.

The first technique applied to the in vivo evaluation of dosage forms was roentgenography. By incorporating barium sulfate into a pharmaceutical dosage form, it is possible to follow its passage through the GI tract using continual x-ray procedures. Movement, location, and integrity of the radiopaque dosage form after administration was determined by placing the subject under a fluoroscope and taking a series of x-rays at various time points. The wide use of this technique, however, has declined due to the large radiation dose the subject receives and the ease and accuracy of more modern methods such as external scintigraphy.

The string technique was first applied in 1958 by Gruber et al. [54] and by Steinberg et al. in 1965 [55]. In these studies, a tablet was attached to a piece of string 90 cm (3 ft) in length. The subject swallowed the tablet, leaving the free end of the string hanging from his mouth. At various time points, the tablets were withdrawn from the stomach by pulling on the string and physically examining the tablet for signs of disintegration. In some studies the tablets were recovered by inducing a vomiting reflex.

The endoscope technique has also been applied to the evaluation of the in vivo behavior of dosage forms. This is an optical technique in which a fiber scope (gastroscope) is used to directly monitor the behavior of the dosage form after ingestion. It requires administration of a mild sedative to facilitate the swallowing of the endoscopic tube. The sedative itself may alter gastric emptying and GI motility.

The radiotelemetry technique involves the administration of a capsule that consists of a small pH probe interfaced with a miniature radio transmitter which is capable of sending a signal (indicating the pH of the environment) to an external antenna attached to the body of the person or animal that swallowed the capsule. To evaluate dosage forms by this technology, it is necessary to physically attach the dosage form of interest to the capsule, which in turn may affect the behavior of the dosage form being studied.

All of these techniques, roentgenography, the string technique, endoscopy, and radiotelemetry have numerous disadvantages. For example, in the case of the x-ray technique, the radiation dose to the subject is very high in comparison to other techniques. With the string and endoscope techniques, a foreign object is placed in the stomach or GI tract which can alter its motility and the physiochemical environment. Gastrointestinal motility may also be affected by the psychological stress and anxiety associated with these methods.

The inherent disadvantage of radiotelemetry is the necessity for the dosage form to be physically attached to the pH capsule, which could lead to a change in the in vivo behavior of the dosage form. Furthermore, the dosage forms being evaluated must contain significant amounts of buffer salts, preventing the evaluation of commercially marketable products. It is the release of these buffer salts from the dosage form that produces a change in the gastrointestinal pH which is detected by the pH capsule and therefore indicates a change in the dosage form.

The most useful technique, to date, to evaluate the in vivo behavior of dosage forms in animals and humans is external scintigraphy. Work in this area began in the 1970s under the direction of Digenis and his group at the University of Kentucky [56]. Through the modification of standard nuclear medicine methods they were able to monitor the in vivo behavior of dosage forms.

External scintigraphy requires in the dosage form the presence of a gamma-emitting radioactive isotope that can be detected by a gamma camera. The dosage form in question can be radiolabeled using conventional labeling or neutron activation (both of which are discussed later). Since its initial application in the early 1970s, external scintigraphy has been applied to the in vivo evaluation of most pharmaceutical dosage forms currently on the market.

The advantages of external scintigraphy are:

1. It produces very little danger to the participating subjects in terms of radiation exposure as compared to roentgenography.
2. Unlike other techniques, it can give both qualitative and quantitative results.
3. It is totally noninvasive, and
4. It allows for the in vivo evaluation of dosage forms under ideal conditions.

Some of the disadvantages of this technique are:

1. Radiation exposure to participating subjects,
2. The inability to accurately quantitate activity in the small bowel, and
3. The inability to label the compound of interest.

An additional disadvantage, associated with the conventional labeling method, is the limitation of being able to label only simple dosage forms under small-scale conditions at the imaging facility. With the application of neutron activation to radiolabel dosage forms, more complex and sophisticated dosage forms can be labeled and manufactured under industrial-scale conditions.

The gamma-emitting isotopes commonly used in the pharmaceutical industry are listed in Table 5. Two of the most commonly used radioactive isotopes within nuclear medicine, Tc-99m and In-111, have also been used to evaluate the in vivo behavior of dosage forms and correlate gastrointestinal behavior with pharmacokinetic parameters (i.e., correlation of location of dosage form in a certain region of the GI tract to maximum plasma concentration). Using these two isotopes and the conventional labeling process, simple pharmaceutical dosage forms, such as direct compression tablets and capsules can be quickly radiolabeled. More sophisticated dosage forms (sustained-released tablets and capsules) can be radiolabeled with barium-139, erbium-171, and samarium-153 employing the neutron-activation radiolabeling method [59].

The other isotopes listed in Table 5 are also used to evaluate dosage form behavior in vivo in the same fashion as Tc-99m and In-111. For example, the radioactive isotopes of iodine (I-123 and I-131) can be used to radiolabel dosage forms and active drug moieties such as peptides as well as other compounds that are easily iodinated, permitting the in vivo evaluation of both the dosage form and the drug. However, prior to extensive studies involving these iodinated compounds, preliminary studies should be undertaken to ensure that the iodination process has not changed the ADME characteristics of the original compound.

The cyclotron-produced nuclides are more difficult to work with but are more applicable to determining the distribution of the drug in vivo and its site of action. As indicated in Table 5, these cyclotron-produced nuclides have very short half-lives and therefore require a cyclotron facility in very close proximity to the imaging facility. They also require a PET scanner, a special camera designed to image these types of isotopes. Since these nuclides have short half-lives and are incorporated directly into the active drug molecule, the synthesis and purification of the radiolabeled molecules must be done in a very short period of time. Positron emitters have the advantages of isotopic radiolabeling of the drug and the generation of a 3-D image. The disadvantage are the cost of the isotopes and imaging equipment and the short imaging time available.

Labeling Procedures

Conventional Method

The conventional labeling method consists of incorporating a gamma-emitting isotope into the dosage form of interest prior to its manufacture. The nuclide (Tc-99m or In-111) is added, in a liquid form, to an aliquot of one of the excipients present in the formulation. The resulting mixture is dried to remove the excess liquid. The dried radiolabeled excipient is incorporated into the formulation in the usual manner. The radiolabeled dosage form is administered via its appropriate route and followed with a gamma-scintillation camera. This method is nonspecific and does not involve the direct radiolabeling of the drug molecule. Therefore, in vitro studies must be undertaken to determine that release of the radioactive marker from the dosage form correlates with the drug release. This method has been used to radiolabel tablets, capsules, suppositories, aerosols, liquids, and enemas since its introduction by Casey et al. [56] in 1976. Although the labeling method is easy, its application is limited to simple dosage forms made in small-scale batches.

Neutron Activation

The conventional method is very effective for radiolabeling simple pharmaceutical dosage forms such as direct-compression tablets and capsules. However, it cannot be readily used to radiolabel more complex dosage forms such as sustained-release or delayed-release dosage forms. These more complex dosage forms may require long manufacturing times or the need for unique manufacturing equipment that is not available at the imaging facility. Additionally, the conventional radiolabeling method cannot be used to radiolabel production-scale batches because of the large amount of radioactive isotopes needed and the radiation exposure to manufacturing personnel.

An alternative method was developed by Parr et al., using neutron activation to radiolabel intact dosage forms [57]. This method, which was initially developed as an analytical tool in 1936, converts stable nuclides to gamma-emitting nuclides which can be easily followed with a gamma-scintillation camera. The nuclides used in this procedure are carefully chosen in such a way that pharmaceutical dosage forms can be safely radiolabeled intact and with a high degree of purity. The isotopes of interest are listed in Table 5. The original work was done with the barium, erbium, and samarium isotopes, but just recently Sandefer et al. reported the use of ytterbium as another viable isotope [58]. The flexibility of this labeling method is based on Eq. (1)

$$A = nfX(1 - e^{-\lambda t_i})e^{-\lambda t_d}$$

where

A = activity (counts per second)
n = number of target atoms
f = neutron flux ($n \cdot cm^2/s$)
X = neutron capture cross-section (units in barns)
λ = decay constant for isotope of interest
t_i = irradiation time
t_d = decay time

Parameters A, n, f, t_i, and t_d can be varied, thus permitting the method to be adapted to the radiolabeling of even complex dosage forms. An example of this is the ability to use two different isotopes to radiolabel different parts of the same dosage form. This is possible by using appropriate quantities of any two of the three isotopes (Ba-138, Er-170, Sa-152) as well as appropriate irradiation and decay times. This way the same dosage form can be radiolabeled (i.e., tablet core with one isotope and the coating with a second isotope) and the in vivo behavior of each evaluated simultaneously. Along with varying the above parameters, the inherent range of radionuclide parameters of each of the isotopes adds flexibility to this method. For example, by using sufficient quantities of the samarium isotope and appropriate irradiation time it is possible to label dosage forms containing sodium or potassium salts. The problem with radiolabeling dosage forms that contain sodium and potassium is that these isotopes become radioactive when the dosage form is irradiated. However, by using sufficient quantities of samarium and appropriate irradiation time, it is possible to let the sodium and potassium isotopes decay to background levels and still have sufficient levels of samarium to image with.

The only requirement for radiolabeling intact dosage forms with these isotopes is the incorporation of a small amount (μg to mg) of the appropriate stable isotope (Ba-138, Sa-152, Er-170) into the formulation prior to the manufacture of the dosage form. This stable isotope is added in the same way as any other bulk excipient. Once manufactured, the dosage form is exposed to a neutron source (nuclear reactor) and the stable isotope is converted to a radioactive gamma-emitting isotope that can be easily followed by a gamma camera. This procedure therefore permits the labeling of industrial-scale batches without the risk of contamination of facilities and equipment or high radiation exposure to personnel. As with conventional labeling, this is a nonspecific method, and in vitro studies need therefore to be undertaken to ensure that release of the radioactive marker correlates with release of drug from the dosage form.

Studies undertaken by Parr et al. have shown that this procedure does not affect the physical parameters of dosage forms, such as hardness, dissolution, and disintegration when concentrations of less than 1% of stable isotopes are used with irradiation times of less than 2 min [59]. The irradiation procedure does not affect the chemical stability of drugs such as erythromycin and ibuprofen [60,61].

Applications

Since its initial application, the external scintigraphy technique has been applied to the in vivo evaluation of tablets, capsules, pellets, suppositories, enemas, aerosols, and parenteral preparations such as iv emulsions, and liposomes. The in vivo information that can be obtained from these studies includes:

- Transit time through various regions of the GI tract,
- In vivo disintegration of dosage forms,
- The ability of a dosage form to target drug delivery to specific regions of GI tract, and
- The ability to predict or explain unusual pharmacokinetic results.

Parr et al. used external scintigraphy to correlate the GI transit of an ibuprofen tablet preparation with its pharmacokinetic results [61]. The study showed a strong correlation ($r = 0.892$) between total area under the curve and total GI transit time. It also indicated that the largest percentage of ibuprofen absorption occurs in the colon. Finally, the researchers used the data to predict and explain unusual pharmacokinetic results such as poor bioavailability (rapid GI transit time), and double peaks observed in the plasma profile (the second peak was associated with the complete disintegration of the dosage form and the complete release of drug).

In a similar vein, Digenis et al. demonstrated the ability for dual-isotope studies [62]. They labeled the pharmaceutical dosage form with two different isotopes, Sa-153 for one half of a bilayer tablet and Er-171 for the other half. Since both isotopes can be monitored by the gamma camera simultaneously, it is possible to evaluate the behavior of both parts of the tablet at the same time. This dual-label system can also be used to evaluate two different dosage forms administered to the same subject at the same time.

External scintigraphy has also been used to evaluate how specific physical properties of the dosage form and certain environmental factors (e.g., food) affect gastric emptying and GI transit time of dosage forms. For example, investigators have reported the effect of dosage form size, shape, weight, and specific gravity on gastric retention time. The technique has also been applied to the evaluation of various environmental factors on gastric emptying, such as food intake, smoking, age, and menstrual cycle.

Outlook

Future trends in this area include the combination of radioisotopes with other analytical methods. For example, external scintigraphy and mass spectrometry can be combined to evaluate calcium absorption. The scintigraphic technique permits the in vivo evaluation of the dosage form and therefore correlation of in vivo behavior to pharmacokinetic parameters. The mass spectroscopy technique permits the monitoring of calcium plasma levels. Although calcium is found in large amounts in the plasma, and can therefore be easily analyzed by more conventional methods, the sophisticated technique of mass spectroscopy is needed to determine calcium levels because the source of the calcium (i.e., dietary intake, bone resorption) cannot be easily determined by standard methods. Therefore, by using mass spectroscopy and an enriched form of calcium it is possible to determine the source of calcium in the plasma. Combining these two techniques could thus give better insight to the site of calcium absorption. It would also permit the evaluation of two different dosage forms in the same subject at the same time. Again, the scintigraphy technique is used to evaluate the in vivo behavior of the dosage forms, and mass spectroscopy is used to evaluate the ratio of drug A and drug A_1 (the same drug labeled with an enriched isotope) in a plasma sample. If the dosage forms behave differently in vivo, as indicated by scintigraphy, then the ratio of A to A_1 may or may not be different as well.

The combination of nuclides with various radiotelemetry devices will also be useful. Work has already begun in combining scintigraphy with a pH-monitoring system to more accurately monitor GI physiology. Work has also begun in combining remote drug-delivery systems (capsule designed to release drug in a specific area of the GI tract) with scintigraphy to more accurately evaluate regional drug absorption sites.

Bibliography

Cannon, J., Hui, H. W., and Adjei, A., Monoclonal Antibodies for Drug Delivery, In: *Encyclopedia of Pharmaceutical Technology* (J. S. Swarbrick, and J. C. Boylan, eds.), Vol. 10, Marcel Dekker, Inc. New York, 1994, pp. 83–120.

Burns, H. D., and Gibson, R. E., Nuclear Imaging in Pharmaceutical Research. In: *Encyclopedia of Pharmaceutical Technology* (J. S. Swarbrick and J. C. Boylan, eds.), Vol. 10, Marcel Dekker, Inc, New York, 1994, pp. 303–334.

Gottschalk, A., Hoffer, P. B., and Potchen, E. J., eds., *Diagnostic Nuclear Medicine*, 2nd ed., Vol 1, Williams and Wilkins, Baltimore, MD, 1988.

Kowalsky, R. J., and Perry, J. R., Radiopharmaceuticals. In: *Nuclear Medicine Practice*, Appleton and Lange, Norwalk, CT, 1987.

References

1. Neirinckx, R. D., Burke J. F., Harrison, R. C., et al., *J. Cereb. Blood Flow Metab.*, 8:S4–S12 (1988).
2. Baldwin, R. M., and Wu, J. L., *J. Nucl. Med.*, 29:122–124 (1988).
3. Kung, H. F., *Semin. Nucl. Med.*, 20:150–158 (1990).
4. Kuhl, D. E., Phelps, M. E., Kowell, A. P., et al., *Ann. Neurol.*, 8:47–60 (1980).
5. Wong, D. F., Wagner, H. N., Jr., Dannals, R. F., et al., *Science*, 226:1393–1396 (1984).
6. Partain, C. L., Alderson, P. O., Donovan, R. L., et al. In: *Radiopharmaceutical Dosimetry Symposium* (R. J. Cloutier, J. L. Coffey, W. S. Synder, and E. E. Watson, eds.), HEW Publication (FDA) 76–8044, Oakridge, 1976, pp. 404–414.
7. Curnes, J. T., Vincent, L. M., Kowalsky, R. J., et al., *Radiology*, 154:795–799 (1985).
8. Nunn, A. D., *Semin. Nucl. Med.*, 20:111–118 (1990).
9. Schelbert, H. R., *Semin. Nucl. Med.*, 17:145–181 (1987).
10. Pohost, G. M., Alpert, N. M., Ingwall, J. S., et al., *Semin. Nucl. Med.*, 10:70–93 (1980).

11. Bonow, R. O., Dilsizian, V., Cuocolo, A., et al., *Circulation*, 83:26–37 (1991).
12. Alazraki, N., Nuclear Imaging of the Cardiovascular System. In: *Cardiac Imaging in Infants, Children, and Adults* (L. P. Elliot, ed.), J. B. Lippincott Co, Philadelphia, 1991, pp. 41–55.
13. Buja, L. M., Tofe, A. J., Kulkarni, P. V., et al., *J. Clin. Invest.*, 60:724–740 (1977).
14. Volpini, M., Giubbini, R., Gei, P., et al., *Am. J. Cardiol.*, 63:7–13 (1989).
15. Alderson, P. O., Biello, D. R., and Gottschalk, A., *Radiology*, 153:515–521 (1984).
16. Davis, M. A., and Taube, R. A., *J. Nucl. Med.*, 19:1209–1213 (1978).
17. Kowalsky, R. J., *J. Nucl. Med. Tech.*, 10:223–227 (1982).
18. Dworkin, H. J., Gutkowski, R. F., Porter, W., et al., *J. Nucl. Med.*, 18:260–262 (1977).
19. Loberg, M. D., Porter, D. W., and Ryan, J. W., Review and Current Status of Hepatobiliary Imaging Agents. In: *Radiopharmaceuticals* II. Proceedings of the 2nd International Symposium on Radiopharmaceticals (J. A. Sorenson, ed.), Society of Nuclear Medicine, New York, 1979, pp. 519–543.
20. Davis, M. A., Jones, A. G., and Trindade, H. J., *Nucl. Med.*, 15:923–928 (1974).
21. Weissman, H. S., Gliedman, M. L., Wilk, P. J., et al., *Semin. Nucl. Med.*, 12:27–52 (1982).
22. Weissman, H. S., Badia, J., Sugarman, L. A., et al., *Radiology*, 138:167–175 (1981).
23. Atkins, H. L., Goldman, A. G., Fairchild, R. G., et al., *Radiology*, 136:501–504 (1980).
24. Eckelman, W., and Richards, P., *J. Nucl. Med.*, 11:761 (1970).
25. McAfee, J. G., Gagne, G., Atkins, H. L., et al., *J. Nucl. Med.*, 20:1273–1278 (1979).
26. Arnold, R. W., Subramanian, G, McAfee, J. G., et al., *J. Nucl. Med.*, 16:357–367 (1975).
27. deKievit, W., *J. Nucl. Med.*, 22:703–709 (1981).
28. Lee, H. B., and Blaufox, M. D., *J. Nucl. Med.*, 26:1308–1313 (1985).
29. Yee, C. A., Lee, H. B., and Blaufox, M. D., *J. Nucl. Med.*, 22:1054–1058 (1981).
30. Van Luyck, W. H. J., Piers, D. A., Beekhuis, H., et al., *J. Nucl. Med.*, 27:1943 (1986).
31. Dubovsky, E. V., and Russell, C. D., *Semin. Nucl. Med.*, 12:308–329 (1982).
32. Eshima, D., Fritzberg, A. R., and Taylor, A., Jr., *Semin. Nucl. Med.*, 20:28–40 (1990).
33. Blaufox, M. D., *J. Nucl. Med.*, 32:1301–1309 (1991).
34. Davis, M. A., and Jones, A. G., *Semin. Nucl. Med.*, 6:19–31 (1976).
35. Subramanian, G., McAfee, J. G., Blair, R. J., et al., *J. Nucl. Med.*, 16:744–755 (1975).
36. Littlefield, J. L., and Rudd, T. G., *J. Nucl. Med.*, 24:463–466 (1983).
37. Thakur, M. L., Coleman, R. E., Welch, M. J., et al., *J. Lab. Clin. Med.*, 89:217–228, (1977).
38. Alavi, A., *Semin. Nucl. Med.*, 12:126 (1982).
39. Winzelberg, G. G., McKusick, K. A., Froelich, J. W., et al., *Semin. Nucl. Med.*, 12:139 (1982).
40. Christian, P. E., Datz, F. L., Sorenson, J. A., et al., *J. Nucl. Med.*, 24:264–268 (1983).
41. Sfakianakis, G. N., and Conway, J. J., *J. Nucl. Med.*, 22:647–654, 732–738 (1981).
42. Ege, G. N., *Radiology*, 118:101–107 (1976).
43. Keenan, A. M., *Semin. Nucl. Med.*, 19:322–331 (1989).
44. Wieland, D. M., Brown, L. E., Tobes, M. C., et al., *J. Nucl. Med.*, 22:358–364 (1981).
45. Kohler, G., and Milstein, C., *Nature*, 256:495–497 (1975).
46. Keenan, A. M., Harbert, J. C., and Larson, S. M., *J. Nucl. Med.*, 26:531–537 (1985).
47. Zuckier, L. S., Rodriguez, L. D., and Scharff, M. D., *Semin. Nucl. Med.*, 19:166–186 (1989).
48. Bhargava, K. K., and Acharya, S. A., *Semin. Nucl. Med.*, 19:187–201 (1989).
49. Westerberg, D. A., Carney, P. L., Rogers, P. E., et al., *J. Med. Chem.*, 32:236–243 (1989).
50. Eckelman, W. C., Paik, C. H., and Steigman, J., *Nucl. Med. Biol.*, 16:171–176 (1989).
51. DePuey, E. G., and Rozanski, A., *Semin. Nucl. Med.*, 21:92–102 (1991).
52. Fink-Bennett, D., *Semin. Nucl. Med.*, 21:128–139 (1991).
53. Fine, E. J., *Semin. Nucl. Med.*, 21:116–127 (1991).
54. Gruber, C. M., Ridolfo, A. A., and Tosick, W. A., *J. Am. Pharm. Assoc., Sci. Ed.*, 47:862–866 (1958).

55. Steinberg, W. H., Frey, C. H., Masci, J. N., et al., *J. Pharm. Sci.*, 54:747–752 (1965).
56. Casey, D. L., Beihn, R. M., Digenis, G. A., et al., *J. Parm. Sci.*, 65:1412–1413 (1976).
57. Parr, A., Jay, M., Digenis, G. A., et al., *J. Pharm. Sci.*, 74:590–591 (1985).
58. Sandefer, E. P., Digenis, G. A., and Beihn, R. M., *Pharm. Res.*, 8:S133 (1991).
59. Parr, A., and Jay, M., *Pharm. Res.*, 4:524–526 (1987).
60. Parr, A., Digenis, G. A., Sandefer, E. P., et al., *Pharm. Res.*, 7:264–269 (1990).
61. Parr, A., Beihn, R. M., Franz, R. M., et al., *Pharm. Res.*, 4:486–489 (1987).
62. Digenis, G. A., Sandefer, E. P., Beihn, R., et al., *Pharm. Res.*, 8:1335–1340 (1991).

RICHARD J. KOWALSKY
ALAN F. PARR

Ocular Drug Formulation and Delivery

Introduction

Except for the skin, the eye is the most easily accessible site for topical administration of medication. Topical administration is preferred over the systemic mode for treating ocular diseases and conditions. The most commonly used dosage form is an eyedrop, an aqueous solution of drug. It is simple to manufacture and administer, relatively inexpensive, and does not obscure vision. A typical time course of drug release in the eye from an eyedrop follows a pulsed entry, that is, a peak and valley, pattern. It initially shows a very high drug concentration, the peak, followed by a rapid decline in the drug concentration (representing the valley) until the next eyedrop is administered. The transient peak can represent an overdose of the applied ocular drug, whereas the valley generally represents a period of underdosing. Ocular bioavailability of drugs from eyedrops is poor, due to precorneal loss factors, including tear dynamics, nonproductive absorption, transient residence time in the cul-de-sac, and the relative impermeability of the corneal epithelial membrane. Only a small fraction of a topically applied dose reaches the inner eye, with the actual amount dependent on the physicochemical properties of the drug and its vehicle. To overcome the limitation of using eyedrops, multiple administrations (typically four times a day) are often required, frequently leading to patient noncompliance.

An ideal ocular drug-delivery system should be able to control the delivery of drugs of varying physicochemical properties and provide sustained therapeutic action in the eye with once-a-day administration. It should be nonirritating, nonsensitizing, sterile, and stable in order to allow multiple dosing from a packaged container. It should be biodegradable, easy to manufacture and administer, relatively inexpensive, and cause no foreign-body sensation or interference with vision. Over the last two decades considerable efforts have been made in the field of ocular formulation research and development to overcome some of the limitations of eyedrops. This has led to the introduction of several improved ocular dosage forms such as Pilopine HS gel, Betoptic S, Ocusert, and others. Despite this progress, the currently available ocular drug delivery systems and formulations are far from ideal. This article focuses on dosage forms designed to deliver drugs to the eye for their local effects and on methods for improving their delivery. Its goal is to give to the reader an overview of the issues involved in the research and development of ocular drug delivery systems and formulations.

Anatomy and Physiology of the Eye

The anatomy and physiology of the eye is described only briefly here. For additional information about the subject the reader is referred to several excellent literature sources [1–7].

The eye is one of the most vital organs in the body and provides one of humans' most treasured senses: vision. The eye consists of two spheres, one placed inside the other. The outer smaller sphere is covered by a transparent membrane, the cornea, which is the window of the eye. The outermost layer surrounding the larger posterior sphere is the sclera. The eye is covered externally by the upper and lower eyelids which protect it from injury and excessive light. They also spread the tears over the cornea and reduce their evaporation. The triangular space found on either side of the cornea is called the canthus. The space nearest the nose is called the medial canthus and the space farthest from the nose the lateral canthus. The canthi are formed by the union of the upper and the lower eyelids. A transverse section of the eyeball is shown in Fig. 1.

The Conjunctiva

The conjunctiva is a thin, filmy, moist mucous membrane that originates at the cornealscleral junction. The portion of the conjunctiva that forms the inner lining of the upper and the lower eyelids is called the palpebral conjunctiva. The portion that covers the eye itself, except for the cornea, is called the bulbar conjunctiva. The area where the two conjunctivae meet is called the fornix. The epithelium of the conjunctiva is continuous with that of the cornea and the lacrimal drainage system.

Outer Coat of the Eye

The outer coat of the eye consists of a relatively tough fibrous tissue divided into segments of two spheres. The white opaque sclera constitutes the posterior five-sixth of the globe, and the transparent cornea makes up the anterior one-sixth of the globe. The junction of the cornea and sclera is called the cornealscleral junction or limbus.

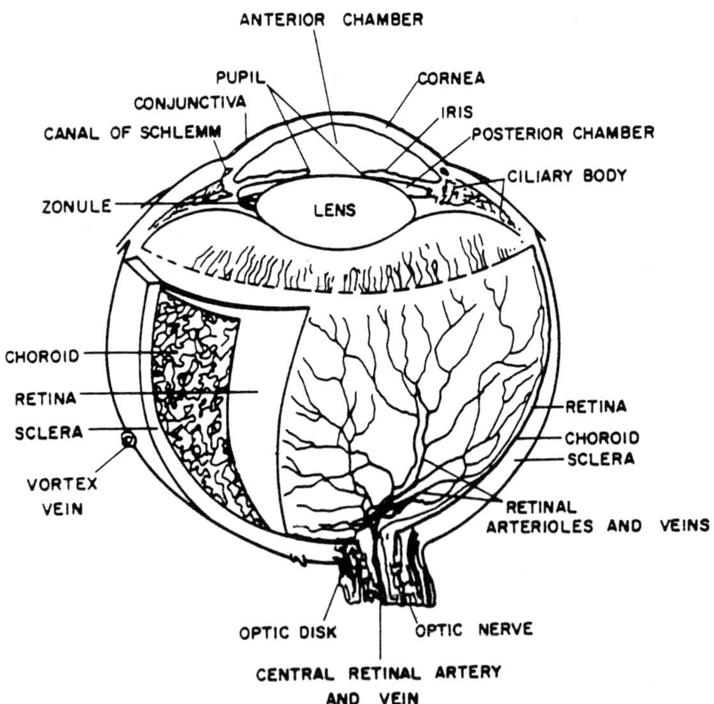

FIG. 1. Transverse section of the eyeball. (From Mitra, A. K. In: *Opthalmic Drug Delivery, Drug Delivery Devices* (P. Tyle, ed.), Marcel Dekker, Inc., New York, 1988, p. 455)

Sclera

The sclera is a dense, fibrous structure that contains few blood vessels. The anterior portion of the sclera, called the white of the eye, is covered with Tenon's capsule and the portion of the conjunctiva through which blood vessels can be seen. The sclera consists of three layers: the episclera, the sclera proper, and the lamina fussa.

Cornea

The cornea is the transparent membrane which forms the anterior one-sixth of the eyeball. It fits into the beveled edge of the sclera like a watch glass. The cornea is composed of five layers, as shown in Fig. 2:

1. the epithelium,
2. Bowman's membrane,
3. the substantia propria (stroma),
4. Descemet's membrane, and
5. the endothelium.

The corneal epithelial layer is five to seven cells thick; it covers the stroma and is continuous with the conjunctival epithelium. This superficial layer is shed every 5 to 8 days. Descemet's membrane is a glossy membrane lying just outside of the endothelium. Near the edge of the cornea the membrane becomes perforated by the openings of the trabecular meshwork. The corneal endothelium is composed of a single layer of flat cells which form the most posterior layer of the cornea. The endothelium is continuous with the endothelium covering the iris.

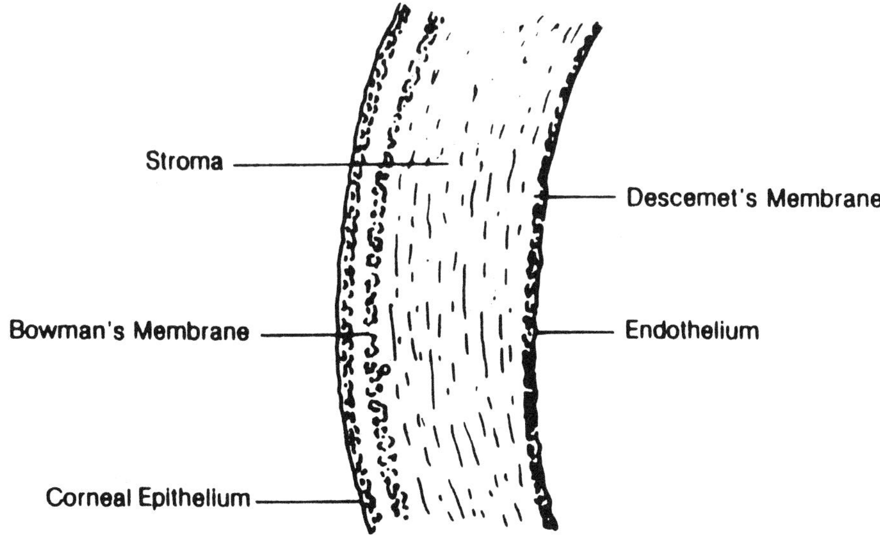

FIG. 2. Cross-section of the cornea. (From Ref. 5, reprinted with permission of American Pharmaceutical Association, Washington.)

Although the central portion of the cornea is avascular, the cornealscleral region is generally supplied with the conjunctival branches of the anterior ciliary arteries.

Cornealscleral Limbus

The cornealscleral limbus or junction includes the trabecular meshwork and the canal of Schlemm which forms the drainage system of the anterior chamber. It has two layers, the epithelium and the stroma. The trabecular meshwork, which connects the anterior chamber and the canal of Schlemm, is located in the central portion of the cornealscleral limbus.

Trabecular Meshwork

The trabecular meshwork surrounds the circumference of the anterior chamber. It is a porous-like structure with openings 2–3 μm in diameter through which the aqueous humor flows into the canal of Schlemm.

Canal of Schlemm

The canal of Schlemm is an oval-shaped channel that covers the entire circumference of the anterior chamber. On its inner side, it communicates with the anterior chamber through the trabecular meshwork. It is connected to the venous system through 25 to 35 collector channels.

Middle Coat of the Eye

The middle or uveal coat of the eyeball consists of the choroid, the ciliary body, and the iris. The ciliary body secretes aqueous humor and contains the smooth muscles responsible for accommodation, which is defined as the ability of the eye to adjust to distant objects in order to obtain a clear image on the retina.

Choroid

The choroid is a vascular layer providing the blood supply to the part of the retina adjacent to the eye. It is composed of an inner layer of capillaries and an outer layer of collecting veins. It extends from the optic nerve posteriorly to the ciliary body anteriorly.

Ciliary Body

The ciliary body extends from the iris to the choroid. It is divided into two portions, the uveal portion (located near the sclera) and the epithelial portion (adjacent to the posterior chamber). The ciliary muscle is the most prominent structure of the uveal portion of the ciliary body. It consists of three groups of smooth muscle fibers. It is believed that during accommodation the ciliary muscle contracts, causing the zonule (i.e., the suspensory ligaments of the lens) to relax and this, in turn, permits the lens to become more convex (thicker).

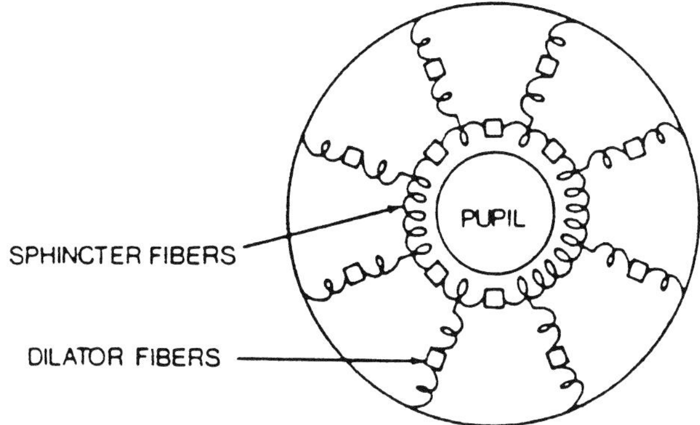

FIG. 3. Diagrammatic representation of the iris musculature in the eye.

Iris and Pupil

The iris is a diaphragm-like structure located in front of the lens and the ciliary body. It separates the anterior and posterior chambers. The iris functions as the shutter mechanism of the eye, controlling the amount of light entering the eye to ensure clear vision.

A central opening in the iris is the pupil which reflexly controls the amount of light admitted to the eye. The iris is composed of two layers: the anteriorly located stroma, and the posteriorly located pigmented epithelium.

The color of the iris depends on the amount of melanin in its stroma.

The iris is composed of two types of muscles, the sphincter muscles and the dilator muscles, which are also called radial muscles. A diagrammatic representation of the iris musculature is shown in Fig. 3. The sphincter muscle is a layer of smooth muscle, one millimeter thick and located in the pupillary zone of the posterior stroma. It forms a sphincter around the pupillary margin. The sphincter muscles are innervated by the parasympathetic (i.e., cholinergic) nerve fibers. The contraction of the sphincter muscles, resulting from their stimulation, constricts the pupil [7–9] producing miosis (i.e., a reduction in pupil diameter). Acetylcholine and other cholinergic drugs (e.g., pilocarpine) produce miosis in the eye and hence are called miotics [9].

The dilator or radial muscle is located between the stroma and the pigmented epithelium and extends as a thin sheet of smooth muscle from the ciliary body to the sphincter muscle. The sympathetic nerve fibers (which are adrenergic in nature) innervate the dilator (radial) muscles of the iris. The stimulation of the dilator muscles of the iris causes them to contract. This, in turn, relaxes the pupil [7–9], resulting in mydriasis (i.e., an increase in pupil diameter). Adrenergic drugs (e.g., epinephrine) cause relaxation of the pupil (mydriasis) and are therefore termed mydriatics [9].

If the amount of light entering the eye is low, the pupil relaxes by a reflex mechanism, and vice versa.

Lens

The lens is a crystalline, transparent biconvex structure located behind the iris and the pupillary aperture and in front of the vitreous body. It is suspended by zonular fibers and is about 4 mm thick and 10 mm in diameter. Like the cornea it does not have any blood vessels, nerve fibers, or connective tissue, and is nourished by the aqueous humor surrounding it.

Inner Coat of the Eye

The inner coat of the eye is called the retina. It contains two types of photoreceptor cells (i.e., light-sensitive receptors) called rods and cones, which transfer impulses from the retina to the brain via the optic nerve. The human eye contains 125 million rods and seven million cones. The rods function best during dim light. A loss of the rods renders a person almost blind at night, although she or he can see very well during the day. The cones function best in daylight and are also responsible for color vision. A partial loss of the cones can result in a loss of visual acuity and color blindness.

Optic Nerve

The optic nerve is a portion of a white fiber tract of the central nervous system consisting of axons of retinal ganglion cells together with nerve fibers that extend from the brain to the eye.

Chambers of the Eye

Internally the eye is made up of two unequal compartments: a smaller compartment that lies anterior to the eye lens termed the aqueous compartment, and a larger (vitreous) compartment that lies behind the lens. The aqueous compartment is further divided into an anterior and a posterior chamber by the iris. The anterior chamber is bounded anteriorly by the cornea and posteriorly by the front surface of the iris and pupillary aperture. The anterior chamber is deepest in the central portion and shallowest near the iris and has a volume sufficient to hold about 0.1 mL of fluid. The posterior chamber is surrounded by the iris anteriorly and the front surface of the zonular fibers posteriorly. It can hold up to 0.06 mL of fluid. The aqueous humor is secreted by the ciliary process and flows through the pupil into the anterior chamber.

The vitreous compartment is bounded by the retina and the optic nerve posteriorly, and by the zonule, ciliary body, and the posterior surface of the lens anteriorly; its volume is 4.5 mL.

Tear Drainage Pathway of the Eye

The anterior surface of the eye is kept moist by tears which are formed by the secretion of the lacrimal fluid and the accessory lacrimal glands located in the superior and inferior fornices. The tears or lacrimal fluid cover the cornea in the form of the tear film.

The tear film consists of three distinct layers:

- The posterior layer rich in glycoprotein derived from the goblet cells of the conjunctival epithelium,

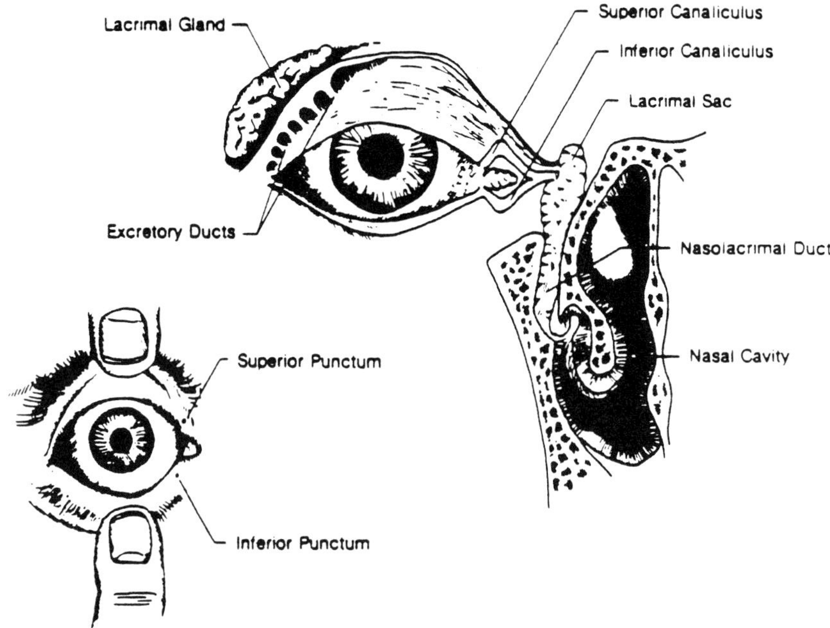

FIG. 4. Tear-drainage apparatus of the eye. (From Ref. 5, reprinted with permission of American Pharmaceutical Association, Washington.)

- The middle watery layer containing lysozyme, with antibacterial activity secreted by the lacrimal glands, and
- The outer oily layer which minimizes the evaporation of the tears and is secreted by the Meibomian gland and the glands of Zeis and Moll [2].

The normal rate of tear secretion is 1.2 μL/min [10].

The tiny opening at the medial or nasal portion of the eyelids is called the punctum. The punctum is the opening of a small canal that drains into the lacrimal sac, which, in turn, drains into the nose (the inferior nasal passage) through the nasolacrimal duct. The drainage of the tears is mediated by the pumping action of the eyelids through the punctum into the lacrimal sac, then through the nasolacrimal duct, and eventually into the nose [11]. Figure 4 shows the tear-drainage apparatus of the eye.

The tears are lost from the cul-de-sac by evaporation and drainage through the nasolacrimal duct. The thickness of the tear film is reported to be 6.5 μm [12]. The normal evaporation rate of the tears with intact oily layer is 3 $\mu L/h/cm^2$ [12]. The main force affecting tear drainage is attributable to the pumping action of the lacrimal sac associated with blinking [10,11]. The tears are spread over the surface of the eye by periodic involuntary blinking. The normal blinking rate in humans is 16 per minute. The tears maintain the optical clarity of the cornea by constantly irrigating the eye and preventing it from becoming dry and inflamed. The normal volume of tears in humans is 7μL, and the normal tear turnover rate is 16%/min [10]. The tears are an isotonic solution (0.9–0.96% NaCl equivalent) with a pH ranging from 7.2 to 7.4 [2,10]; they are not produced during sleep.

A serious concomitant of the elimination of topically applied drugs from the precorneal cavity into the nasal cavity is that the surface area and the permeability of the nasal mucosal membrane are large compared to those of the cornea. Therefore, ocular drugs are prone to absorption into the systemic circulation through the nasal mucosal lining. As much as 74% of the timolol applied in eye drops has been shown to be absorbed into the systemic circulation [13,14]. Systemic absorption of timolol can cause severe respiratory and cardiovascular problems, especially in patients with predisposing respiratory and cardiovascular disease [15].

Vision

In humans the two eyes function as if they were one. Both project at the same point in time and fuse their image in such a way that a single mental impression is created or felt. The ability of the eyes to fuse two images into a single one is called binocular vision. Accommodation refers to the ability of the two eyes to adjust in order to focus on distant objects.

Glaucoma

The aqueous humor found between the lens and the cornea is a clear, colorless, watery fluid. It is formed by an active secretion from the ciliary processes and, to a lesser extent, by diffusion from the blood vessels of the iris. The aqueous humor is in continuous circulation and it flows from the posterior chamber through the pupil into the anterior chamber. It leaves the inner eye via the trabecular meshwork, the canal of Schlemm, and the aqueous vein, into the venous system. The inflow of the aqueous humor into the eye is faster than its outflow. This leads to pressure within the eye which is called the intraocular pressure. If for any reason this pathway for exit of aqueous humor from the eye is blocked, accumulation of the fluid in the eye results. If the intraocular pressure is persistently elevated above the normal value (21 mm Hg), it often leads to glaucoma in which there is a progressive cupping and atrophy of the optic nerve, deterioration of visual fields, and ultimately blindness [16,17]. Glaucoma is one of the leading causes of blindness in the United States. It threatens to affect the vision of one out of every 50 people over the age of 35 [16]. If left untreated, it can lead to irreversible optic nerve damage and eventually blindness. Glaucoma is regarded as a leading cause of irreversible blindness throughout the world [16,17].

Topical Ocular Drug Delivery

For diseases and conditions affecting the eye, topical or local administration is preferred over systemic administration for obvious reasons, for example, the systemic toxicity of many ophthalmic drugs, the rapid onset of action, and the smaller dose required compared to the systemic route. Various types of ophthalmic dosage forms are commercially available, but the most commonly used are aqueous solutions (eyedrops). However, the time course of drug delivery from an eyedrop shows a typical ''pulse-entry'' pattern with a transient increase in the tear concentration of the drug (sometimes exceeding the desired therapeutic concentration), followed by a rapid decline in its concentration in the tears. Adequate therapy from eyedrops can be achieved by providing a pulse of sufficient magnitude, or by more frequent application of a dilute pulse. Additionally, a medication instilled into the eye as an aqueous solution is subject to the negative influence exerted by the normal protective physiological mechanisms present in the eye, such as drainage, dilution, spillage, and other factors, including tear turnover, aqueous humor turnover, drug–protein interactions, and ocular metabolism.

The cul-de-sac has a maximum capacity to hold 30 μL of tears in the upright position [10]. The normal dropper used with commercial ophthalmic solutions delivers about 50–75 μL per drop [18]. Therefore, the excess instilled solution is spilled out onto the cheek. Furthermore, the instilled drop is diluted by the constant tear production and it is also drained away by the very efficient lacrimal-drainage system of the eye. It has been reported that the rate of drainage of an instilled solution is linearly related to the instilled volume and rate of tear secretion [18,19]. Therefore, the volume of tear fluid does not normally exceed its average value [10]. Thus the volume instilled has a definite influence on the quantity and rate of drug solution lost via the drainage apparatus. A drop of an aqueous solution, irrespective of the instilled volume, is eliminated completely from the eye and the eye returns to the normal lacrimal lake volume within 5–6 min of its application. This results in a very short period during which the drug has access to the ocular tissues [18,19].

Corneal Permeation

Most topically applied ocular drugs have to reach the inner parts of the eye to be effective. Transcorneal penetration is believed to be the major route for drug absorption into the eye. Unfortunately, the corneal epithelium is relatively impermeable to most ocular drugs. Due to its structure and composition, the cornea offers a barrier to the passage of many drugs, particularly those with high molecular weight or polarity, including salts. Therefore, one of the suggested ways to improve ocular bioavailability of a drug is to increase its corneal permeability. The cornea is a trilaminate structure consisting of a hydrophilic stroma located between the outermost highly lipophilic epithelial layer (five to seven cells thick) and the endothelial layer (one cell thick) which is less lipophilic. The resistance to corneal penetration offered by these three layers varies, depending upon the physicochemical properties of the drug. The corneal epithelium contributes about 90% of the corneal resistance for hydrophilic drugs, 50% for moderately lipophilic drugs, and less than 10% for lipophilic drugs [20]. Due to the amphiphilic nature of the cornea with a lipophilic epithelium and a hydrophilic stroma, the corneal epithelium appears to rate-limit the movement of hydrophilic drugs, whereas the stroma is rate-limiting for lipophilic drugs.

Most ocular drugs seem to penetrate the cornea by diffusion and none appear to transfer by carrier-mediated transport or endocytosis. The paracellular (i.e., through intercellular space) and transcellular pathways (i.e., through intracellular space) are the two mechanisms for drug transport across the cornea. The former is the primary route of passive permeation for ions and low molecular weight nonelectrolytes (ethanol, glycerol, etc.) in the corneal epithelium.

The principal drug properties influencing drug absorption via the transcellular pathway are the lipophilicity, as reflected by the octanol/buffer or octanol/water partition coefficient, the pK_a which determines the percentage of the preferentially absorbed unionized form of the drug present at a given pH, the solubility, and the molecular size. Among the above-mentioned drug properties, the effect of lipophilicity on corneal drug absorption has been the best documented [20]. The extent of corneal drug absorption appears to vary parabolically with the partition coefficient of the drug [20]. This type of correlation has been shown for several classes of drugs [21–24], including steroids [22] and beta blockers [23]. The corneal permeability of drugs increases with increasing partition coefficient, reaches a maximum that corresponds to the optimum partition coefficient, and then declines with further increase in the partition coefficient (i.e., higher lipophilicity). The decline in the corneal permeability is due to the decrease in drug solubility with increasing lipophilicity. Thus, maintaining a proper balance between hydrophilicity and lipophilicity is a prerequisite for the corneal penetration of drugs [24].

Noncorneal Penetration

Although corneal penetration has been traditionally considered to be the major route of drug entry into the eye, a minor route through the sclera and conjunctiva has recently been reported [25–29]. This alternative route by which drug may penetrate into the eye is called the noncorneal route [20]. It has been shown to be important for the delivery of ocular drugs that are poorly absorbed across the cornea (e.g., inulin, a linear, polar macromolecule with molecular weight of about 5000 Daltons) because of their physicochemical properties [26–28]. Doane et al. [25] determined that the contribution of scleral penetration of hydrocortisone or pilocarpine into the aqueous humor or the iris–ciliary body is relatively minor. The noncorneal route may be a less significant route of ocular penetration than the traditional corneal route, partially because of the heavy vascularization of underlying sclera through which most drugs are lost into the systemic circulation [25,26]. There is no conclusive evidence about the usefulness of this route. Therefore, further studies are needed to fully characterize and understand the utility and significance of the noncorneal route in ocular drug absorption.

Ocular Pharmacokinetics

Ocular pharmacokinetics refers to the study of the time course of absorption, distribution, metabolism, and excretion of an administered drug in the tissues and fluids of the eye. Of major concern is the fact that pharmocokinetic studies cannot be conducted routinely on the intact human eye because of the impossibility of sampling internal tissues or fluids without the risk of severe damage [30]. In recent years, the traditional view of the cornea as a barrier to drug transport has been expanded to include its capacity to metabolize ocular drugs and also peptides [31–36]. It has been reported that about 45% of the chloramphenicol recovered in the aqueous humor of the albino rabbit 2 h after administration was in a metabolized form [36]. Drug metabolism and drug binding to the proteins in the ocular fluids and pigments in the iris, ciliary body, and uveal tract should be considered in the design and evaluation of ocular drug-delivery systems.

Pharmacokinetic models have been developed for several drugs, including pilocarpine [37–40], fluoromethalone [41], timolol [42], and clonidine [43]. Ocular pharmacokinetics is described in detail in several review articles [30, 44–47]. Most of the models and the resulting equations are rather complex. A simplified model, describing the movement of a topically applied drug to the front of the eye, as shown in Scheme 1, has been used [44].

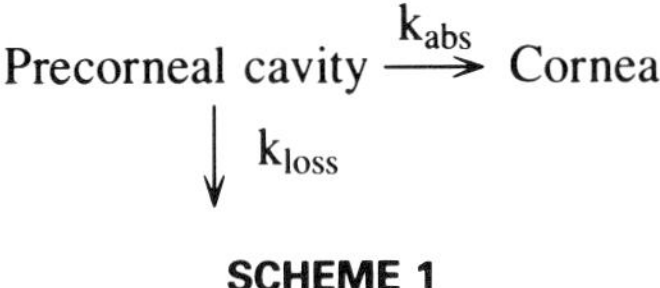

SCHEME 1

In the above model, k_{loss} represents the elimination process operating in the precorneal cavity which is responsible for removal of a topically applied drug by lacrimal drainage, tear turnover, protein binding, "nonproductive" absorption via the scleral and conjunctival routes, and metabolism, and k_{abs} represents absorption of the drug into the cornea. Corneal absorption is a much slower process than elimination [30]. For many drugs k_{loss} is approximately 0.5–0.7/min and k_{abs} is about 0.001/min [44]. Thus, there is a vast difference in the magnitudes of the two rate constants. It is the sum of these two rate constants that controls the fraction of the applied dose absorbed into the eye [44]. The ocular bioavailability of topically applied ocular drugs can be increased significantly by decreasing k_{loss} or by increasing k_{abs}. The former can be achieved by modifying the ocular dosage form and the latter by formulating ocular dosage forms containing lipophilic prodrugs or by adding penetration enhancers.

Desirable Properties of Ophthalmic Dosage Forms

A number of factors must be considered in preparing ophthalmic dosage forms. These include sterility, preservation, clarity, pH, buffering, tonicity, viscosity, additives, and appropriate packaging. Many of these factors are interrelated, and often a compromise among optimal properties and components is necessary. For example, for some drugs that are heat stable at acidic pH but unstable near eye pH (about 7.4) it may be necessary to sterilize the unbuffered solution in an autoclave and add any necessary buffering agents aseptically later [48]. Typical "inactive" ingredients that may be present in ophthalmic products to achieve these properties include preservatives, viscosity-increasing agents, antioxidants, wetting agents, buffers, and tonicity-adjusting agents [49].

Several newer ophthalmic dosage forms (e.g., solid inserts, liposomes, nanoparticles, etc.) are currently in use or under development as well as a wide variety of contact lenses, lens-care products, artificial tear products, etc. This section will focus on the more conventional topical ophthalmic products, such as solutions, suspensions, and ointments, with particular emphasis on ophthalmic solutions since they are the most widely used of the topical products.

Sterility

Probably the most important property of ophthalmic formulations is that they be sterile. The *USP XXII–NFXVII* (1990) lists five methods of achieving sterility:

- Steam sterilization at 121°C,
- Dry-heat sterilization,

- Gas sterilization using ethylene oxide (due to environmental concerns the use of ethylene oxide is being phased out wherever possible),
- Sterilization using ionizing radiation, e.g., radioisotope decay (gamma radiation) and electron beam radiation, and
- Sterilization by filtration.

The method chosen is often dictated by the resistance of the active ingredient and the resultant product to heat and to the type of packaging (i.e., container) used.

The USP permits ophthalmic solutions for use in eyes with intact corneal membranes to be packaged in multiple-dose containers. Each solution must contain a preservative or mixture of preservatives to prevent the growth of microorganisms accidentally introduced into the product during use. The risk of serious ocular infection resulting from the use of contaminated ophthalmic solutions is well-documented. The organism most commonly encountered is *Staphylococcus aureus*. A less frequently observed, though much more dangerous and opportunistic contaminant, is *Pseudomonas aeruginosa*. In the presence of a corneal abrasion, this organism (and others) can pass through this barrier freely and rapidly proliferate in the cornea, producing ulceration and possibly complete loss of vision in 24–48 h. Other organisms that have been encountered less frequently include *Bacillus subtilis*, *Aspergillus fumigatus*, and certain viruses [50].

Preservatives

The selection of a preservative for ophthalmic solutions is not an easy task, with very few candidates to choose from. The following criteria are important [50,51]:

1. Broad spectrum of activity against both Gram-positive and Gram-negative organisms and fungi.
2. The agent should rapidly kill virulent organisms such as the various strains of *Pseudomonas aeruginosa*.
3. Satisfactory chemical and physical stability over a wide range of pH and temperature.
4. Compatibility with formulation components and container materials.
5. Nontoxic and nonirritating during use.

There are relatively few agents which meet enough of the above criteria to be of use in ophthalmic solutions. The classes of such compounds which have been used at one time or another in the past are given in Table 1 [51]. Each of these has certain limitations due to instability, incompatibility with other formulation ingredients, or antibacterial activity. It appears that the formulation must often be designed to accommodate the requirements of the preservatives desired [52]. In fact, an FDA Advisory Review Panel on OTC Ophthalmic Products published the much shorter list of potentially acceptable preservatives shown in Table 2 [53].

By far the most widely used ophthalmic preservative is the quaternary ammonium compound, benzalkonium chloride (BAK), with has excellent chemical stability and antimicrobial activity. Its limitations include its incompatibility with salicylates, nitrates,

TABLE 1 Ophthalmic Preservatives[a]

Type	Concentration Range (%)	Incompatibilities	Remarks
Quaternary ammonium compounds	0.004–0.02 0.01 most common	Soaps, anionic materials, salicylates	Benzalkonium chloride is the single most frequently used ophthalmic preservative; EDTA increases effectiveness[b]
Organic mercurials	0.001–0.01	Certain halides with phenylmercuric acetate	Typically used as substitute for benzalkonium where latter is incompatible
Parahydroxybenzoates	0.1 maximum	Adsorpion by macromolecules	Infrequently used; activity limited to bacteriostasis
Chlorobutanol	0.5	Stability is pH-dependent; active concentration is near solubility maximum	Diffuses through low-density polyethylene containers
Aromatic alcohols	0.5–0.9	Low solubility in water	As above; occasionally used in combination with other preservatives

[a]Adapted from Ref. 51, with permission of Mack Publishing Co.
[b]Ethylenediaminetetraacetic acid.

and anionic compounds. Other, less widely used quaternary ammonium agents include benzethonium chloride and cetylpyridinium chloride.

In the past, when benzalkonium chloride could not be used due to an incompatibility, one of the organic mercurials (phenylmercuric nitrate, phenylmercuric acetate, or thimerosal) was often employed. Although they have been used effectively in some formulations, their bacteriocidal action is relatively weak and slow. Their application is generally restricted to solutions that vary from slightly acidic to alkaline. The possibility of mercury deposits in the lens resulting from their use severely reduces their appeal compared to other preservatives available. Because of environmental concerns their use is gradually being phased out as existing products are reformulated.

The parahydroxybenzoic acid esters, typically mixtures of the methyl and propyl esters, are severely limited in their use by their low aqueous solubility and the fact that they

TABLE 2 Suitable Ophthalmic Preservative Agents and their Maximum Recommended Concentrations for Safe Use in the Eye[a]

Preservative	Maximum Recommended Concentration (%)
Benzalkonium chloride	0.013 (1:7,500)
Benzethonium chloride	0.01 (1:10,000)
Chlorobutanol	0.5 (1:200)
Phenylmercuric acetate	0.004 (1:25,000)
Phenylmercuric nitrate	0.004 (1:25,000)
Thimerosal	0.01 (1:10,000)

[a]From Ref. 53.

are believed to cause stinging and irritation in the eye. They have been used primarily to prevent mold growth and possess a weak antibacterial activity with the result that an FDA expert panel evaluating OTC drugs for ophthalmologic use found them to be unacceptable as preservatives [50]. Despite this, a recent monograph [54] noted that the parabens are "nontoxic and . . . viable preservatives" which "probably approach utopia."

Chlorobutanol has been shown to be an effective preservative for ophthalmics and is still found in some products. It has a relatively slow antimicrobial action and rapidly decomposes when autoclaved. This hydrolytic process may occur (albeit more slowly) at lower temperatures in unbuffered solutions that were originally neutral or alkaline with the formation of hydrochloric acid. This may render the solution susceptible to microbial growth and can alter the pH of an unbuffered or lightly buffered solution to an extent that the stability and physiologic activity of the active ingredient is compromised [48]. It is therefore important to buffer ophthalmic solutions preserved with chlorobutanol at a pH of 5.0–5.5 [50]. Chlorobutanol is also volatile and can readily permeate many of the current polyolefin plastic ophthalmic containers, thereby limiting its use to formulations packaged in glass.

Of the aromatic alcohols, only phenylethyl alcohol has been used to any degree, primarily in combination with other preservatives. Like chlorobutanol, its antimicrobial activity is relatively weak, and it is sufficiently volatile to permeate through typical plastic packaging materials. Its limited aqueous solubility increases the possibility of it being "salted out" of solution in the formulation or in the eye. It can also reportedly produce stinging and burning sensations in the eye.

A preservative whose use in ophthalmics is currently under investigation, is polyquat, also known as polyquaternium-1 [55,56]. Up to now the use of this agent has been confined to several soft contact lens care products because of its very low sensitization potential and insignificant adsorption to the eye lens. It has been shown to be ten times less toxic than BAK at equivalent preservative concentrations [57].

All of the previously listed preservatives (including BAK) are ineffective against some resistant strains of *Pseudomonas aeruginosa* in concentrations tolerated by ocular tissues. However, the acquired resistance could be overcome by the addition of ethylenediaminetetraacetic acid (EDTA), 0.01–0.1%, to benzalkonium chloride (0.01%). EDTA is a chelating agent capable of binding divalent cations which are apparently responsible for the resistant strains of *Pseudomonas* [52]. An alternative formulation which has been suggested to be effective against most resistant *Pseudomonas* strains is a mixture of 0.01% BAK and 1000 USP units/mL of Polymyxin B sulfate [48].

Preservatives as Penetration Enhancers

An additional aspect of some ophthalmic preservatives which has recently received attention is the beneficial effect in increasing corneal epithelial permeability [54,58]. The rationale for his approach is based on the fact that an increase in corneal permeability is one important means of increasing the ocular bioavailability of drugs [59].

The effects of the various preservatives on corneal permeability are given in Table 3. These data pertain to results obtained at preservative concentrations within the normal ranges found in ophthalmic solutions. Any potential permeability enhancement by these agents gained as a result of increasing their concentrations beyond the normal range needed for preservation would in all probability be negated by increased toxicity.

TABLE 3 Effect of Ophthalmic Preservatives on Corneal Permeability[a]

Preservative	Uses	Effect on Corneal Permeability
Benzalkonium chloride		Causes a significant increase in permeability for a variety of agents
Cetylpyridinium chloride		Increased corneal permeation of penicillin and fluorescein
Thimerosal		Only a minimal effect at normal preservative concentration
Chlorobutanol		Increased corneal permeability for some drugs at normal preservative concentrations
Parahydroxybenzoates		Minimal data available indicate that corneal permeation enhancement is unlikely
Chlorhexidine digluconate	In contact lens solutions	Can cause increased permeability of drugs
Hydrogen peroxide (H_2O_2)	Contact lens cleaner	Appears unlikely to have any effect
Sorbic acid	Care of contact lenses	Scanty available data are inconclusive
Sodium bisulfite	Antioxidant	Scanty available data are inconclusive
Ethylenediaminetetraacetic acid	Chelating agent	Limited data available indicate an increased permeability for some molecules

[a]From Refs. 54 and 58.

Nevertheless, this often overlooked aspect of preservatives may be worthy of future investigation as a means of improving the permeability of drugs with a low ocular bioavailability.

Clarity

The official definition of ophthalmic solutions requires that they be free of particulate matter. Solution clarity is usually achieved by filtration, either with a clarifying filter or as part of a sterile filtration procedure. It is essential that these procedures be performed in a ''clean-room'' environment, for example, in a laminar-flow hood, with personnel properly attired in nonshedding clothing. The filtered solution must be filled into appropriate glass or plastic containers which are scrupulously clean. The container must then be sealed by means of an inert closure device which does not generate particulates over the intended shelf-life of the product. The degree of clarity of the finished product can be monitored by means of various instruments capable of detecting any light scattering or blockage resulting from the presence of particulate matter [50,51]. Recently proposed limits on particulate matter in ophthalmic preparations are as shown in Table 4 [60]. Subsequent discussion indicated that these limits would require considerable revision before they could be adopted and implemented [61].

TABLE 4 Proposed Limits on Particulate Matter in Ophthalmic Preparations

Particle Size (μm)	Limits Proposed, Particles per mL
≥10	≤50
≥25	≤5
>50	None allowed

Stability

The stability of the active ingredient in an ophthalmic solution depends upon the chemical nature of the active ingredient, pH, manufacturing procedure, type of additives, and type of container. The maintenance of a pH that is consistent with acceptable stability is often in conflict with a pH that would provide optimum corneal penetration of the drug in question and optimum patient acceptance of the product.

The maintenance of stability may also dictate the type of packaging employed. For example, epinephrine salts are sensitive to air oxidation, thereby precluding the use of the air-permeable plastic containers that many patients find convenient to use. Epinephrine-containing formulations typically require antioxidants such as sodium bisulfite or sodium metabisulfite or, more recently, combinations of antioxidants such as ascorbic acid and acetylcysteine, sodium bisulfite and 8-hydroxyquinoline, or isoascorbic acid and polyvinylpyrrolidone [50,52].

pH Adjustment and Buffers

The adjustment of ophthalmic solution pH by the appropriate choice of a buffer is one of the most important formulation considerations. Buffers may be used in an ophthalmic solution for one or more of the following reasons: to maintain the physiologic pH of the tears upon administration in order to minimize tearing and patient discomfort (and in so doing enhance patient compliance); to optimize the therapeutic activity of the active ingredient by altering corneal penetration through changes in the degree of ionization; and to optimize product stability [48,58].

The tear fluid pH is reported to vary between 6.9 and 7.5 during the waking hours of the day [62]. The most common active ingredients found in ophthalmic solutions are acid salts of weak bases which are most stable at an acidic pH. Thus the formulator is often faced with the need to choose a pH which does not compromise the stability of the product but is still acceptable to the patient. The solution to this dilemma is usually maintenance of the product at an acid pH with a buffer of low capacity. Provided the drug itself has a weak buffering effect, for example, the alkaloidal salts, and the volume instilled is small, the tears should be able to rapidly adjust the pH to a value near 7.4, thereby minimizing any discomfort. However, occasionally the drug itself may exert a significant buffering effect (e.g., epinephrine bitartrate) and thus a different salt form (epinephrine hydrochloride) may be necessary [52].

Recently, Ahmed and Chaudhuri [63] illustrated that the pH achieved by the buffer may not be the only factor influencing ocular bioavailability. Using pilocarpine nitrate as a model drug, they instilled solutions buffered at pH 4.0 with equimolar concentrations of acetate, phosphate, or citrate buffers into rabbits eyes and measured the in vivo tear pH-vs.-time profiles. The ocular bioavailability was assessed from miosis-vs.-time profiles. Analysis of these two profiles indicated that the relative order of efficacy for these buffers, compared to an unbuffered system, was unbuffered > acetate > phosphate > citrate. Their most interesting finding was that the bioavailability of pilocarpine was greater from the acetate buffered formulation than from the phosphate buffered formulation, even though the acetate-containing formulation was more strongly buffered at the pH formulated and caused more tearing. The authors attributed this effect to the high residual buffer capacity of the phosphate buffer, exerting a resistance to pH reequilibration near the pKa of pilocarpine. This study underscores the fact that the time course of lacrimal-fluid pH change (and hence the activity of the active ingredient) may be influenced by both precorneal-fluid dynamics (i.e., the rate of drainage, tear, turnover, and extent of induced lacrimation) and concentration (i.e., buffer capacity) as well as the type of buffer.

Tonicity

Tonicity refers to the osmotic pressure exerted by a solution due to the solutes (drugs, additives, etc.) present. Osmotic pressure is a colligative property and therefore its magnitude depends upon the number of "particles" present in the solution, irrespective of whether they are molecules or ions. Thus a uni-univalent electrolyte such as sodium chloride contributes nearly twice the number of "particles" to the solution as an equimolar concentration of a nonelectrolyte such as glucose. Tears and other body fluids exert an osmotic pressure of 302 to 318 mOsm/kg [62] which is approximately equivalent to that of a 0.9% w/v solution of sodium chloride (normal saline). Tear fluid and Normal Saline are said to be isoosmotic, that is, to have equal osmotic pressure. The term isotonic (equal tone) is commonly used interchangeably with isoosmotic. Strictly speaking, the term isotonic should only be used when referring to two solutions consisting of the same solvent separated by a membrane permeable only to the solvent, that is, a semipermeable membrane. Thus it is possible for two solutions to be isoosmotic but not isotonic if one or more of the solutes present can pass through the membrane separating them. Solutions with osmotic pressures lower than that of normal saline are said to be hypotonic, whereas those with higher osmotic pressures are termed hypertonic [48].

In theory, a hypertonic solution placed in the eye tends to draw solvent (water) from its surroundings in order to dilute the instilled solution. In this case, water flows from the aqueous layer through the cornea to the eye surface. Conversely, a hypotonic solution could result in the passage of water from the site of application through the eye tissues. In this case, the epithelial permeability is increased, allowing water to flow into the cornea, the corneal tissue swells, and drug concentration on the ocular surface is temporarily increased [62]. The result of these stimuli could be an increase in lacrimal secretion and blinking which would rapidly wash the instilled solution out of the eye.

In actual practice, it has been observed that the eye can tolerate a range of osmotic pressure values equivalent to 0.6 to 2.0% sodium chloride without marked discomfort [48]. The normal osmolality of the eye is typically restored within 1 to 2 min of instillation of a nonisotonic solution, depending upon the drop size. Thus the adjustment of tonicity becomes a more important consideration for eye washes where the volume of solution in contact with the ocular surface is increased considerably. Nevertheless, the adjustment of solution tonicity is generally advisable and can be accomplished using a variety of approaches described in detail elsewhere [48,50,51,64,65].

Recently, Meyer and McCulley [66] developed an in vitro bioassay procedure using stratified rabbit corneal epithelial cultures to evaluate the tolerance of the corneal epithelium to the combined effects of pH and osmotic pressure changes. Four different vehicles were evaluated: balanced salt solution, physiological saline, phosphate buffered saline, and acetate–citrate. Their results indicated that balanced salt solutions at pH 5 all caused significant tissue damage which was inversely proportional to the osmolality of the vehicle, that is, the hypotonic and isotonic solutions were much more damaging than the corresponding hypertonic formulations. Balanced salt solutions buffered at pH 6 and 7 were nontoxic, indicating that osmolality is not a critical factor as long as the solution pH is maintained near neutral. The differential impact of pH on the biotolerance of unbuffered salines was less striking, even though the acidic (pH 5) hypotonic vehicles were, once again, the most damaging.

The acetate–citrate buffered vehicles that are more typically used commercially, resulted in the highest toxicity, with acidic solutions (pH 5) being more toxic than vehicles near neutral pH; hypotonic solutions were more toxic than the corresponding isotonic and hypertonic solutions; and acidic hypotonic vehicles were by far the most damaging. For these vehicles the tolerable range of pH and osmotic pressure of the tissue was much more restricted. These properties were largely attributed to the chelating properties of the citrate present in the formulation. In contrast, the phosphate-buffered saline vehicles were much better tolerated, suggesting that they may be more appropriate for commercial formulations.

In a closely related study employing the same four buffer systems examined at pH 5.0 and 7.5, these authors [67] examined the effect of EDTA on corneal epithelial biocompatibility. The effect of EDTA on the toxicity of balanced salt solutions (BSS) was negligible at both pH values studied. EDTA moderately reduced the toxicity of the acetate-citrate buffered vehicles at pH 5, but increased the toxicity considerably at pH 7.5. On the other hand, EDTA had little effect on the toxicity of the physiological saline and phosphate-buffered saline (PBS) vehicles at pH 5.0, but it considerably increased the toxicity of these vehicles at pH 7.5. These data illustrate once again the differential effect of chelation, pH, and buffer type on rabbit corneal epithelium in tissue culture.

Viscosity

The viscosity of ophthalmic solutions is often increased in order to prolong the corneal contact time, decrease the drainage rate, and increase the bioavailability of the active ingredient. The polymers used to increase viscosity may also lower the frictional resistance between the cornea and the eyelid which occurs with each blink, thereby exerting a lubricating effect that may be of benefit for some patients. Numerous studies [52] have demonstrated that the increased contact time and the resultant increases in pharmacologic effect observed as viscosity is increased reaches a plateau, at which point further increases in viscosity produce no increase in response. This may be due to two factors. First, tears have a normal viscosity varying between 1.05 and 5.98 mPa·s [62]. They exhibit pseudoplastic flow behavior and have a yield value of about 0.032 Pa·s. During a normal blink, a force of 0.2 N is required to move the eyelids, with a forceful blink requiring 0.8 N. A blink requiring a force greater than 0.9 N produces pain which may, in turn, cause reflex blinking and tearing, resulting in the rapid elimination of solution present on the ocular surface. A second consideration is due to the fact that if the viscosity of an instilled solution is too high, it may obstruct the puncti and the canaliculi which are subjected to much lower shear rates than the eye surface during a blink. In order to ensure proper drainage of the tear fluid, it is important that the viscosity of ophthalmic solutions not exceed 40 to 50 mPa·s. The primary viscosity-increasing agents used commercially in ophthalmic solutions are polyvinyl alcohol (Liquifilm) and hydroxypropyl methylcellulose (Isopto). The Liquifilm products generally have viscosities in the range of 4 to 6 mPa·s, whereas those of the Isopto products range from 10 to 30 mPa·s [52]. Newer viscolyzing agents, which have shown some promise in increasing ocular bioavailability, include Carbopol 940 and sodium hyaluronate [62].

Additives

Stabilizers

The use of stabilizers is permitted in ophthalmic solutions when necessary. Epinephrine hydrochloride and bitartrate solutions undergo oxidative degradation and an antioxidant such as sodium bisulfite or metabisulfite is commonly added up to a 0.3% concentration. Epinephrine borate stabilization requires special consideration, and mixtures of ascorbic acid and acetylcysteine or sodium bisulfite and 8-hydroxyquinoline have been used for this purpose. Isoascorbic acid and polyvinylpyrrolidone combinations have also been used to stabilize this compound.

Surfactants

The addition of surfactants to ophthalmic solutions is permitted, even though their use is greatly restricted. The toxicity of surfactants is on the order anionic > cationic > nonionic. Nonionics are used in low concentrations to increase the dispersion of suspended drugs, such as steroids, and thereby improve solution clarity. The ability of these compounds to bind and thereby inactivate certain preservatives [68], coupled with their irritation potential, limits their use to low concentrations. For example, the FDA limits the concentrations of Tween 20 and Tween 80 to 1% [64].

Packaging

Ophthalmic solutions should be packaged in such a way that they are easy to administer and maintain in a sterile condition. Other considerations include the protection of light-sensitive drugs from exposure to light, and the use of an "inert" container which does not allow material to leach out. Such materials may affect product stability (e.g., leaching of alkaline materials from certain types of glass) or patient acceptance by generating particulate matter or other irritants [65]. Originally, ophthalmic solutions were packaged in glass containers with an accompanying glass dropper. Since the introduction of the low-density polyethylene Droptainer in the 1950s, glass containers have largely been replaced, except where stability considerations dictate their use. The advantages of the Droptainer include a lower contamination potential, increased convenience of use, lower weight, and lower cost. Since the dispensing tip is an integral part of the package, the solution remaining in the bottle after use is not exposed to airborne contaminants during use as occurs with the glass bottle with a separate dropper.

The primary disadvantages of the polyethylene plastic containers are their sorption and permeability characteristics. Materials contained in the plastic such as plasticizers, stabilizers, antioxidants, pigments, lubricants, etc., may leach from the container into the solution. Label components such as glue, inks, adhesives, and dyes may also penetrate the polyethylene container. Conversely, volatile solution components (chlorobutanol or phenylethyl alcohol) can migrate into or through the plastic container. To address these potential problems the *USP XXII–NFXVII* [69] specifies an eye irritation test to monitor leachable materials as well as a moisture permeation test for plastic ophthalmic containers. The regulatory agencies are currently focusing on the interaction of the formulations with the containers over an extended time period. This is a difficult task, since it requires a comprehensive knowledge of the container composition, and manufacturers are often reluctant to divulge this proprietary information. Low-density polyethylene plastics are translucent, and for light-sensitive drugs, additional packaging (e.g., an opacifying agent such as titanium dioxide) or an opaque external cardboard package may be necessary. Low-density polyethylene plastic containers cannot be autoclaved and are usually sterilized with ethylene oxide or by gamma or cobalt-60 irradiation.

Glass dropper–bottle containers (type I glass) are still used for ophthalmic solutions prepared extemporaneously. These containers are also used for products that are highly susceptible to oxidative degradation or contain components that are too volatile to package in plastic. Powders to be reconstituted also require glass containers since they have the appropriate heat-transfer properties required during the lyophilization process.

Like most consumer products today, some form of tamper-evident packaging is mandatory to ensure product safety. The most common type of tamper-evident packaging of ophthalmic solutions is a moisture- or heat-sensitive shrink band at the cap-and-bottle junction. These bands are usually clearly identified, and their rupture or absence constitutes a clear warning that the package has been opened [50,52].

Formulation Approaches to Improve Ocular Bioavailability

For two reasons there is a growing interest in developing new and more efficient ocular drug-delivery systems for providing the continuous and controlled release of drugs for a longer period of time. One is the introduction of newly developed drugs with shorter biological half-lives, and the second is the introduction of drugs which have significant systemic side effects. Ocular bioavailability from topically applied traditional drug-delivery systems is poor. The fraction of a topically applied dose of pilocarpine nitrate absorbed into the anterior chamber and the aqueous humor is in the range of 0.01–0.1 and 0.0002–0.003, respectively. This is due, in part, to the negative influence of the physiological constraints imposed by the eye through such factors as tear turnover [18,19, 70–72], drug–protein interaction [73,74], aqueous humor turnover [70,75], instilled fluid drainage [18,19,70–72], the relative impermeability of the cornea [70,76–79], corneal metabolism [31–36], and drug absorption into the conjunctiva and the sclera [80,81]. Drugs absorbed via the conjunctiva (which is a vascularized tissue) can get into the systemic circulation and eventually return to the eye by the uveal or choroid tissue. However, it has been demonstrated that this route is only of minor importance [82].

The challenge faced by scientists involved in opthalmic pharmaceutical research is to improve ocular drug bioavailability from less than 1–3% to at least 15–20%. The ocular bioavailability of several drugs can be improved by prolonging their residence time in the cul-de-sac and by increasing their corneal permeability [83].

To date, ophthalmic drugs have been marketed in four different dosage forms: aqueous solutions, suspensions, ointments, and solid ocular inserts. The various approaches that have been attempted to increase the bioavailability and the duration of therapeutic action of ocular drugs can be divided into two categories. The first is based on maximizing corneal drug absorption and minimizing precorneal drug loss. The second involves the use of drug-delivery systems which provide the controlled and continuous delivery of ophthalmic drugs to the pre- and intraocular tissues.

Maximizing Corneal Drug Absorption and Minimizing Precorneal Drug Loss

Viscosity-Imparting Agents

There have been several claims of improvement in ocular bioavailability of drugs based on the increased residence time in the eye due to the addition of viscosity-building soluble polymers to aqueous formulations [84–86]. It is reasoned that the solution drainage would be reduced by the increased solution viscosity. The polymers used include polyvinyl alcohol, polyvinylpyrrolidone, methylcellulose, hydroxyethylcellulose, and hydroxypropyl methylcellulose. However, as studies to date indicate, this approach has only limited value as the formulations are liquid and therefore subject to elimination from the eye by all of the factors discussed previously.

Polymer solutions generally exhibit two types of flow behavior, Newtonian and non-Newtonian. The former show constant viscosity (i.e., independent of the rate of applied shear) and are poorly tolerated in the eye because of the shear forces associated with blinking and rapid eye movement. Newtonian solutions feel uncomfortable because of the resistance they offer to the movement of the eyelids over the globe during blinking [87]. Conversely, polymeric solutions that display pseudoplastic flow behavior, in which viscosity decreases with increasing rate of shear (shear thinning), offer less resistance to the eyelid movement and hence are better accepted by the patients [87].

Prodrugs and Ion Pairs

Another useful method for increasing the ocular absorption of poorly absorbed drugs involves prodrugs. Prodrugs are chemical drug derivatives which are sensitive to chemical or enzymatic cleavage. They are designed to alter a specific property of the parent drug molecule, such as absorption, solubility, taste, volatility, or stability. An example of a commercially available ocular prodrug is dipivalyl epinephrine (Propine, Allergan Pharmaceuticals). Owing to its increased lipophilicity, the prodrug penetrates the corneal epithelium 10 times faster than the parent drug, epinephrine. The active parent drug is regenerated in vivo upon absorption by the cleavage of the ester linkage by esterases in the cornea and iris. The regenerated pivalic acid is nontoxic.

Ion-pair association, a coulombic association between large organic ions of opposite charge, can also increase the ocular absorption of poorly absorbed drugs. The ions are transferred better when associated (paired) than individually. In animals, the method had been used with success to transfer the anti-inflammatory agent sodium chromoglycate (the di-anion) across the cornea by coupling it with a quaternary ammonium cation such as dodecylbenzyldimethylammonium chloride [88].

Penetration Enhancers

The corneal epithelial membrane is a significant barrier to the passage of drug molecules. The transport characteristics across the cornea can be enhanced or maximized by changing the physicochemical properties of a drug or by increasing the permeability of the corneal epithelial membrane. Inclusion of 0.02% cetylpyridinium chloride with pilocarpine nitrate applied topically to the rabbit eye caused a miotic effect 10 times that obtained in the absence of cetylpyridinium [89]. In another study, cetylpyridinium chloride was shown to enhance penicillin penetration across the isolated rabbit cornea [90]. Mitra [91] showed that an ionophore such as lasalocid can be used to enhance the corneal permeability of pilocarpine; drug absorption was significantly higher. Benzalkonium chloride has also been reported to increase the corneal penetration of ^{14}C-inulin by tenfold and eighteenfold, at 0.01 and 0.02% concentrations, respectively, of the preservative [92]. Tween 20, a nonionic surfactant, increased the corneal penetration of fluorescein fivefold [93]. Due to the sensitive nature of the ocular tissues involved in the passage of ocular drugs to the inner parts of the eye, the use of chemicals to increase penetration of topically applied ocular drugs has not been very successful. Agents like benzalkonium chloride and cetylpyridinium chloride, at concentrations at which they significantly enhance corneal drug absorption, are toxic to the ocular tissues. In a recent study, the absorption of insulin through the rabbit eye with various penetration-enhancing agents was investigated [94]. Among the seven enhancers tested, saponin showed the highest potency to increase insulin absorption and to reduce blood glucose level [94]. The effects of long-term use of any penetration enhancers on the ocular tissues remain to be studied. The usefulness of penetration enhancers to improve the corneal absorption of topically applied ocular drugs will be limited until agents are identified which alter the corneal permeability reversibly (i.e., do not inflict permanent damage to the rather sensitive ocular tissues) and are safe for chronic use in humans.

Aqueous Suspensions

Aqueous suspensions contain a sparingly soluble drug as finely divided particles dispersed in a saturated solution of the drug with a suspending agent dissolved in the medium. The advantage of suspensions over solutions is that the suspended particles are better retained in the cul-de-sac [95,96]. Retention increases with an increase in the particle size as does the irritation of the eye. The rate of dissolution of the suspended drug increases with decreasing particle size. Thus, an optimum particle size exists for ocular suspensions.

Ocular suspensions, however, have the following disadvantages: shaking is required which can lead to inconsistency in the administered dose if not done properly; a fine sediment may form which can be difficult to disperse with gentle shaking; and seldomly occurring, but of serious consequence, is a polymorphic change in the suspended drug to form a less soluble or inactive form of the drug. In addition, suspensions are prone to elimination by the previously discussed physiological mechanisms.

Ointments

Ointments are useful as drug carriers for improving bioavailability and sustaining drug release. An attractive feature of ointments is their entrapment in the fornices which thereby serve as a reservoir [97]. Drug bioavailability is usually higher from an ointment than from an aqueous solution or suspension [95]. The superior bioavailability of drugs from ointments is due to their increased resistance to nasolacrimal drainage, higher tissue concentration, inhibition of dilution by the tears, and increased contact time, all of which can lead to increased ocular drug absorption. Interference with vision and esthetic considerations are obvious disadvantages associated with the use of ocular ointments.

Nanoparticles

Nanoparticles are colloidal particles 10-1000 nm in size in which drug can be dispersed, encapsulated, or absorbed [98]. Wood et al. [99] demonstrated that a 0.385% suspension of polyhexyl-2-cyanoacrylate nanoparticles, like neutral liposomes, disappeared from the tear pool almost as rapidly as aqueous solutions. Although this approach shows promise for delivering lipophilic drugs, it would not likely be beneficial for incorporating drugs that are water soluble as these drugs are released from the nanoparticles more rapidly than the rate at which the nanoparticles themselves are eliminated from the precorneal cavity (see the article Nanoparticles in this volume, pp. xx–xx).

Aqueous Gels

The poor patient acceptability of ocular ointments has led researchers [100–106] to investigate aqueous gels as vehicles to improve ocular bioavailability of both hydrophilic and lipophilic drugs. These gels typically utilize polymers, such as polyvinyl alcohol, polyacrylamide, polymethyl–vinyl ether–maleic anhydride, poloxamer, carbopol (also called carbomer), hydroxyethylcellulose, hydroxypropylcellulose, and hydroxypropyl methylcellulose. Overall, three- to fivefold increases in corneal absorption of drugs have been reported. The mechanism of drug release from gels involves a combination of drug diffusion within the gel and erosion (dissolution) of the gel surface. The disadvantage associated with aqueous gels for ocular delivery is due to their hydrophilic nature. Tears diffuse into the gel interior quickly and therefore rapidly leach out water-soluble drugs such as pilocarpine and prednisolone sodium phosphate [83].

Liposomes

Liposomes, first described by Bangham [107], are biocompatible and biodegradable phospholipid microcapsules. Liposomes consist of membrane-like vesicles made up of a concentric series of alternating lipid bilayers with an aqueous compartment in between two layers (see the article Liposomes as Pharmaceutical Dosage Forms, Vol. 10, pp. 1–40, of this encyclopedia.) In addition to their application as model biological membranes, liposomes have been used for administering bioactive agents orally [108] and topically to the skin [109] and the eye [110–112]. Smolin et al. [110] were among the first to demonstrate the usefulness of a liposomal ocular delivery system for enhancing corneal drug absorption. They reported that idoxuridine entrapped in liposomes was more effective than a comparable therapeutic regimen of idoxuridine alone in the treatment of acute and chronic herpetic keratitis. Schaeffer and Krohn [111] showed that the transcorneal flux of penicillin-G and indoxol doubled when these drugs were topically applied to the cornea in liposomal form. They also reported that the liposomal entrapment of a drug is prerequisite to enhanced corneal transport. According to Schaffer and Krohn [111], the interaction between liposomes and the corneal surface may be due to electrostatic adsorption, and positively charged liposomes are absorbed to the greatest extent. Taniguchi et al. [113] have shown that the addition of stearylamine, which confers a positive charge, increases the corneal absorption of dexamethasone valerate. In a study of precorneal factors influencing the ocular distribution of topically applied liposomal inulin, Lee et. al [114] concluded that, for liposomes to be effective in ocular drug delivery, they must not only show affinity for and be bound to the corneal surface but, in addition, must release their contents at an optimal rate. Positively charged liposomes are more effective than neutral or negatively charged liposomes in enhancing the corneal absorption of some ocular drugs. The reason for this apparent difference is not clear, but it is known that the corneal epithelium is thinly coated with negatively charged mucin to which the positive surface charge of the liposomes may adsorb more strongly [115].

Liposomes can enhance or reduce the ocular absorption of topically applied drugs [116]. The nature and extent of altered ocular uptake of liposome-associated agents appear to depend on a number of factors, such as physicochemical properties of the entrapped drug, chemical composition and physical characteristics of the liposomes, and the method of ocular administration of the liposomal formulation.

Liposomes are a potentially useful ocular drug-delivery system, but suffer from the disadvantage of instability due to the hydrolysis of phospholipids normally used in their preparation, limited drug loading capacity, and technological difficulties in obtaining a sterile liposomal preparation [117]. Thus, there is a definite need to further optimize liposomal preparations in order to use them effectively for delivering ocular drugs.

Bioadhesive Polymers

Bioadhesion refers to the process of attaching a drug to a specific biological surface or fluid. Mucin is a thin film of glycoprotein which forms the bottom layer of the tear film adjacent to the corneal epithelium. Mucin acts as a wetting agent, serving as a bridge between the hydrophobic corneal epithelial surface and the aqueous layer of the tear film which lies immediately above the mucus layer. Without the mucus layer, the corneal surface would not be wetted by the aqueous layer of the tear film, and instead of forming a thin film, the tears would form into discrete drops.

The success of ocular drug-delivery systems depends on their retention in the eye. Improved retention can be obtained by incorporating bioadhesive polymers into formulations. These polymers attach to conjunctival mucin by noncovalent bonds (hydrogen bonding) and remain in contact with the precorneal tissue until eliminated by mucin turnover. Hui and Robinson [118] demonstrated that mucoadhesive polymers are better retained in the albino rabbit eye and can provide a sustained release of progesterone.

Polyacrylic acid has been proposed as a potential mucoadhesive polymeric agent by Park and Robinson [119] and Smart et al. [120]. Saettone et al. [121] reported a moderate increase (1.6-fold compared to a solution) in the ocular bioavailability of pilocarpine in the albino rabbit eye using Carbopol 941, which is a lightly cross-linked polyacrylic acid. However, rapid leaching of drug from this delivery system appears to reduce its utility.

Systems that Undergo Phase Transition

A major recent advance in the field of ocular drug delivery is the development of several polymeric systems that undergo phase transition. These systems are liquid under certain conditions, and therefore are easy to administer as eyedrops. They undergo a sol-to-gel-phase change leading to an increase in viscosity when their local environment is changed in the cul-de-sac. Such a phase transition can be mediated by a change in temperature, a change in pH, or by electrolyte or ion activation.

Poloxamer 407 is a thermally reversible gel-forming polymer. In concentrations of 20% w/v and higher, aqueous solutions remain as a liquid at low temperature (4°C) and yield a highly viscous semisolid gel upon instillation into the cul-de-sac. The phase change is mediated by the temperature increase upon instillation. The gel so formed, is retained longer in the albino rabbit eye. It cannot easily be drained away and significantly increases the ocular bioavailability of pilocarpine compared to isotonic solutions of pilocarpine [122,123].

Gurny [124] described the use of pH-sensitive latex particles for sustained delivery of pilocarpine to the eye with cellulose acetate hydrogen phthalate at a 30% w/w polymer concentration. The latex is a free-flowing liquid at a formulation pH of 4.4; it gels at physiological pH 7.4 in the eye. When placed in the cul-de-sac, the pH change due to neutralization by tears causes gelation of the latex. Pilocarpine, 2% w/v, adsorbed onto the latex maintained miosis in the rabbit eye for 10 h as compared to 4 h with pilocarpine solution [124,125].

Gelrite is a cation-selective heteropolysaccharide, low-acetyl gellan gum that undergoes phase transition to a clear gel in the presence of mono- and divalent cations [126]. The ion concentration of sodium ions in human tears (2.6 g/L) is sufficient to induce gelation when Gelrite is topically instilled into the eye. Gellan, 0.6% w/v, forms a gel in the cul-de-sac within a few seconds due to the diffusion of cations present in tears [127]. In rabbits, the gel so formed increased the bioavailability of 0.35% timolol maleate (equivalent to 0.25% timolol-free base), compared with an equiviscous solution of the more conventional vehicle hydroxyethylcellulose [127]. The enhanced drug bioavailability was explained by the longer residence time in the cul-de-sac. In another study, the contact time or residence time was measured by gamma scintigraphy with $^{99}Tc^{m}$-labeled diethylenetriaminepentaacetic acid ($^{99}Tc^{m}$-DTPA) as the tracer in humans and rabbits. In humans, the gellan gum formulation provided significantly longer retention compared to that provided by hydroxyethylcellulose (HEC) [128]. However, in rabbits the HEC solution was retained longer than the gellan formulation [128].

The temperature-sensitive poloxamer 407 system and the pH-sensitive cellulose acetate–hydrogen phthalate system both require a high polymer concentration in order to gel in the precorneal cavity (25 and 30%, respectively). The gellan gum system Gelrite gels at a much lower concentration (0.6%) in the eye.

In addition to the above-mentioned ocular dosage forms, presoaked matrices, such as drug-loaded soft contact lenses [129,130], emulsions [131], and soluble, solid hydrophilic inserts [132,133], have been employed to deliver ophthalmic drugs and can often improve corneal absorption.

Drug-Delivery Systems that Provide Controlled and Continuous Ocular Delivery

Solid-state ocular inserts represent another category of dosage form. Based on this approach, dosage forms can overcome the disadvantages reported with more traditional ophthalmic systems like aqueous solutions, suspensions, and ointments. The typical pulse-entry-type drug-release behavior observed with ocular aqueous solutions (eyedrops), suspensions, and ointments is replaced by more controlled, sustained, and continuous drug delivery, using a controlled-release ocular drug-delivery system (e.g., Ocusert, Alza). These systems can achieve therapeutic action with a smaller dose and fewer systemic and ocular side effects. Atropine-containing gelatin wafers called ''Lamellae'' were described in the *British Pharmacopoeia* as early as 1948. Solid wafers of solubilized collagen containing ^{14}C-gentamicin afforded higher drug concentrations in tears, sclera, and cornea in rabbits than eyedrops and ointments [134].

Ocusert

Ocusert (Alza) is an example of an ocular delivery system providing the controlled and continuous delivery of pilocarpine at a constant (zero-order) rate of 20 or 40 μg/h around the clock for seven days [135]. It is a membrane-reservoir type device, containing pilocarpine and alginic acid in the core reservoir, which is placed between a transparent, lipophilic ethylene–vinyl acetate rate-controlling membrane.

A survey among ophthalmologists [136] revealed that, in the opinion of physicians, the Ocusert is of value for younger patients who have the necessary motivation and energy to handle this system. They are less popular and useful among the elderly who have difficulty with insertion, do not retain the device well, and often do not seem to notice if it falls out. Many patients feel a foreign body sensation in the eye. A significant drawback of Ocusert therapy is its high cost due to its complicated fabrication procedure. Furthermore, replacing a contaminated device with a fresh one after loss from the eye socket increases the cost of an already expensive therapy. Finally, Ocusert is a nonbiodegradable system and must therefore be removed at the end of its therapeutic life (seven days).

Soluble Ophthalmic Drug Insert (SODI)

A soluble ophthalmic drug insert (SODI), first described by Maichuk [137,138] was originally introduced for the delivery of pilocarpine in the former USSR. The SODI is a small oval wafer composed of copolymers of acrylamide, vinylpyrollidone, and ethyl acrylate and impregnated with a drug. Maichuk and Erichev [139] showed that the SODI with 2.7 mg pilocarpine, administered once-a-day, effectively reduced the intraocular pressure in 155 glaucoma patients. The SODI was brought to the United States by Diversified Technology which has exclusive rights to market the technology.

Ocular Therapeutic System or Minidisc

Bawa et al. [140,141] developed a controlled-release device for the eye, known as the ocular therapeutic system (OTS) or minidisc, a monolithic matrix-type device. It consists of a contoured disc with a convex front and concave back surface in contact with the eyeball [141]. Its principal component is α,ω-bis(4-methacryloxybutyl)-polydimethylsiloxane (M_2D_x), where M represents the methacryloxybutyl and D represents the dimethylsiloxane functionalities. The OTS can be made hydrophilic or hydrophobic to permit extended release of both water-soluble as well as water-insoluble drugs. Hydrophilic OTS released sulfisoxazole for 118 h, and hydrophobic OTS released gentamicin for longer than 320 h. In three volunteer subjects, sulfisoxazole was released from the hydrophilic OTS over three days [140,141].

New Ophthalmic Drug-Delivery System (NODS)

The New Ophthalmic Drug-Delivery System (NODS), developed by Smith and Nephew, is another example of an ophthalmic insert designed to deliver a precise amount of an ocular medication for an extended period [142]. The device is made of water-soluble polyvinyl alcohol with a median molecular weight of 98,000. In a recent scintigraphy study, the ocular retention of the NODS radiolabelled with a soluble marker comprised of $^{99}Tc^{m}$-labeled diethylenetriaminepentaacetic acid ($^{99}Tc^{m}$-DTPA) was compared in human volunteers with a solution of the marker. The solution was cleared much more rapidly than the NODS (3 s vs. 7 min) [143].

Kelly et al. [144] found that the NODS containing 67 μg of pilocarpine nitrate gave a dose response equivalent to a conventional 2% w/v pilocarpine nitrate solution (517 μg of the drug). The results of this study suggest that ocular bioavailability of pilocarpine is eightfold higher when administered with the NODS compared to a pilocarpine solution administered in a conventional way. The delivery of an insoluble drug, tropicamide, in the NODS has also shown higher ocular bioavailability compared with that of an aqueous suspension of the drug [145].

The anhydrous nature of the NODS system can be advantageous for water-sensitive drugs which can be formulated under aqueous conditions without risking a significant drug loss. The NODS system is well received by patients and physicians in terms of ease of administration, comfort, and effectiveness. However, once in the cul-de-sac, the system begins to hydrate and soften and may release the drug too fast. Since it does not have a prolonged residence time in the precorneal cavity, the NODS may fall short of achieving the goal of once-a-day therapy. The advantages of solid inserts in ocular therapy are great, but it should be noted that their future development must overcome some problems that are less likely to occur with the more traditional ocular dosage forms available on the market, that is, solutions, suspensions, or ointments. Polymer inserts often retain ingredients used in their manufacture, such as plasticizers, antioxidants, or cross-linking agents which may have toxic effects. The manufacturing cost of solid inserts may be exceptionally high, since it often involves a specialized process. Because of interference with vision and other problems, these solid and semisolid delivery systems have not been well accepted by patients [83].

The previous discussion of the current concepts and recent developments in the field of ophthalmic pharmaceutical research, development, and delivery systems is only an introduction. The reader seeking detailed information is directed to the huge compilation of excellent articles, textbook chapters, and reviews on the subject found in the literature [146–158].

Future Trends

A primary consideration in the design and development of new and improved ocular drug formulations and delivery systems should be ease of use and comfort to the patient. The ultimate aim of an ocular drug-delivery system is to achieve an effective drug concentration at the target tissues for an extended period while minimizing the number of required administrations.

Although attempts to maximize the bioavailability of topically applied ocular drugs have been ongoing for the last two decades, this goal remains difficult to accomplish. Ocular bioavailability from conventional eyedrops is poor and only a fraction of an administered dose (typically less than 1 to 3%) reaches the intraocular tissues. It is clear that ocular drug-delivery systems based on the above approaches are inefficient and far from ideal. Based on patient-acceptance considerations alone, future efforts to improve ocular delivery systems should focus primarily on liquid systems.

The following are future challenges in the development of topical ocular drug-delivery systems:

- Ocular bioavailibility should be increased from its typical value of 1–3% of an administered dose to 15–20%.
- The ocular and systemic side effects of ocular drugs are primarily related to overdosing and result from the absorption of ocular drugs through the nasal mucosal lining. In the future, ocular drugs and prodrugs should be designed that will be absorbed preferentially through the ocular tissues rather than through the nasal mucosa, in order to reduce side effects, some of which can be life threatening,
- Recent developments in the field of biotechnology have resulted in a dramatic increase in the number of proteins and peptides of potential therapeutic importance. There is thus a need to design efficient delivery systems for ocular use in order to evaluate their therapeutic potential in treating various conditions of the eye.
- Many of the currently marketed ocular drugs were initially developed for nonocular applications. It is therefore imperative to develop new drug candidates primarily intended for ocular use. Although there is no conclusive evidence about the usefulness of the noncorneal route, further studies are needed to fully characterize and understand the significance of this route in the overall scheme of ocular drug absorption.

Future strategies in ocular drug development should focus on ocular drug-delivery systems which can provide a controlled and sustained release of drugs to ocular tissues. To date, very few ocular dosage forms provide once-a-week, or even once-a-day, therapy. As a result, ophthalmic pharmaceutical scientists continue to seek improved ocular drug-delivery systems which will have the ease of administration of eyedrops and the prolonged residence time of Ocusert.

References

1. Moses, R. A., *Adler's Physiology of the Eye*, 7th ed., C. V. Mosby Co., St. Louis, 1981.
2. Scheie, H. G., and Albert, D. M., *Textbook of Ophthalmology*, 9th ed., W. B. Saunders Co., Philadelphia, 1977.
3. Miller, D., *Ophthalmology, the Essentials*, Houghton Mifflin Professional Publishers, Boston, 1979.
4. Fatt, I., *Physiology of the Eye. An Introduction to the Vegetative Functions*, Butterworths, Boston, 1978.
5. Cummings, S. J., Relevant Anatomy and Physiology of the Eye. In : *Ophthalmic Drug Delivery Systems* (J. R. Robinson, ed.), Am. Pharmaceutical Assoc., Washington, 1980, pp. 1–27.

6. Prince, J. H., *The Rabbit in Eye Research*, Charles C Thomas Publishing Co., Springfield, IL, 1970.
7. Kaufman, P. L., Wiedman, T., and Robinson, J. R., Cholinergics. In: *Handbook of Experimental Pharmacology: Pharmacology of the Eye*, Vol. 69 (M.L. Sears, ed.), Springer-Verlag, Berlin, 1984, pp. 149–168.
8. Guyton, A. C. The Eye: II. Neurophysiology of Vision. In: *Human Physiology and Mechanisms of Disease*, 5th ed., W. B. Saunders Co., Philadelphia, 1992, pp. 380–391.
9. Theodore, K., *Manual of Glaucoma: Diagnosis and Management*, Chap. 7, Pharmacology, Churchill Livingstone, New York, 1988, pp. 115–118.
10. Mishima, S., Gasset, A., Klyce, S. D., and Baum, J. L., *Invest. Ophthalmol.*, 5:264–276 (1966).
11. Maurice, D. M., *Int. Clin. Ophthalmol.*, 13:103–116 (1973).
12. Mishima, S., *Arch. Ophthalmol.*, 73:233–241 (1965).
13. Chang, S. C., and Lee, V. H. L., *J. Ocul. Pharmacol.*, 3:159–167 (1987).
14. Akingebehin, T., and Raj, S. P., *J. Toxicol.-Cut. Ocular Toxicol.*, 9:131–147 (1990).
15. Nelson, W. L., Fraunfelder, F. T., Sills, J. M., Arrowsmith, J. B., and Kuritsky, J. N., *Am. J. Ophthalmol.*, 102:606–611 (1986).
16. Rubin, I., *Wellcome Trends in Pharmacy*, June 2–6 (1989).
17. Shields, B. M., *Textbook of Glaucoma*, 3rd ed., Williams & Wilkins, Philadelphia, 1992.
18. Chrai, S. S., Patton, T. F., Mehta, A., and Robinson, J. R., *J. Pharm. Sci.*, 62:1112–1121 (1973).
19. Chrai, S. S., Makoid, M. C., Eriksen, S. P., and Robinson, J. R., *J. Pharm. Sci.*, 63:333–338 (1974).
20. Lee, V. H. L., *J. Control. Rel.*, 11:79–90 (1990).
21. Kishida, K., and Otori, T., *Jap. J. Ophthalmol.*, 24:251–259 (1980).
22. Schoenwald, R. D., and Ward, R. L., *J. Pharm. Sci.*, 67:786–788 (1981).
23. Schoenwald, R. D., and Huang, H. S., *J. Pharm. Sci.*, 72:1266–1272 (1983).
24. Burstein, N. L., and Anderson, J. A., *J. Ocular Pharmacol.*, 1:309–326 (1985).
25. Doane, M.G., Jesse, A. D., and Dohlman, C. H., *Am. J. Ophthalmol.*, 85:383–386 (1978).
26. Ahmed, I., and Patton, T. F., *Invest. Ophthalmol.Vis. Sci.*, 26:584–587 (1985).
27. Ahmed, I., and Patton, T. F., *Int. J. Pharm.*, 38:9–21 (1987).
28. Ahmed, I., Gokhale, R. D., Shah, M. V., and Patton, T. F., *J. Pharm. Sci.*, 76:583–586 (1987).
29. Ashton, P., Podder, S. K., and Lee, V. H. L., *Pharm. Res.*, 8:1166–1174 (1991).
30. Schoenwald, R. D., *Clin. Pharmacokinet.*, 18:255–269 (1990).
31. Wood, R. W., and Robinson, J. R., *Int. J. Pharm.*, 29:127–135 (1986).
32. Anderson, J. A., Davis, W. L., and Wei, C .-P., *Invest. Ophthalmol. Vis. Sci.*, 19:817–823 (1980).
33. Lee, V. H. L., Carson, W. L., Kashi, S. D., and Stratford, R. E., Jr., *J. Ocul Pharmacol.*, 2:345–352 (1986).
34. Lee, V. H. L., Hui, H.-W., and Robinson, J. R., *Invest. Ophthalmol. Vis. Sci.*, 19:210–213 (1980).
35. Southern, A. L., Altman, K., and Vittek, J., *Invest. Ophthalmol. Vis. Sci.*, 15:222–228 (1976).
36. Green, K., and Mackeen, D. L., *Invest. Ophthalmol. Vis. Sci.*, 15:220–222 (1976).
37. Himmelstein, K. J., Gurvenir, I., and Patton, T. F., *J. Pharm. Sci.*, 67:603–606 (1978).
38. Lee, V. H. L., and Robinson, J. R., *J. Pharm. Sci.*, 68:673–684 (1979).
39. Makoid, M. C., and Robinson, J. R., *J. Pharm. Sci.*, 68:435–443 (1979).
40. Miller, S. C., Himmelstein, K. J., and Patton, T. F., *J. Pharmacokin. Biopharm.*, 9:653–677 (1981).
41. Sieg, J. W., and Robinson, J. R., *J. Pharm. Sci.*, 7:1026–1029 (1981).
42. Francouer, M. L., Sitek, S. J., Costello, B., and Patton, T. F., *Int. J. Pharm.*, 25:275–292 (1985).

43. Chiang, C. H., and Schoenwald, R. D., *J. Pharmocokin. Biopharm.*, 7:453–462 (1986).
44. Lee, V. H. L., and Robinson, J. R., *J. Ocular Pharmacol.*, 2:67–108 (1986).
45. Shell, J. W., *Surv. Ophthalmol.*, 26:207–218 (1982).
46. Maurice, D. M., and Mishima, S., Ocular Pharmacokinetics. In : *Handbook of Experimental Pharmacology: Pharmacology of the Eye*, Vol. 69 (M. L. Sears, ed.), Springer-Verlag, Berlin, 1984, pp. 19–116.
47. Maurice, D. M., Kinetics of Topically Applied Ophthalmic Drugs. In: *Ophthalmic Drug Delivery: Biopharmaceutical, Technological, and Clinical Aspects*, Vol. 11 (M. F. Saettone, M. Bucci, and P. Speiser, eds.), Livinia Press, Springer-Verlag, Berlin, 1987, pp. 19–26.
48. Ansel, H. C., and Popovich, N. G., *Pharmaceutical Dosage Forms and Drug Delivery Systems*, 5th ed., Lea and Febiger, Philadelphia, 1990, pp. 347–372.
49. Kastrup, E. K., ed., *Facts and Comparisons*, J. B. Lippincott Co., Philadelphia, Aug. 1989, pp. 477a–477b.
50. Mullins, J. D., and Hecht, G., Ophthalmic Preparations. In: *Remington's Pharmaceutical Sciences*, 18th ed. (A. R. Gennaro, ed.)., Mack Publishing Co., Easton, PA, 1990, pp. 1581–1595.
51. Cadwallader, D. E., EENT Preparations. In: *Dispensing of Medication*, 9th ed. (R. E. King, ed.), Mack Publishing Co., Easton, PA, 1984, pp. 140–164.
52. Hecht, G. A., Roehrs, R. E., Cooper, E. R., Hiddemen, J. W., and Van Duzee, B. F., Design and Evaluation of Ophthalmic Pharmaceutical Products. In: *Modern Pharmaceutics*, 2nd ed. (G. S. Banker and C. T. Rhodes, eds.), Marcel Dekker, Inc., New York, 1990, pp. 539–603.
53. *Federal Register*, Vol. 45, No. 89, Tues., May 6, 1980.
54. Green, K., The Effect of Preservatives on Corneal Permeability of Drugs. In: *Biopharmaceutics of Ocular Drug Delivery* (P. Edman, ed.), CRC Press, Boca Raton, FL, 1993, pp. 43–59.
55. Stark, R. L., U.S. Pat. 4,407,791 (Oct. 4, 1983).
56. Nikitakis, J. M., ed., *Cosmetic Ingredient Dictionary*, Cosmetic, Toiletry and Fragrance Assoc., Washington, 1988, p. 245.
57. Bapatla, K. M., and Lorenzetti, O. J., Development of Ophthalmic Formulations. In: *Pharmaceutical Dosage Forms, Parenteral Medications*, Vol. 2 (K. E. Avis, H. A. Lieberman, and L. Lachman, eds.), Marcel Dekker, Inc., New York, 1992, pp. 541–581.
58. Olejnik, O., Conventional Systems in Ophthalmic Drug Delivery., In: *Ophthalmic Drug Delivery Systems* (A. K. Mitra, ed.), Marcel Dekker, Inc., New York, 1993, pp. 177–198.
59. Keister, J. C., Cooper, E. R., Missel, P. J., Lang, J. C., and Hager, D. F., *J. Pharm. Sci.*, 80:50–53 (1991).
60. Anon., *Pharmacopeial Forum*, 16:107–108 (Jan.-Feb. 1990).
61. Anon., *Pharmacopeial Forum*, 18:2953–2957 (Jan.-Feb. 1992).
62. Van Ooteghem, M. M. M., Formulation of Ophthalmic Solutions and Suspensions—Problems and Advantages. In: *Biopharmaceutics of Ocular Drug Delivery* (P. Edman, ed.), CRC Press, Boca Raton, FL, 1993, pp. 27–42.
63. Ahmed, I., and Chaudhuri, B., *Int. J. Pharm.*, 44:97–105 (1988).
64. Robinson, J. R., and Goshman, L. M., Topical Drug-Delivery Systems (Eye, Ear, Nose). In: *Pharmaceutics and Pharmacy Practice* (G. S. Banker and R. S. Chalmers, eds.), J. B. Lippincott Co., Philadelphia, 1984, pp. 312–352.
65. Jenkins, G. L., Sperandio, G. J., and Latiolais, C. J., *Clinical Pharmacy, A Text for Dispensing Pharmacy*, McGraw-Hill, New York, 1966, pp. 181–194.
66. Meyer D. R., and McCulley, J. P., *J. Toxicol.-Cut. Ocular Toxicol.*, 10:79–94 (1991).
67. Meyer, D. R., and McCulley, J. P., *Ophthalmic Res.*, 23:204–212 (1991).
68. Blanchard, J., *J. Pharm. Sci.*, 69:169–173 (1980).
69. *USP XXII-NF XVII*, United States Pharmacopeial Convention, Inc., Rockville, MD, 1990, pp. 1495–1500 and pp. 1573–1575, respectively.

70. Havener, W. H., *Ocular Pharmacology*, 5th ed., C. V. Mosby Co., St. Louis, MO., 1983, pp. 18–43.

71. Patton, T. F., and Robinson, J. R., *J. Pharm. Sci.*, 62:267–71 (1975).

72. Patton, T. F., and Robinson, J. R., *J. Pharm. Sci.*, 65:1295–1301 (1976).

73. Mikkelson, T. J., and Robinson, J. R., *J. Pharm. Sci.*, 62:1648–1653 (1973).

74. Chrai, S. S, and Robinson, J. R., *J. Pharm. Sci.* 65:437–439 (1976).

75. Conrad, J. M., and Robinson, J. R., *J. Pharm. Sci.* 66:219–224 (1977).

76. Harris, J. E., Problems in Drug Penetration. In: *Symposium on Ocular Therapy*, Vol. 3 (I. H. Leopold, ed.), C. V. Mosby Co., 1973. Through *J. Parent. Sci. Technol.*, 32:149–161 (1978).

77. Sieg, J. W., and Robinson, J. R., J. Pharm. Sci., 65:1816–1822 (1976).

78. Chrai, S. S., and Robinson, J. R., *Am. J. Ophthalmol.*, 77:735–739 (1974).

79. Benson, H., *Arch. Ophthalmol.*, 91:313–327 (1974).

80. Ahmed, I., and Patton, T. F., *Invest. Ophthalmol. Vis. Sci.*, 26:584–587 (1985).

81. Maurice, D. M., and Polgar, J., *Exp. Eye Res.*, 25:577–582 (1977).

82. Doane, M. G., Jensen, A. D., and Dohlman, C. H., *Am. J. Ophthalmol.*, 85:383–386 (1978).

83. Lee, V. H. L., and Robinson, J. R., *J. Ocul. Pharmacol.*, 2:67–108 (1986).

84. Patton, T. F., and Robinson, J. R., *J. Pharm. Sci.*, 64:1312–1316 (1978).

85. Chrai, S. S., and Robinson, J. R., *J. Pharm. Sci.*, 63:1218–1223 (1974).

86. Kassem, M. A., Attia, M. A., Habib, F. S., and Mohmed, A. A., *Drug Develop. Ind. Pharm.*, 13:1447–1469 (1987).

87. Greaves, J. L., Olejnik, O., and Wilson, C. G., *S.T.P. Pharm. Sci.*, 2:13–33 (1992).

88. Davis, S. S., Tomlinson, E., and Wilson, C. G., *Br. J. Pharmacol.*, 64:444–445 (1978).

89. Mikkelson, T. J., Chrai, S. S., and Robinson, J. R., *J. Pharm. Sci.*, 62:1942–1945 (1973).

90. Godbey, R. E. W., Green, K., and Hull, D. S., *J. Pharm. Sci.*, 68:1176–1178, (1979).

91. Mitra, A. K., *Passive and Facilitated Transport of Pilocarpine Across the Corneal Membrane of the Rabbit*, Ph.D. Thesis, University of Kansas, Lawrence, 1983.

92. Marsch, R. J., and Maurice, D. M., *Exp. Eye Res.*, 11:43–48 (1971).

93. Keller, N., Moore, D., Carper, D., and Longwell, A., Exp. Eye Res., 30:203–210 (1980).

94. Chiou, G. C. Y., and Chuang, C. A., *J. Pharm. Sci.*, 78:815–818 (1989).

95. Sieg, J. W., and Robinson, J. R., *J. Pharm. Sci.*, 64:931–936 (1975).

96. Sieg, J. W., and Triplett, J. W., *J. Pharm. Sci.*, 69:863–864 (1980).

97. Norn, M. S., *Acta Ophthalmol.*, 50:206–209 (1972).

98. Oppenheim, R. C., Nanoparticles. In: *Drug Delivery Systems. Characteristics and Biomedical Applications* (R. J. Juliano, ed.), Oxford University Press, New York, 1980, pp. 177–188.

99. Wood, R., Li, V. H. K., Kreuter, J., and Robinson, J. R., *Int. J. Pharm.*, 23:1175–1183 (1985).

100. Schoenwald, R. D., and Boltralik, J. J., *Invest Ophthalmol. Vis. Sci.*, 18:61–66 (1979).

101. Bottari, F., Giannaccini, B., Preverni, D., Saettone, M. F., and Tellini, N., *Can J. Pharm. Sci.*, 14:39–43 (1979). Through Ref. 83.

102. Miller, S. C., and Donovan, M. D., *Int. J. Pharm.*, 12:147–152 (1982).

103. Goldberg, I., Ashburn, F. S., Kass, M. A., and Beckner, B., *Am. J. Ophthalmol.*, 88:843–846 (1979).

104. Saettone, M. F., Giannaccini, B., Guiducci, A., and Savigni, P., *Int. J. Pharm.*, 31:261–270 (1986).

105. March, W. F., Stewart, R. M., Mandell, A. I., and Bruce, L. A., *Arch. Ophthalmol.*, 100:1270–1271 (1982).

106. Schoenwald, R. D., Ward, R. L., DeSantis, L. M., and Roehrs, R. E., *J. Pharm. Sci.*, 67:1280–1283 (1978).

107. Bangham, A. D., *Prog. Biophys. Mol. Biol.*, 18:29–95 (1968).

108. Patel, H. M., and Ryman, B. E., *Biochem. Soc. Trans.*, 5:1054–1055 (1977).

109. Mezei, M., and Gulsekharam, V., *Life Sci.*, 26:1473–1477 (1980).

110. Smolin, G., Okumoto, M., Feiler, S., and Condon, D., *Am. J. Ophthalmol.*, 91:220–225 (1981).

111. Schaeffer, H. E., and Krohn, D. L., *Invest. Ophthalmol. Vis. Sci.*, 22:220–227 (1982).

112. Singh, K., and Mezei, M., *Int. J. Pharm.*, 16:339–344 (1983).

113. Taniguchi, K., Yamamoto, Y., Itakura, K., Miichi, H., and Hayashi, S.-I., *J. Pharmacobio-Dyn.*, 11:607–611 (1988).

114. Lee, V. H. L., Takemoto, K. A., and Iimoto, D. S., *Curr. Eye Res.*, 3:585–591 (1984).

115. Shek, P. N., and Barber, R. F., *Biochim. Biophys.. Acta*, 902:229–236 (1987).

116. Stratford, R. E., Jr., Yang, D. C., Redell, M. A., and Lee, V. H. L., *Int. J. Pharm.*, 13:263–272 (1983).

117. Lee, V. H. L., Urrea, P. T., Smith, R. E., and Schanzlin, D. J., *Surv. Ophthalmol.*, 29:335–348 (1985).

118. Hui, H.-W., and Robinson, J. R., *Int. J. Pharm.*, 26:203–213 (1985).

119. Park, H., and Robinson, J. R., *Int. J. Pharm.*, 19:107–127 (1984).

120. Smart, J. D., Kellaway, I. W., and Worthington, H. E. C., *J. Pharm. Pharmacol.*, 36:295–299 (1984).

121. Saettone, M. F., Chetoni, P., Torracca, M. T., Burgalassi, S., and Giannaccini, B., *Int. J. Pharm.*, 51:203–212 (1989).

122. Miller, S. C., and Donovan, M. D., *Int. J. Pharm.*, 12:147–152 (1982).

123. Desai, S. D., *Formulation of Controlled Release Ocular Delivery Systems of Pilocarpine*, Ph.D. Dissertation, University of Arizona, Tucson, 1992.

124. Gurny, R., *Pharm. Acta Helv.*, 56:130–132 (1981).

125. Gurny, R., Ocular Therapy with Nanoparticles. In: *Polymeric Nanoparticles and Microspheres* (P. Guiot and P. Couvreur, eds.), CRC Press, Boca Raton, FL, 1986, pp. 127–136.

126. Moorhouse, R., Colegrove, G. T., Sandford, P. A., Baird, J. K., and Kang, K. S., PS-60: A New Gel-Forming Polysaccharide. In: *Solution Properties of Polysaccharides* (D. A. Brandt, ed.), American Chemical Society, Washington, 1981, pp. 111–124.

127. Rozier, A., Mazuel, C., Grove, J., and Plazonnet, B., *Int. J. Pharm.*, 57:163–168 (1989).

128. Greaves, J. L., Wilson, C. G., Rozier, A., Grove, J., and Plazonnet, B., *Curr. Eye Res.*, 9:415–420 (1990).

129. Becker, B., Assef, C., Hartstein, J., and Podos, S., *Am. J. Ophthalmol.*, 73:336–341 (1972).

130. Waltman, S. R., and Kaufman, H. E., *Invest. Ophthalmol.*, 9:250–255 (1970).

131. Ticho, U., Blumenthal, M., Zonis, S., Gal, A., Blank, I., and Mazor, Z. W., *Br. J. Ophthalmol.*, 63:45–47 (1979).

132. Maichuk, Y. F., *Invest. Ophthalmol.*, 14:87–90 (1975).

133. Saettone, M. F., Chetoni, P., Torracca, M. T., Giannaccini, B., Naber, L., Conte, U., Sangalli, M. E., and Gazzaniga, A., *Acta. Pharm. Technol.*, 36:15–19 (1990).

134. Bloomfield, S. E., Miyata, T., and Dunn, M. W., *Arch. Ophthalmol.*, 87:210–214 (1979).

135. Zaffaroni, A., *Drug Metab. Rev.*, 8:191–221 (1978).

136. Conn, H., and Langer, R. S., Ocular Applications of Controlled Release. In: *Medical Applications of Controlled Release* (R. S. Langer, and D. L. Wise, eds.), CRC Press, Boca Raton, FL, 1984.

137. Maichuk, Y. F., *Antibiotiki*, 5:435 (1967).

138. Maichuk, Y. F., Polymeric Drug Delivery Systems in Ophthalmology. In: *Ocular Therapy* (I. H. Leopold and R. P. Burns, eds.), John Wiley and Sons, New York, 1976, pp. 1–16.

139. Maichuk, Y. F., and Erichev, V. P., *Glaucoma*, 3:239–242 (1981).

140. Bawa, R., Dais, M., Nandu, M., and Robinson, J. R., New Extended Release Ocular Drug Delivery System: Design, Characterization and Performance Testing of Minidiscs Inserts.

In: *Proceedings of the 15th International Symposium on Controlled Release of Bioactive Materials*, Controlled Release, Inc., Lincolnshire, IL, 1988, pp. 106a–107b.

141. Bawa, R., and Nandu, M., *Biomaterials*, 11:724–728 (1990).

142. Bentley, P. H., A New Ophthalmic Delivery System (NODS). In: *Proceedings of 9th Pharmaceutical Technology Conference*, Abstract Vol. 2, Vendhoven, Holland, 1990, p. 7.

143. Greaves, J. L., Wilson, C. G., Birmingham, A. T., Richardson, M. C., and Bentley, P. H., *Br. J. Pharmacol.*, 33:603–609 (1992).

144. Kelly, J. A., Molyneux, P. D., Smith, S. A., and Smith, S. E., *Br. J. Ophthalmol.*, 73:360–362 (1989).

145. Richardson, M. C., An Investigation of Tropicamide NODS Compared with Tropicamide Solution in Human Volunteers. In: *Proceedings of 9th Pharmaceutical Technology Conference*, Abstract Vol. 2, Vendhoven, Holland, 1990, p. 307.

146. Shell, J. W., *Surv. Ophthalmol.*, 29:117–128 (1984).

147. Shell, J. W., *J. Toxicol.-Cut. Ocular Toxicol.*, 1:49–63 (1982).

148. Lee, V. H. L., *Pharmacy International*, pp. 135–138, June (1985).

149. Lee, V. H. L., *J. Ocular. Pharmacol.*, 6:157–168 (1990).

150. Lesar, T. S., and Fiscella, R., *Drug Intell. Clin. Pharm.*, 19:642–654 (1985).

151. Robinson, J. R., *Wellcome Trends in Pharmacy*, pp. 10–11, June (1989).

152. Mackeen, D. L., *Int. Ophthalmol. Clin.*, 20:79–92 (1980).

153. Chien, Y. W., *Novel Drug Delivery Systems: Fundamentals, Development Concepts and Biomedical Assessments*, Marcel Dekker, Inc., New York, 1982.

154. Gurny, R., Ibrahim, H., Aebi, A., Buri, P., Wilson, C. G., Wahington, N. Edman, P., and Camber, O., *J. Control. Rel.*, 6:367–373 (1987).

155. Shell, J. W., and Baker, R. W., *Ann. Ophthalmol.*, 6:1037–1045 (1974).

156. Dohlman, C. H., Pavan-Langston, D., and Rose, J., *Ann. Ophthalmol.*, 2:823–832 (1972).

157. Nagataki, S., and Mishima, S., *Int. Ophthalmol. Clin.*, 20:33–49 (1980).

158. Shell, J. W., *Surv. Ophthalmol.*, 26:207–218 (1982).

SUKETU D. DESAI
JAMES BLANCHARD

Optimization Techniques in Formulation and Processing

Introduction

Most pharmaceutical products for therapeutic use are available in solid dosage forms for oral application. This is, however, a very heterogeneous group, including uncoated or (enteric) coated tablets, controlled-release tablets, effervescent tablets, (micro) granules, and capsules. The requirements concerning the release of the active ingredients differ from immediate release (fast disintegration, fast dissolution) to (very) slow release (e.g., matrix tablets). They also differ in intended route of absorption via the mouth (sublingual absorption), stomach, or intestine.

The quality of these dosage forms can be defined as the reproducibility of the optimized pharmaceutical availability profile of the drug in vivo for the intended route of administration. Quality in this context also applies to other dosage forms, such as formulations for parenteral, transdermal, rectal, vaginal, or nasal application. Molecular or colloidal solutions, emulsions, suspensions, and carriers for drugs like liposomes must equally fulfill the requirements of variability, long-term chemical and physical stability, and many other relevant properties.

Within pharmaceutical development this ultimate quality is expressed in product specifications to expiration date for the relevant product properties. Requirements or specifications may be of statistical nature (variability of content), physical nature (crushing strength, physical stability), physicochemical nature (in vitro release, stability of emulsions or suspensions), or chemical nature (chemical stability). For some products an optimum value of a specific property is most relevant, but more often ranges can be designated within which a set of properties by preference should fall.

All properties of the dosage form depend on the following important factors upon which they depend in a very complex way by mutual interaction of some or all of them.

1. The characteristics of the drug and the selected excipients,
2. Their relative and/or absolute concentration,
3. Type of processing,
4. Processing conditions, and
5. The packaging properties of the final product.

Obviously, a number of requirements have to be defined to ensure optimized availability at the site of application, and it can be stated that the development of a high quality product is a very complex process.

Before the advent of operations research techniques and the availability of fast computers, formulation research was based on experience and experimenting by trial and error. At best the influence of composition and process factors on dosage form properties was evaluated by changing factors one by one, keeping the other factors constant. In this pragmatic approach, optimization of a specific problematic property could be achieved, thus solving a pharmaceutical development problem. However, attainment of an optimum

ROYAL PHARMACEUTICAL SOCIETY LIBRARY
1, LAMBETH HIGH STREET, LONDON SE1 7JN

composition or process could never be guaranteed, because it was not recognized that the effect of one factor might depend on the level of the other factors or, stated otherwise, the possibility of interacting factors was not recognized.

It was not until the 1950s that, based on the work of Box [1–4], statistical experimental design came to the attention of a broader scientific community. But even then it took almost 20 years before these techniques were applied in pharmaceutical technology (Leuenberger [5], Schwartz [6,7], Sucker [8], and Gurny [9–11]). This is remarkable because quality requirements were steadily increasing and a systematic approach to built-in quality with the help of statistical design techniques for optimization purposes, along with the methods used so far, could offer considerable advantages.

In the following discussions attention will be paid to many aspects of systematic optimization; goals, methods, and strategies will be discussed, concepts explained, and definitions given. No attention will be paid to operations research techniques in general; the interested reader is refered to the literature or, for pharmaceutical applications, to a series of papers by Altenschmidt [12].

Optimization

Optimization may be interpreted as the way to find those values of controllable independent variables that give the most desired value of the dependent variable, the objective. This, however, is a product- or system-centered definition, the system consisting of composition and process variables and the properties of the product. In innovative pharmaceutical companies, the manufacture of production batches is preceded by extensive pharmaceutical development effort on small-scale batches for clinical studies only. Quality of design and product quality in terms of product specifications, composition, and type of manufacturing process are set in the early phase of pharmaceutical development. Factors like production costs are also taken into account. Further pharmaceutical development, including scale-up, is focused on the already defined quality standards in order to ensure bioequivalency of the commercial product and the product used in clinical studies. Therefore, optimization in the early preclinical stage of pharmaceutical development is considered essential; one must be aware, however, that the system consisting of composition and process variables and the product properties is a subsystem only and can be, to some extent, different where large-scale processing is concerned.

Before any experiment is conducted at the preformulation stage, the following questions should be answered:

1. What is the goal? What are the objectives? The strategy to be chosen may depend on the character of the problem and on the required quality of the answer.
2. What is already known about the system.
3. What is not known?
4. What must be known to be able to solve the problem?

Only when the problem is analyzed in sufficient depth, can experiments be designed to fill the gap between necessary and a priori knowledge.

TABLE 1 Quantitative Variables and Objectives in a Tablet Formulation for Direct Compression

Factors	Objectives
Compression force	Crushing strength
Relative humidity	Friability
Concentrations	
Disintegrant	Weight variability
Filler-binder	Disintegration time
Lubricant	Dissolution
Glidant	Robustness (for each response)
Drug	

With respect to the above questions, some complicating problems must be considered. It is often not known beforehand which variables will significantly influence the response(s). This problem can be solved by using screening designs and ANOVA, explained later.

A second serious complication may arise with new excipients or new process factors. Their qualitative or quantitative effects are not known, nor are they predictable. The following questions must be answered: Which part of the factor space should be chosen for the experiments? Are there constraints to be put on the levels of the variables?

These questions do not arise solely for new factors, since also for well-known factors the feasible factor space may not be thoroughly known. An educated guess may limit the number of experiments, but the question may arise if a systematic approach will be possible; if so, what is the best strategy?

The third complication is that formulated products, in particular dosage forms, with only one desirable property are rare; most dosage forms have to conform to several requirements, very often competing, as can be seen for tablets from Table 1. The formulator has to trade off objectives (e.g., crushing strength for disintegration time) and choose a compromise.

For the moment it is assumed that optimization is pursued for one property (objective) only. An optimal value of this property may be a maximum or a minimum. Very often a value within the product specifications instead of the optimum is sufficient. These different optimization goals can be dealt with by response surface methodology.

A fourth problem is the lack of insight in the balance between the needed a priori knowledge to perform an adequate optimization study and the gain in knowledge obtained by this study. Will the acquired knowledge justify the experimental effort?

It should be emphasized that in the performance of an optimization study the development scientist can also be a factor; reliable a priori experience and knowledge is a prerequisite.

Concepts and Definitions

A product (formulation) can be considered as a system consisting of input variables X, a transfer function (sometimes called a "black box"), and output Y (Fig. 1); the uncontrollable variables U are also shown. The black box should be given this name only when the transfer function is not known; if it is (partially) known, the term "grey box" is appropriate. The term "white box" may be used only for a mechanistic model. In formu-

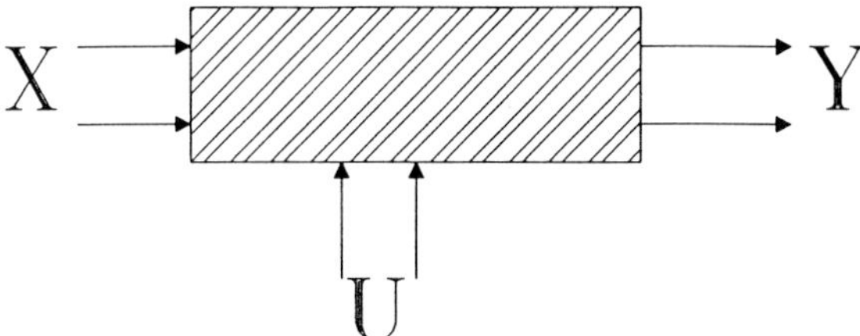

FIG. 1. System with controlled input variables X, uncontrolled input variables U, black box ▨, and output variables Y.

lation studies, the transfer function is usually a black box, that is, the effect of changing the input variables on the output is not predictable from theory.

In the following discussion the different parts of the systems under study will be indicated and definitions will be given. The distinction between objective, criterion, and response, all related to the dependent variable and thus to the goal(s) of the optimization, will be made clear as well as the distinction between variable and factor and the phenomenon of interaction of factors. The difference in the handling of process variables and compositional or mixture variables has to be explained.

If more than one property of a product has to be optimized (several objectives), decisions must be made about their relative importance with the help of multiple-objective methods. By empirically modeling the output of the system with respect to the input, the transfer function may be estimated, resulting in a better understanding of the system. Last but not least, the importance of the robustness of the system against controlled or uncontrollable changes of the input variables for the ultimate quality of the product or the process will be discussed.

Objective, Criterion, and Response

There is some confusion in the literature regarding these concepts. The term "objective" has been used with the mathematical meaning (objective function), but also to indicate a property of a procedure or a product, or as the goal of an optimization experiment. The term "criterion" has been used to indicate a property, but also as a measure to judge the realization of a target value of that property. The term "response" is mostly interpreted as the outcome of an experiment or the set of outcomes of experiments, arranged according to some design. Sometimes "response" is used in a broader sense for the objective mathematical relationship between the controllable factors and the estimate of the outcome, that is, the response surface. Some authors do not discriminate between objective and criterion, others use criterion for desirable value, a means to judge the success of an optimization. Other authors do not discriminate at all and use only the term "response."

In this article, the term "objective" is used to indicate the property of interest; "criterion" as a measure of judgment, the required value or required range; and "response" as the outcome of a measurement or a set of outcomes. Thus a "response" is the value an objective acquires, depending on the values a set of input variables is given. Therefore, a response is a dependent variable. An example is the value (the response) the crushing strength (objective) of a tablet attains when a mixture of constituents (compositional variables) is compressed with a specified compression force (a process variable).

Objectives that will be met in the following discussion are crushing strength, disintegration time, weight variability, storage-to-initial ratio (STIR) (of tablets). In the literature of formulation research a large number of objectives can be found, depending on the product or process under study. Some examples for tablets are given in Table 1. Examples for capsules are powder-blend homogeneity and release characteristics; for suspensions, chemical and physical stability; for eye drops, viscosity; for film-coated tablets, resistance to disintegration and physical appearance. More extensive lists are given later (Tables 13 and 14).

An important objective that is often not appreciated is robustness as a tool for constant quality. If the response surface is known, it is not difficult to identify optima or acceptable ranges of properties under consideration. It also gives insight in the robustness of these properties as a criterion for product quality.

Robustness as a Criterion for Quality

For pharmaceutical products and processes a large number of objectives can be found in the literature (Tables 13 and 14). When speaking about optimization of a formulation, one almost always has that property in mind. There is another important desirable property of formulations that is seldom the object of optimization, namely, robustness toward deviations in process conditions or a mixture of variable settings. Good robustness (also called ruggedness) means that despite (small) deviations or errors in the compositional and process variables, the values of the responses considered remain at almost the same level or within an acceptable range. Low robustness can potentially result in production batches below specifications. Robustness can be extended to environmental factors like temperature and humidity. Shelf life of a formulation that withstands temperature and humidity can be guaranteed with better reliability.

It can easily be seen that robustness depends on the form of the response surface. A steep slope of the response surface means that in that area of the factor settings a small deviation results in considerable increase or decrease of the objective under consideration, whereas a flat response surface means good robustness (Fig. 2).

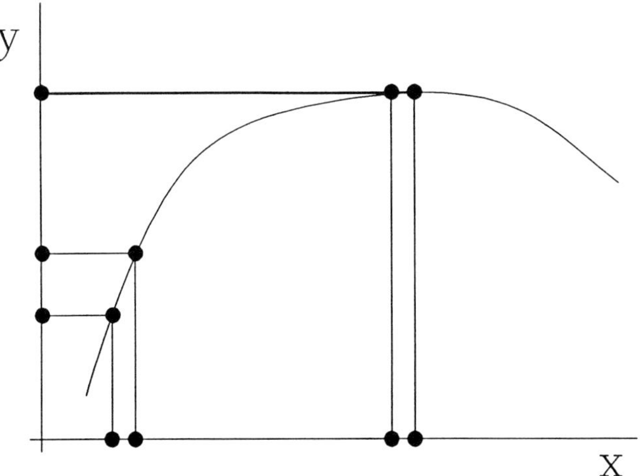

FIG. 2. Response surface on variable x with optimum and different slopes $\Delta y/\Delta x$.

To judge robustness, all relevant variables and the response surface of each of the main properties of the product or process must be known. If constant quality is an important aim of the optimization, robustness should be added to the list of objectives.

A thorough discussion of robustness in pharmaceutical development can be found in the papers by de Boer [13,14]. Robustness measures can be implemented in strategies for multicriteria decision making.

Multiple Objectives

A product has often to comply with more than one requirement. Criteria can be set, such as dissolution rate, crushing strength, and weight variance. Combining criteria into the "combined criterion" makes it possible to use sequential optimization methods. This pathway is, however, not straightforward and has several disadvantages, the most important being that it obscures the influence that the separate criteria have on the resulting number and thus lead to ambiguous results. More feasible is the application of methods especially developed for decision making in multiple-objective problems; two important categories are overlay diagrams and trade-off methods.

Variables and Factors

The term "variables" comprises dependent and independent variables alike. The term "factor" is in general restricted to independent variables, in particular those that have been found to influence the response. Noninfluential variables should not be called factors. It cannot be excluded, however, that they are factors in a so-far not explored area of the experimental domain. The experimental domain is that part of variable space which is limited by natural or practical constraints imposed on the independent variables. Natural limits may be of physical nature (e.g., negative temperature or time, negative amount or concentration of a filler–binder, or a negative compression force). Practical limits may be of instrumental nature, for example, the compression force may be limited by the design of a specific tableting machine.

Practical constraints may also be known from previous experience, such as a lower limit of the disintegrant in a tablet or an upper limit of a lubricant.

Variables may be continuous (quantitative) or discrete (qualitative). Quantitative variables can be set to all possible values (real numbers) within their constraints. Examples are again temperature, the amount of disintegrant, the amount of lubricant, the applied compression force, and the moisture content or the relative humidity in the processing area, although it is not always possible to set these variables precisely at the desired value. Repeating experiments with the same variable settings thus may lead to variance of the response.

Each of these variables can be projected onto one of the coordinate axes of the system, together with its response axis, spanning a multidimensional space. Two variables and one response can span a three-dimensional space (Fig. 3). Higher dimensional spaces are more difficult to imagine but mathematically they can be treated analogously.

Qualitative variables include the type of disintegrant, lubricant, and tableting machine. They can be treated or their influence can be evaluated in almost the same way as quantitative variables by giving them dummy values.

Up to this point, it was assumed that the variables influencing the response are under control, which, however, is never perfect. This gives rise to variance on the response, also

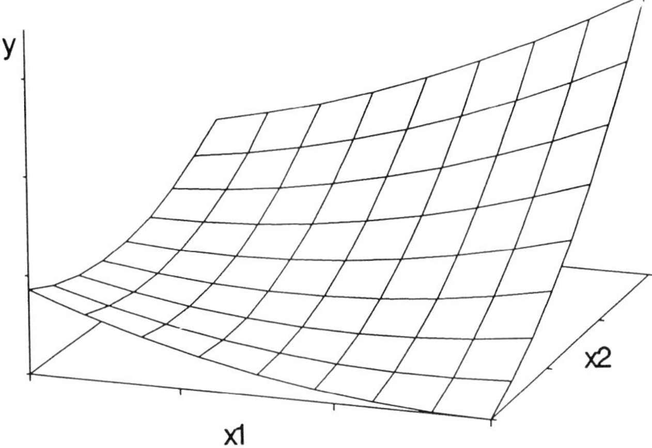

FIG. 3. A system with two independent variables x_1 and x_2 and one response y; x_1 = compression force, x_2 = mixing time; y = crushing strength.

called noise, and observed as decreased reproducibility. Noise cannot be eliminated but its development into bias can be prevented by the randomization of experiments.

Interaction of Variables

The effect of a factor on a response may be linear, at least within the experimental region. This means that if the factor level is repeatedly increased by a constant amount, the response changes also by a constant amount. A well-known example is the linear calibration graph. With some factors the effect may be nonlinear in part or all of the experimental domain. Moreover it occurs often that the effect of factor A depends on the level given to factor B, which has not been recognized in the past. Then it is said that factors A and B interact (two-factor interaction). Both factors may interact with factor C giving rise to a three-factor interaction. This simply means that the effect of each of these factors depends on the levels of the two other factors. In the case of interaction, the measured property depends on a fundamental variable that in some way is composed of the interacting variables. In this way the phenomenon interaction can be considered as a tool to a better understanding of the fundamentals of the process. A well-known example is the effect of the interaction of temperature and reaction time on the yield of a chemical reaction [15]. Here the essential parameter may be the amount of energy supplied to the system.

Models and the Response Surface

Both physics and chemistry provide many examples of functional relationships between a dependent variable η and independent variables x_1, x_2, x_3, etc., which are based on well-proven theories, although they were initially based on repeated experimenting, for example, Beer's law on absorption of light. Such relations may be represented as in Eq. (1).

$$\eta = f(x_1, x_2, x_3, \ldots . x_k) \tag{1}$$

The outcome y of a single measurement on a process with a set of specific settings of the factors $x_1 \ldots x_k$ is an estimate y of η, as shown in Eq. (2),

$$y = \eta + e \tag{2}$$

where e is the residual error in which the effect of the lack of absolute control of all factors x_i and noise (due to uncontrollable factors) and lack of fit is summed. Combining Eqs. (1) and (2) gives Eq. (3).

$$y = f(x_1, x_2, x_3 \ldots x_k) + e \tag{3}$$

If the function $f(x_i)$ is known from theory, it is called a mechanistic or analytical model. In formulation research (and in other branches of science such as analytical chromatography) the relation between a response and the influential variables is often complex and at best known only approximately. But an empirical model may be postulated and evaluated by (multiple) linear regression, using experimental data obtained by changing factor settings and measuring responses y.

Both types of model are mathematical descriptions of the responses over the variables space. The concept of response surface has led to response surface methodology, described by Box and Draper [16] as follows:

> Response surface methodology comprises a group of statistical techniques for empirical model building and model exploitation. By careful design and analysis of experiments, it seeks to relate a response or output variable to the levels of a number of predictors or input variables that affect it.

In this article different types of models are described for formulation problems with only process variables, only mixture variables, or problems in which both types of variables influence a response. These different types arise from the fact that compositional variables (the fractions of the components of a mixture) are subject to the special constraint that the sum of the fractions equals unity, so that they cannot be chosen freely; the number of degrees of freedom is one less than the number of variables. All models described here are linear polynomial models in the sense that they are linear in the coefficients (but not necessarily in the factors x_i).

Optimization, a Strategy

Before starting with optimization studies, one should have a clear picture of the possible approaches, from the nonsystematic method of "trial and error" to the univariate and multivariate systematic ones, the sequential "hill climbing," and the simultaneous "response surface" methods, and several possible combinations. It must be emphasized that there is no "best" strategy. The strategy to be chosen depends not only on the character of the problem and the required quality of the answer, but of importance is also the justification of the experimental effort in view of the gained information.

Under the heading "optimization," it is often suggested that a choice should be made between a sequential method and a simultaneous method or eventually a combination of both. The concept "strategy" is however more complex. A strategy consists of a number of successive steps to approach an optimization problem. These steps have been visualized and numbered in the flow diagram.

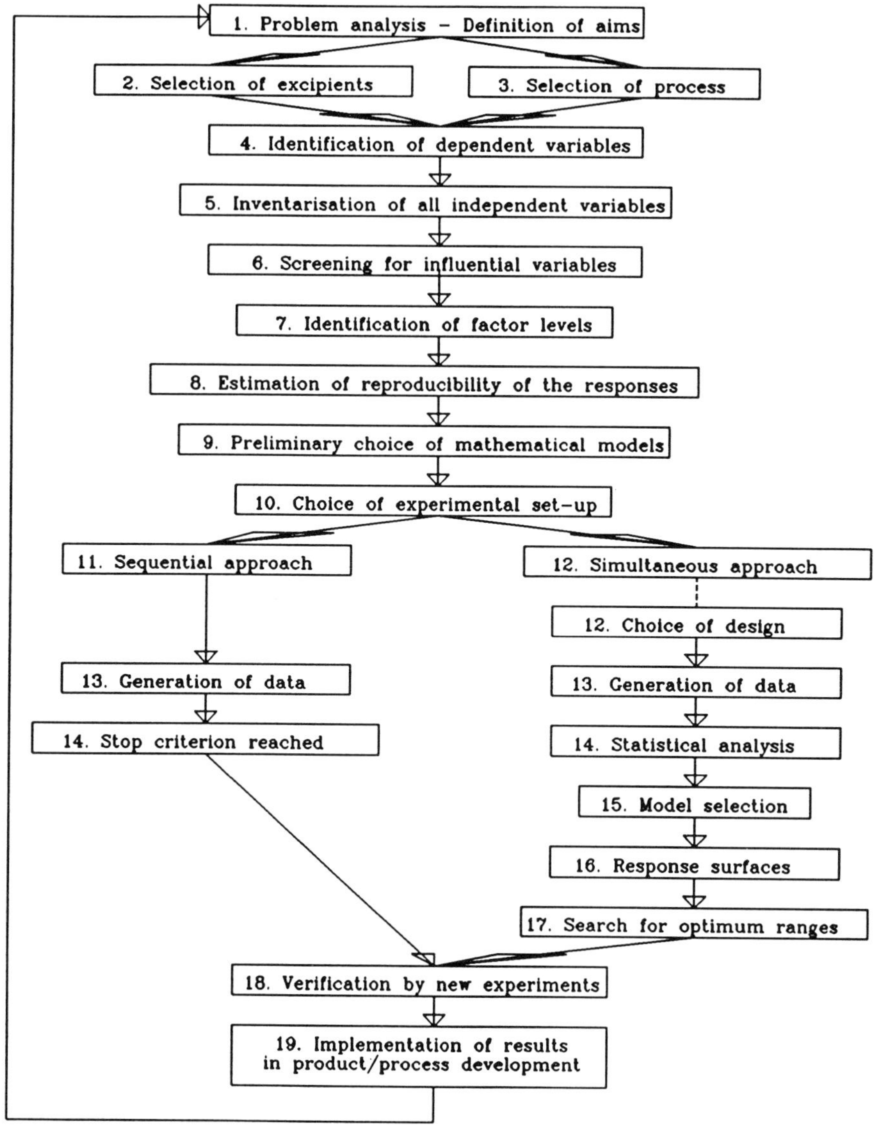

1. Analysis and definition of the problem:
What are the objectives; what is the nature of the problem?
What is already known about the system?
What is not known?
What must be known to allow solving the problem?

2 and 3. Based on previous knowledge, a preliminary choice can be made: which processes and which excipients are expected to lead to a possibly, not yet optimal, but at least acceptable solution of the defined problem (Step 1)?

4. The objectives are identified. Will there be one objective or more? What must be the specifications of the product in terms of required crushing strength, weight variance, etc.? Are specifications required for the robustness with respect to several objectives?

5. Based on a priori knowledge, what are the expected independent variables affecting the relevant objectives? A list of all variables involved should be prepared. What is the range of settings of the independent variables?

6. To reduce experimental effort, it is desirable to identify the influential variables (factors). This can be done with a screening design like the Plackett-Burman, described later.

7. Is it possible to constrain the variable space for compositional and process variables, identified as factors, from a priori knowledge or from preliminary experiments?

8. Reproducibility Study. In order to check whether all factors for relevant responses are controlled within the system, the reproducibility of the responses should be determined at an early stage. The variables that are expected to affect the response(s) can be tuned at "average settings." In this way, it can be ascertained whether the system to be optimized is completely controlled or not.

9. A preliminary model is chosen, based on the results of the factor screening, but preferably with the possibility of extension to a higher-order model.

10–12. A choice has to be made now between a sequential approach (Step 11), a simultaneous approach (Step 12), or a combination of both, and between the several designs possible, preferable fractional designs that can be easily extended if necessary.

13. If a sequential approach is chosen, data are generated and analyzed. This process is repeated until the results are satisfactory and can be implemented. In the case of a simultaneous approach, data are generated and preprocessed; abnormal values must be detected.

14. Following a simultaneous approach a statistical analysis by ANOVA, tests on lack of fit, and tests on predictive performance like R^2_{adj}, Pc, and c_p are performed. If a sequential approach is chosen, the analysis is limited to a judgment on the stop criterion (Simplex) or a judgment of a simple local model (steepest ascent).

15. Further evaluation leads to the selection of the preferred model (for each of the objectives a separate model may be adequate). This also leads to the definitive identification of influential variables and interactions.

16. By scanning the response surfaces for each of the objectives, feasible regions can be found, be it optima or acceptable ranges, for one or more objectives.

17. Identification of optima or ranges, aided by multicriteria decision making, if there are multiple objectives.

18. With both the simultaneous and the sequential approach (be it only on the local model) the existence of optima and their quality in terms of robustness must be checked by performing experiments in selected regions. This may lead to a new design or extra experiments, but if the checks are satisfactory the outcomes can be implemented (Step 19).

Models

Empirical Models

Empirical models provide a way to describe the relation between variable settings and a response. Assuming a smooth empirical function *f* (most often justified if the variables are quantitative), this function may be approximated by a Taylor expansion, most conveniently rewritten as in Eq. (4),

$$E(y) = \beta_0 + \sum_{i=1}^{k} \beta_i x_i + \sum_{i=1}^{k-1} \sum_{j=i+1}^{k} \beta_{ij} x_i x_j + \sum_{i=1}^{k} \beta_{ii} x_i^2 + \text{third-order terms} + \text{fourth-order terms} + \ldots + R(x) \quad (4)$$

where $R(x)$ becomes negligibly small if sufficient higher-order terms are included.

The (linear) parameters β of the model may not be known precisely, but their estimates b can be found, by fitting the polynomial to the data by multiple linear regression. The data are the set of y values experimentally obtained by changing the factor settings $x_1 \ldots x_k$. How to change these factors efficiently is discussed later. By statistical means (comparing the variance of the estimated parameters β with pure error), it can be decided which terms are not significant and thus can be omitted.

The set of response values pertaining to this empirically evaluated polynomial (and also its graphical representation, possibly as a contour plot) is called the response surface. It may show maxima, minima, saddles, and/or ridges. From these the desired optimum or the desired range of y can be read or, in multidimensional space, be calculated. Calculation can be performed by classical calculus, but today is most often done by grid search of the response surface, a "brute force" method.

In most areas of chemistry and pharmacy, polynomial models of the general form, given in Eq. (5), can be used.

$$E(y) = \beta_0 + \sum_{i=1}^{k} \beta_i x_i + \sum_{i=1}^{k-1} \sum_{j=i+1}^{k} \beta_{ij} x_i x_j + \sum_{i=1}^{k} \beta_{ii} x_i^2 + \sum_{i=1}^{k-2} \sum_{j=i+1}^{k-1} \sum_{k=i+2}^{k} \beta_{ijk} x_i x_j x_k + \sum_{i=1}^{k} \beta_{iii} x_i^3 \quad (5)$$

The fourth- and higher-order terms are always omitted, and indeed almost always also the third-order terms. Most response surfaces are smooth; higher-order terms predominantly describe error variance which is nonproductive. This is avoided with simple models where fewer experiments are needed. With multiple linear regression at least as many response values must be measured as there are parameters to be estimated in the model.

In a second-order model with three factors, ten parameters must be estimated. To estimate pure error, some measurements must be duplicated; a realistic number of experiments may thus be 13 to 15. If third-order terms are retained (with three factors there are ten of these), at least 23–25 experiments must be performed. With more factors, the experimental effort increases rapidly. In particular, if the experimental domain is only a small part of the variable space, the response surface may be approximated by a second-order, or even a first-order model. With a priori knowledge, the advice is to start with a small experimental domain in an area where the optimum is probably situated. In the absence of a priori knowledge, a sequential approach may be advantageous.

Some commonly used models are shown in Eqs. (6) to (11),

$$E(y) = \beta_0 + \beta_1 x \tag{6}$$

$$E(y) = \beta_0 + \beta_1 x_1 + \beta_2 x_2 \qquad \text{(Fig. 4)} \tag{7}$$

$$E(y) = \beta_0 + \beta_1 x_1 + \beta_2 x_2 + \beta_3 x_3 \tag{8}$$

$$E(y) = \beta_0 + \beta_1 x_1 + \beta_2 x_2 + \beta_{12} x_1 x_2 \qquad \text{(Figs. 5 and 6)} \tag{9}$$

$$E(y) = \beta_0 + \beta_1 x_1 + \beta_2 x_2 + \beta_3 x_3 + \beta_{12} x_1 x_2 + \beta_{13} x_1 x_3 + \beta_{23} x_2 x_3 \tag{10}$$

$$E(y) = \beta_0 + \beta_1 x_1 + \beta_2 x_2 + \beta_3 x_3 + \beta_{12} x_1 x_2 + \beta_{13} x_1 x_3 + \beta_{23} x_2 x_3 + \beta_{11} x_1^2 + \beta_{22} x_2^2 + \beta_{33} x_3^2 \tag{11}$$

where y = measured response
x_i = values of the factors
β_0 = a constant, the intercept
β_i = coefficients of first-order terms
β_{ii} = coefficients of second-order quadratic terms
β_{ij} = coefficients of second-order interaction terms

Equations (6)–(10) are linear in the variables, but Eq. (11) is not. Nevertheless, these six equations are all linear models because they are linear in the coefficients. Equation (6) describes a straight line and Eq. (7) a plane, a flat surface in 3D space. Equation (8) describes a flat hyperplane in 4D space because there are three factors. Equations (6) to (8) are linear first-order models. Equation (9) describes a twisted plane in 3D space; it is a linear second-order model. Equation (10) is a linear second-order model that describes a twisted hyperplane in 4D space. Equation (11) is a linear second-order model that describes a twisted plane with curvature, arising from the quadratic terms. It would have been of third order if cross-product terms between the quadratic terms and the remaining variables had not been omitted.

From Eqs. (9) and (10) the meaning of interaction can be demonstrated mathematically. After grouping of the x_1 terms and taking the first partial derivative, it can be seen that the slope s of the effect of factor x_1 depends on the level of factor x_2.

$$E(y) = \beta_0 + (\beta_1 + \beta_{12} x_2) x_1 + \beta_2 x_2 \tag{9}$$

$$s_{x1} = \beta_1 + \beta_{12} x_2 \tag{10}$$

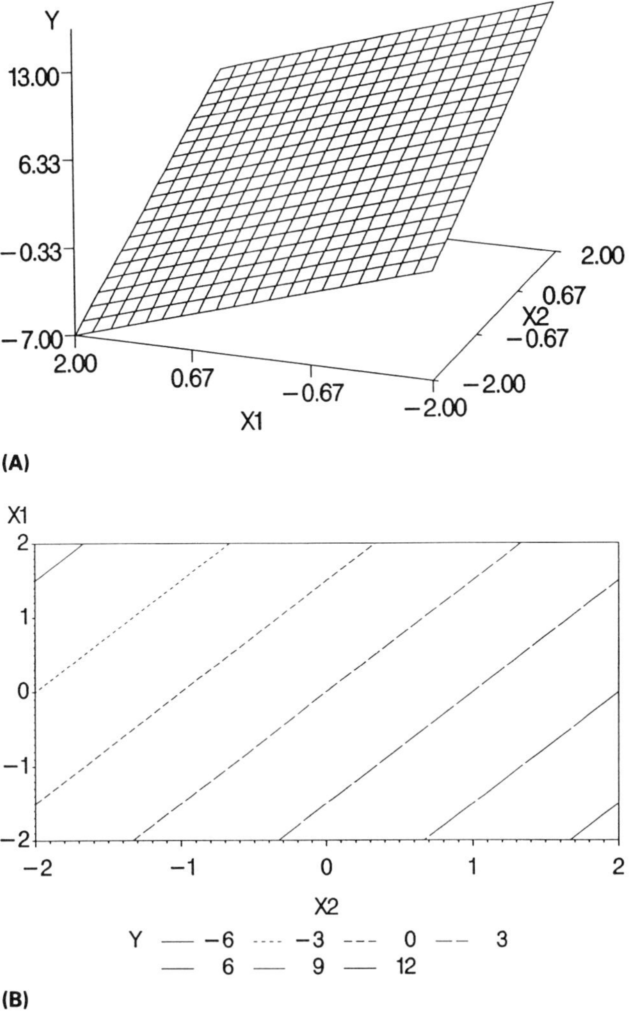

FIG. 4. Response surface and contour diagram of Eq. (7) with parameters $\beta_0 = 3$, $\beta_1 = -2$, and $\beta_2 = 3$. (A). Response surface. (B). Contour diagram.

Now it is clear that once a model has been found by regression on experimental data, one could find optima by analytical evaluation of the model or by a grid search over the experimental domain. This ''brute force'' method means that a grid of variable settings is scanned by the computer and responses predicted by these grid points. The outcomes are evaluated for the overall optimum, local optima, or acceptable ranges. If the experimental data are measurements of the response for several objectives at each set of factor settings, regression can produce a model and a response surface for each of the responses. Then it is possible to have the computer compare these responses and advise on a composite criterion or a compromise with one of the multiple-objective techniques. This also holds for mixture models and models combining mixture and process variables. Once a model is selected and the coefficients of the model are found by multiple linear regression, optima or a feasible region for one or more responses can be found.

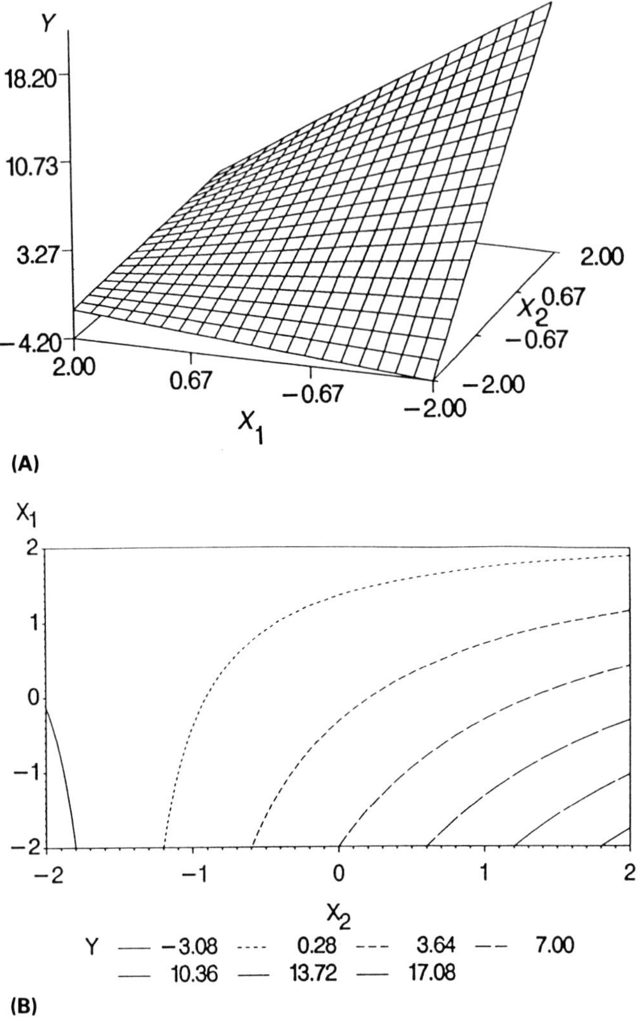

FIG. 5. Response surface and contour diagram of Eq. (9) (two-factor interaction term added) with parameters $\beta_0 = 3$, $\beta_1 = -2$, $\beta_2 = 3$, $\beta_{12} = -1.3$. (A). Response surface. (B). Contour diagram.

Models for Mixtures

When experimenting with mixtures, as is often the case in formulation research but also in thin-layer chromatography, HPLC, or solubility studies in mixed solvents, special constraints are placed on the compositional variables, that is, the sum of the fractions of all the mixture components equals 1, as shown in Eq. (12). Moreover, none of the fractions can be negative.

$$\sum_{i=1}^{k} m_i = 1 \tag{12}$$

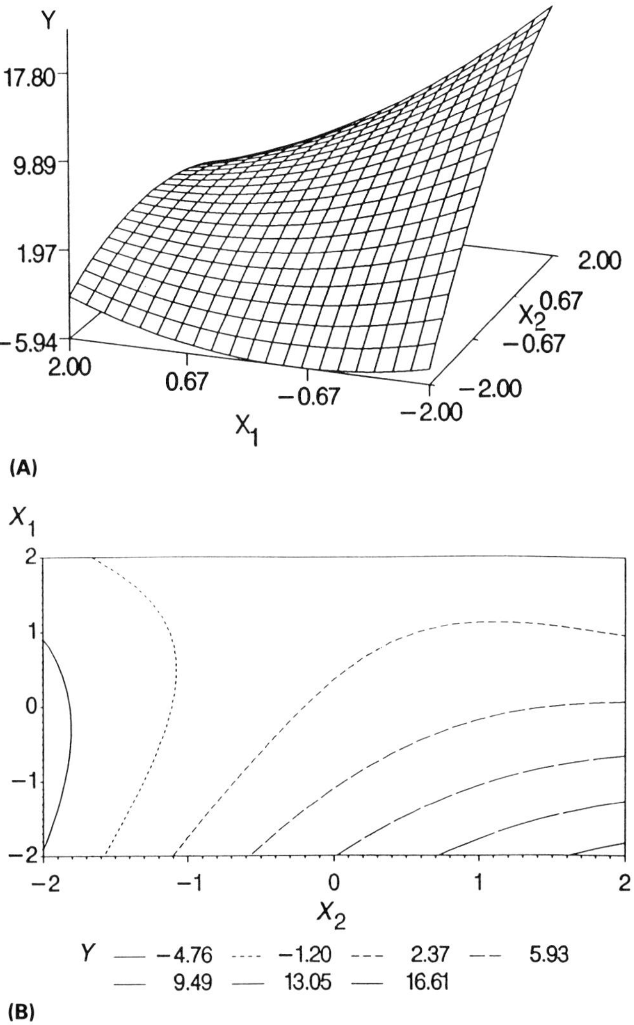

FIG. 6. Response surface and contour diagram of Eq. (9) (quadratic terms added) with parameters β_0 = 3, β_1 = −2, β_2 = 3, β_{12} = −1.3, β_{11} = 0.6, β_{22} = −0.7. (A). Response surface. (B). Contour diagram.

The first constraint, graphically depicted in Figs. 7, 8, and 9 results in a special type of polynomials, as has been derived by Scheffé. Because a change of one fraction m_i in a mixture implies a change of another fraction, there are no quadratic (e.g., $m_1 * m_1$) interaction terms in these polynomials. The two-factor, second-order, polynomial model, shown in Eq. (13),

$$E(y) = \beta_0 + \beta_1 x_1 + \beta_2 x_2 + \beta_{12} x_1 x_2 + \beta_{11} x_1^2 + \beta_{22} x_2^2 \tag{13}$$

with six parameters to be estimated, using the constraint $m_1 + m_2 = 1$, yields a new polynomial with three new parameters β^*, given in Eq. (14). Response surface is shown in Fig. 10.

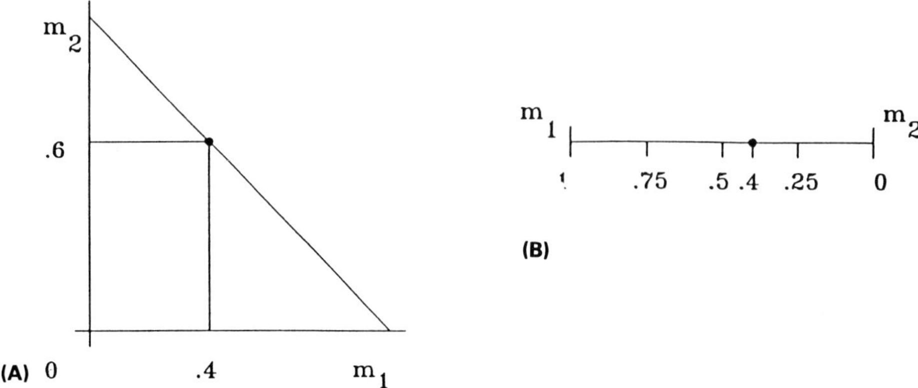

FIG. 7. The mixture constraint for a binary mixture. (A). Two axes and the constraint; point m_1 = 100% of component m_1, point m_2 = 100% of component m_2. (B). The variable space is a line; points m_1 and m_2 as in (A).

$$E(y) = \beta_1{}^*m_1 + \beta_2{}^*m_2 + \beta_{12}{}^*m_1m_2 \tag{14}$$

The three-factor second-order polynomial, depicted as Eq.(11), has ten parameters to be estimated. Using the constraint $m_1+m_2+m_3 = 1$, it yields a new polynomial with six new parameters β^*, as in Eq. (15). Response surface is shown in Fig. 11.

$$E(y) = \beta_1{}^*m_1 + \beta_2{}^*m_2 + \beta_3{}^*m_3 + \beta_{12}{}^*m_1m_2 + \beta_{13}{}^*m_1m_3 + \beta_{23}{}^*m_2m_3 \tag{15}$$

For three-factor third-order polynomials more terms have to be added; a three-factor, full cubic Scheffé model has ten terms. A frequently used "special cubic" Scheffé model consists of the terms given in Eq. (15) to which the special cubic three-factor cross-product term has been added in Eq. (16).

$$E(y) = \beta_1{}^*m_1 + \beta_2{}^*m_2 + \beta_3{}^*m_3 + \beta_{12}{}^*m_1m_2 + \beta_{13}{}^*m_1m_3 + \beta_{23}{}^*m_2m_3 + \beta_{123}{}^*m_1m_2m_3 \tag{16}$$

It should be noted that in these models the intercept, present in normal model equations, has disappeared. As a consequence it is not possible to evaluate Scheffé models with linear regression, using standard regression software. Special regression algorithms can, however, be implemented in some software packages, for example, SAS. Algorithms for implementation in SAS have been given by Cornell (see Bibliography).

Because of the mixture constraint, the number of parameters to be estimated (and thus the number of experiments that are minimal necessary for regression analysis) has decreased considerably. Whereas in normal polynomials the cross-product terms describe the interaction of factors, in Scheffé polynomials these terms are said to describe "nonlinear blending." This phenomenon should not be termed an interaction, because as a consequence of the mixture constraint it is not possible to vary the components and thus to evaluate their effects independently.

In most articles on mixture models the symbol x_i is used. This author prefers m_i to draw a distinction from the normal variables. Whatever symbol is used, it does not rep-

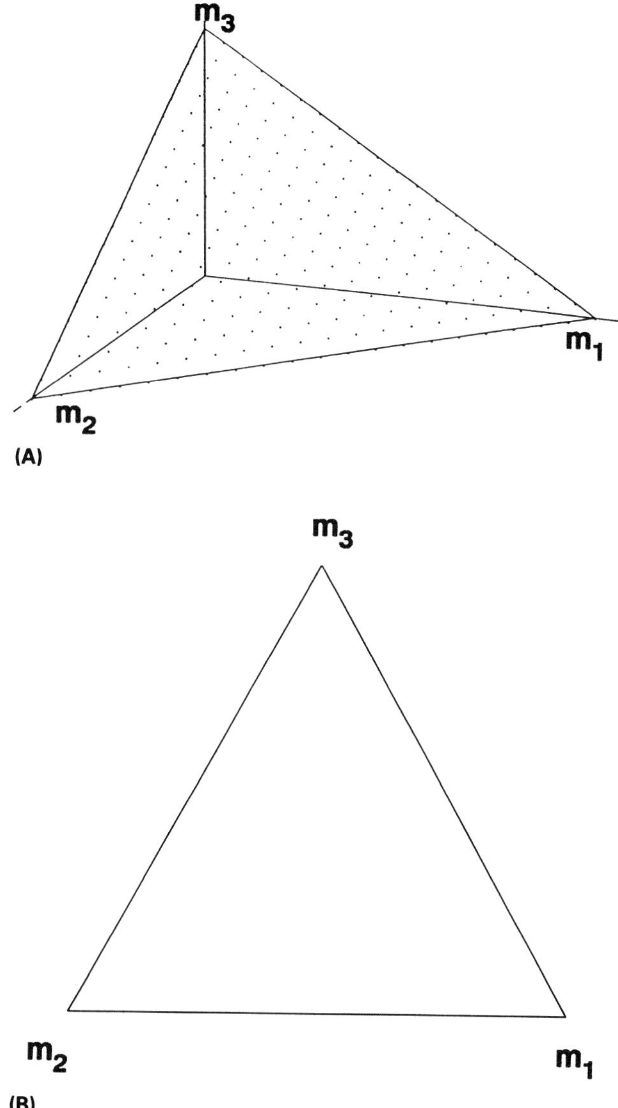

FIG. 8. The mixture constraint for a ternary mixture. (A). Three axes and the constraint; m_1, m_2, and m_3 represent the pure components (100% m_1, m_2, and m_3). (B). The variable space can be represented by a triangle; at the vertices the pure components m_1, m_2, and m_3.

resent a variable expressed in normal quantities but in fractions of the components in the mixture. In the following discussion the asterisk from β^* is omitted and β is used whenever this does not cause confusion.

Models Combining Mixture and Process Variables

In the foregoing discussion models have been described for "normal" variables and for those subject to the mixture constraint. The mixture model is more efficient because

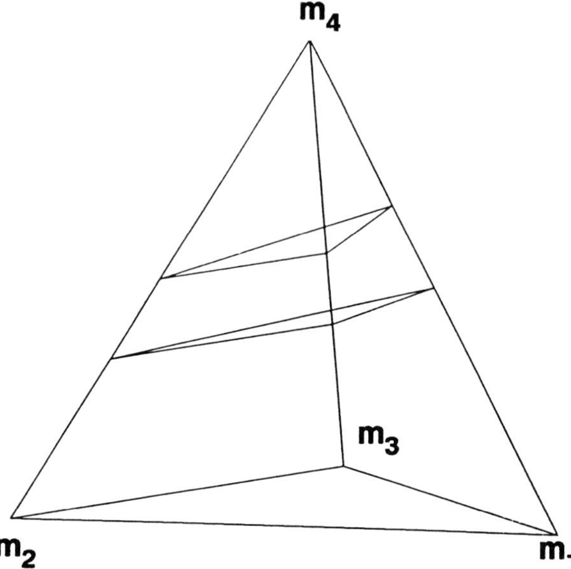

FIG. 9. The mixture space for a quaternary mixture: tetrahedron and feasible design space with upper and lower restrictions.

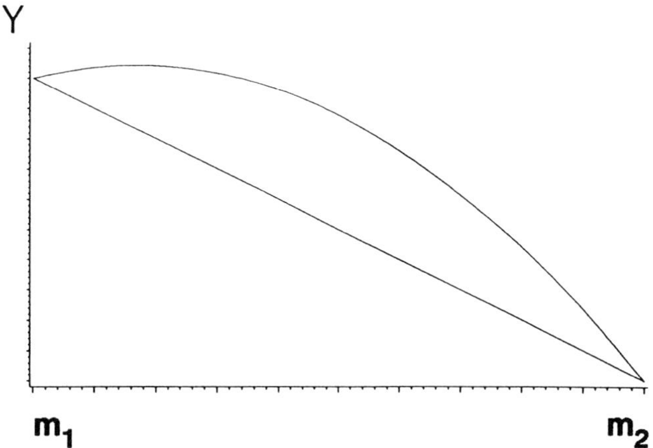

FIG. 10. Response surface belonging to Eq. (14), a binary mixture model with blending term, with parameters $\beta_1 = 2$, $\beta_2 = 3$, $\beta_{12} = 1.5$.

fewer experiments are required for model evaluation by regression analysis. For mixtures of more than two components or pseudo-components the Scheffé models should always be used; the normal polynomial models should be reserved for process factors.

Formulation research presents many problems where both process variables and compositional variables influence the objective(s). Moreover, these two types of variables may interact. It would be advantageous to have models in which both types of variables occur and yet the advantage of the mixture model can be preserved. These models and the pertaining experimental designs have been developed and are described below.

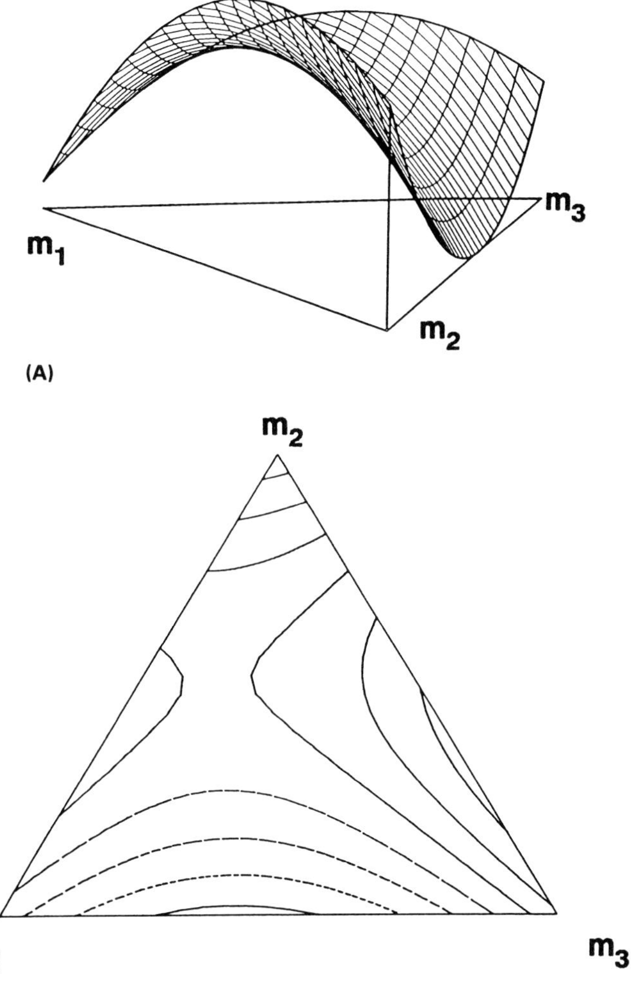

FIG. 11. Response surface belonging to Eq. (15), a ternary mixture model with binary blending terms, with parameters $\beta_1 = 2$, $\beta_2 = 3$, $\beta_3 = 4$, $\beta_{12} = 5$, $\beta_{13} = 6$, $\beta_{23} = -7$. (A). Response surface. (B). Contour diagram.

Assuming a problem where an objective y depends on three mixture variables m_i and two process variables p and t (e.g., tableting with three excipients—two filler binders and a disintegrant—and the process factors of compression force and mixing time). If it is expected that a special cubic model for the mixture would suffice and that there is an interaction of mixture variables with linear and quadratic process variables, the model could be illustrated by Eq. 17.

$$\begin{aligned} E(y) = {} & \beta_1^* m_1 + \beta_2^* m_2 + \beta_3^* m_3 + \beta_{12}^* m_1 m_2 + \beta_{13}^* m_1 m_3 + \beta_{23}^* m_2 m_3 \\ & + \beta_{123}^* m_1 m_2 m_3 + \gamma_1^{1} m_1 p + \gamma_2^{1} m_2 p + \gamma_3^{1} m_3 p + \gamma_1^{11} m_1 p^2 + \gamma_2^{11} m_2 p^2 \\ & + \gamma_3^{11} m_3 p^2 + \gamma_1^{2} m_1 t + \gamma_2^{2} m_2 t + \gamma_3^{2} m_3 t + \gamma_1^{22} m_1 t^2 + \gamma_2^{22} m_2 t^2 + \gamma_3^{22} m_3 t^2 \\ & + \gamma_1^{12} m_1 pt + \gamma_2^{12} m_2 pt + \gamma_3^{12} m_3 pt \end{aligned} \tag{17}$$

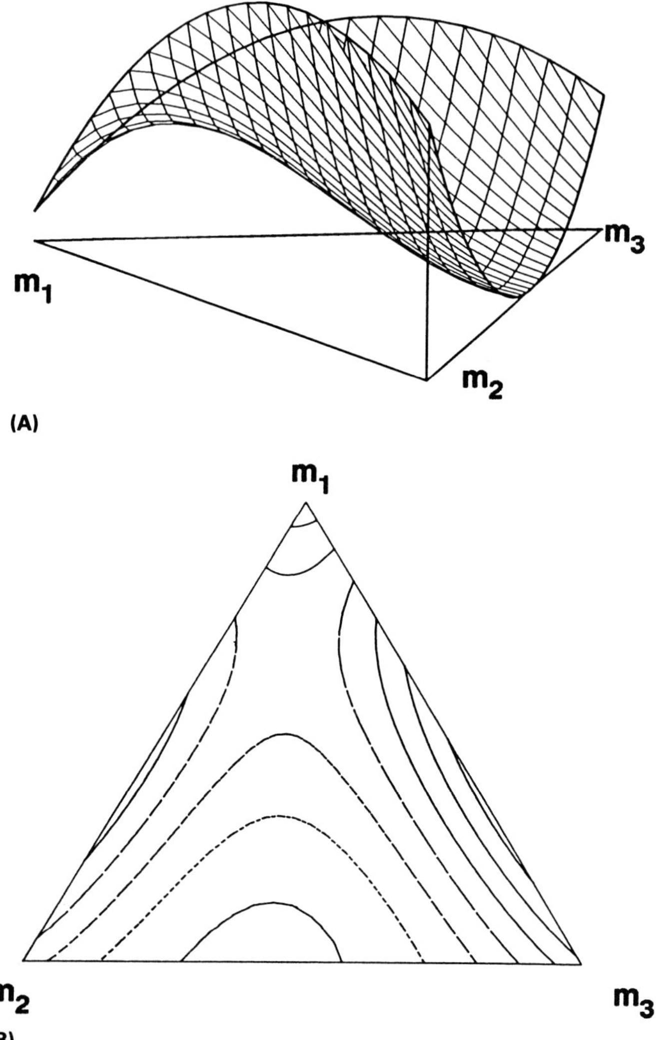

FIG. 12. Response surface belonging to Eq. (16), a ternary-mixture model with binary and ternary blending terms with parameters $\beta_1 = 2$, $\beta_2 = 3$, $\beta_3 = 4$, $\beta_{12} = 5$, $\beta_{13} = 6$, $\beta_{23} = -7$, $\beta_{123} = -29$. (A). Response surface. (B). Contour diagram.

As usual, β represents the parameters of the mixture part of the model, and γ the parameters of the interaction terms between mixture and process variables; subscripts refer to the mixture variables involved, superscripts to the process variables. The model can be more easily constructed using the general representation given in Table 2, from which it can be seen if the chosen model is well defined and symmetrical in the mixture variables. To be well defined, a certain hierarchy in model terms is required. This means that all mixture terms of the same order are introduced at the same time, and higher-order blending effects are only used if the concomittant lower-order blending terms have been adopted.

TABLE 2 Schematic Representation of Eq. (17)[a,b]

Mixture Variable	1	p^c	t^c	p^2	t^2	$p*t$
m_1	■	■	■	■	■	■
m_2	■	■	■	■	■	■
m_3	■	■	■	■	■	■
m_1m_2	■					
m_1m_3	■					
m_2m_3	■					
$m_1m_2m_3$	■					

[a]From Ref. 30.
[b]■ = Presence of term.
[c]Process variables.

Choice of Models

A choice must be made between an essentially unlimited number of models of different type and order. The choice depends on the type of variables and the use that will be made of the model. Will it be used for description of a system or for prediction of optima or feasible regions? The choice also depends on the a priori knowledge of the experimenter about possible interactions and quadratic effects. Model choice before design construction and model validation after experimenting according to the chosen design is by no means simple. If the model chosen is too simple, higher-order interactions and effects may be missed because the relevant terms are not part of the model. Model validation may reveal this, and terms may be added, provided the design and data permits this.

If the model selected is too complicated, overfitting of the data may occur. The effect is a larger variance in the predictions, and reliability of the predicted optimum would be too low.

Experimental Design

Simultaneous Methods

The tuning of variables that affect a property of interest in such a way that an optimum value for this property is attained, is an often occurring problem in many branches of technology. Because of the economical importance, a number of experimental optimization techniques have been developed. Response surface methodology, based on statistical experimental design and data modeling, is the most widely used technique in areas where a theoretical model relating a response to the independent variables does not exist or has not yet been found, as is most often the case in formulation research.

Statistical designs prescribe or advise a set of variable combinations. The number and layout of these design points within the experimental region depend on the number of regression coefficients that must be estimated, and thus depend on the postulated model. This, in turn, depends on the number of factors, their levels and possible interactions, and the order of the model (or models) that the experimenter postulates. The whole set of experiments is thus planned and subsequently performed and evaluated; this is the reason for the designation simultaneous. The pertaining response surface spans part of or the entire experimental domain.

Statistical designs require careful planning and adherence to statistical rules, for example, randomizing the experiments and/or blocking. When the design has the property of orthogonality, it is possible to evaluate the significance of all model terms independently (main effects of all factors, interaction effects), except when fractional designs have been used. (Although these designs are also orthogonal, some effects will be confounded, but still the aliased duplets, triplets, etc. can be estimated independently from the other aliased duplets, etc.)

With sound statistical designs, the design points are distributed within the experimental region in such a way that the regression coefficients can be estimated with equal accuracy. When the model is used for the prediction of responses within the experimental region in points where no experiments were laid out, the predictions have also a reasonably homogeneous distributed accuracy. (Outside the experimental region, extrapolation gives unreliable results.)

Sequential Methods

It may be advantageous not to plan all the experiments at once but to adopt an interactive strategy. The response surface is a surface that exists, but is unknown to the experimenter as long as no experiments have been performed. It should be possible to plan a small number of experiments, starting in an arbitrary part of the experimental region, evaluate a gradient on that part of the response surface, climb uphill, plan some more experiments, and so on, until the response does not improve anymore. Several of such sequential or interactive methods, called "hill-climbing" methods, have been developed, including the method of steepest ascent, the simplex method, the modified simplex, and the supermodified simplex. They work efficiently, provided there are no multiple optima. However, they climb only one specific response surface and cannot be used on multiple-objective problems.

Factorial Designs

Each experiment can be represented as a point within the experimental domain, the point being defined by its coordinates, that is, the values given to the variables. A set of such points, the design points, constitute the experimental design. Its basic problem is how to distribute the design points over the design space. If the response surface would be known, it could be decided which design points would be the most informative, but since the response surface is mostly unknown, there is a problem of circularity, described by Box [17] as follows: "The situation relates to the paradox that the best time to design an experiment is after it is finished, the converse of which is that the worst time is at the beginning, when least is known," and this ". . . points to the desirability of a sequence of moderately sized designs and reassessment of the results as each group of experiments becomes available."

The simplest factorial design is for two factors, each at two levels; without replication, four (2^2) experiments, situated in 2D factor space at the corners of a rectangle, are performed. If there are three factors, each at two levels, eight (2^3) experiments are necessary, situated at the corners of an orthogonal prism in 3D factor space (Fig. 13). For k factors, the notation is a 2^k factorial design; experiments must be performed with all possible combinations of two different levels of the k factors. The number of experiments is

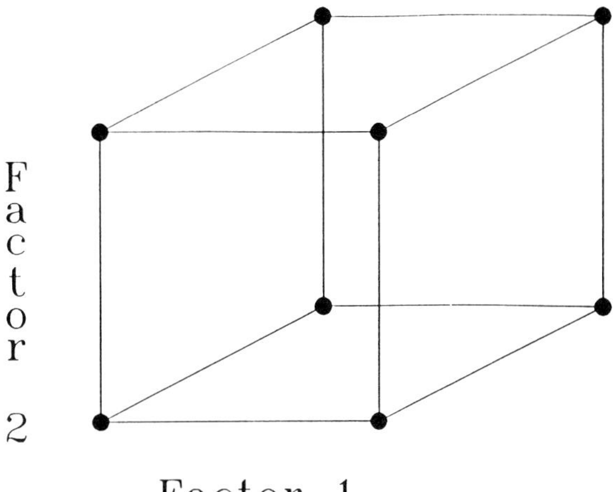

FIG. 13. Two-level factorial design for process variables.

simply obtained by evaluating the expression n^k arithmetically, where n = number of levels, and k = number of factors. The following example of a 2^3 factorial design illustrates the design representation after centering and scaling of the factors.

TABLE 3 Data from a 2^3 Factorial Design Pilot-Plant Example[a]

Run	Temp T (°C)	Concentration, C (%)	Catalyst K (A or B)	Yield y (g)
1	160	20	A	60
2	180	20	A	72
3	160	40	A	54
4	180	40	A	68
5	160	20	B	52
6	180	20	B	83
7	160	40	B	45
8	180	40	B	80

[a]From Ref. 18 with permission.

Table 3 shows the yield of a chemical reaction that has been studied at varying temperatures (160 or 180°C), concentrations (20 or 40%), and the type of catalyst (A or B). The first two factors are of quantitative nature, whereas the catalyst is a qualitative factor. The entries in Table 3 are the real values. In Table 4 the quantitative factors have been centered and scaled, using Eqs. (18) and (19).

Centering $$T' = T_i - T_{av} \quad \text{and} \quad C' = C_i - C_{av} \tag{18}$$

Scaling $$T'' = T'/(T_i - T_{av}) \quad \text{and} \quad C'' = C'/C_i - C_{av} \tag{19}$$

The results are −1 and +1, abbreviated to − and +; the qualitative factor has arbitrarily been given the values −1 and +1 (− and +). The design is written in a convenient order, but the experiments numbered 1–8 in Table 3 should be performed in randomized

TABLE 4 The Data of Table 3 with Coded Units of the Variables

Run	T	C	K	Y
1	−	−	−	60
2	+	−	−	72
3	−	+	−	54
4	+	+	−	68
5	−	−	+	52
6	+	−	+	83
7	−	+	+	45
8	+	+	+	80

order to exclude bias. If they cannot be performed in one day, they should not only be randomized but also blocked. Attention is required for column K, which because it is a qualitative factor is given a dummy value, + or −.

Orthogonality

Table 4 shows the usual representation of a factorial design; coding the factors in this way is notationally convenient and very useful for calculations and for the construction of fractional factorial designs. Moreover, it makes the design orthogonal. Two columns (T,C; C,K; T,K), each of which can be seen as a vector, are orthogonal if they have the property that the multiplied entries sum up to zero. For columns T and C, it can be seen that

$$(-1)(-1)+(+1)(-1)+(-1)(+1)+(+1)(+1)+\ .\ .\ .\ .\ .\ =0$$

Thus, they are orthogonal. The same holds for the other combinations. A design is orthogonal if and only if each pair of columns in that design is orthogonal. Stated in terms of linear algebra: the inner product of the column vectors $\Sigma x_i y_j = 0$. The advantage of orthogonal designs is that the effects can be estimated independently of each other, and that the estimated effects have good statistical properties.

Curvature

If a factor has two levels, it is possible to detect only a linear effect. To detect curvature, a factor must have at least three levels. In a neat 3^k factorial design, the intermediate level should be the average of the extremes; in a coded table, it appears as a zero. Other notations (e.g., 0, 1, 2) can be found in the literature but they are less sound if one bears the coding operation in mind.

It is possible, of course, to choose two levels for one factor and three or four levels for other factors. Regression can be used equally well, although the number of experiments increases and fractional factorial designs are not easy to construct.

Calculations of 2^k Factorial Designs

There are three ways to calculate effects of factors and interactions from the experimental results: by the Yates algorithm, by constrasts, and by multiple linear regression.

The Yates algorithm is not discussed here [19,20]; it can be used for 2^k and 3^k factorial designs and also for 2^{k-p} fractional factorial designs.

Contrasts

In principle, calculations using contrasts can be used for an unlimited number of factors, but only at two levels each. They are simple and direct, as will be demonstrated by expanding Table 4 to Table 5 with columns of + and − signs for interactions T*C, T*K, C*K, and T*C*K. The signs in these interaction columns are obtained by multiplying the appropriate entries in the T,C, and K columns. A column with only + signs is added and the heading "mean"; it is not part of the experimental design. A row is added for the divisors. The added columns do not disturb the orthogonality of the design. The orthogonality property provides that the contrasts can be used to calculate the effects and interactions independently.

TABLE 5 Table 4 Expanded by the Addition of Interaction Columns[a]

Run	Mean	T	C	K	TC	TK	CK	TCK	y
1	+	−	−	−	+	+	+	−	60
2	+	+	−	−	−	−	+	+	72
3	+	−	+	−	−	+	−	+	54
4	+	+	+	−	+	−	−	−	68
5	+	−	−	+	+	−	−	+	52
6	+	+	−	+	−	+	−	−	83
7	+	−	+	+	−	−	+	−	45
8	+	+	+	+	+	+	+	+	80
Div	8	4	4	4	4	4	4	4	

[a]Effect of T: $(-60+72-54+68-52+83-45+80)/4 = 23$
Effect of K: $(-60-72-54-68+52+83+45+80)/4 = 1.5$
Interaction TK: $(+60-72+54-68-52+83-45+80)/4 = 10$

It can be seen that the effects of the qualitative factors were calculated in exactly the same way as those of the quantitative ones. There is a difference, however, in interpretation. With quantitative factors interpolation (on the continuous response surface) between the + and − level is meaningful, whereas this is not the case with qualitative factors. This has an implication for calculations using regression; models for regression should not contain qualitative factors.

Calculations by the Yates algorithm and by contrasts both rely on the assumption that the experiments can be conducted exactly as was specified by the sign tables of the design. In practice, however, this is almost never the case in chemical and pharmaceutical experimenting; the theoretical level may be approached but not reached. It can, nevertheless, be read accurately. Therefore it is better to use the factor value read and multiple linear regression that can handle the actual factor settings.

The question remains if the calculated effects and interactions are statistically significant in view of the experimental error. As usual, this depends on the (residual) error itself.

Factorial designs because of the internal replication of the experiments are more efficient than designs in which not all factor combinations are explored, resulting in a smaller variance and thus sharper tests of significance. A first impression of the significance of effects and interactions can be obtained by transforming them and entering the results on normal probability paper [21]. A serious deviation of some entries from the straight line (provided that there is a sufficient number of entries left that do lie on a straight line) indicates a significant effect of the pertaining factors or interactions. This is very useful for screening experiments.

Regression

Regression is the most widely used method for quantitative factors. It cannot be used for qualitative factors, because interpolation between discrete (dummy) factor values is meaningless, as has been stated before.

In linear-regression analysis (also called ordinary least-squares regression or OLS), a linear model like that shown in Eq. (20),

$$E(y) = \beta_0 + \beta_1 x \quad \text{or} \quad E(y) = \beta_0 + \beta_1 x + \beta_{11} x^2 \tag{20}$$

is fitted to experimental data, that is, estimating values b_i for β_i in such a way that the sum of squared differences between $\hat{y}$ and y_i, $\Sigma(\hat{y} - y_i)^2$ is minimized.

The same holds for multiple linear regression; which treats models with more factors x_i or interactions $x_i x_j$ or higher-order terms, as shown in Eq. (21).

$$E(y) = \beta_0 + \beta_1 x_1 + \beta_2 x_2 + \beta_1 \beta_2 x_1 x_2 + \ldots . \tag{21}$$

Regression analysis can only be performed after one or several models have been postulated, the choice being based on some expectation of the response surface. Then a design must be chosen with enough design points to evaluate these models and to permit decisions about the definitive model, that is, the significance of terms.

If coded variables are used, the effects and interactions found with regression can be compared with those calculated by contrast. They are very much the same, and the mean found by contrasts is the same as the intercept found by regression, whereas the effects and interactions found by contrasts are seemingly twice as much as the coefficients b estimated by regression. This factor of 2 is explained by the fact that the effect by contrasts is measured over the range of -1 to $+1$ (two units), whereas the regression coefficient b represents the effect of a factor if the change is one unit in the coded variable. If the variables were not coded, b would represent the effect for a change of one unit in the original physical units.

Screening for Influential Variables

At the start of a study, one should always screen (in one design or in several consecutive smaller designs to restrict experimental effort) possible input variables of the system under study to see if they are factors. An input variable identified as a factor increases the chance of success. An input variable that is not a factor and is not identified as such, has no consequence. There are two other possibilities: If an input variable is not a factor but is falsely identified as such, the factor will be unnecessarily included in the experimental setup, unduly increasing the effort and costs. If, on the other hand, an input variable is a factor but not recognized as such, an incomplete picture of the response surface results and a true optimum may be missed. Of the four possibilities the last situation has the most serious consequences. Screening experiments may reduce the risk of missing an influential variable. This may be accomplished with the help of normal probability plots. This method must be used if no replicates are available and no prior knowledge of interactions justifies neglecting higher-order terms.

Another way to answer the question what factors have a significant effect on a response y, requires some statistical insight. The question can be reformulated: which effects (and interactions) show deviation from noise, the noise level being the measurement error of y? An estimate s_{pe} of σ_{pe} can be obtained by replicating the experiment at all or some of the design points. If all the design points are replicated, ANOVA can be used to calculate the significance of the effects [22,23]. Background of the use of ANOVA is the partitioning of the total sum of squares SS_T into sum of squares of the mean, sums of squares due to factor influences (e.g., SS_C, SS_T, SS_{TC}), sum of squares of the residuals (SS_r), sum of squares due to lack of fit (SS_{Lof}), and sum of squares due to pure error (SS_{pe}) in a "sums of squares and degrees of freedom tree," as shown in Fig. 14.

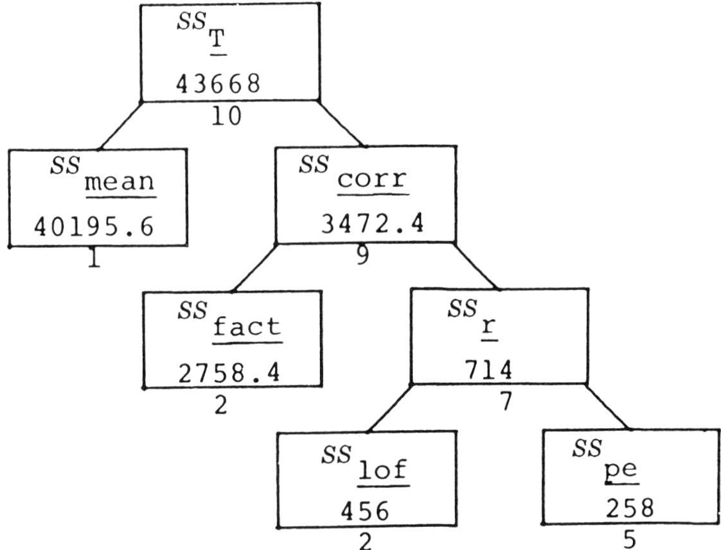

FIG. 14. Sum of squares and degrees of freedom tree for a one-factor quadratic model. (Reprinted with permission from Ref. 22, p. 167.)

For the purpose of screening the main effects of factors alone, the number of experiments can be reduced (replication is not necessary) by neglecting higher-order terms. Lack of fit and effects of interactions then are confounded with pure error. The background is given in the ANOVA equality by Eq. (22).

$$x_{ij} - \bar{x}_{..} = (\bar{x}_{i.} - \bar{x}_{..}) + (\bar{x}_{.j} - \bar{x}_{..}) + (x_{ij} - \bar{x}_{i.} - \bar{x}_{.j} + \bar{x}_{..}) \tag{22}$$

The difference between an individual outcome (x_{ij}) and the design average ($\bar{x}_{..}$) can be explained by the effects of factor C ($\bar{x}_{i.} - \bar{x}_{..}$) and factor T($\bar{x}_{.j} - \bar{x}_{..}$). The rest is supposed to be unexplained. The last term of Eq. (22) would estimate interaction and pure error, but if interaction is assumed to be zero, this term can be used to estimate noise (pure error). Squaring and summing of Eq. (22) gives the partition in sum of squares (SS), as in Eq. (23).

$$\sum\sum(x_{ij} - \bar{x}_{..})^2 = \sum\sum(\bar{x}_{i.} - \bar{x}_{..})^2 + \sum\sum(\bar{x}_{.j} - \bar{x}_{..})^2 + \sum\sum(x_{ij} - \bar{x}_{i.} - \bar{x}_{.j} + \bar{x}_{..})^2 \quad (23)$$

Division by the appropriate degrees of freedom gives the mean sums of squares associated with the factors T and C and with the residuals (in this case LOF, confounded with pure error).

Another way of screening for factor effects is the use of fractional factorial designs (FDs), in particular ''saturated,'' that is, highly fractionated FDs.

Fractional Factorial Designs

The literature of formulation research gives a number of examples of fractional factorial designs. Unfortunately, in most papers experimental details are lacking, and therefore they are not suitable to explain the technique.

If in a full factorial design the number of factors becomes larger, the number of experiments increases rapidly, as can be seen from Table 6. However, with a large number of factors it is plausible that highest-order interactions have no significant effect. In such a case factorial designs have a poor experimental efficiency and the number of experiments could be reduced in a systematic way. This has been explored for designs on two levels and the resulting designs are called fractional factorial designs (FFD).

A FFD is a fraction (1/2, 1/4, etc., in general $1/(2^p)$ of a complete or ''full'' FD. The notation for FFDs (all factors at two levels) is $2^{(k-p)}$, where 2 = number of levels, k = number of factors in the FFD, and p = degree of fractionation. An example demonstrates this: A complete 2^5 FD requires 32 experiments; 32 main effects and the interactions of five factors are estimated. A $2^{(5-1)}$ FFD consists of 16 experiments; 16 effects are estimated but they are combined effects of factors and interactions. A $2^{(5-2)}$ FFD has eight experiments; eight (combined) main effects and interactions of five factors are estimated.

The drawback of reducing the number of experiments is that effects can no longer be uniquely estimated. In the case of a half fraction of a full FD ($2^{(k-1)}$), every estimated (combined) effect is a summation of two effects, in the case of a quarter fraction ($2^{(k-2)}$), a summation of four effects. The technique of fractionation allows prediction which effects will be combined (confounded). When applying FFDs, it must be assumed (or known) that at most one of the factors, confounded in the calculated effect, has an influence on the response. The effect can then be allocated to that factor.

The FFD is called ''saturated'' if the number of factors plus the mean equals the number of effects that can be calculated. It is assumed implicitly that every effect relates to one and only one factor; the effects confounded with this factor are neglected.

TABLE 6 Minimum Number of Experiments According to a Factorial Design, Depending on Number of Factors and of Levels

	Factors					
Levels	2	3	4	5	6	7
2	4	8	16	32	64	128
3	9	27	81	243	729	2187

TABLE 7 Variables from the Reactor Example[a]

Run[b]	Variable	−	+
1	Feed rate (L/min)	10	15
2	Catalyst (%)	1	2
3	Agitation rate (rpm)	100	120
4	Temperature (°C)	140	180
5	Concentration (%)	3	6

[a]Reprinted with permission from Ref. 21.
[b]From Table 8.

As an example, a $2^{(7-4)}$ FFD is taken. Whereas the 2^7 FD requires 128 experiments and estimates one mean, seven main effects and 120 higher-order effects, the $2^{(7-4)}$ FFD requires only 2^3 or eight experiments. Each combined effect is a summation of 16 main and interaction effects. A design can be constructed in such a way that the effect of each of the original seven factors can be estimated in a separate combined effect, confounded with 15 interactions, but not with the other factors. This special design is known as the Plackett-Burman design; it is one of a group that is very well suited for screening purposes. A larger fractionation is undesirable, because in that case factors would be confounded not only with interactions but also with other factors.

A second example shows how FFDs can be constructed, in a $2^{(5-1)}$ design [21] which has been used in several formulation studies. The original 2^5 FD (Tables 7 and 8) contains 32 experiments and estimates 32 effects, which are:

- one mean
- five main effects of factors (1,2,3,4,5)
- ten 2-factor interactions (12,13,14,15,23,24,25,34,35,45)
- ten 3-factor interactions (123,124,125,134,135,145,234,235,245,345)
- five 4-factor interactions (1234,1235,1245,1345,2345)
- one 5-factor interaction (12345)

If it is assumed that 3-, 4-, and 5-factor interactions are nonsignificant, a half fraction of the 2^5 FD can be chosen in such a way that these higher-order interactions are 1-to-1 mixed (aliased) with the factors, 2-factor interactions, and the mean. Given this assumption, each of the 16 combined effects (which contains two original effects from the 2^5 FD) contains at least one nonsignificant effect. Therefore, a significant combined effect can only be produced by a main effect or a 2-factor interaction.

The generation of an FFD and the choice of the 16 experiments (and the belonging alias structure, i.e., the prescribed confounding pattern) can be chosen within certain limits. Instead of the chosen half fraction of the FD, the other complementary half fraction could have been chosen. This would have made no difference for the estimation of the effects. The complementary parts, of course, form the complete 2^5 FD.

If all 32 experiments were performed and the responses evaluated (e.g., by plotting on normal probability paper), it would have been found that only factors 2, 4, and 5 and interactions 24 and 45 are significant. If this had been known beforehand, eight experiments would have been sufficient (a 2^3 FD in factors 2, 4, and 5). Instead, in this reactor example, the number of experiments is limited to 16, arranged in a $2^{(5-1)}$ FFD. The experiments selected in Table 8 are marked with an asterisk; they seem to be arbitrarily chosen, but that is not the case, as will be seen below.

TABLE 8 Results of the Reactor Example Given in Table 7

Run	Mean	1	2	3	4	5	y(%)
1	+	−	−	−	−	−	61
*2	+	+	−	−	−	−	53
*3	+	−	+	−	−	−	63
4	+	+	+	−	−	−	61
*5	+	−	−	+	−	−	53
6	+	+	−	+	−	−	56
7	+	−	+	+	−	−	54
*8	+	+	+	+	−	−	61
*9	+	−	−	−	+	−	69
10	+	+	−	−	+	−	61
11	+	−	+	−	+	−	94
*12	+	+	+	−	+	−	93
13	+	−	−	+	+	−	66
*14	+	+	−	+	+	−	60
*15	+	−	+	+	+	−	95
16	+	+	+	+	+	−	98
*17	+	−	−	−	−	+	56
18	+	+	−	−	−	+	63
19	+	−	+	−	−	+	70
*20	+	+	+	−	−	+	65
21	+	−	−	+	−	+	59
*22	+	+	−	+	−	+	55
*23	+	−	+	+	−	+	67
24	+	+	+	+	−	+	65
25	+	−	−	−	+	+	44
*26	+	+	−	−	+	+	45
*27	+	−	+	−	+	+	78
28	+	+	+	−	+	+	77
*29	+	−	−	+	+	+	49
30	+	+	−	+	+	+	42
31	+	−	+	+	+	+	81
*32	+	+	+	+	+	+	82
Div.	32	16	16	16	16	16	

If it is assumed that the four-factor interaction (1234) does not exist (or is highly improbable), it can be confounded with one of the factors (e.g., factor 5). Then the 16 experiments are set up in standard 2^4 FD order for factors 1, 2, 3, and 4 (see Table 9). A fifth column is added for factor 5, which is confounded with interaction 1234. The signs in this columns are found by multiplying the entries in columns 1-4. The "equation" 5 = 1234 (which means that the effect of factor 5 is chosen to be confounded with the interaction 1234) is called the "design generator." The signs of column 5 are the same as those of column 1234, and the product 5*1234 results in a column of + signs (mean column, now designated with the symbol I). The "equality" I = 12345 is called "the defining relation"; I and 12345 are called the "words" of the defining relation. One may also say that the mean is "aliased" with the 5-factor interaction 12345.

A column I with only + signs can also be generated by multiplying the columns of each factor with itself; thus I = 1*1 = 2*2 = 3*3 = 4*4 = 5*5. To find the con-

TABLE 9 Interaction Effects of the Reactor Example Given in Table 8

Run	I	1	2	3	4	5 = 1234	12	13	23	145	245	y
17	+	−	−	−	−	+	+	+	+	+	+	56
2	+	+	−	−	−	−	−	−	+	+	−	53
3	+	−	+	−	−	−	−	+	−	−	+	63
20	+	+	+	−	−	+	+	−	−	−	−	65
5	+	−	−	+	−	−	+	−	−	−	−	53
22	+	+	−	+	−	+	−	+	−	−	+	55
23	+	−	+	+	−	+	−	−	+	+	−	67
8	+	+	+	+	−	−	+	+	+	+	+	61
9	+	−	−	−	+	−	+	+	+	+	+	69
26	+	+	−	−	+	+	−	−	+	+	−	45
27	+	−	+	−	+	+	−	+	−	−	+	78
12	+	+	+	−	+	−	+	−	−	−	−	93
29	+	−	−	+	+	+	+	−	−	−	−	49
14	+	+	−	+	+	−	−	+	−	−	+	60
15	+	−	+	+	+	−	−	−	+	+	−	95
32	+	+	+	+	+	+	+	+	+	+	+	82
Div	16	8	8	8	8	8	8	8	8	8	8	

founding of factor 1, every "word" in the defining relation is multiplied by 1; thus 1*I = 1*12345. With 1*I = 1 and 1*1 = I (can be removed), there remains 1 = 2345. In the same way, the confounding of the other main effects can be found: 2 = 1345, 3 = 1245, 4 = 1235, 5 = 1234.

By comparing the rows of signs in Table 8 with those in Table 9, the necessary runs in the $2^{(5-1)}$FFD can be identified; in Table 8 they are marked with an asterisk.

For demonstration purposes in Table 9, columns for some two- and three-factor interactions and their signs have been added. By searching for identical columns the confounded effects can be identified. For example, 13 is confounded (or "aliased") with 245, and 23 with 145; they are aliases of each other, as we have seen already for 2 and 1345, etc. Searching the columns is a tedious operation, and fortunately there is a simple way via the defining relation I = 12345; when searching for the alias of 24, both sides of the defining relation are multiplied by 24: 24I = 1223445. With 2*2 = I and 4*4 = I and omitting I, the result is 24 = 135, and effect 24 is confounded with 135, etc.

The effect of factor 1 (which is, however, confounded with the effect of interaction 2345) can be found using contrasts, as shown earlier; in Eq. (24), l_1 estimates the sum of the effects 1 and 2345.

$$l_1 = (-56+53-63+65-53+55-67+61-69+45-78+93-49+60-95+82)/16 = -2.0 \quad (24)$$

The effect of, for example, interaction 13 (but confounded with 245), the notation being l_{13}, can be found in the same way by Eq. (25).

$$l_{13} = (+56-53+63-65 \ldots\ldots -49+60-95+82)/8 = 0.5 \quad (25)$$

Analogously to l_1, the value 0.5 found for l_{13} estimates the sum of the effects 13 and 245.

The complementary half fraction of this $2^{(5-1)}$ FFD can be found by changing the design generator in 5 = −1234; the defining relation then changes into I = 12345. In the example given, this means that column 5 is inverted and the entries change signs.

It is possible to reduce the experimental effort even more by taking higher fractions, for example, $2^{(5-2)}$ FFD. The complexity of the confounding pattern will increase. Fortunately, many software packages have modules for the construction and evaluation of FFDs. The general rules are as follows:

1. The fewer interactions there are to be expected, the higher the degree of fractioning one can choose.
2. If no interactions are expected (or for screening purposes interactions are neglected), a "saturated" (highly fractionated) design can be chosen.
3. If two-factor interactions are expected, a design has to be chosen which allows the calculation of these effects alongside (but not confounded) with the main effects.

Plackett-Burman Designs

In the foregoing, screening for influential variables using FFDs has been described. With FFDs the experimental effort can be limited at the cost of information about higher interaction effects. In the above examples, the two-factor interactions were maintained. Although normal FFDs have 2^{n-p} (4, 8, 16, 32 . . .) experiments, Plackett and Burman [24] developed special FFDs with $k = m*4$ experiments, $m = 1 \ldots 25$ (4, 8, 12, 16, 20, 24, 28, 32 . . .) for the screening of $(k - 1)$ variables. Their use is mostly limited to $k \leq 16$. The main effects may of course be confounded with interactions.

Plackett and Burman found a way to construct the first row of − and + signs in such a way that the following rows could be formed by cyclic permutation of the signs from the first row. The following method is employed:

The first (+ or −) sign of the first row is moved to the end of that row, and the row is shifted one position to the left. This cycle is repeated until the $(k - 1)^{th}$ row has been completed; for the design of a last row, only minus signs are added.

Inasmuch as the first row always has one plus sign more and thus the first $(k - 1)$ rows have an excess of plus signs, this is balanced by adding a last row of minus signs. This makes the design orthogonal.

The k experiments are performed in randomized order. Table 10 gives the result of the operation for $k = 8$; Table 11 shows the first rows to be used for constructing Plackett-Burman (PB) designs. If nine or ten factors are to be screened, for which there is no PB design (and the same holds for 13 or 14 factors, etc.), the PB design with $k = 12$ (or $k = 16$) can be used by the addition of dummy factors for the remaining variables. These can be interpreted as interactions, but since the alias structure of PB designs is not as straightforward as that of normal FFDs, the responses will be used mostly for the estimation of experimental error.

Calculations can be performed on PB designs by contrasts or by regression analogously to those on FFDs; the model is given in Eq. (26).

$$E(y) = \beta_0 + \sum \beta_i x_i \tag{26}$$

TABLE 10 A Plackett-Burman Design for Seven Variables[a]

Run	1	2	3	4	5	6	7	y
1	+	+	+	−	+	−	−	
2	+	+	−	+	−	−	+	
3	+	−	+	−	−	+	+	
4	−	+	−	−	+	+	+	
5	+	−	−	+	+	+	−	
6	−	−	+	+	+	−	+	
7	−	+	+	+	−	+	−	
8	−	−	−	−	−	−	−	

[a] $k = 8$.

TABLE 11 First Rows Used for the Construction of Plackett-Burman Designs

k	Variables																						
8	+	+	+	−	+	−	−																
12	+	+	−	+	+	+	−	−	−	+	−												
16	+	+	+	+	−	+	−	+	+	−	−	+	−	−	−								
20	+	+	−	−	+	+	+	+	−	+	−	+	−	−	−	−	+	+	−				
24	+	+	+	+	+	−	+	−	+	+	−	−	+	+	−	−	+	−	+	−	−	−	−

Special Designs for Process Variables

A described above, by the use of (fractional) factorial designs main effects and interactions can be evaluated, but it is not possible to detect a curvature of the response surface as long as no more than two levels for a factor are chosen. A simple solution seems to be to augment the design with experiments at the center point of the factorial design (Fig. 15). Then not only the average, linear, and interaction effects, but also a combined quadratic effect can be estimated simply by comparing the prediction at the center point (based on contrasts or regression using only the experimental points of the 2^n FD) with the mean of the center-point measurement(s). If there is any curvature in either one of the independent variables or in both, this effect can be found with the help of this design. The source of the effect in terms of a specific variable, however, cannot be detected.

Star Design

For two factors the star design is simply a 2^2 FD, rotated over 45° (Fig. 16). A center point is usually added, which may be replicated to estimate experimental error. Then each factor has three levels, and for each factor a quadratic effect can be estimated, but interactions cannot be measured.

In the star designs, 2^k FDs are rotated over 45° in $(k-1)$ directions in k-dimensional space with a replicated center point. They consist of $(2k+r_c)$ experiments, r_c being the number of replicates at the center. The design is rotatable; orthogonality depends on the number of replicates r_c.

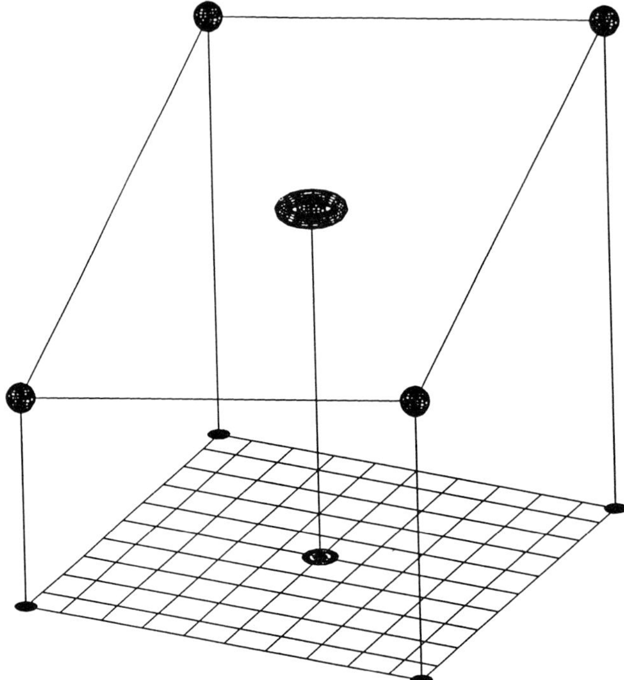

FIG. 15. A 2^2 factorial design with replicated center point.

Central Composite Design

A better solution that combines the advantages of the FD (or FFD) and the star design, is the central composite design (CCD) (Fig.17), developed by Box and Wilson [1]. It is composed of [25]:

- a 2^k FD($n_c = 2^k r_c$ experiments) or $2^{(k-p)}$) FFD ($n_c = 2^{(k-p)} r_c$ experiments), where r_c is the number of replicates of the FD part of the design,
- a $2*k$ star design ($2k$ axial points, $n_s = 2kr_s$ experiments), where r_s is the number of replicates of the star part of the design, and
- n_o center points.

This design allows the estimation of a full second-order model. The case of two factors is given by Eq. (27).

$$E(y) = \beta_0 + \beta_1 x_1 + \beta_2 x_2 + \beta_{12} x_1 x_2 + \beta_{11} x_1^2 + \beta_{22} x_2^2 \quad (27)$$

If the coordinates of the FD part of the design are of the type ($\pm 1, \pm 1, \ldots \pm 1$), the axial points of the star design are chosen with coordinates ($\pm\alpha, 0, \ldots, 0$), ($0, \pm\alpha, 0, \ldots 0$), $\ldots$, ($0, 0, \ldots \pm\alpha$). To a certain extend, one has the freedom to choose a value for α. For $\alpha = 1$, the result is a standard 3^k FD with a replicated center point (Fig. 17). There is one value, $\alpha = (n_c/r_s)^{1/4}$ that gives the design the highly desirable property of rotatability [25]

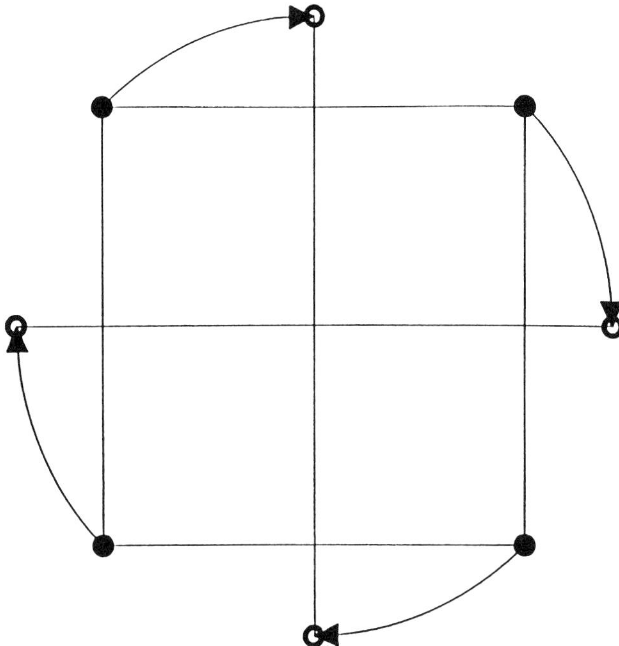

FIG. 16. A star design, derived from the factorial design by rotation over 45°; ● = factorial design, ○ = axial points, star design.

Rotatability

A response surface model, determined by regression to experimental data, can be used for the prediction of responses for any combination of factor settings within the experimental domain. As the experimental error is in general reflected in the precision of the coefficients in the model, the error of prediction is not the same in all directions over the response surface.

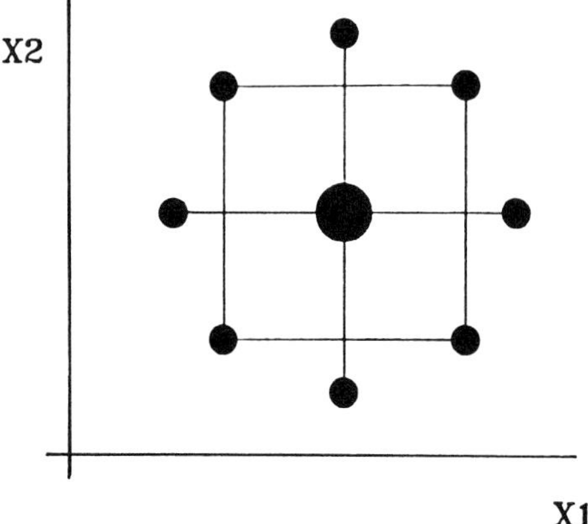

FIG. 17. The central composite design, a 2^2 factorial design, augmented with a star design and replicated center point ($\alpha = 1.414$).

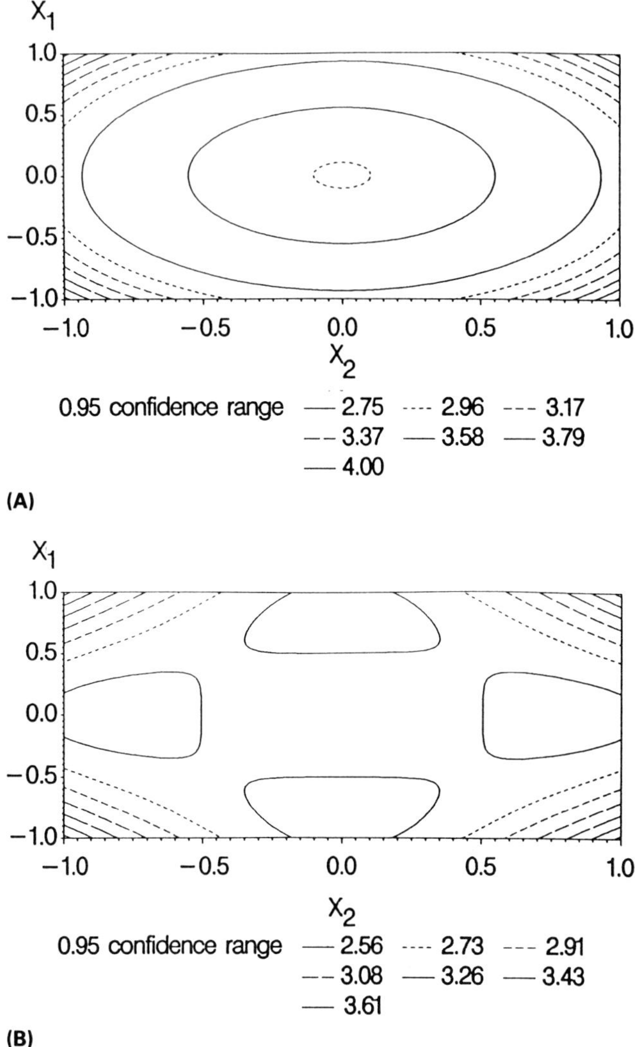

FIG. 18. Distribution of prediction error for (A) a rotatable CCD ($\alpha = 1.414$), and (B) a nonrotatable CCD ($\alpha = 2.00$).

A design is rotatable when the prediction error, although variable over the response surface, is independent of the direction taken from the center point of the design. This is illustrated in Fig. 18 for a two-factor central composite design (CCD) with $\alpha = 2$ (not rotatable) and $\alpha = 1.414$ (rotatable). Values of α for rotatable CCDs for 2, 3, and 4 factors, with only replicated center points, replicated central and ''cube'' points, and replicated center and star points are given in Table 12. Orthogonality of the CCD again depends on the number of replicated center points. Data can be found in Refs. 26 and 27.

TABLE 12 Values of α^a for a Central Composite Design

Conditions	Number of Factors			
	2	3	4	5
None or only center point	1.414	1.682	2.000	2.378
Center + FD points	1.682	2.000	2.378	2.828
Center + axial star points	1.189	1.414	1.682	2.000

[a]Given in three decimal places.

Box-Behnken Design

In central composite designs each factor has five levels. If the number of factors increases, the number of experiments may become too high. The Box-Behnken (BB) designs for three or more factors are an economical alternative in which each factor is given three levels. The design is called an orthogonal balanced incomplete block design. It can be split into a set of incomplete blocks, which means that every effect is not estimated in every block but every factor effect is measured an equal number of times with a balanced partition over the different blocks.

The design for the three-factor case is shown in Fig. 19, where it is compared to the face-centered CCD. The design points in the BB design are at the midst of the edges of the cube instead of at the corners and the centers of the sides. No design points are placed on the extreme points of the (hyper)cube which spans the complete design space. This can be advantageous when physical–chemical problems arise under these extreme conditions. Rotatability and orthogonality depend on the number of replicates at the center point.

Doehlert Hexagon or Uniform Shell Design

Doehlert [28] proposed uniform shell designs, starting with an equilateral triangle, mirrored in one side to a hexagon, as in Fig. 20 A. The hexagon is expandable in 2D space by mirroring of the center point in the outward sides. The equally spaced design points are uniformly distributed in concentric circles, as can be seen from Fig. 20 B. It is also expandable in 3D to concentric spherical shells. Due to the uniform distribution, models based on this design provide a good basis for interpolation. A disadvantage may be that the number of levels is not the same for all factors. If the experimenter has prior knowledge of the relative importance of the factors, the design may be started with one side of the hexagon parallel to this most important axis.

Mixture Designs

For mixtures of components (e.g., in formulations of drugs and excipients), special models have been derived, based on the mixture constraints: A fraction cannot be negative, and the sum of the fractions of the components equals one. An important property is that the number of coefficients to be estimated is reduced. Many papers describing this type of design can be found in the literature on formulation research.

The mixture constraint has consequences for the experimental designs. Factors cannot be chosen freely. In a two-component mixture only one fraction (variable) can be chosen,

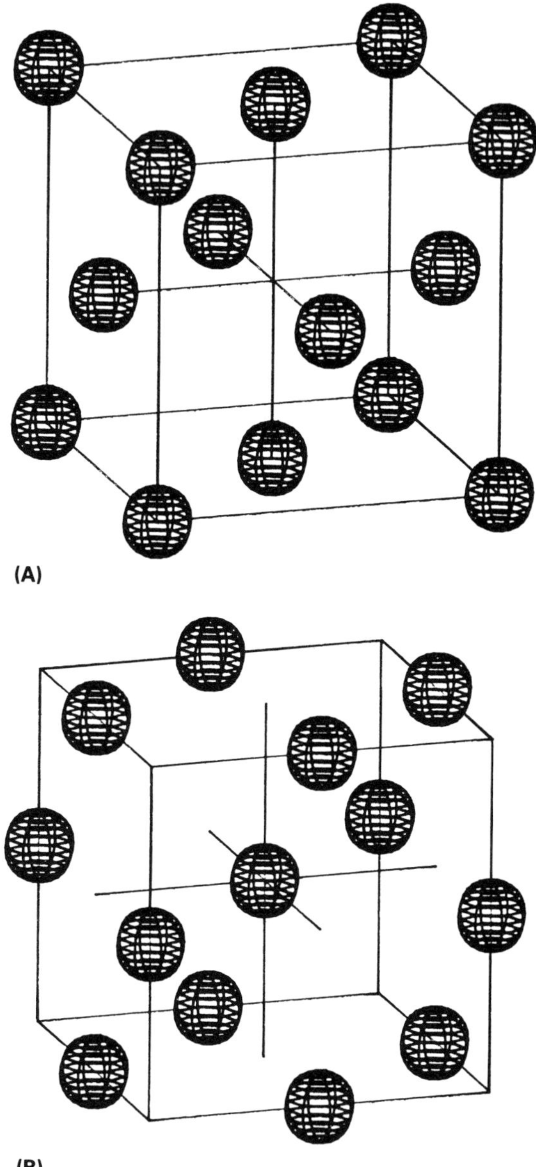

FIG. 19. (A) Face-centered CCD and (B) a Box-Behnken design; three factors.

in a three-component mixture only two fractions. The remaining fraction completes the sum to one. This implies a dimension reduction. For k variables the factor space can be represented geometrically by a $(k-1)$ dimensional regular simplex: for two components a line, for three a triangle, and for four a tetrahedron. For a ternary mixture, this is illustrated in Fig. 21. Figure 22 shows how the coordinates of a point P (the composition of a mixture associated with point P) can be found. Every point within a mixture triangle has a one-to-one relation with a three-component composition which can be described by a

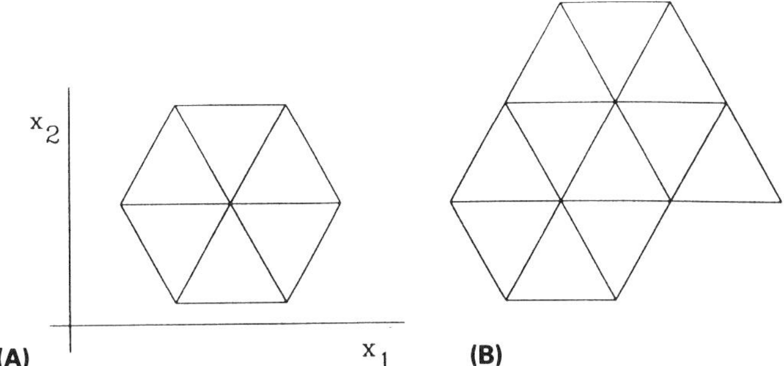

FIG. 20. Doehlert design. (A). Construction starting from an equilateral triangle; (B). Expansion of the hexagon in 2D space.

special coordinate system. The corners correspond to a fraction of 1 and the opposing base line to a fraction of zero of the associated compound. Inside the triangle, lines parallel to the edges are depicted where the component associated with the opposing corner has a constant concentration. Any point in the mixture triangle is determined by two of these lines, the third being fixed by the first two because of the mixture restriction. The levels of these lines indicate the coordinates of the point. Analogously, the vertices of a tetrahedron represent the pure components, the edges binary mixtures, the faces ternary mixtures. The inner space of the tetrahedron represents the set of mixtures of four components. The coordinates of any point within the tetrahedron can now be found as the intersection of three planes parallel to the faces of the tetrahedron (the fourth plane fixed by the levels of the other three).

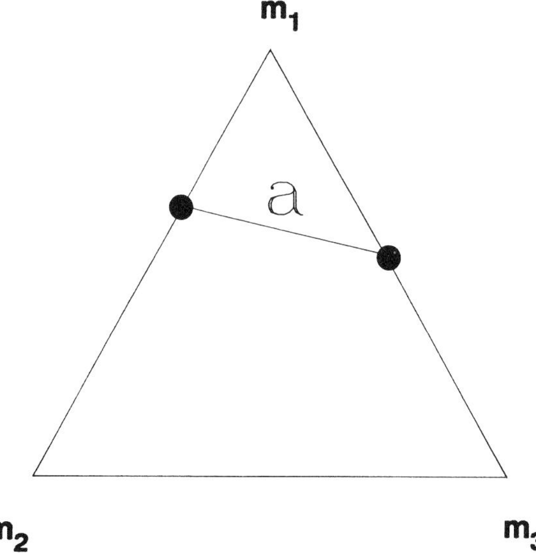

FIG. 21. The mixture space is a triangle. Line a represents ternary mixtures, composed of the binary pseudo-components, represented by the intersections of the line with the sides of the triangle.

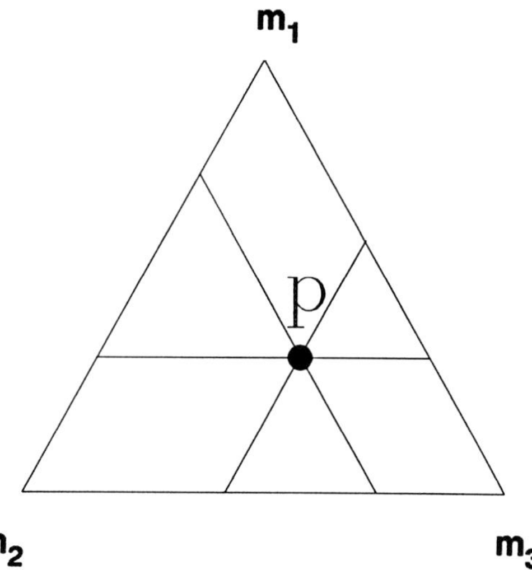

FIG. 22. The mixture triangle and the coordinates of point P.

Simplex Lattice Designs

Simplex lattice designs are used to explore the interior and the boundaries of the simplex; its dimensions are determined by the number of factors. The pattern of the design points in the factor space and their number depend on the degree (the term of highest order) of the model that is postulated. The points are distributed orderly over the factor space, forming a lattice. Arrangements for three factors are shown in Fig. 23. If factors can be controlled accurately and precisely the coefficients of the model equations can be calculated manually as was the practice before computers became available. This can easily be shown by Eq. (28) for the three-factor special cubic model.

$$E(y) = \beta_1^* m_1 + \beta_2^* m_2 + \beta_3^* m_3 + \beta_{12}^* m_1 m_2 + \beta_{13}^* m_1 m_3 + \beta_{23}^* m_2 m_3 + \beta_{123}^* m_1 m_2 m_3 \quad (28)$$

The values of m_1, m_2, and m_3 in each design point are substituted successively in Eq. (27), resulting in seven equations with seven coefficients to solve. Nowadays calculations are performed by regression analysis. Simplex lattice designs, however, have exactly as many design points as there are coefficients in the model, and it is not possible to estimate residual error. Replication of measurements allows estimation of pure error. Extra design points and replication of some measurements give an estimation of residual and pure errors and thus make it possible to estimate the lack of fit (see Fig. 14).

Often three extra design points, halfway to the vertices and the center point, as indicated in Fig. 23 C, are added. In this augmented simplex centroid design, the design points are distributed as uniformly as possible. It has the advantage over the seven-point simplex lattice design that information about blending effects of three components is provided by four design points instead of one. Replication, however, is still necessary, because an estimate of pure error is needed for the estimation of lack of fit.

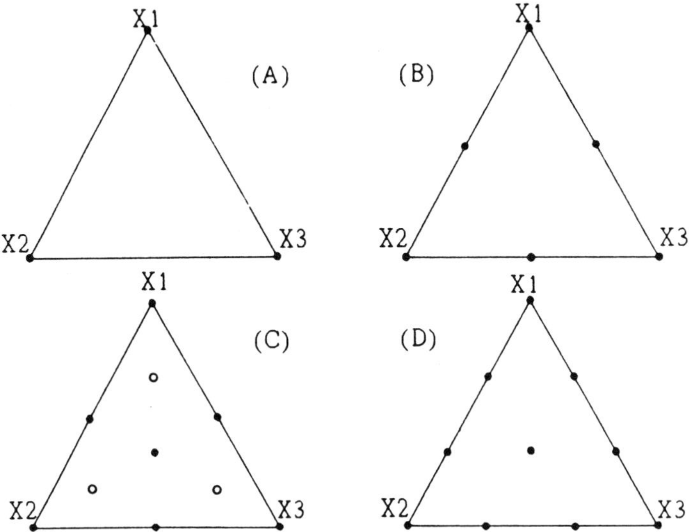

FIG. 23. Simplex lattice designs. (A). Linear model; (B). Quadratic model; (C). Special cubic model; the augmented simplex centroid design, where three extra design points have been added. (D). Cubic model.

Extreme-Vertices Design

It often occurs in formulation studies that not the whole factor space is accessible for experiments or that some areas are expected not to give useful responses, for example, mixtures with more than 1% of lubricant or more than 30% of disintegrant in tablet formulations for direct compression. The factor space can then be restricted, as shown for a three-component mixture in Figs. 24 and 25. In the general case, restrictions on upper limits (u_i) as well as lower limits (l_i) exist for all components, $l_i \leq m_i \leq u_i$ (Fig. 24). These limits can best be shown as lines with the border value. In a special case, only a lower

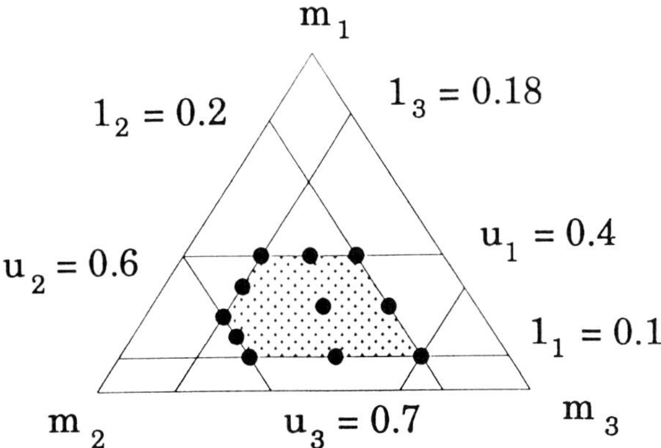

FIG. 24. Extreme-vertices design for a three-component mixture. Because of upper and lower restrictions only ternary mixtures exist in the feasible region.

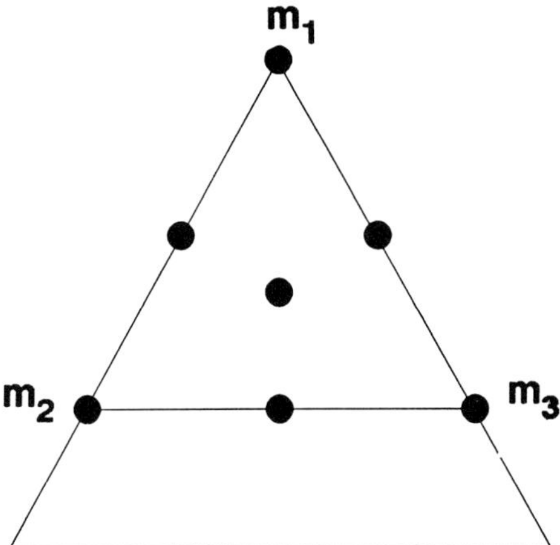

FIG. 25. Extreme-vertices design for a three-component mixture. Binary and ternary mixtures can be composed from the pure component and pseudo-components.

restriction is set on one component (Fig. 25), $l_i \leq m_i$. In this case, the compositions at the corners can be used as pseudo-components.

In an extreme-vertices design, observations are made at the corners of the bounded design space, at the middle of the edges, and at the center of the design space. These designs are most useful. They can be used for mixture compositions as well as in combination with (fractional) factorial designs. They can be evaluated only with regression. Dedicated software (OMEGA, the Fortran routines CONVRT, or CONACV given by Cornell, see Bibliography) facilitates the calculation of the design points.

Pseudo-components

Figures 24 and 25 show the situations where only a part of the mixture space is feasible. With four-component mixtures an analogous situation may occur. If one of the components has a fixed concentration in the final mixture, the feasible region is restricted to the set of design points in a triangular cross-section of the tetrahedron. This component may be the active substance itself or one of the excipients, such as 0.5% lubricant (or eventually both). The compositions in this cross-section can be calculated as linear combinations of pseudo-components, being binary mixtures themselves. Another example is shown in Fig. 25 for a ternary mixture with a lower restriction on the component m_1. The restricted mixture can be represented in a smaller triangle within the original, one with vertices m_1, m_2, and m_3. Two of these, m_2, and m_3, are binary mixtures themselves. The composition of the mixtures in the design points can be calculated as linear combinations of the pure component m_1 and the pseudo-components m_2 and m_3. Dedicated software, such as OMEGA, can be very helpful.

Designs Combining Process and Mixture Variables

In formulation studies properties frequently depend on mixture as well as process variables. For example, in tableting by direct compression, the mixture variables are the drug, disintegrant, binder, and lubricant, and the process variables the compression force

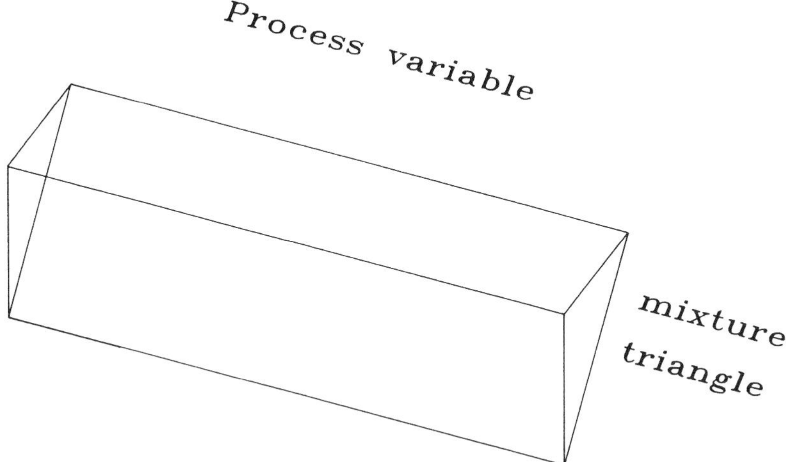

FIG. 26. Representation of a combined design for three mixture variables and one process variable.

and mixing time. In film coating, the mixture variables are plasticizers, polymers, and pigments, and the process variables the spraying rate, nozzle type, and temperature.

In a simple case, there are two mixture components and several process variables. The mixture variables reduce to one variable (the fraction or the amount of one of the mixture components) that in a normal (fractional) factorial design can be combined with the process variables. Another simple case is the combination of three mixture components with one process variable. The design space then can be depicted as a prism (Fig. 26).

A mixture design can be combined with a factorial design, as shown in Fig. 27 A and B for two process variables and three mixture components (or pseudo-components). These combined designs may look different but are equivalent; that is, the design points are exactly the same. In each design point of the factorial design for the process variables, a complete mixture design must be implemented or vice versa. Instead of the pictured special cubic mixture design an extreme-vertices design can be chosen, and the 2^2 factorial design can be equally well replaced by any other design for process variables.

The number of experiments, although limited because of the properties of the mixture design, is rather high (4*9 or more) if a 2^2 FD is combined with an extreme-vertices design. The experimental effort may become prohibitive if three or more process factors are studied and more levels are needed for the evaluation of the postulated model, possibly with quadratic terms for the process variables.

In those cases, the mixture design can be combined with a $2^{(k-1)}$ fractional factorial design instead of a full 2^k design, and the number of experiments can be halved; a choice can be made between two complementary half-fractions.

Instead of fractioning the factorial design, methods have been developed recently to fractionate both, the mixture design part and the process design part, by treating all factors initially as unconstrained variables [29, 30]. Interesting propositions are the "projection–contraction" procedure, the "projection–flexible contraction" procedure, and the "projection–rotation–contraction" procedure [31–33]. To understand these, the way the mixture triangle was developed from the factorial representation of the component fractions (see Fig. 8(A)) must be kept in mind. The set of unconstrained variable settings of the mixture design is projected to the diagonal plane of the 2^3 factorial design

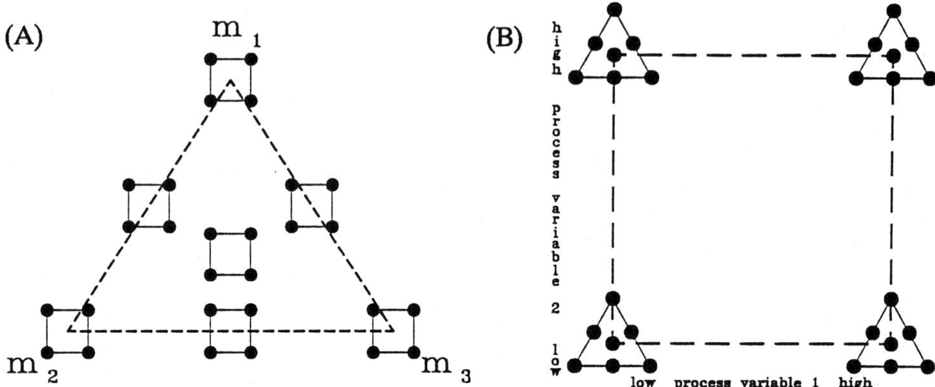

FIG. 27. Two equivalent representations of a combined design for three mixture and two process variables: a mixture design with seven mixture compositions and a full 2^2 factorial design. A. In each design point of the mixture design a 2^2 factorial design is implemented. B. In each design point of the 2^2 factorial design a mixture design is implemented.

cube (Fig. 28A). The resulting projections are shown in Fig. 28B. Part of the projections fall outside the mixture triangle (Fig. 28B). This means that these compositions do not comply to the mixture constraints, that is, the sum of the fractions equals 1 and the non-negativity of the fractions. Several solutions have been proposed (Fig. 29 A,B,and C). The first is contraction of all projections toward the center of the triangle, resulting in an insufficient coverage of the mixture variable space. The second is a flexible contraction, where only the points outside the triangle are subjected to contraction. The whole mixture triangle is now covered. The third is a combined rotation-contraction procedure, where all projected points are rotated over 30° and subsequently contracted toward the center until they comply again with the mixture constraint. In general, the flexible contraction gives the best results, but the quality of the result depends on the chosen model [33].

After this mixture design construction, a half-fraction can be chosen and combined with a factorial design as depicted in Fig. 30. Although it seems that in this representation only the mixture design is fractionated, careful inspection of the design points reveals that the factorial design is fractionated as well.

Optimal Design Theory

The "optimal design" method is generally applicable for the construction of designs. The theory was summarized in 1969 by Fedorov in Russian. A translation in English appeared in 1972 (see Bibliography). A review by Atkinson [34] provides references to the whole field of optimal experimental design.

The optimal design method requires that a model is postulated, the variable space defined, and the number of design points fixed. A further requirement is that the model is correct. The chosen number of design points is distributed in the variable space in such a way that the selected criterion has the optimal value.

In general a relatively complex model is chosen. For the selection of the algorithm two approaches can be used: The first allows not only integer design points, but also fractional points, for example, a 0.5 design point at one setting of variables, and 0.3 at another, up to the preselected total number of design points. This is called a continuous

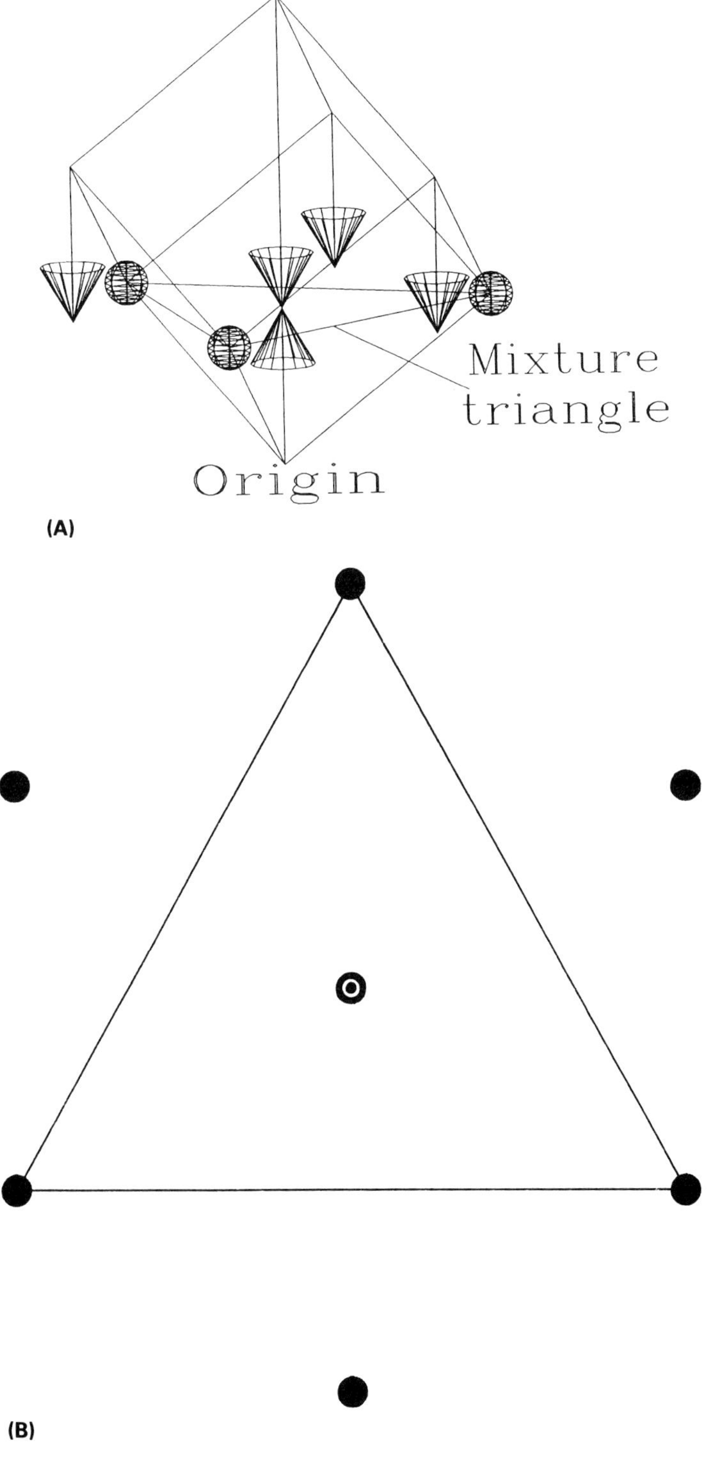

FIG. 28. (A) Projection of unrestricted mixture variable settings to the diagonal plane of the cube formed on the three mixture variable axes. The tops of the cones indicate the projections. (B) The projected points and the mixture triangle.

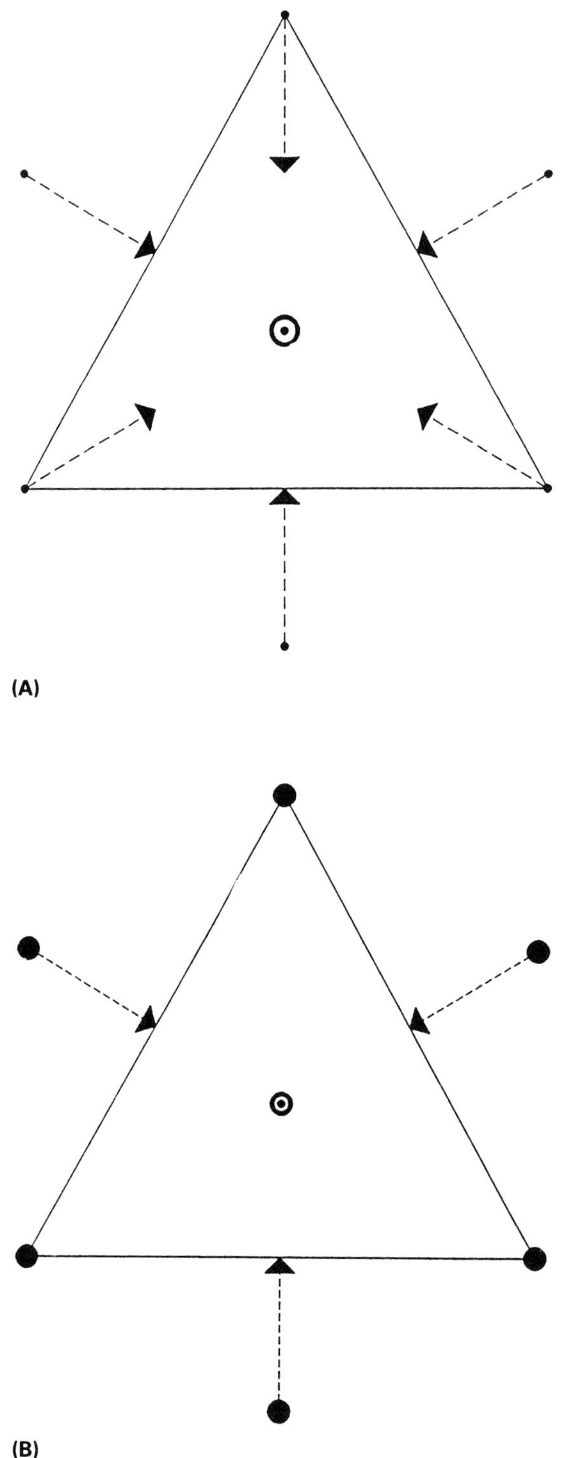

FIG. 29. Manipulation of the projected points: A. Contraction, B. Flexible contraction, C. Rotation and contraction.

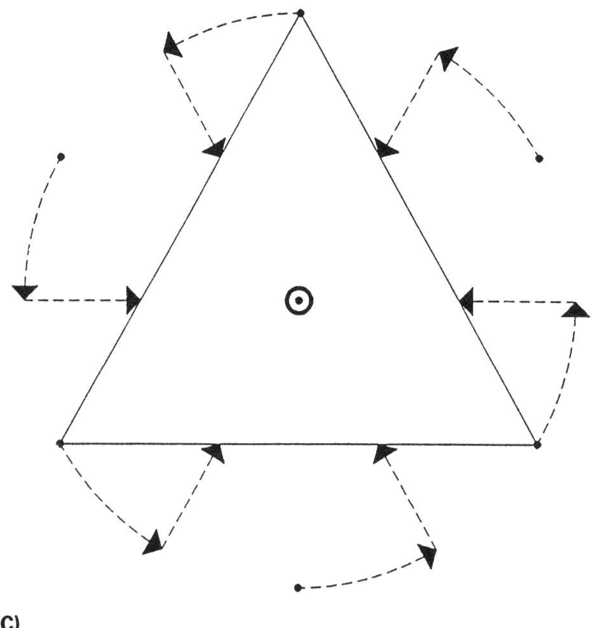

FIG. 29 (C). Manipulation of the projected point. Rotation and contraction.

design. It must be followed by a step in which a design is constructed consisting of integer points, the selected number of design points. The second approach uses only integer values for design points. The result is called an exact design. Several methods are used to construct an exact design, the most common is Detmax.

Several design properties can be optimized, related to the purpose for which the design will be used. A critical discussion can be found in Ref. 33. The D-criterion minimizes the variance and the covariance of the parameters. With the G-criterion, the maximum variance of prediction in all design points is calculated. A design is selected where the maximum variance is minimal. If a design is D-optimal it is also G-optimal and vice-versa.

With the A-criterion, the variance of the parameters is minimized without consideration of their covariance, whereas the V-criterion minimizes the average prediction error.

The differences between the D and A criteria and between the V and G criteria are observed easily. The D and A criteria both give some measure for the variance of the parameters. The D-criterion includes the covariance between the parameters, the A-criterion does not. The difference between a design I, which performs better on the A criterion and worse on the D-criterion, and a design II, which performs better on the D-criterion but worse on the A-criterion, can best be explained as follows. Design I has model terms with a lower variance and therefore with a higher significance. The model terms have a higher covariance, which means that if model terms are incorrect the other model terms are more influenced by that than with design II. On the basis of design II, the parameters are estimated with a higher variance, but lower covariances, and are therefore more independently estimated.

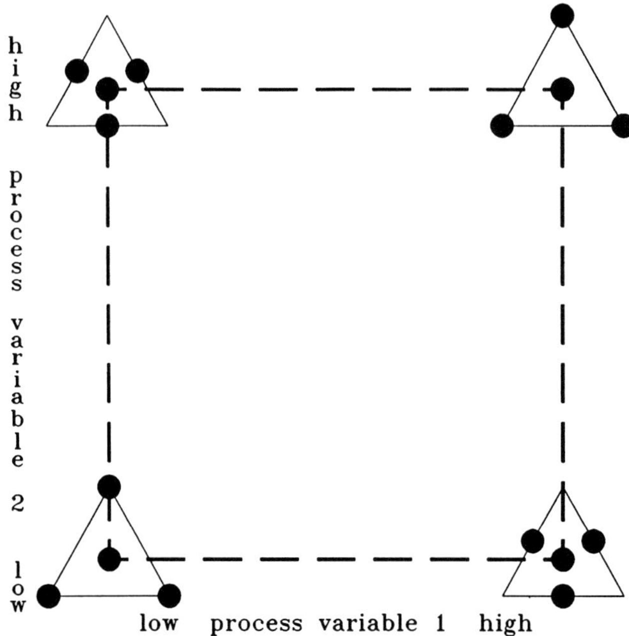

FIG. 30. One of two representations of a fractionated combined designs for mixture- and process variables. See also Fig. 27.

The G- and V-criteria operate on the variance of predictions instead of parameters. If the experimenter chooses the G-criterion, he or she knows the maximum variance of the predictions over the design space; in other words, he or she knows that the prediction is at least as good as a certain value. This is a minimax strategy, that is, the maximum loss is minimized, and the experimenter plays it safe. In the other approach, the V-criterion, the average variance of prediction is known over the design space. At most factor settings the variance is smaller; at some settings it is larger than with the G-criterion, but it is not known where this occurs. The criterion that has been used most frequently is the D-criterion.

Response Surface Methodology

Response surface methodology (RMS) was defined by Box and Draper [16] as ". . . a group of statistical techniques for empirical model building and model exploitation. By careful design and analysis of experiments, it seeks to relate a response, or output variable to the levels of a number of predictors, or input variables, that affect it."

In the course of the essentially iterative process, knowledge of influential factors is acquired, such as the location of the experimental region, appropriate scaling and transformations (e.g., logarithmic) for input and output variables, and the degree of complexity of the empirical model and hence the designs needed. Building blocks of RSM are a priori knowledge of the experimenter, screening designs, and simple two-level factorial designs, but also of the more complex designs, discussed above. In a simultaneous strategy, empirical models and their statistical evaluation are important.

Model Choice and Validation

Model choice is like sailing between Scilla and Charybdis. Some models are too simple, others are too complex. A too simple model certainly results in considerable bias in the predicted optima or ranges. Models too complex always carry the risk of overfitting, in-particular if the number of experiments is close to the number of model coefficients. Predictions will then be too optimistic. Because of their large variance, the confidence interval of the predicted value is larger than in a smaller model.

A model must be selected in accordance with the intended application, that is, will it be used for description or prediction. For optimization purposes, the quality of a model should be judged on its predictive potential. The problem of model selection for prediction is how to discard all model terms which, when included, increase the variance more than they reduce the bias when they are excluded.

The first step in model validation is the performance of ANOVA calculations. Cornell (see Bibliography) has given ANOVA algorithms, in particular for mixture problems, as the normal ANOVA does not give reliable results because of the missing intercept. The second step is the estimation of the pure measurement error. This is only possible if at some design points several independent measurements are performed. To be independent, they must be randomized. The variance of these observations, pooled over all design points, is an estimate of pure error variance. If the residual variance of the model is much higher than the pure error variance, there are obviously systematical deviations of the model; this is tested with an F-test on lack of fit.

There are many other criteria [33] for model validation, but not one can do the job alone. One of the best known criterion is the coefficient of multiple determination, the correlation coefficient given by Eq. (29),

$$R^2 = \frac{SSR}{SST} \tag{29}$$

where *SSR* is the sum of squares due to regression and *SST* the total sum of squares (see also Fig. 14). It can be interpreted as the part of the variation which is explained, but since it does not contain a penalty for a too complex model it is not feasible for the purpose here. Somewhat better is the adjusted correlation coefficient $R^2{}_{\text{adj}}$, given by Eq. (30),

$$R^2_{\text{adj}} = 1 - \frac{SSE/(n-p)}{SST/(n-1)} \tag{30}$$

where *SSE* is the sum of squares due to residual error (SS_r in Fig. 14) and both sums of squares are divided by their respective degrees of freedom.

The adjusted correlation coefficient does not include a consideration of the loss associated with choosing an incorrect model. Therefore other criteria have been devised. Very useful are Mallow's C_{p} and the prediction criterion *Pc* of Amemiya, shown in Eqs. (31) and (32), respectively, cited in Ref. 33,

$$C_{\text{p}} = \frac{SSE}{\hat{\sigma}^2} + 2p - n \tag{31}$$

$$Pc = \frac{SSE}{n-p}\left(1 + \frac{p}{n}\right) \tag{32}$$

where p is the number of parameters and n the number of observations; $\hat{\sigma}^2$ is model independent. The loss by using too small a model is included in C_p. A disadvantage may be that an estimate of error variance is needed. The Pc can be interpreted as an estimator of the mean square prediction error.

The above mentioned criteria use some function of the residual variance to obtain a measure for goodness of fit of a model. If the model has to be used for predictive purposes, the data-splitting approach is more feasible, where a training set is used to obtain the parameters of the model and a test set to assess its predictive quality. This method has the disadvantage that only part of the data is used to estimate the parameters. As a consequence, these are inferior to those obtained by using all data. A better approach is cross-validation, where the data are split in a test set (mostly one point), and the remainder in a training set. All points, in turn, are entered in the test set and the total prediction error on these subsequent test sets (PRESS) or its mean (mean PRESS) is used as the criterion for model selection. This predictive error sum of squares (PRESS) is a cross-validation method that is calculated as in Eq. (33).

$$PRESS = \sum_{i=1}^{n} (y_i - \hat{y}_{\backslash i})^2 \tag{33}$$

The "back slash" means that a predicted value of y is calculated without observing i.

The F-tests on regression and lack of fit (LOF) perform well for judging descriptive properties of a model and can very well be used for judging the significance of model terms; R^2_{adj} is useful but C_p, Pc, and $PRESS$ are better for model selection with the purpose of prediction.

Predictions Using the Selected Model

Once a model has been selected and validated, how is it used for prediction? Since fast computers and dedicated software became available, the "brute force" method is applied most frequently. The response surface is scanned according to a grid by changing the input variables x_i with small increments, that is, 1, 2, 5, or 10%, of the range of each variable. With two factors, a 3D response surface or a 2D contour diagram can be drawn in x_1 and x_2, and with three factors a series of contour diagrams at selected values of one of the input factors. With more factors, drawing diagrams is not feasible, but just as in the former cases, the computer can select ranges of the input factors that give a maximum or adequate response values. In the case of multiple objectives, all response surfaces can be calculated separately. Contour diagrams can be drawn separately or overlayed, or the computer can identify ranges for the factors where all responses have the required values.

The following questions can be answered at the end of the calculations:

- What input variables influence the response, and to what extent do they interact?
- What response can be expected (predicted) for some specified region of interest of the input variables?

- To what extent changes the response with limited changes in the input variables or, stated otherwise, how robust is the response?
- What settings of the input variables will yield a maximum or minimum or a desirable range of the response?
- If there are multiple responses, will there be a region where they all show a desirable value?

A response surface model, by nature of its derivation from a Taylor series and due to experimental uncertainty, is an approximation of the true model. Moreover, it provides only a local model in the experimental region and should not be extrapolated outside this region.

Visualization by graphical representation of systems with multiple input greatly enhances the interpretation of the empirical models. A two-factor system can be pictured with its output in 3D space. By taking slices of the response surface at various levels parallel to the plane of the factors, a contour diagram is obtained in 2D space. It is also possible to construct 3D contour diagrams of a three-factor system with one response. An alternative is keeping each factor in turn at a constant level and constructing a series of 2D contour diagrams.

In Figs. 31 A–C contour diagrams are shown, taken from a study on tableting by direct compression [35]. In Fig. 32 the contours are overlaid to find an overall acceptable region.

Multiple Responses

Sometimes only one response is measured, but more often a product has to meet more requirements. A tablet should meet requirements of crushing strength, friability, weight variation, disintegration time, content uniformity, and of course robustness of one or more of these objectives. With an appropriate design, these properties can be measured in each design point, provided sufficient tablets are produced. The measurements also can be replicated to have a measure of pure analytical error available. The appropriate models may differ in these properties, and each property will have its own response surface and model. The design chosen should make possible the evaluation of the most complex model. It is, however highly improbable that the optimum for all responses will be found at one and the same factor setting. Moreover, the criteria may conflict. For the tablet example, high crushing strength and short disintegration time will require differing settings of both compression force and composition. Hence there is a demand for decision making to find an overall optimum situation that may deviate from the optima of one or more of the single criteria, that is, the best compromise must be found.

Combined Criteria

In analytical chemistry, particularly liquid chromatography, a large number of criteria have been studied that combine the characteristics of a chromatogram, such as the number of peaks, the resolution of all peak pairs, and the analysis time, eventually weighted, into one number; this is called a combined criterion. The general conclusion is that a noninterpretable number results that almost never gives a correct impression of the analytic quality.

ROYAL PHARMACEUTICAL SOCIETY LIBRARY
1, LAMBETH HIGH STREET, LONDON SE1 7JN

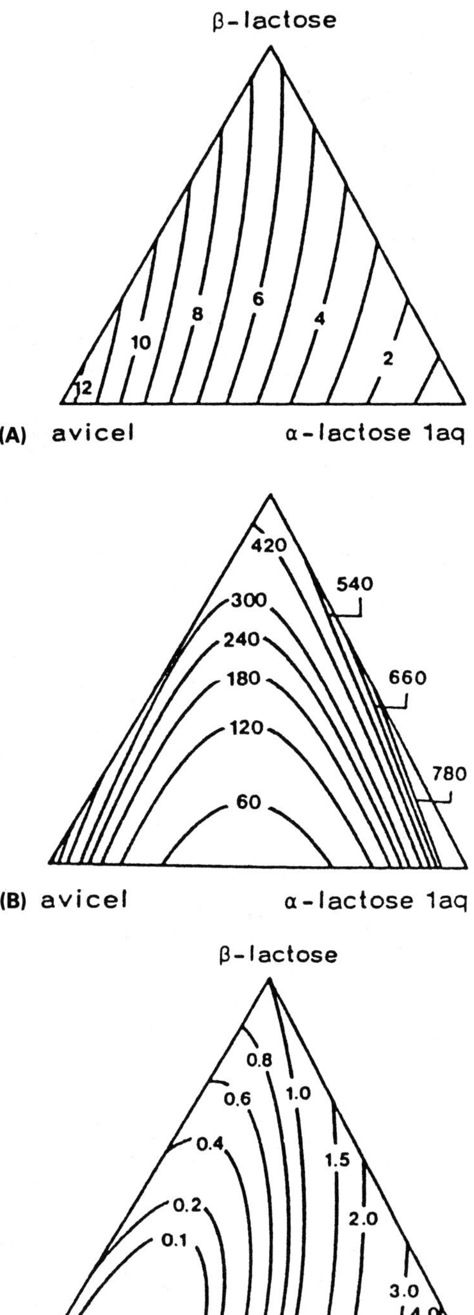

FIG. 31. Contour diagrams and levels of: (A) Crushing strength (kg); (B) Disintegration time (s), logarithmic transformed; (C) Friability (%). No disintegrant added. Compression force 10 kN. Reprinted with permission from Ref. 35.

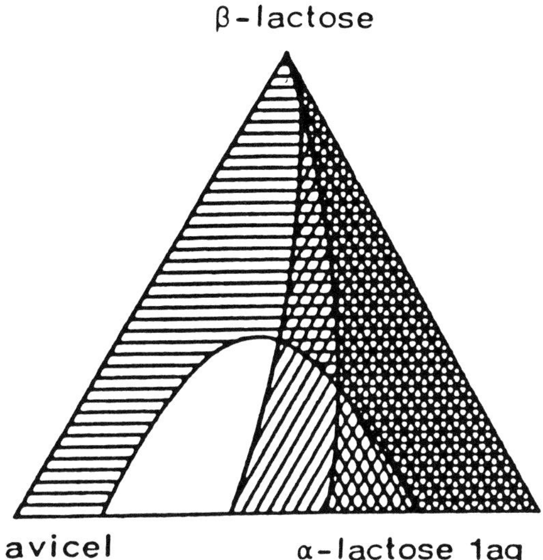

FIG. 32. Overlay diagram of the contours from Figs. 31 A, B, and C. Crushing strength < 6 kg; Disintegration time > 120 s; friability > 1.0- %. The blank area represents compositions that conform to all three requirements. (Reprinted with permission from Ref. 35).

In formulation research weighted combinations of criteria have been used, but only in a sequential (hill-climbing) strategy where, by nature of this strategy, it is the only possibility. For simultaneous methods the combination of criteria into one new criterion must be strongly discouraged. It does not give good results and far better methods are available.

Contour Overlay Diagrams

Once a model has been chosen for each of the objectives, the response surfaces can be scanned in small steps. A contour diagram can be drawn for each objective on transparent sheets or overlaid in one figure. Minimum and maximum boundaries must be set for acceptable objective values and marked in the separate contour diagrams. Then the region can be sought where all responses are acceptable; within that area an optimum can be found, trading off the different responses. The use of contour overlay diagrams is limited to three or four factors. Examples can be found in Refs. 36–38. Overlay diagrams are shown in Fig. 32.

Trade-off Methods

Although the combined-objective method and overlay-contour diagrams are essentially trade-off methods, they have been treated above separately because they rely on prior information and decisions with regard to weights and boundaries. A number of methods that do not require prior decisions are based on Pareto optimality (MCDM plots, biplots), desirability functions, and outranking methods (Promethee, Electre, Oreste, Gaia).

A tutorial on these methods, including contour-overlay plots and utility functions and a comparison of these methods, has been given by Hendriks et al. [39]. They conclude that all methods, except overlay-contour diagrams, perform well in multiobjective problems, the performance with many objectives being best for Promethee/Gaia and worst with Pareto optimality and overlay diagrams. The addition of biplots or stacked MCDM plots, however, makes Pareto optimality useful in higher dimensional problems. Together with the overlay diagrams the Pareto optimality concept is the most comprehensible; computations and interpretation are relatively simple.

Pareto Optimality

It is assumed that the factors are mixture variables (this explanation is also valid for process factors) and that for each of the objectives to be optimized a model is fitted with which the considered formulation properties can be predicted for every mixture composition in the factor space.

In the multicriteria decision-making (MCDM) approach, an MCDM plot is created from the predicted values of both objectives. The predictions are made at points in a regular grid in the factor space, using a fixed-scan percentage (1, 2, or 5%). Each scan point represents a specific mixture composition; it is entered in a graph with its two coordinates, the predicted values of the objectives. The space occupied by the resulting cloud of points is called the feasible criteria space. A special subset of the points (forming a shell partly around the cloud) are the pareto-optimal (PO) points, marked in Fig. 33.

A PO point is defined as a point in the feasible criteria space, if there exists no other point in that space which yields an improvement in one criterion without causing a degradation in the other. The set of PO points (in a table or in a graph) is the output of the MCDM method. This method does not result in any further reduction or selection; the

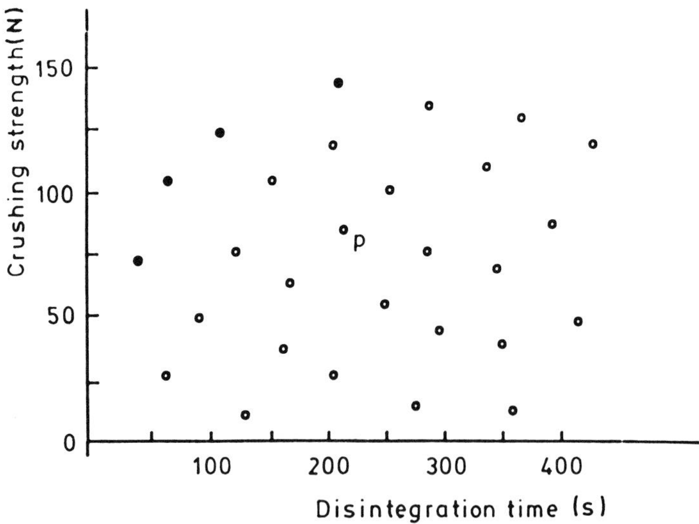

FIG. 33. Plot of the feasible criteria space of the crushing strength and the disintegration time; · = pareto optimal point; o = inferior point. (Reprinted with permission from Ref. 37).

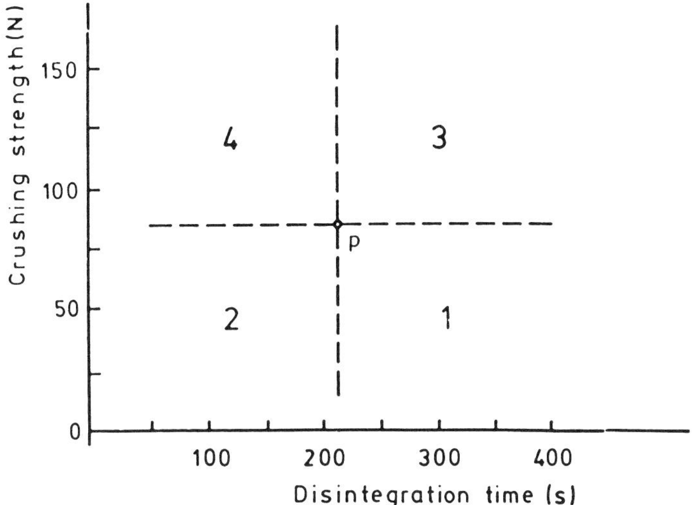

FIG. 34. Point p from Fig. 33, with an illustration of the four quadrants. (Reprinted with permission from Ref. 37).

experimenter has to make a choice, trading off one objective for other(s), according to acceptability, that is, the relative importance of the objectives considered.

For illustrative purposes, point p (Fig. 33) is depicted in Fig. 34 and the space around it is divided in four quadrants. The following deductions can be made about these quadrants.

Quadrant 1. All the points falling in this quadrant are inferior to point p, the considered mixtures having a larger disintegration time and a smaller crushing strength.

Quadrants 2 and *3.* Point p is incomparable to the points falling in these regions. Points in quadrant 2 have a lower crushing strength compared to point p but a better disintegration time; for quadrant 3 the reverse is true.

Quadrant 4. Point p is inferior to any point falling in quadrant 4 because it has a lower crushing strength and an inferior disintegration time.

Taking every point in Fig. 33 successively as a point p, all the inferior points can be removed by applying those three rules. Thus, only the noninferior (PO) points remain.

From the PO points shown in Fig. 35 identified in this way, the experimenter makes a choice. Thereafter, the selected PO points are traced back to the respective mixture compositions. For the example given in Fig. 33, these compositions are depicted in Fig. 36.

The experimenter can also take into account a preference for a specific mixture, that is, a binary over a ternary or quaternary. The MCDM procedure can equally well be used with process variables. It can easily be extended to more objectives [13, 39]. The MCDM/PO approach for up to six objectives is one of the options in the OMCA software package.

Designs for Hill Climbing

The aim of factorial and other experimental designs and of response surface methodology is to obtain insight into the behavior of a system, in this case a formulation or a process.

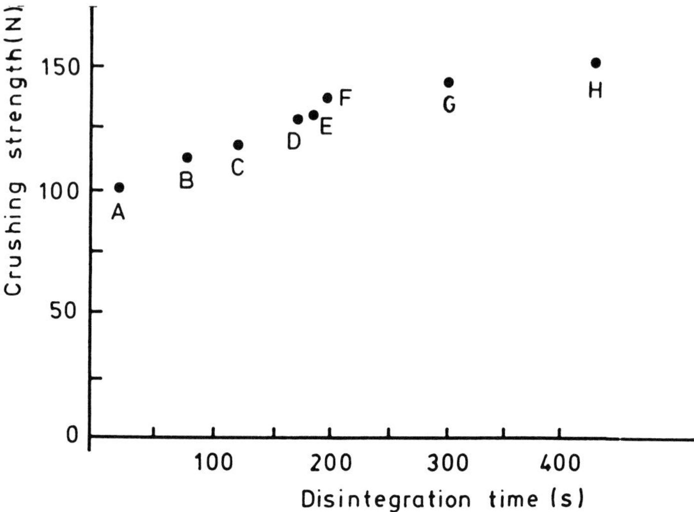

FIG. 35. MCDM plot of crushing strength and disintegration time. The points A-H are the Pareto optimal points. (Reprinted with permission from Ref. 37).

From that it can be learned which variables are factors, what are their effects on the responses, do interactions exist, and what is the range for a factor to give an acceptable or optimum response. In the case of a multivariable multiobjective problem, it can be learned which variable settings give acceptable or optimum values for all objectives.

The aim of sequential (hill-climbing) methods is more limited. It is primarily to find the optimum, not to model the response. No model is assumed, although a response surface exists. The only assumption is that the response surface is continuous.

There is also a practical difference. If the location of the acceptable response in factor space is not known, a sequential approach might lead very efficiently to the right

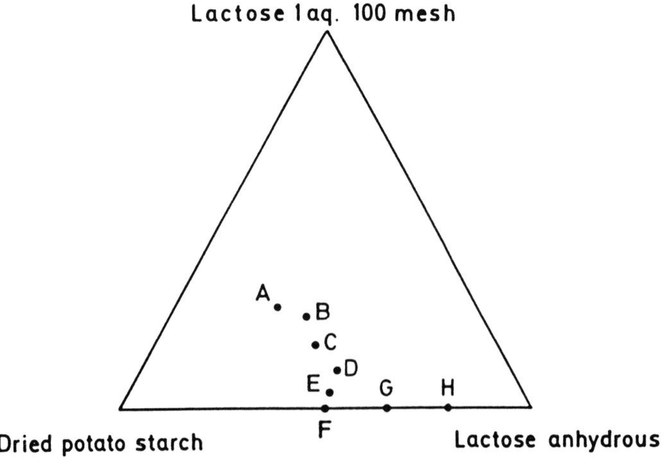

FIG. 36. PO-plot. The points A-H correspond to those in Fig. 35. (Reprinted with permission from Ref. 37).

area. If from a priori knowledge the interesting area is approximately known, an FD or CCD would give the desired information about the system with a limited number of experiments.

Sequential methods have in common that a small number of experiments are designed, the outcomes are evaluated, and new experiments are designed according to an algorithm that directs these new experiments toward the optimum. Although the optimum may not be a maximum but a minimum, the general term is hill climbing. The assumption is that the optimum will be found with the help of a sequential method with a minimum number of experiments. It is recommended that once an optimum has been found, new experiments around that optimum are performed according to a central composite design to obtain an impression of the robustness of the optimum. This information can then be used to establish tolerances for the factors.

Sequential methods can be applied only if

- the response surface is continuous,
- the factors are under reasonable control,
- the factors are continuously adjustable, and
- the experiments can be performed in a relatively short time.

Sequential methods in general cannot easily handle multimodal response surfaces (surfaces with several maxima or minima); the optimum found is not necessarily the global (overall) optimum. This problem can be solved by locating the small start design successively in different parts of the variable space. Thus the number of experiments will increase and the supposed advantage over simultaneous methods will be lost.

There are other drawbacks. Although it is possible to find a response surface by multiple linear regression on the experiments performed during hill climbing, this only gives information about the immediate neighborhood of the uphill path; no reliable knowledge can be obtained about the remaining part of the factor space. Furthermore, each objective has its own response surface. The sequential method is guided uphill by the slope of this single-response surface. It is inherently impossible to optimize several objectives at the same time. Combining objectives, eventually by assigning weight factors, gives numbers that are not interpretable unambiguously and should be discouraged. In addition, sequential methods are sensitive to experimental errors (noise), unless measurements are duplicated, but then an assumed advantage is lost.

Although most emphasis is on multivariate methods (optimizing more factors at a time) because of the interaction phenomenon, it should be recognized that even in univariate cases (optimizing one single factor at a time), there are other strategies than trial and error. These "univariate search" methods comprise binary search, single-step search, Fibonacci search (named after Leonardo Fibonacci of Pisa who lived from 1175–1230), and golden section search. These strategies have not found application so far in formulation research and are not discussed here. They have in common that they offer a method to place experiments efficiently in factor space, which in the one-factor case is a line segment.

Steepest Ascent

This method is easily visualized for the two-factor case (see Fig. 37). A starting area is chosen where a two-factor two-level factorial design is laid out, preferably with a repli-

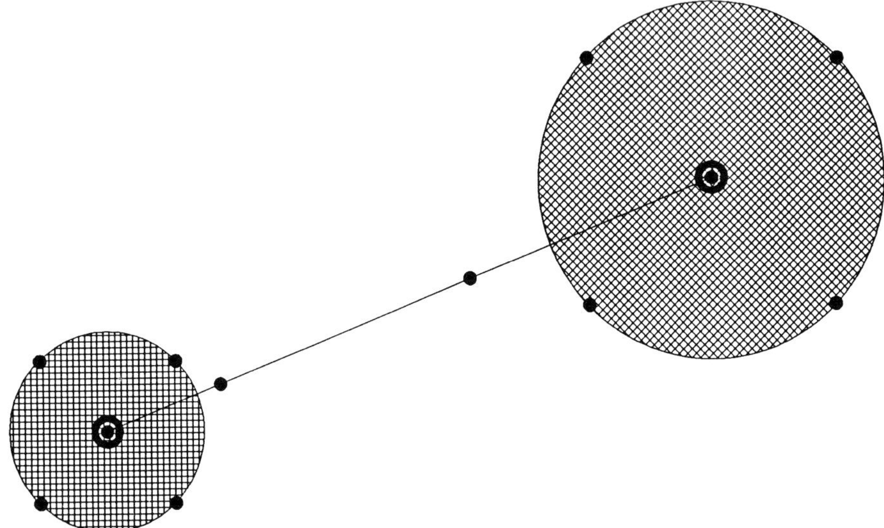

FIG. 37. Factorial design for steepest ascent (two factors); path uphill and second factorial design. (Reprinted with permission from Ref. 33).

cated center point. It is assumed that in this small part of the factor space the response surface can be approximated by a planar model, expressed by Eqs. (34).

$$E(y) = \beta_0 + \beta_1 x_1 + \beta_2 x_2 \quad \text{and} \quad y = b_0 + b_1 x_1 + b_2 x_2 + e \tag{34}$$

The measurements at the center point are used to estimate experimental error and, although this is not essential, to detect curvature. The other design points are used to calculate the direction in which the response surface rises most steeply. The assumption is, of course, that in that direction the optimum will most probably be found.

Using contrasts, E_i, as was explained earlier under Factorial Designs, values for b_i, the slopes in the directions x_i, are calculated as in Eqs. (35),

$$E_1 = (y_2 - y_1 + y_4 - y_3)/2 \quad \text{and} \quad E_2 = (y_3 - y_1 + y_4 - y)/2 \tag{35}$$

where E_i is average effect of changing factor x_i from the low to the high level, followed by $b_i = E_i/\Delta x_i$, the average effect per unit of x_i. Then the direction k of steepest ascent can be calculated with the help of Eq. (36).

$$k = \text{tg}\, \alpha = b_2/b_1 \tag{36}$$

Starting from the centerpoint, experiments are performed in the direction of steepest ascent until the response does not improve significantly anymore. Around this temporary optimum a new local factorial design is constructed to estimate the effect of the variables. The response will at least be closer to the maximum or minimum (provided there is only one optimum); the local design may even contain the optimum. If this is not the case, a new direction of steepest ascent can again be calculated and steps along this path taken until no improvement is attained anymore. There is a good chance that the response surface in that area will have less curvature. It thus may be advantageous to broaden the design to avoid the blurring effect of experimental error. In the neighborhood of the optimum, the system can be studied in more detail by adding a star design, together with the FD forming a central composite design, to detect curvature and estimate the optimum and its robustness more precisely.

As Forster and Bathe [40] have recently shown, in many textbooks that appeared between 1971 and 1990 an incorrect algorithm is given for the calculation of k, shown in Eq. (37).

$$k = E_2 \Delta x_2 / E_1 \Delta x_1 \tag{37}$$

This algorithm gives the correct direction of steepest ascent only if $\Delta x_1 \approx \Delta x_2$. Presumably this has been the cause of disappointment in the method of steepest ascent.

Sequential Simplex and Modifications

The original sequential simplex method (SM), first described by Spendley et al. [41] (not to be mistaken for the simplex lattice design), is a gradient method like the steepest ascent, but the progression rules are different. Details can be found in many publications (e.g., [42]).

The simplex is a geometrical figure with $(k + 1)$ vertices in k-dimensional factor space. In many applications in chemistry and pharmacy $k = 2$, and the simplex is an equilateral triangle, with a 3D response surface and 2D contour diagrams. With $k = 3$, the simplex is a tetrahedron, the response surface in 4D space, and the contour diagrams in 3D space.

The main progression rule is reflection of the vertex, with the worst response in the centroid of the opposing edge (of the triangle) or side (of the tetrahedron). For details the reader is referred to Ref. 42 or manuals of software (e.g., Elsevier's COPS).

A two-factor simplex can end up circling around one common vertex. This phenomenon is not observable when dealing with systems of higher dimensions. If circling is found around that vertex, a central composite design can be constructed to study the response surface in the neighborhood of the optimum in more detail.

Using the simplex method, a stop criterion must be formulated beforehand. It should be related to the standard deviation (SD) of the measurement in the region of the optimum, for example, twice the SD.

Only in the method of Spendley et al. [41] is the simplex a regular figure during the whole optimization process; the modification of Nelder and Mead [43], the modified simplex method (MSM), uses expansion and contraction in the direction of reflection to improve speed and decrease the number of experiments. Regularity is destroyed and the danger of degeneration arises. Routh et al. [44] developed the supermodified simplex (SMS), applying a more advanced strategy for expansion and contraction. Through the responses W, P (the centroid), and R, a quadratic model is fitted and the optimum O is estimated analytically. This estimated optimum is the new vertex. Modified and supermodified simplex are programmed for up to ten factors in Elsevier's software package COPS (formerly named CHEOPS).

Software for Designs and Optimization

Many commercial software packages are available which are either dedicated to experimental design or are of a more general statistical nature but have modules for experimental design.

Experimental Designs

Design Ease and Design Expert
OMEGA
COED
NEMROD

Programs of General Statistical Nature

SAS
SPSS
Statgraphics
Systat

Programs for sequential optimization, in particular sequential simplex, include COPS and simplex V.

A most important criterion for judgment of the utility of a program for design and data analysis is sound statistics, which is sufficient for the above programs as far as normal designs are concerned. For mixture designs, only Design Ease/Expert and OMEGA have special statistical facilities that take into account the mixture constraint and the absence of the intercept. SPSS, Statgraphics, and Systat have numerous statistical facilities, not only for experimental design and regression, but one should study the manuals carefully to ascertain if these also apply to mixture designs.

A special case is SAS, a very large package consisting of SAS-Base, the basic and excellent statistical core, and a large number of modules, of which in particular SAS-STAT, SAS-Quality Control (for generation of designs), and STAT-Graph (for graphs and figures) are excellent for optimization techniques. Moreover, SAS gives the possibility to program any algorithm and add them to the standard program, for example, the algorithms given by Cornell (see Bibliography) for the evaluation of mixture designs or the algorithms for calculating an "optimal design." A welcome feature for the pharmaceutical industry is that the FDA considers SAS a well-validated statistical package.

Design Ease, Design Expert, and OMEGA are much more dedicated. It is not possible to add algorithms, but in many cases this is not necessary.

Design Ease and Design Expert are very user friendly. They can be employed for all types of factorial designs and contain advisory schemes for fractional factorial designs down to Placket-Burmann designs (Design Ease) and for response surface methodology and mixture designs (Design Expert). They support several types of diagnostic statistical plots.

Omega is more limited, and supports only mixture designs, but within this restriction it is very user friendly, has good statistics (e.g., Pc, PRESS that are not included in other programs), good graphical facilities (in particular for overlay-contour plots for up to six objectives in which a trade off between objectives can be made visible), and extensive possibilities for designs in mixture components and pseudo-components. Moreover, it is the only program that supports multicriteria decision making by Pareto optimality, up to six objectives. COED (computer optimized experimental design) is the only program in this group that supports "optimal design."

Both COPS and SIMPLEX-V are directed only to sequential simplex. They perform well, although it is a handicap that graphical representation of the progress of simplex by nature is limited to the three-factor case. COPS has the advantage that a choice can be made between the original simplex method, the modified simplex [43], and two modifications of the supermodified simplex. Extensive descriptions of these packages can be found in the user manuals.

Optimization of Processes and Formulations

Applications are presented here of various methods for optimizing pharmaceutical formulations by experimental design methods or for determining the effect of the variables on the properties of the product. In several of the examples, a systematic search is conducted for the best formulation for products, representing an effective compromise under a given set of restrictions. Optimization in pharmaceutical development is most often focused at producing any combination of independent variables imparting desirable attributes to the final product. Process optimization is, therefore, indistinguishably linked to product optimization. For this reason, applications of optimization techniques are categorized into various types of pharmaceutical dosage forms, where process optimization is sometimes accomplished.

Examples of objectives for pharmaceutical preparations and processes described in experimentally designed studies are given in Tables 13 and 14 for illustrative purposes. Uniformity of the drug content and release characteristics, for examples, are of importance for most of these preparations.

TABLE 13 Objectives of Pharmaceutical Preparations

Form	Objectives
Tablets (general)	Crushing strength, weight uniformity, disintegration time, physical-chemical stability, thickness, porosity, content uniformity, in vitro dissolution
CR[a] tablets	release parameters, bioavailability
Effervescent tablets	chemical and physical stability
Hard gelatin capsules	Powder blend homogeneity, flow, weight, dissolution rate
Soft gelatin capsules	Solubility, release characteristics, chemical-physical stability
Suspensions	Chemical and physical stability
Spheroidal granules	In vitro release, flow rate, bulk density, friability, mean particle size
Microcapsules	In vitro release rate, size distribution, drug entrapment, surface-associated drug
Injectable solution	Solubility, stability
Eye drops	Viscosity, chemical stability
Film-coated products	Resistance to drug–water vapor permeability, resistance to disintegration, physical appearance (mottling, picking, peeling, cracking)

[a]Controlled release.

TABLE 14 Process Objectives for the Manufacture of Pharmaceutical Preparations

Process	Objectives
Synthesis of nanoparticles	Particle diameter, yield, composition, release characteristics
Film coating	Mechanical properties, release characteristics, resistance to disintegration, pitting and pin-hole formation
Microencapsulation	Polydispersity, micrometric properties, yield, release properties
Extrusion	Granulate hardness, porosity
Extrusion–spheronization	Yield, size distribution of spheres, granule friability, flow rate, mean particle size
Tableting	Lubrication, weight variation, efficient processing parameters, surface free energy
Granulation	Heat production, specific particle fraction, compaction rate of granules, particle size distribution, change in rotation rate, impellor shaft, distribution, flowability, median granule diameter, powder content

Tablets

Wet granulation, a procedure commonly used in the manufacture of tablets, is one of the most widely used technologies of size enlargement adopted by the pharmaceutical industry. Its objectives are, besides size enlargement, to overcome adverse electrostatic properties of a dry powder blend; to improve cohesion, flow, and density; and to prevent segregation of starting materials during processing. The granulation process is recognized for its complexity, due to the huge amount of variables that can affect the properties which are pertinent to the granular powder state, particularly physical and technological characteristics. The granulate properties can have an important influence on the processing of tablets and on their final quality.

Variables in the process of preparation of essentially spherical, free-flowing pellets on the properties of tablets were studied by Malinowski et al. [45]. The effects of extruder speed, screen size, spheronizer speed, spheronizer time, and water content at two levels on the crushing strength of the tablets, friability, disintegration time, and dissolution rate were assessed in a 2^5 full-factorial design. Evaluation of the results by analysis of variance showed, among other conclusions, that crushing strength increases by increasing extruder screen size and by reducing the other three independent variables. The dissolution rate was found to decrease as the amount of granulating solvent was increased. More information about the main and interaction effects could have been obtained from their experiments by regression analysis, fitting a second-order polynomial.

A systematic approach for granulation in a pilot-scale high shear mixer was presented by Holm et al. [46], illustrating the effect of process variables in the liquid addition phase of the granulation process with respect to the initial granule growth and the liquid distribution, using water-soluble (lactose) and insoluble (calcium hydrogen phosphate) excipients as starting materials. For both excipients, a 3×2^3 factorial design without replicates was applied and variables responsible for the observed differences were identified qualitatively by analysis of variance. The growth rate of the granules for both substances appeared to be determined mainly by the impeller speed, whereas the moisture distribution and the amount of lumps were affected primarily by both the impeller speed and the method of liquid addition. In a second paper Holm et al. [47] investigated the influence of kneading time, intensity of kneading, and atomization of binder on further granule

TABLE 15 Experimental Design for Two Factors[a]

Form No.	x_1(mL)[b]	x_2[c]
1	1	1
2	1	−1
3	−1	1
4	−1	−1
5	0	0
6	1.414	0
7	0	1.414
8	−1.414	0
9	0	−1.414

[a]From Ref. 49 with permission.
[b]Total amount of ethanol and water.
[c]Volume ratio of ethanol to water.

TABLE 16 Translation of Experimental Conditions to Units[a]

Factor	1.414	1	0	−1	−1.414
x_1[b](mL)	880	851	780	709	680
x_2[c]	0.4414	0.4	0.3	0.2	0.1586

[a]From Ref. 49 with permission.
[b]Total amount of ethanol and water.
[c]Volume ratio of ethanol to water.

growth and liquid distribution. The factorial experiments allowed to clearly distinguish between the granule growth processes of lactose and calcium hydrogen phosphate.

Paschos et al. [48] performed a granulation study with a high-speed mixer-granulator-dryer, in which drying was achieved by partial vacuum and increasing temperature. Starting with a 2^4 factorial design for determining a simplified empirical relationship and for screening the four independent variables for influence on granule and tablet properties, they found the ratio between the volume of binder solution and powder mass and the gelatin concentration of the binder solution to be the main factors for most of the objectives. Validity of the model was tested by performing a second factorial study. Factor effects on selected objectives provided insight in the applied granulation system.

The optimal conditions for preparing tablets by wet granulation in a high-speed mixer–granulator with variable amounts of granulating solution and volume ratio of ethanol to water in this solution was investigated by Shirakura et al. [49], using response surface methodology (Tables 15 and 16). Several responses, including disintegration time, crushing strength, and the physical stability during storage were obtained in a 2^2 factorial design augmented with a star design ($\alpha = 1.414$) and a center point and fitted by a second-order polynomial regression model with interaction term, shown in Eq. (38).

$$E(y) = \beta_0 + \beta_1 x_1 + \beta_2 x_2 + \beta_{12} x_1 x_2 + \beta_{11} x_1^2 + \beta_{22} x_2^2 \tag{38}$$

After defining the restrictions on the characteristics of interest, the optimal formulation was found by a computer optimization technique. The predicted values correlate well with the experimental data. Three-dimensional response surface plots for all responses are given; they show the quadratic and interaction effects except for tablet hardness which is nearly linear dependent on both factors (Figs. 38 and 39).

Gordon et al. [50] studied in a high shear mixer the effect of incorporating croscarmellose sodium at various concentrations intragranularly, extragranularly, or distributed equally between the two phases, and the effect of the granulation moisture content on the friability and the dissolution of a poorly soluble drug at high concentration. It should be emphasized that the use of crushing strength as independent variable is not quite straightforward. For statistical significant characterization of the independent variables, 24 batches of tablets were prepared. The design was determined according to optimal design theory by a computer program (computer-optimized experimental design, COED). It was not indicated which algorithm was used. Dissolution efficiency was increased by incorporating the superdisintegrant intragranularly rather than extragranularly.

In their proposal for a general procedure for computer optimization of pharmaceutical formulations, Schwartz et al. [51] focused on the optimization of a tablet with four independent formulation variables and one process variable:

x_1 = diluent ratio, calcium phosphate–lactose
x_3 = disintegrant level, starch, 1 exp. unit = 1 mg
x_4 = binder level, gelatin, 1 exp. unit = 0.5 mg
x_5 = lubricant level, magnesium stearate, 1 exp. unit = 0.5 mg
x_2 = compressional force, a process variable

The sum of the mixture components (the total mass) was not kept constant and all variables were treated as unconstrained factors within the experimental region. A $2^{(5-1)}$ fractional factorial design was constructed, but no indication was given which factor was aliased with the four-factor interaction. The 16-point design was expanded with a star design to a five-factor orthogonal central composite design without replicated center point (27 batches). The value 1.547 for α was not disputed, but certainly would not lead to a rotatable design. The values for the responses (disintegration time, crushing strength, dissolution rate, friability, weight, thickness, porosity, and mean pore diameter) were fitted by a second-order polynomial with quadratic and only two-factor interaction terms. The lack of fit for three of the responses was larger than desirable. Constrained linear programming was used to find a feasible region for a number of formulations. In the feasibility region, a grid search was performed and the most suitable formulation was selected. In a second paper, Schwartz et al. [52] applied the results of the previous computer optimization technique for troubleshooting. Their objective was to increase the dissolution response of a production tablet without sacrificing other tablet properties.

A wide variety of materials have been introduced as excipients for direct compression. The application of a simplex lattice mixture design in the development and optimization of the composition of direct compression mixtures has been demonstrated by Huisman et al. [53]. The mixtures of α-lactose monohydrate, α-lactose anhydrous, and dried potato starch were not constrained and allowed measurements of disintegration time and crushing strength at all design points. The responses of the crushing strength were best fitted with the special cubic model by multiple linear regression analysis. Areas of interest for selecting the best formulation were obtained by superimposing the contour plots of the responses (see Figs. 31 and 32).

In a series of papers, Bos et al. [54, 55] studied the influence of several process and formulation variables on α-lactose monohydrate–rice starch tablets, with emphasis on the physical stability in storage at two temperatures and humidities. Bos [56] used a combined design (Fig. 27(A)) for identifying tablet formulations with acceptable physical sta-

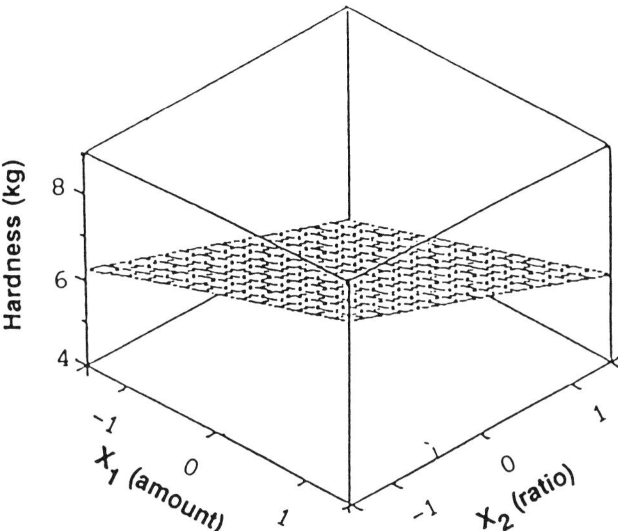

FIG. 38. Three-dimensional plot of disintegration time of tablets as function of x_1 and x_2. (Reprinted with permission from Ref. 49.)

bility: at each point of a mixture design (three components) the process parameters compression load and mixing time with magnesium stearate were varied according to a 2^2 factorial design. The physical stability of the tablets after storage was assessed with the selection criteria storage-to-initial ratio (SIR) of the crushing strength and of the disintegration time. The author, however, does not disclose the evaluation of the performed statistical analysis.

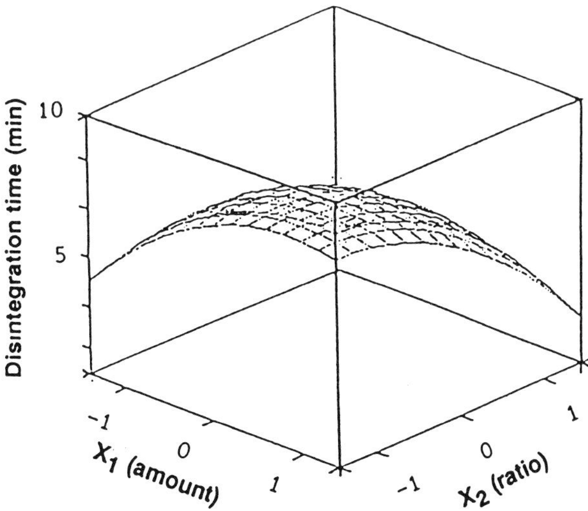

FIG. 39. Three-dimensional plot of tablet hardness as function of x_1 and x_2. (Reprinted with permission from Ref. 49.).

Fenyvesi et al. [57] assessed the effectiveness of cyclodextrin polymer in tablets as an additive to improve the dissolution parameters of the formulation with a poorly soluble drug as the most important response. Moreover, stability of crushing strength, disintegration time, and weight increase of the tablets were included. By varying the content of microcrystalline cellulose and cyclodextrin in the direct compression mixtures in a 2^2 factorial design augmented to a central composite design (nine batches of tablets; $\alpha = 2$, indicating a poor rotatability of the design), they found by regression analysis with a quadratic model that the dissolution rate of furosemide was completely determined by the linear and quadratic terms of cyclodextrin concentration. At the end of the optimization procedure, minimum specifications were set for all objectives, weights were given to the objectives, and the constraints relaxed until a solution was found that was judged to be optimum.

Controlled-Release Tablets

Hydrophilic matrix tablets, comprising fractions of microcrystalline cellulose, lactose, dicalcium phosphate dihydrate, and a fixed amount of basic granulate with drug and gums have been optimized by Waaler et al. [58], using the three-pseudo-component simplex centroid design. The pseudo-components can be imagined as microcrystalline cellulose, lactose, and calciumphosphate, each mixed with the same amount of the base granulate. The simplex centroid design can be pictured as a triangular cross-section parallel to the base of a trigonal pyramid, with the base granulate at the top. Quadratic and special cubic models were fitted to the response's release rate, weight variation, friability, and crushing strength by means of regression analysis. For both models almost identical adjusted coefficients of determination R^2_{adj} were calculated. Evaluation of the contour plots clearly showed, as an example, the lowering effects of dicalcium phosphate on the release characteristics from the matrix systems. The conclusion was that the simplex centroid design is applicable in tablet optimization when a wet massing step is a part of the process; the conclusion can be extended to all types of mixture designs.

Franz et al. [59] evaluated the in vitro release characteristics and physical properties of mixed polymeric matrix systems for sustained oral delivery of a benzodiazepine derivate. The key variables identified in preliminary experiments included the ratio of different viscosity grades of hydroxypropyl methylcellulose, the ratio of sodium carboxymethylcellulose to lactose in the formulation, and the matrix drug loading. The three-factor uniform precision rotatable central composite design (Table 17) was selected for the response surface study; the rotatability is connected with the value chosen for $\alpha = 1.682$ (see Table 12).

Second-order regression models with quadratic and two-factor interaction terms were applied to describe the physical parameters of the matrix (crushing strength, thickness, moisture uptake, and drug uniformity) as well as the various delivery parameters derived from the cube-root dissolution model and the frequently used exponential model. The predicted responses of the optimal matrix formulation obtained by constrained optimization agreed fairly well with the experimentally obtained responses.

Perez-Marcos et al. [60] studied hydrophilic drug-delivery systems with three types of carboxyvinyl polymers, together with the polymer concentration in the formulation and compression force at two levels in a 3×2^2 factorial design for their impact on dissolution

TABLE 17 Uniform Precision Rotatable Central Composite Design for Three Variables[a]

Trial Formulation Number[b]	Variable Level in Coded Form		
	x_1	x_2	x_3
1	−1	−1	−1
2	+1	−1	−1
3	−1	+1	−1
4	+1	+1	−1
5	−1	−1	+1
6	+1	−1	+1
7	−1	+1	+1
8	+1	+1	+1
9	−1.682	0	0
10	+1.6582	0	0
11	0	−1.682	0
12	0	+1.682	0
13	0	0	−1.682
14	0	0	+1.682
15	0	0	0
16	0	0	0
17	0	0	0
18	0	0	0
19	0	0	0
20	0	0	0

[a]From Ref. 59 with permission.
[b]Formulations were randomized during actual experimentation.

efficiency and the tablet parameters crushing strength, friability, and porosity. The influences of the variables on the observations were identified by variance analysis. Regression analysis quantification of the factor effects on the dissolution efficiency of the water-soluble drug showed that the polymer concentration was the only factor of importance.

An extreme-vertices design (Fig. 40) for three formulation factors (polyvinyl pyrrolidone (PVP), carboxyvinyl polymer, and crystalline cellulose) and one process factor (tablet dimension) was applied by Hirata et al. [61] to optimize the parameters of a simple exponential equation for the in vitro release of chlorpheniramine maleate from matrix tablets. By multiple regression analysis with a modified special cubic model, taking into account the process factor, it was demonstrated that the predicted values of the release parameters showed good agreement with the experimental data.

Silicone elastomer latex as wet granulation agent in controlled-release matrix tablets has been evaluated by Li and Tu [62] in a $2^{(5-1)}$ fractional factorial design with compression force, drying temperature, drug-to-polymer ratio, silicone-to-silica ratio, and pH of the dissolution medium as independent variables. Factors and factor interactions affecting the slope of the plot of the cumulative percent drug released vs. the square root of time have been detected by variance analysis.

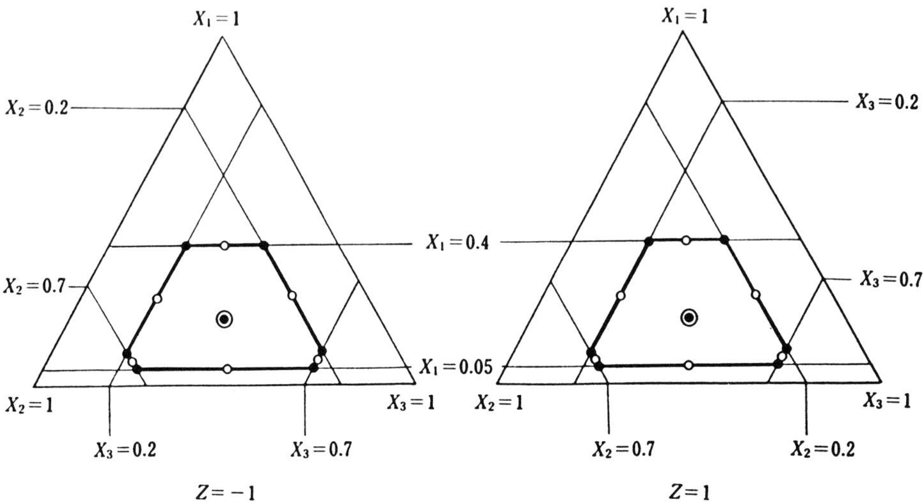

FIG. 40. Extreme-vertices design for three components and one process factor (not fractionated). (Reprinted with permission from Ref. 61.)

Effervescent Tablets

A full 2^3 factorial design was employed by El-Banna et al. [63] to find a regression equation expressing the effects of compression force, aspirin content, and particle size of ingredients on the crushing strength of effervescent tablets prepared by direct compression. This approach cannot separate the impact of variable tablet weight on the crushing strength, indicating that for this problem a combined mixture and factorial design would be preferable. In a second paper, El-Banna et al. [64] optimized the hardness of effervescent acetylsalicylic acid tablets using the percentage of the drug, the particle size of the ingredients, the solvent composition, the dipping time, and finally the compression force as independent variables. After regression analysis of the results, arranged according to a $2^{(5-2)}$ fractional factorial design with design generators $x_4 = x_1x_2x_3$ and $x_5 = x_2x_3$, the steepest ascent method was applied to find the optimum conditions for preparing the effervescent tablets.

Devay et al. [65] performed an optimization study on the operational parameters in fluidized-bed granulation of effervescent tablets. The effects of two independent formulation variables and two technological variables,

x_1 = citric acid–sodium bicarbonate ratio,
x_2 = PVP content of granulating liquid,
x_3 = air temperature, and
x_4 = air velocity,

on granule size, powder content, and dissolution rate of the tablets have been studied with a $2^{(4-1)}$ factorial design in which x_4 was confounded with the four-factor interaction term. After defining the appropriate quality properties in terms of constraints on the criteria, the optimal settings of the independent variables were found by the method of steepest ascent.

The effects of temperature and humidity on the stability of four commercially available effervescent and dispersable aspirin tablet products were determined by Bulut et al.

[66] at two levels in a 2^2 factorial design. Variance analysis showed that the impact of temperature is different for the various products, whereas the effect of humidity significantly depended on the packaging quality.

Capsules

Operating with a semiautomatic capsule machine, Reier et al. [67] investigated the mean capsule-fill weight and weight variation by preparing powder blends varying in mean particle size, particle size distribution, specific volume, and flowability. The excipients microcrystalline cellulose, dicalcium phosphate, lactose, talc, and magnesium stearate were incorporated at various concentrations. In addition, three operating speeds and three capsule sizes were included. By combining the number of blends and taking one third replicates of the different filling conditions, the experimental effort was considerably reduced. For different operating conditions, the mean gross capsule weight, capsule weight standard deviation, and coefficient of variation could be predicted by simplified quadratic equations.

The effect of additives on the in vitro release of drugs from hard gelatin capsules was the subject of a series of papers by Newton and co-workers. For the drugs nitrofurantoin, nitrofurazone, oxytetracycline dihydrate, and tetracycline hydrochloride, Newton and Razzo [68] applied a 3×2^3 factorial design for the qualitative factor diluent (three levels, lactose, Primojel, and Dry Flow Starch) and three quantitative factors (diluent, 20 or 80%, magnesium stearate, and sodium lauryl sulfate, for both presence or absence at 1% level). The surfactant did not significantly enhance drug release. Moreover, the authors concluded that the impact of additives on drug release cannot be always anticipated. The data in their paper are insufficient, however, to check their conclusions.

A predetermined set of constrained objectives for the compaction rate and the amount of drug dissolved at 8 and 30 min of a capsule formulation was aimed for in the study of Shek [69], employing the simplex method of optimization. Independent variables included drug concentration, disintegrant, and lubricant, and the total capsule weight. The three dependent variables were combined into one response. After the optimum had been reached, a second-order polynomial equation was fitted to the observations to estimate the response surface. During the simplex procedure, measurements were taken at 45 vertices (of which three were replicates). It is questionable if the simplex is a good choice for this problem as well because of the combined criteria and the number of experiments.

Controlled-Release Capsules

In the design of a controlled-release hydrophilic matrix capsule containing blends of anionic and nonionic cellulose ether polymers, Hussain et al. [70] compared an artificial neural network technique with response-surface methodology in their precision of prediction of the in vitro release performance (release exponent and dissolution half time). Factor effects were studied with the help of the four-pseudo-component simplex centroid mixture design shown in Fig. 41. Evaluation of the mean sum of squared residuals for a validation data set revealed that for both release parameters the neural computing method predicted the response values more precisely than the response-surface method applying the special quartic equation.

Ortigosa et al. [71] performed two 2^3 factorial designed studies, focusing on the effects of the properties of lipophilic material on the in vitro release kinetics of theophylline

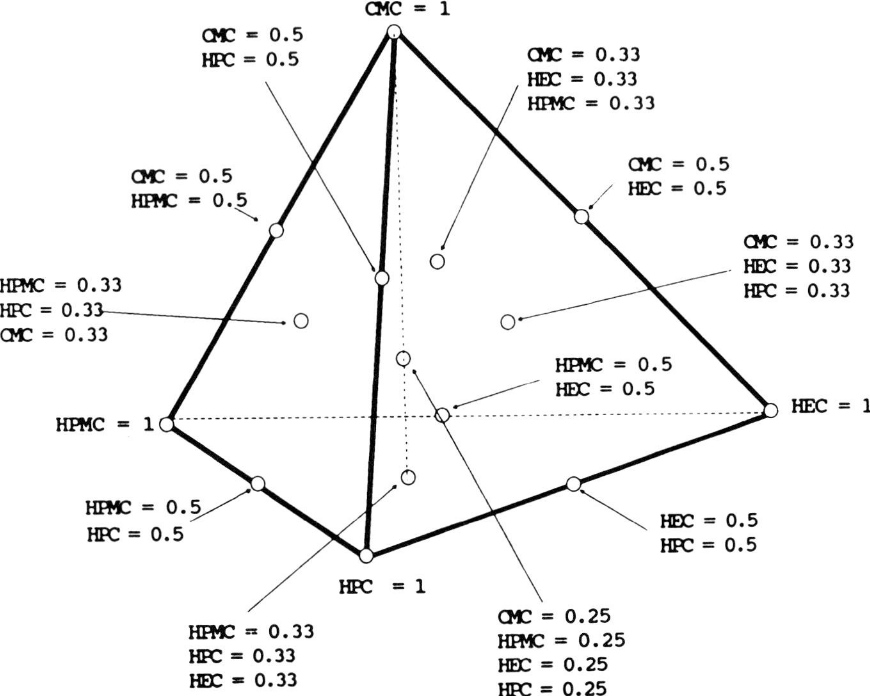

FIG. 41. The four- (pseudo)-component simplex centroid design. The drug-to-polymer ratio is kept constant at 1:3. (Reprinted with permission from Ref. 70.)

in semisolid matrix capsules. The variables pH of the dissolution medium and speed of paddle rotation were successively combined with the melting point and hydrophile-lipophile balance (HLB) value of the excipient for controlled drug delivery. The in vitro release points after 2 h were fitted with second-order polynomial equations.

Spherical Granules

Uniform, free-flowing granulations prepared by extrusion-spheronization, as described in Ref. 45, were investigated by Malinowski and Smith [72], defining relevant capsule-fill parameters such as flow rate, bulk density, granule friability, and mean particle size as dependent variables. A 2^5 full factorial design was used for the independent variables water content, extruder speed, extruder screen size, spheronizer speed, and spheronizer residence time. Only qualitative estimation of main effects, first-order and second-order interactions have been assessed. A small increase in experimental effort by adding star design points and regression analysis on the data would have permitted a quantitative evaluation.

Hileman et al. [73] used a 12-run Plackett-Burman screening design in the characterization of the main effects of eight formulation and process variables on the final pellet drug content, density, and roundness in an extrusion-spheronization process. The high drug-loaded pellets were intended to be appropriate for controlled-release coating and for filling particularly sized capsules. The independent variables studied were the type of

TABLE 18 Levels and Variation Intervals of Factors Under Investigation[a]

Factors	Base Level (0)	High Level (+1)	Low Level (−1)	Variation Interval (I)
x_1, Phase ratio	12.5:1	15:1	10:1	2.5
x_2, Temperature (°C)	75	90	60	15
x_3, Speed of rotation (s^{-1})	12.5	15	10	2.5
x_4, Time of rotation (s)	240	360	120	120

[a]From Ref. 75 with permission.

microcrystalline cellulose (Avicel RC581 or RC591, a qualitative factor), Avicel concentration, extruder screen size, spheronizer speed, residence time, water concentration, feeder speed, and plate rotational speed. Only the first six factors appeared to be of importance for the final product. It would have been of interest to extend the study to a less fractionated factorial design, retaining the influential factors and study interactions.

Microcapsules

Hassan et al. [74] applied a four-factor central composite design (27 experimental batches) to develop magnetic drug-containing chitosan microspheres with optimal characteristics in a combined emulsion–polymer cross-linking–solvent-evaporation technique. By regression analysis, relationships were obtained between drug entrapment, surface-associated drug, an overall desirability function for simultaneous evaluation of several responses, and four independent variables (amount of drug added, cross-linking time, glutaraldehyde concentration, and amount of Arlacel-83 in the emulsification step). Conditions for the manufacture of microcapsules with high drug entrapment and low surface-associated drug were derived by response-surface graphic analysis.

In the preparation of microcapsules by melt dispersion, Devay and Racz [75] focused on the average particle size as a function of four operational variables: phase ratio, temperature, speed of rotation, and time of rotation (Tables 18 and 19).

Analysis of the responses in the $2^{(4-1)}$ fractional factorial design showed that the model for the particle size was linear and that the factor interactions were not significant. Devay and Racz [76] also studied the effect of four independent variables (acetylsalicylic acid content, ethylcellulose viscosity, agitation speed, and rate of hexane addition) on particle size and particle size distribution of microcapsules of ethylcellulose prepared by phase separation. In this process, recrystallization of the active compound occurred before coacervation. The observations obtained in a $2^{(4-1)}$ fractional factorial design were described by polynomials and the sequence of effectiveness of the factors was determined. Significant positive two-factor interactions between the first three factors were found; the rate of hexane addition was not significant.

Nanoparticles of poly(D,L-lactide/glycolide) (PLA/GA) were produced by Julienne et al. [77] using a solvent-evaporation method. After screening the technological and formulation variables, a three-factor rotatable central composite design ($\alpha = 1{,}682$) was chosen to evaluate simultaneously the most relevant factors for controlling mean particle size, coefficient of variation, and polydispersity of the particle size distribution; these factors include phase volume ratio, polymer concentration, and homogenization pressure

TABLE 19 Matrix of Factorial Design with Experimental and Calculated Response and Regression Coefficients[a]

	Factors								Particle Size (mm)	
Trial	x_0	x_1	x_2	x_3	x_4 $(x_1x_2x_3)$	x_1x_2	x_1x_3	x_2x_3	Exp.	Calcd.
1	+	+	+	+	+	+	+	+	0.403	0.409
2	+	+	−	+	−	−	+	−	0.511	0.508
3	+	−	+	+	−	−	−	+	0.518	0.523
4	+	−	−	+	+	+	−	−	0.549	0.545
5	+	+	+	−	−	+	−	−	0.512	0.506
6	+	+	−	−	+	−	−	+	0.524	0.527
7	+	−	+	−	+	−	+	−	0.547	0.542
8	+	−	−	−	−	+	+	+	0.638	0.642
bj	0.5253	−0.0378	−0.0303	−0.0291	−0.0195	−0.0003	−0.0005	−0.0045		

[a]From Ref. 75 with permission.

TABLE 20 Real Values Corresponding to the Three-Variables Central Composite Design and Particle Size Distribution Parameters[a]

	Independent Variables[b]						Response Values[c]		
	Orthogonal Values			Real Values			Size	C.V.	Polydispersity,
Formulation	x_1	x_2	x_3	x_1	x_2	x_3	(nm)	(%)	MU2/ Gamma SQ
1	−1	−1	−1	15.00	2.50	100.00	178	22	0.080
2	1	−1	−1	35.00	2.50	100.00	325	22	0.081
3	−1	1	−1	15.00	7.50	100.00	268	27	0.062
4	1	1	−1	35.00	7.50	100.00	406	33	0.142
5	−1	−1	1	15.00	2.50	200.00	188	38	0.090
6	1	−1	1	35.00	2.50	200.00	332	18	0.080
7	−1	1	1	15.00	7.50	200.00	236	25	0.097
8	1	1	1	35.00	7.50	200.00	466	34	0.178
9	−1.682	0	0	8.18	5.00	150.00	177	32	0.088
10	1.682	0	0	41.82	5.00	150.00	616	40	0.143
11	0	−1.682	0	25.00	0.79	150.00	220	31	0.126
12	0	1.682	0	25.00	9.20	150.00	343	25	0.105
13	0	0	−1.682	25.00	5.00	65.90	312	22	0.107
14	0	0	1.682	25.00	5.00	234.10	273	24	0.107
15	0	0	0	25.00	5.00	150.00	279	21	0.046
16	0	0	0	25.00	5.00	150.00	289	21	0.068
17	0	0	0	25.00	5.00	150.00	308	31	0.055
18	0	0	0	25.00	5.00	150.00	294	22	0.063
19	0	0	0	25.00	5.00	150.00	291	23	0.059
20	0	0	0	25.00	5.00	150.00	278	22	0.065

[a]From Ref. 77 with permission.
[b]x_1 = Phase volume ratio (percent v/v); x_2 = PLA/GA concentration in organic phase (percent w/v); x_3 = homogenization pressure (bars).
[c]Of mean particle size, coefficient of variation, and polydispersity.

(see Table 20). The two most influential factors were studied in depth by employing a 3^2 factorial design and evaluating the results with variance and regression analyses.

El Banna and Efimova [78] employed a $2^{(6-3)}$ fractional factorial design for microencapsulation in a fluidized bed. They assessed the influence of the relative mean diameter and of x_1 = particle size of core material, x_2 = feeding rate volume, x_3 = ratio shellac–polyvinyl pyrrolidone, x_4 = volume of the coating solution, x_5 = pressure of compressed air, and x_6 = temperature of fluidizing air on the amount of sodium chloride released in the acidic solution after 1-h exposure. As can be seen from Table 21, x_4 was combined with x_1x_2, x_5 with x_2x_3, and x_6 with $x_1x_2x_3$. The authors draw the firm conclusions that factor x_4 has the strongest influence, but that the influences of x_3 and x_5 are also highly significant. They do not mention, however, the possibility that this influence (except that of x_3) might be also caused by the aliased interactions.

Solutions

In the optimization of a solution for oral administration with a slightly water-soluble drug and a nonionic surfactant, Senderak et al. [79] defined the cloud point and turbidity as the dependent variables. In a sequential approach, a 2^4 factorial design with four center

TABLE 21 Matrix of the Fractional Factorial Design for the Eight Treatment Combinations and the Resulting Responses[a]

	Factors								Responses			
									1[b]		2[c]	
Exp. No.	X_0	X_1	X_2	X_3	X_4 (X_1X_2)	X_5 (X_2X_3)	X_6 ($X_1X_2X_3$)	X_1X_3	Experim.	Predicted	Experim.	Predicted
1	+	−	−	−	+	+	−	+	15.77	15.77	2.26	2.15
2	+	+	−	−	−	+	+	−	68.12	68.11	1.09	1.02
3	+	−	+	−	−	−	+	+	58.15	58.17	1.37	1.44
4	+	+	+	−	+	−	−	−	8.06	8.07	1.63	1.74
5	+	−	−	+	+	−	+	−	16.64	16.63	1.65	1.57
6	+	+	−	+	−	−	−	+	68.47	68.45	1.01	0.88
7	+	−	+	+	−	+	−	−	84.00	84.03	1.17	1.30
8	+	+	+	+	+	+	+	+	18.67	18.69	1.07	1.15

[a]From Ref. 78 with permission.
[b]Amount of sodium chloride released in the acidic dissolution medium (%).
[c]Relative mean microcapsule diameter.

TABLE 22 Sample Composition[a]

Component	Concentration (% w/v)
Drug 1 (slightly water soluble)	0.3
Drug 2 (water soluble)	0.6
Drug 3 (water soluble)	0.3
Butylated hydroxytoluene	0.01
Oleic acid	0.25
Lactic acid 50%	0.06
Alcohol USP	2.0
Sodium hydroxide 50% solution	qs[b] to pH 5.3–5.5
Purified water	qs[b]

[a]Adapted from Ref. 79 with permission.
[b]Quantity sufficient.

points for screening purposes was set up first. All components of the solution were kept constant except alcohol (1 or 5%), polysorbate 80 (2 or 4%), propylene glycol (5 or 25%), and sucrose invert medium (25 or 65%). The solution was brought to the desired volume with purified water. The factorial design was followed by a central composite design with six center points (see Tables 22 and 23) in which the alcohol was kept constant at 2%, whereas the factor ranges were focused on the region where turbidity was no more than 4 ppm and the cloud point was no less than 60° C. The CCD was evaluated with a second-order model.

Since a typical mixture problem is described here, the appropriate approach would have been to screen for relevant composition variables and subsequently to use an extreme-vertices design with four (pseudo)components, that is, polysorbate, propylene glycol, and invert sugar medium.

An extreme-vertices design (Fig. 42) with 14 points was derived by Anik and Sukumar [80] for a solubility study on butoconazole nitrate, an antifungal agent, in a multicomponent system comprising polyethylene glycol 400, glycerin, polysorbate 60, water, and one component, poloxamer 407, fixed at 10%. An estimation of the response surface was provided by regression analysis with a quadratic mixture model, resulting in an adequate equation for calculating solubilities in any formulation of interest.

A 2^3 factorial design was used by Karabit et al. (81), who screened the variables pH, tonicity of the solution, and presence of EDTA on the preservative efficacy of phenol. The slopes of the survivor curves were subjected to variance analysis, and a qualitative insight was obtained on the effects of the formulation variables and their interactions.

Patel et al. [82] assessed the effects of pH, ethylenediaminetetraacetic acid (EDTA), and PVP in ophthalmic solutions of Enalkiren on aqueous humor drug levels in the rabbit eye. The in vivo data obtained by arranging the experiments according to a 2^3 factorial design were statistically evaluated with ANOVA. From the results it was difficult to identify the only significant terms, pH and the interaction between pH and PVP. Nevertheless, the factorial experimental setup allowed screening for the best of the ophthalmic solutions by comparison of the mean responses.

Gupta et al. [83] applied a 2^4 x 3 factorial design in a stability study of doxorubicin hydrochloride in solution. The independent variables were temperature, light, composition of the medium, ionic strength, and pH. Qualitative factor effects on the values of a

TABLE 23 Composition of Samples for the Second-Order Experimental Design[a]

	Concentration (% w/v)			Response Variables	
Preparation Order	Polysorbate 80	Propylene Glycol	Sucrose Invert Medium	Turbidity (ppm)	Cloud Point (°C)
12	3.7	17	49	3.1	75.7
7	4.3	17	49	2.8	73.5
5	3.7	23	49	3.9	80.5
4	4.3	23	49	3.1	83.7
2	3.7	17	61	6.0	62.0
11	4.3	17	61	3.4	69.5
8	3.7	23	61	3.5	69.9
9	4.3	23	61	1.8	70.8
17	3.5	20	55	4.9	73.4
16	4.5	20	55	3.3	74.6
13	4.0	15	55	4.5	81.9
15	4.0	25	55	5.1	69.5
18	4.0	20	45	3.3	80.7
14	4.0	20	65	3.2	59.9
1	4.0	20	55	2.3	67.7
3	4.0	20	55	3.8	74.9
6	4.0	20	55	2.9	72.7
10	4.0	20	55	2.4	74.8
19	4.0	20	55	3.5	70.4
20	4.0	20	55	3.2	72.8

[a]From Ref. 79 with permission.

parameter for drug loss were found by variance analysis. Besides the main factor effects, a two- and a three-way interaction were found to be significant. Regression analysis could have provided more quantitative insight in the effects of the various variables on the stability of the drug in solution.

Film-Coated Products

Dincer and Ozdurmus [84] reported empirical relationships between four independent process and formulation variables (concentration of the film-forming methacrylic acid–methyl methacrylate copolymer, x_1; concentration of the plasticizer dibutylphthalate, x_2; total spraying time of coating solution, x_3; and length of drying interval, x_4) and the disintegration time of the film-coated tablets in simulated intestinal fluid. A second objective was the investigation of the resistance to disintegration of the coated film in simulated gastric fluid. A preliminary tolerance study defined the suitable levels of the independent variables. A $2^{(4-1)}$ fractional factorial design with four replicated center points was used; x_1 was confounded with the three-factor interaction $x_2x_3x_4$. The responses could be fitted adequately by first-order polynomials, but curvature was not tested for, although that would have been possible because of the replicated center point. ANOVA results demonstrated that the regression coefficients of the main effects of all variables were significant. With the help of the steepest descent method, various combinations of variable levels were found, resulting in coated tablets with responses in the restricted region.

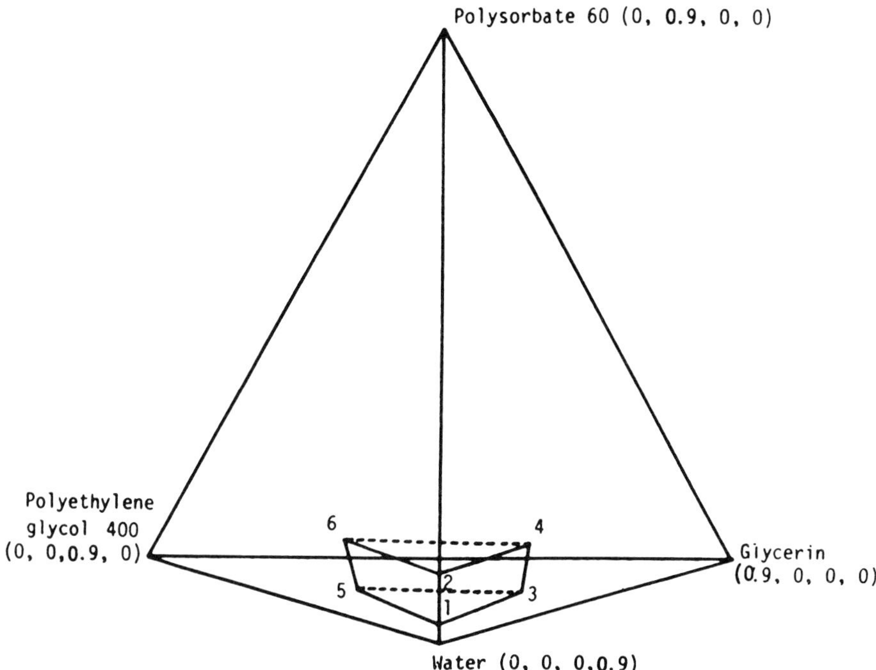

FIG. 42. Region defined by the extreme vertices to which the face centroids, overall centroid, and midpoints of the edges are added. (Reprinted with permission from Ref. 80.)

Devay et al. [85] studied the effect of four independent variables in tablet coating on the quality of enteric coated tablets in terms of resistance to acidic conditions, disintegration time in simulated intestinal fluid, and crushing strength. The observations obtained in a $2^{(4-1)}$ fractional factorial design with three center points were subjected to regression analysis. Resistance to acidic conditions and to simulated intestinal fluid proved to be linearly dependent on x_1 (the ratio Eudragit/talc) and x_2 (the amount of coating); crushing strength was only dependent on the amount of coating. Resistance was optimized by using the method of steepest ascent with the most important factors, the ratio between polymer and talc and the quantity of applied coating material.

For an aqueous film-coating process in a production-size tablet coating pan, Stetsko et al. [86] applied a second-order polynomial with five main factor terms, all two-factor interaction terms, and five quadratic terms for explaining changes in the water removal efficiency (WRE) with changes in the five process variables. The process variables included: solution spraying rate, pan rotational speed, inlet air temperature, exhaust air flow, and tablet surface area. A $2^{(5-1)}$ fractional factorial design was combined with a star design without replicated centerpoint to a five-factor orthogonal central composite design. It is not clear why $\alpha = 1.547$ was chosen. They made 27 observations; at four factor settings, experiments were repeated for the estimation of experimental error.

Osmotic devices with microporous coatings prepared from aqueous-based cellulose acetate latex in a pancoater were investigated by Appel et al. [87] for their release properties and burst strength. The variables plasticizer level, pore-former level, cure time, and cure temperature were incorporated in a full 2^4 factorial design. The most suitable formulation was obtained by evaluation of the response surfaces generated by regression analysis on the experimental values.

Arwidsson et al. [88] compared films of two types of ethylcellulose dispersions for their mechanical properties (free films) and barrier properties for drug release (films on compacted drug surface). The variables in the coating conditions included spraying distance, flow rate of dispersion, atomizing air pressure, solids concentration, plasticizers, and air drying temperature. Experiments were performed according to a matrix of two combined fractional factorial $2^{(6-3)}$ designs with reversed signs. No indications were given of the aliasing structure. Relevant conclusions were obtained from the main effects on the various responses concerning differences in film-forming behavior of the two types of ethylcellulose dispersions.

Thoennes and McCurdy [89] determined the moisture resistance of film coatings by incorporating a hygroscopic anionic exchange resin into tablet cores. They studied the effects of six independent formulation variables (concentration of magnesium stearate, talc, polyethylene glycol, hydroxypropyl methylcellulose, and the products Opaspray and Eudragit E30D) on the dependent variables of moisture resistance, disintegration time, and physical appearance. Moreover, and not simultaneously, the impact of the core characteristics on the properties of the final product was illustrated. A geometrical variable-size sequential simplex design, using COPS software and an arbitrarily combined criterion for coating quality, was selected. This problem-solving approach with all factors simultaneously varied required no more than 14 experiments. The optimized formulation of the film coating was resistant to environmental moisture, maintaining desirable disintegration properties.

With the aid of three operating variables (spray rates of the binding solution, powder addition, and rotation speed) Gajdos [90] evaluated the process technology of granulation in a Wirbelschicht (WS) rotor granulator and a centrifugal–fluidizing (CF) granulator. Data on yield, density, hardness, quality of pellet geometry, and surface were collected in two separate 2^3 factorially designed experiments. Factor effects and interactions for both granulators were calculated, allowing further comparison of their performance.

Dietrich and Brausse [91] investigated three critical operational coating process variables. In order to obtain essential information for installation and operational qualifications, as defined by Pharmaceutical Inspection Convention (PIC) and GMP guidelines, they used for an automated fluid-bed coating apparatus a 2^3 factorial design extended to a central composite design (α = 1,215, whereas for rotatability α = 1.682 would be needed). The effects of spraying temperature, air velocity, and humidity on in vitro release parameters for the coated pellets (amount of active compound released after one hour and the slope of the curve from the first to the third hour) were evaluated qualitatively by variance analysis and quantitatively by regression analysis. Recommendations for the ranges of the independent variable settings, within which a product conforming with the specifications (with respect to in vitro release) can be manufactured, have been defined.

In the optimization of the aqueous film coating of theophylline granules in a rotary fluidized-bed process, Turkoglu and Sakr [92] used a three-factor three-level Box-Behnken design (15 experiments). Variables included polymer amount, coating temperature, and spray nozzle pressure. A second-order model with two-factor interaction terms and quadratic terms was used to fit the data of the six dependent variables present in the in vitro release profiles by regression analysis. Along with the judgment of the six response surfaces resulting from the regression analyses based on the data of the Box-

Behnken design, a sequential simplex optimization procedure was applied to optimize a theophylline release of more than 80% after 11 h.

Conclusions and Outlook

Optimization methods have found extended applications in a wide variety of formulation and process problems. Papers have been published mostly by university groups, but a considerable number eminated from industrial research. It may be assumed that this constitutes only a minor part of the industrial development effort. A recent survey [93] on excipients for tableting and encapsulation and the use of direct compression vs. wet tableting massing and of computer optimization in formulation development was send to 68 pharmaceutical companies in the United States. Of these, 58 companies responded; their answers showed that 13.8% of the respondents always, and 34.5% occasionally, used computer optimization in formulation development. Thus, computer optimization techniques are known and used by 48.3% of the respondents. By the others they are not used for some reason, may be because the technology is not available within the company. However, a large number of academic courses in experimental design and statistics have been announced in recent years, and lack of knowledge should be no longer an excuse.

Another reason may be that pharmaceutical development personnel are not well-trained in statistics. Looking at university curricula, there is certainly reason for concern. Universities should be encouraged to teach statistics and experimental design in the pharmaceutical curriculum to keep pharmacy abreast of new developments for the benefit of the industry and the patients.

Bibliography

Box, G. E. P., Hunter, W. G., and Hunter, J. S., *Statistics for Experimenters. An Introduction to Design, Data Analysis and Model Building*, John Wiley & Sons, New York, 1978.

Box, G. E. P., and Draper, N. R., *Empirical Model-Building and Response Surfaces*, John Wiley & Sons, New York, 1987.

Carlson, R., *Design and Optimization in Organic Synthesis*, Elsevier Science Publishers B.V., Amsterdam, 1992.

Cornell, J. A., *Experiments with Mixtures: Designs, Models and the Analysis of Mixture Data*, 2nd ed., John Wiley & Sons, New York, 1990.

Deming, S. N., and Morgan, S. L., *Experimental Design: A Chemometric Approach*, Elsevier Science Publishers B.V., Amsterdam, 1987.

Draper, N. R., and Smith, H., *Applied Regression Analysis*, John Wiley & Sons, New York, 1981.

Fedorov, V. V., *Theory of Optimal Experiments*, Academic Press, New York, 1972.

References

1. Box, G. E. P., and Wilson, K. B. On the experimental attainment of optimum conditions, *J. Roy. Stat. Soc.*, 13(1):1–45 (1951).

2. Box, G. E. P., Statistical design in the study of analytical methods, *Analyst*, 77:879–891 (1952).
3. Box, G. E. P., The exploration and exploitation of response surfaces: some general considerations and examples, *Biometrics*, 10:16–60 (1954).
4. Box, G. E. P, and Youle, P. V., The exploration and exploitation of response surfaces. An example of the link between the fitted surface and the basic mechanism of the system. *Biometrics*, 11:287–323 (1955).
5. Leuenberger, H., Guitard, P., and Sucker, H., Mathematische Modellierung and Optimierung Pharmazeutisch-technologischer Qualitätsmerkmale fester Arzneiformen, *Pharmazie in unserer Zeit*, 5(3):65–76 (1976).
6. Schwartz, J. B., Flamholz, J. R., and Press, R. H., Computer optimization of pharmaceutical formulations. I: General procedure, *J. Pharm. Sci.*, 62(7):1165–1170 (1973).
7. Schwartz, J. B., Flamholz, J. R., and Press, R. H., Computer optimization in pharmaceutical formulations. II: Application in troubleshooting, *J. Pharm. Sci.*, 62(9):1518–1519 (1973).
8. Sucker, H., Methoden zum Planen und Auswerten von Versuchen. 1. Factorial Design, eine Einführung, *APV-Informationsdienst*, 17:52–68 (1971).
9. Gurny, R., Buri, P., Sucker, H., Guitard, P., and Leuenberger, H., Réalisation et développement de formes médicamenteuses a libération contrôlée par des films méthacryliques; 2e communication. Étude par analyse orthogonale des facteurs influencant le transport a travers un film plan, *Pharm. Acta Helv.*, 52:175–181 (1977).
10. Gurny, R., Guitard, P., Buri, P., and Sucker, H. Réalisation et développement théorique de formes médicamenteuses a libération contrôlée des films méthacrylique; 3e communication. Préparation et characterisation de formes galéniques a libération contrôlée, *Pharm. Acta Helv.*, 52:182–186 (1977).
11. Gurny, R., Buri, P., Sucker, H., Guitard, P., and Leuenberger, H., Réalisation et développement théorique de formes médicamenteuses a libération contrôlée par des films méthacryliques; 4e communication. Étude par régression lineaire de facteurs téchnologiques influencant la libération d'un principe actif a partir de microgranules énrobes par fluidisation, *Pharm. Acta Helv.*, 52:247–251 (1977).
12. Altenschmidt, W., Einsatz von Methoden des Operations Research bei der Pharma Produktion, 1–8, *Pharm. Ind.*, 36 (1974) and 37 (1975).
13. De Boer, J. H., *Chemometric aspects of quality in pharmaceutical technology. The application of robustness criteria and multicriteria decision making in optimization procedures for pharmaceutical formulations*, Ph.D. Thesis, University of Groningen, Groningen, The Netherlands, 1992.
14. De Boer, J. H., Smilde, A. K., and Doornbos, D. A., Introduction of a Robustness Coefficient in optimization procedures: Implementation in mixture design problems. Part III: Validation and comparison with competing criteria, *Chemom. Intell. Lab Syst.*, 15:13–28 (1992).
15. Box, G. E. P., Hunter, W. G., and Hunter, J. S., *Statistics for Experimenters. An Introduction to Design, Data Analysis and Model Building*, Wiley, New York, 1978, Chap. 15.
16. Box, G. E. P., and Draper, N. R., *Empirical Model-Building and Response Surfaces*, John Wiley & Sons, New York, 1987, p. 1.
17. Box, G. E. P., Hunter, W. G., and Hunter, J. S., Statistics for Experimenters. An Introduction to Design, Data Analysis and Model Building, Wiley, New York, 1978, Chap. 9, p. 303.
18. Box, G. E. P., Hunter, W. G., and Hunter, J. S., *Statistics for Experimenters. An Introduction to Design, Data Analysis and Model Building*, Wiley, New York, 1978, Chap. 10, p. 308.
19. Box, G. E. P., Hunter, W. G., and Hunter, J. S., *Statistics for Experimenters. An Introduction to Design, Data Analysis and Model Building*, Wiley, New York, 1978, Chap. 10, pp. 323, 342, 407.
20. Box, G. E. P., and Draper, N. R., *Empirical Model-Building and Response Surfaces*, John Wiley & Sons, New York, 1987, Chap. 4, p. 127, Chap. 6, p. 185, Chap. 7, p. 240.

21. Box, G. E. P., Hunter, W. G., and Hunter, J. S., *Statistics for Experimenters. An Introduction to Design, Data Analysis and Model Building*, Wiley, New York, 1978, Chap. 12.
22. Deming, S. N., and Morgan, S. L., *Experimental Design: A Chemometric Approach*, Elsevier Science Publishers B.V., Amsterdam, 1987, Chap. 9.
23. Box, G. E. P., Hunter, W. G., and Hunter, J. S., *Statistics for Experimenters. An Introduction to Design, Data Analysis and Model Building*, Wiley, New York, 1978, Chap. 6.
24. Plackett, R. L., and Burman, J. P., The design of optimum multifactorial experiments, *Biometrika*, 33:305 (1946).
25. Box, G. E. P., and Draper, N. R., *Empirical Model-Building and Response Surfaces*, John Wiley & Sons, New York, 1987, Chap. 15, p. 508.
26. Box, G. E. P., and Hunter, J. S., *Ann. Math. Statist.*, 28:195 (1957).
27. Box, G. E. P., and Draper, N. R., *Empirical Model-Building and Response Surfaces*, John Wiley & Sons, New York, 1987, Chap. 14, p. 488, Chap. 15, p. 508.
28. Doehlert, D. H., Uniform shell designs, *Appl. Statist.*, 19(3):231–239 (1970).
29. Hau, I., *Constrained experimental designs*, Ph.D. Thesis, University of Wisconsin, Madison, 1990.
30. Duineveld, C. A. A., Smilde, A. K., and Doornbos, D. A., Comparison of experimental designs combining process and mixture variables. Part I: Design construction and theoretical evaluation, *Chemom. Intell. Lab. Syst.*, 19:295–308 (1993).
31. Duineveld, C. A. A., Smilde, A. K., and Doornbos, D. A., Designs for mixture and process variables applied in tablet formulations, *Anal. Chim. Acta*, 277:455–465 (1993).
32. Duineveld, C. A. A., Smilde, A. K., and Doornbos, D. A., Comparison of experimental designs combining process and mixture variables. Part II: Design evaluation on measured data, *Chemom. Intell. Lab. Syst.*, 19:309–310 (1993).
33. Duineveld, C. A. A., *Systematic optimization of tablet formulations; construction and analysis of mixture-process variables design*, Ph.D. Thesis, University of Groningen, Groningen, The Netherlands, 1993.
34. Atkinson, A. C., Recent developments in the methods of optimum and related experimental designs, *Int. Stat. Rev.*, 56(2):99–115 (1988).
35. Van Kamp, H. V., *Optimization of the formulation of fast disintegrating tablets*, Ph.D. Thesis, University of Groningen, Groningen, The Netherlands, 1987.
36. Van Kamp, H. V., Bolhuis, G. K., and Lerk, C. F., Optimization of a formulation based on lactoses for direct compression, *Acta Pharm. Technol.*, 34:11–16 (1988).
37. De Boer, J. H., Smilde, A. K., and Doornbos, D. A., Introduction of multi-criteria decision making in optimization procedures for pharmaceutical formulations, *Acta Pharm. Technol.*, 34:140–143 (1988).
38. Doornbos, D. A., Smilde, A. K., De Boer, J. H., and Duineveld, C. A. A., *Experimental Design, Response Surface Methodology and Multi Criteria Decision Making in the Development of Drug Dosage Forms*, Scientific Computing and Automation (Europe), Elsevier Science Publishers B.V., Amsterdam, 1990, pp. 85–95.
39. Hendriks, M. M. W. B., De Boer, J. H., Smilde, A. K., and Doornbos, D. A., Multicriteria decision making, *Chemom. Intell. Lab Syst.* 16:175–191 (1992).
40. Forster, E., and Bathe, R. V., Avoiding possible confusion in usual methods of steepest ascent calculation, *Chemom. Intell. Lab Syst.*, 9:207–215 (1990).
41. Spendley, W., Hext, G. R., and Himsworth, F. R., Sequential application of simplex designs in optimisation and evolutionary operation, *Technometrics*, 4(4):441–461 (1962).
42. Burton, K. W. C., and Nickless, G., Optimisation via simplex. Part I. Background, definitions and a simple application, *Chemom. Intell. Lab. Syst.*, 1:135–149 (1987).
43. Nelder, J. A., and Mead, R., A simplex method for function minimization, *Computer J.*, 7:308 (1965).
44. Routh, M. W., Swartz, P. A., and Denton, M. B., Performance of the super modified simplex, *Anal. Chem.*, 49(9):1422 (1977).

45. Malinowski, H. J., and Smith, W. E., Effects of spheronization process variables on selected tablet properties, *J. Pharm. Sci.*, 63(2):285–289 (1974).
46. Holm, P., Jungersen, O., Schaefer, T., and Kristensen, H. G., Granulation in high speed mixers, Part 1: Effects of process variables during kneading, *Pharm. Ind.*, 45(8):806–811 (1983).
47. Holm, P., Jungersen, O., Schaefer, T., and Kristensen, H. G., Granulation in high speed mixers, Part 2: Effects of process variables during kneading, *Pharm. Ind.*, 46(1):97–101 (1984).
48. Paschos, S., Cognart, J., Jeannin, C., Ozil, P., and Verain, A., Granulation with a high-speed mixer-granulator-dryer: Optimization of the process, *Acta Pharm. Technol.*, 34(2):80–83 (1988).
49. Shirakura, O., Yamada, M., Hashimoto, M., Ishimaru, S., Takayama, K., and Nagai, T., Effect of amount and composition of granulating solution on physical characteristics of tablets, *Drug Dev. Ind. Pharm.*, 18(10):1099–1110 (1992).
50. Gordon, M. S., Chatterjee, B., and Chowhan, Z. T., Effect of the mode of croscarmellose sodium incorporation on tablet dissolution and friability, *J. Pharm. Sci.*, 79(1):43–47 (1990).
51. Schwartz, J. B., Flamholz, J. R., and Press, R. H., Computer optimization of pharmaceutical formulations, I. General procedure, *J. Pharm. Sci.*, 62(7):1165–1170 (1973).
52. Schwartz, J. B., Flamholz, J. R., and Press, R. H., Computer optimization in pharmaceutical formulations. II: Application in troubleshooting, *J. Pharm. Sci.*, 62(9):1518–1519 (1973).
53. Huisman, R., Van Kamp, H. V., Weyland, J. W., Doornbos, D. A., Bolhuis, G. K., and Lerk, C. F., Development and optimization of pharmaceutical formulations using a simplex lattice design, *Pharm. Weekbl. Sci. Ed.*, 6:185–194 (1984).
54. Bos, C. E., Bolhuis, G. K., Lerk, C. F., De Boer, J. H., Duineveld, C. A. A., Smilde, A. K., and Doornbos, D. A., The use of a factorial design to evaluate the physical stability of tablets prepared by direct compression. I. A new approach based on the relative change in the tablet parameters, *Eur. J. Pharm. Biopharm.*, 37(4):204–209 (1991).
55. Bos, C. E., Bolhuis, G. K., Lerk, C. F., De Boer, J. H., Duineveld, C. A. A., Smilde, A. K., and Doornbos, D. A., The use of a factorial design to evaluate the physical stability of tablets prepared by direct compression. II. Selection of excipients suitable for use under tropical storage conditions, *Eur. J. Pharm. Biopharm.*, 37(4):210–215 (1991).
56. Bos, C. E., Bolhuis, G. K., Lerk, C. F., De Boer, J. H., Duineveld C. A. A., Smilde, A. K., and Doornbos, D. A., Optimization of direct compression tablet formulations for use in tropical countries, *Drug Dev. Ind. Pharm.*, 17(18):2477–2496 (1991).
57. Fenyvesi, E., Takayama, K., Szejtli, J., and Nagai, T., Evaluation of cyclodextrin polymer as an additive for furosemide tablets, *Chem. Pharm. Bull.*, 32(2):670–677 (1984).
58. Waaler, P. J., Graffner, C., and Mueller, B. W., Optimization of a matrix formulation using a mixture design, *Acta Pharm. Nord.*, 4(1):9–16 (1992).
59. Franz, R. M., Sytsma, J. A., Smith, B. P., and Lucisano, L. J., In vitro evaluation of a mixed polymeric sustained release matrix using response surface methodology, *J. Contr. Rel.*, 5:159–172 (1987).
60. Perez-Marcos, B., Iglesias, R., Gomez-Amoza, J. L., Martinez-Pacheco, R., Souto, C., and Concheiro, A., Mechanical and drug-release properties of atenolol-carbomer hydrophilic matrix tablets, *J. Contr. Rel.*, 17(3):267–276 (1991).
61. Hirata, M., Takayama, K., and Nagai, T., Formulation optimization of sustained-release tablet of chlorpheniramine maleate by means of extreme vertices design and simultaneous optimization technique, *Chem. Pharm. Bull.*, 40(3):741–746 (1992).
62. Luk Chiu Li, and Yu-Hsing Tu, In vitro drug release from matrix tablets containing a silicone elastomer latex, *Drug Dev. Ind. Pharm.*, 17(16):2197–2214 (1991).
63. El-Banna, H. M., and Sautin, S. N., Interaction of factors in the factorial design of experiments for preparing effervescent tablets, *Sci. Pharm.*, 48:369–377 (1980).
64. El-Banna, H. M., and Minina, S. A., The construction and uses of factorial designs in the preparation of solid dosage forms. Part 1: Effervescent acetylosalicylic acid tablets, *Pharmazie*, 36(6):417–420 (1981).

65. Devay, A., Uderszky, J., and Racz, I., Optimization of operational parameters in fluidized bed granulation of effervescent pharmaceutical preparations, *Acta Pharm. Technol.*, 30(3):239–242 (1984).
66. Balut, P., Ozer, A. Y., Sumnu, M., and Hincal, A. A., Evaluation of the stability of commercial effervescent and dispersible aspirin tablets by factorial analysis, *S.T.P. Pharma Sci.*, 1(6):357–361 (1991).
67. Reier, G., Cohn, R., Rock, S., and Wagenblast, F., Evaluation of factors affecting the encapsulation of powders in hard gelatin capsules I., *J. Pharm. Sci.*, 57(4):660–666 (1968).
68. Newton, J. M., and Razzo, F. N., The influence of additives on the in vitro release of drugs from hard gelatin capsules, *J. Pharm. Pharmacol.*, 26(Suppl.):30P–36P (1974).
69. Shek, E., Ghani, M., and Jones, R. E., simplex search in optimization of capsule formulation, *J. Pharm. Sci.*, 69:1135–1142 (1980).
70. Hussain, A. S., Xuanqiang, Yu, and Johnson, R. D., Application of neural computing in pharmaceutical product development, *Pharm. Res.*, 8(10):1248–1252 (1991).
71. Ortigosa, C., Gaudy, D., Jacob, M., and Puech, A., The role of gelucire in the availability of theophylline in semisolid matrix capsules. A study of the factors: pH, melting point, H.L.B. and paddle rotation speed, *Pharm. Acta Helv.*, 66(11):311–315 (1991).
72. Malinowski, E. J., and Smith, W. E., Use of factorial design to evaluate granulations prepared by spheronization, *J. Pharm. Sci.*, 64:1688–1692 (1975).
73. Hileman, G. A., Goskonda, S. R., Spalitto, A. J., and Upadrashta, S. M., A factorial approach to high dose product development by an extrusion/spheronization process, *Drug. Dev. Ind. Pharm.*, 19(4):483–491 (1993).
74. Hassan, E. E., Parish, R. C., and Gallo, J. M., Optimized formulation of magnetic chitosan microspheres containing the anticancer agent oxantrazole, *Pharm. Res.*, 9(3):390–397 (1992).
75. Devay, A., and Racz, I., Examination of parameters determining particle size of sulfamethoxazole microcapsules prepared by a new melt-dispersion method, *Pharm. Ind.*, 46(1):101–103 (1984).
76. Devay, A., and Racz, I., Examination of parameters determining particle size distribution: acetylsalicylic acid microcapsules, *J. Microencaps.*, 5:21–25 (1988).
77. Julienne, M. C., Alonso, M. J., Gomez-Amoza, J. L., and Benoit, J. P., Preparation of poly(D,L-lactide/glycolide) nanoparticles of controlled particle size distribution: Application of experimental designs, *Drug Dev. Ind. Pharm.*, 18:1063–1077 (1992).
78. El-Banna, H. M., and Efimova, L. S., The construction and use of factorial design in fluidized bed microencapsulation, *Pharm. Ind.*, 44:641–644 (1982).
79. Senderak, E., Bonsignore, H., and Mungan, D., Response surface methodology as an approach to optimization of an oral solution, *Drug. Dev. Ind. Pharm.*, 19(4):405–424 (1993).
80. Anik, S. T., and Sukumar, L., Extreme vertices design in formulation development: solubility of butoconazole nitrate in a multicomponent system, *J. Pharm. Sci.*, 70:897–900 (1981).
81. Karabit, M. S., Juneskans, O. T., and Lundgren, P., Factorial designs in the evaluation of preservative efficacy, *Int. J. Pharm.*, 56:169–174 (1989).
82. Patel, J. P., Marsh, K., Carr, L., and Nequist, G., Factorial designs in ophthalmic formulation development of Enalkiren, *Int. J. Pharm.*, 65:195–200 (1990).
83. Gupta, P. K., Lam, F. C., and Hung, C. T., Investigation of the stability of Doxorubicin hydrochloride using factorial design, *Drug Dev. Ind. Pharm.*, 14(12):1657–1671 (1988).
84. Dincer, S., and Ozdurmus, S., Mathematical model for enteric film coating of tablets, *J. Pharm. Sci.*, 66(8):1070–1073 (1977).
85. Devay, A., Kovacs, B., Uderszky, J., and Domotor, Z., Optimierung der Verfahrensparameter bei der Herstellung von Filmüberzügen auf Grund eines Mehrfaktoren-Versuchsplanes, *Pharm. Ind.*, 44(8):830–833 (1982).
86. Stetsko, G., Banker, G. S., and Peck, G. E., Mathematical modeling of an aqueous film coating process, *Pharm. Techn.*, 7(11):50–62 (1983).

87. Appel, L. E., Clair, J. H., and Zentner, G. M., Formulation and optimization of a modified microporous cellulose acetate latex coating for osmotic pumps, *Pharm. Res.*, 9:1664–1667 (1992).
88. Arwidsson, H., Hjelstuen, O., Ingason, D., and Graffner, C., Properties of ethyl cellulose films for extended release. III. Influence of process factors when using aqueous dispersions, *Acta Pharm. Nord.*, 3(4):223–228 (1991).
89. Thoennes, C. J., and McCurdy, V. E., Evaluation of a rapidly disintegrating, moisture resistant lacquer film coating, *Drug Dev. Ind. Pharm.*, 15(2):165–185 (1989).
90. Gajdos, B., Rotorgranulatoren—Verfahrenstechnische Bewertung der Pelletherstellung mit Hilfe der factoriellen Versuchsplanung, *Pharm. Ind.*, 45(7):722–728 (1983).
91. Dietrich, R., and Brausse, R., Validation of the pellet coating process used for a new sustained-release theophylline formulation, *Drug Res.*, 38:1210–1219 (1988).
92. Turkoglu, M., and Sakr, A., Mathematical modelling and optimization of a rotary fluidized-bed coating process, *Int. J. Pharm.*, 88:75–87 (1992).
93. Shangraw, R. F., and Demarest, Jr., D. A., A survey of current industrial practices in the formulation and manufacture of tablets and capsules, *Pharm. Technol.*, Jan.:32–44 (1993).

DURK A. DOORNBOS
PIETER DE HAAN

Orphan Drugs

Introduction

Back in the 1960s and 1970s, developers and manufacturers of several potential drugs and biologicals, which were considered medically important but financially unprofitable, faced a difficult dilemma. Should they proceed with development, recognizing that the resources required to develop the product and secure Food and Drug Administration (FDA) approval to market it were not likely to be recovered in anticipated United States sales? This dilemma pertained to a wide range of products for a variety of reasons, some obvious, and some not. The categories of products included those for [1]:

1. Rare diseases (small markets);
2. Chronic diseases (which required sufficient testing periods to assess long-term effects, while the 17-year patent protection clock was ticking);
3. Single administration (vaccines or diagnostic agents, involving relatively small volume and liability risks);
4. Women of childbearing age, children, or elderly (all of whom at the time were excluded from participation in clinical testing, and in the case of the first two, carried high liability risks);
5. Rare or common diseases for which the drugs were not patentable (shelf chemicals, natural substances, drugs known to exist, or drugs already patented for other uses);
6. Substance abuse treatment or relapse prevention (where the target population was likely to be reluctant to enter treatment and might pose liability risks, and where providers and manufacturers were required to keep extensive records); and
7. Developing countries (unable to pay and facing drug distribution problems).

In a few instances, the government developed drugs for some of these categories as a public service. Occasionally commercial manufacturers developed and provided drugs for these situations as a corporate social responsibility that could be entered on the "good will" line of their balance sheets [2]. Recognizing that technological feasibility was not necessarily the limiting factor for the development of some promising therapies, certain of the National Institutes of Health (NIH), most notably the National Cancer Institute and the National Institute of Neurological and Communicative Disorders and Stroke, established federally funded chemical screening programs to identify bioactive compounds that might be tested for various cancers and epilepsy, respectively. Through these programs, the institutes tried to interest pharmaceutical companies in collaborating in investigations of agents that might prove to be therapeutically promising.

During this time, several articles were published by academic researchers who formulated new dosages for available drugs or encapsulated chemical ingredients for tests on patients with rare diseases because pharmaceutical companies had shown no interest in assisting in these efforts [3–9]. One of these researchers, John Walshe of Cambridge University, made and tested the drug trientine on a few patients with Wilson's disease, a disorder of copper metabolism that allows copper deposits to build up in the brain, causing motor and cognitive deficits and eventually death. These patients were not able to tolerate penicillamine, the only chelating agent available for this rare neurologic disease. Walshe finally concluded that this "do it yourself" drug creation had gone on long enough and should be placed on a sound commercial basis [10].

Primarily as a result of the efforts of federal and academic scientists, the FDA identified a growing list of potentially promising therapeutic agents that had no commercial sponsors to initiate larger-scale (Phase III) clinical trials and seek a New Drug Application (NDA) approval from the FDA to market the drug. The FDA convened a Task Force on Drugs of Little Commercial Value in 1979 to find industry sponsors to complete the testing and NDA process for these therapeutic agents which were primarily for diseases that were rare in the United States [11,12]. In the same year, Louis Lasagna, then professor of pharmacology, toxicology, and medicine at the University of Rochester, gave a name to this dilemma in the journal *Regulation* [13] when he asked, who will adopt the "orphan drugs?" Lasagna asserted that at a time when technological innovation was poised for new advances, regulatory requirement costs were pricing important but unprofitable therapies out of the development calculation, and forcing certain groups of patients to become therapeutic "orphans." He used the term about a decade after Provost discussed homeless or orphan drugs in the *American Journal of Hospital Pharmacy* [14]. These were drugs that might be in common use but were not potentially profitable enough to invite commercial introduction. The term became "an idea in good currency," as defined by Schon [15]. The term "orphan drugs" became applied to all drugs and biologicals whose potential development costs were likely, at best, to be covered by profits; that is, companies expected only to be able to break even.

Initially, the term orphan drugs was applied to all seven categories listed above. In the 1980s, however, the term became reserved for drugs for diseases or conditions that were rare in the United States (category 1 above) through the 1983 Orphan Drug Act (Public Law 97–414). For other categories, such as vaccines for children, other legislative approaches have been taken to increase the willingness of pharmaceutical companies to be involved. The National Childhood Vaccine Injury Act of 1986 (Public Law 99–660), for example, established a pooled reserve for vaccine-associated adverse effects. For some of the other categories, such as drugs for the elderly, FDA administrative changes have occurred. The FDA now requires that elderly people be included rather than excluded from clinical trials of agents intended for use in this population.

This article deals exclusively with orphan drugs intended for rare diseases. It describes events leading up to the legislation, passage, and implementation of the 1983 Orphan Drug Act and its subsequent amendments, the current status of the law, of development efforts by industry, and remaining issues.*

Circumstances Leading to the Legislation

Some might argue that the origin of the dilemma for industry in developing drugs for rare diseases goes back to 1790, when the U.S. Patent and Trademark Act established a 14-year period of market protection (changed to 17 years in 1861) [16]. Developers and manufacturers of patentable products could be protected from exact replicas being produced and sold at lower prices during this period of protection in order to facilitate and reward

*The views expressed here are those of the author and no endorsement by The Pew Charitable Trusts is intended or should be inferred.

innovation. The next important event contributing to the orphan-drug dilemma was the introduction of antibiotics in the early 1930s. The discovery of antibiotics confirmed the importance of patents in strengthening the competitive positions among industrial firms. Rather than compete on the basis of price, manufacturers became research-intensive vertically integrated firms. Profits from antibiotics were used to invest in the development of new products which could be protected by patents.

The next developments contributing to the eventual orphan-drug dilemma were the 1938 Food, Drug and Cosmetic Act (FD & C Act) and the 1962 Kefauver-Harris Amendments to it. These required proof of safety and efficacy, respectively, to gain FDA market approval. Both, however, were drafted in response to disasters. The FD & C Act was passed after diethylene glycol, used as a sulfanilamide vehicle, formed lethal quantities of oxalic acid in the body, resulting in 100 fatalities, mostly children [17]. It required manufacturers to provide evidence that the drugs were relatively safe. However, in order to keep a drug off the market, the FDA was required to prove that it was not safe. The 1962 amendments, requiring a demonstration of efficacy from the manufacturer, were added in response to the thalidomide disaster in which birth defects were reported in infants born to women in Europe and Canada who had taken the drug while pregnant. Thalidomide had not been approved by the FDA for sale in the United States, and this fortunate delay resulted in the passage of the 1962 amendments. They strengthened the FDA's authority to place the burden of proof of safety on the manufacturers by requiring approval of an Investigational New Drug (IND) Application, establishing relative safety before clinical trials for efficacy could begin. These amendments also required proof of efficacy through well-controlled clinical trials, presented in the New Drug Application (NDA) for marketing approval [18].

An essential interplay developed between patent protection and regulatory requirements. Patent protection became even more critical for newly emerging products developed by technological innovation by research-intensive, vertically integrated firms that looked to a few major market winners to survive in an era of increased development costs created by regulatory reform [19]. Major market winners generally proved to be drugs for widespread conditions that created large markets and encouraged brand loyalties by prescribing physicians. The reliance on a continual pipeline of promising, therapeutically effective patentable products for large markets, in turn, relegated drugs for rare diseases (small markets) to the outer bounds of development decisions. For example, estimates of drug development costs in the late 1960s and early 1970s before the 1962 FDA Kefauver-Harris amendments were operational, grew from a low of $2.7 to $4.7 million per new chemical entity (NCE) to a high of $16.9 million per NCE [20,21]. By the late 1970s, the estimate had risen to $54 million [22]. In the 1980s the estimate was approximately $124 million, and a 1991 estimate put the development costs of NCEs or new molecular entities (NMEs) at $231 million (including the costs of the estimated four out of five products that undergo clinical testing without reaching commercialization) [23].

While these data on estimated new drug development costs have eluded close scrutiny, the relative costs and anticipated return on investment (ROI) for drugs for rare diseases compared to drugs for large markets have been the critical issue. The first step to address the development needs for these potential products was taken by the NIH. Recognizing a void in the development of therapies for various cancers because of anticipated low ROI, the National Cancer Institute (NCI) established the Cancer Drug Development Program in 1955 to screen for biologically active compounds. The program began with a $5 million appropriation by Congress. In early 1958, a $35 million NCI–industrial contract program was negotiated to preserve the industrial partners' trade secret status of data and ability to seek patent rights for those compounds which screened successfully for bioactivity and which were entered into testing. Grants were used only to coordinate clinical trials. By 1980, these clinical trials were supported by an NCI budget allocation of $117.5 million.

Initially the NCIs clinical testing requirements had not been coordinated with the FDA. This created problems for a few industrial sponsors who unsuccessfully sought NDAs for anticancer drugs developed through this process because the FDA would not accept the clinical trials data. Industry's consternation led to closer coordination between the NCI and FDA on clinical trials requirements [24–26]. Similarly, the Antiepileptic Drug Development program of the National Institute of Neurological and Communicative Disorders and Stroke (NINCDS) thereafter developed a screening program to identify agents with possible anticonvulsant activity. This program was launched because only one new anticonvulsant therapeutic had come on the market since the 1962 Kefauver-Harris amendments [27,28]. Other, less formalized efforts to stimulate industry interest in specific drug categories began to be undertaken in the areas of heart disease, contraceptives, and substance abuse.

The second step was taken by several NIH grantees from academic centers. They expressed concerns over their individual efforts to interest industry in adopting and refining potential drugs emanating from their research. Several researchers demonstrated increasing frustration at their inability to interest commercial sponsors in adopting and further developing promising agents to treat rare diseases. Complications included how to interest industry in taking on the task of securing NDA approval for a drug that industry did not develop (the "not initiated here" often referred to as the "NIH" syndrome), how to preserve the trade-secret status of data if academic research results were published, as is customary, and how to establish market protection in the absence of patentability. The FDA had identified and listed 13 drugs for rare diseases whose sponsors had been awarded INDs to undertake clinical testing. Most of these IND sponsors were academic researchers who had not been able to find pharmaceutical sponsors to support clinical trials and to submit an NDA application to receive marketing approval from FDA [29].

The third step was taken by the FDA when it created the 1978–79 FDA Task Force on Drugs of Little Commercial Value, after some congressmen expressed concern about the lack of effective therapies for Huntington's disease and other rare neurological disorders described in the *Huntington's Disease Commission Report* [30]. The task force recommended that incentives be provided to industry to develop commercially limited drugs, but that any profits from those incentives by returned, in whole or in part, to the government. This arbitration-type approach was based on the assumption that industry would be willing to make trade-offs with the FDA on behalf of these drugs. There was no indication from industry, however, that this was the case [31].

The Evolution of the Orphan Drug Act

In 1980, a researcher at the Mount Sinai School of Medicine (Melvin Van Woert), who was seeking a pharmaceutical sponsor for L-5HTP for myoclonus, appealed to Congresswoman Elizabeth Holtzman of New York for a legislative solution [32]. She introduced

H.R. 7089, to establish an Office of Drugs of Limited Commercial Value to assist NIH in developing drugs of limited commercial interest; no action was taken on this bill. However, the committee heard testimony from a young Californian suffering from Tourettes syndrome, a genetically determined neurological condition causing the exhibition of tics, twitches, and uncontrolled verbal outbursts. Available therapy with haloperidol was not effective, and the patient had not been able to obtain pimozide, a drug available in Europe and Canada [33]. A Los Angeles newspaper carried an account of the testimony which was read by the producer of the television series Quincy. A Quincy episode was devoted to the difficulties Tourettes victims had functioning in society, and to the dilemma industry faced in not having incentives to develop drugs to treat this devastating condition. The program emphasized that there were no villains, but there were no remedies either. In the episode, Quincy delivered an impassioned appeal to Congress to find a solution. Shortly thereafter, Congressman Henry Waxman held a hearing on an orphan drug bill introduced by Representative Ted Weiss of New York in 1981 which was similar to the earlier Holtzman bill. The star of the Quincy show appeared before the congressional subcommittee and delivered the speech that he had delivered in the episode on the air [34–36]. By the end of 1981, Congressman Waxman had introduced H.R. 5238, the Orphan Drug Act [37].

The Orphan Drug Survey

As background to subsequent action on the bill, a survey was undertaken of three groups of drugs:

- Products listed by member companies of the Pharmaceutical Manufacturer's Association (PMA) as drugs for rare diseases that member companies had marketed, or had made available on a compassionate basis to specialists,
- Drugs listed by the FDA as needing a pharmaceutical sponsor, and
- Drugs under development by NIH scientists or grantees.

The latter two gave an indication of the extent and nature of federal involvement in studying or carrying out clinical trials for drugs, most of which were intended for rare diseases. The industry survey provided development and market information on rare-disease drugs and biologicals that were available. It revealed that industry had developed and marketed 34 drugs for rare diseases or conditions over a 17-year period, and had made 24 additional drugs available to specialists on a Compassionate IND basis. Most drugs (82%) were for conditions affecting fewer than 100,000 people in the United States; 10% were for 100,000 to 500,000 people, and the remaining 8% of drugs or biologicals were for up to 1 million people. According to survey responses, substantial federal funds for research and development (R&D) had been provided for all but ten of these industry-sponsored products. An additional 13 rare-disease drugs that were on the market had been developed and sponsored solely by federal agency or academic scientists.

The ROI for 83% of the drugs was lower than the average for these industry-sponsored drugs, whereas development costs were higher than the average for 12% of these drugs. The PMA company sponsors indicated that the FDA clinical trials guidelines were not clear, further complicating their ability to estimate the likely ROI on products under development. On the positive side, one in four PMA company-sponsored orphan products also had a nonorphan (common) indication. This suggested that companies can be successful with one-fourth of their orphan products if these are later found to have a common use and therefore a larger market. Patent time remaining on approved products may be eroded by lengthy premarket development, in part attributed to difficulties in finding sufficient numbers of clinical trials participants and in determining types of trials and total numbers of patients needed to satisfy FDA requirements. Unpatented orphan products were less likely to be submitted for NDA approval in the 1970s (29% of the total) compared to the 1960s (39% of the total), suggesting the increasing importance of patents for marketed orphan products. Moreover, liability claims had been filed against the manufacturers of one-fifth of the marketed orphan drugs [38,39].

Provisions of the Orphan Drug Act

Based largely on congressional testimony and information obtained through the survey, the Orphan Drug Act of 1983 (Public Law 97–414) and subsequent amendments were passed. They apply to drugs, biologicals, and antibiotics for rare diseases and conditions. Initially the establishment of "rare" was to be based on evidence that the prevalence of the disease in the United States was insufficient to generate enough revenues to offset projected development costs. This criterion proved to be not feasible, however, and only a few manufacturers submitted requests to the FDA for orphan designations. A 1984 amendment (Public Law 98–551) defined rare as pertaining to diseases or conditions with a U.S. prevalence rate of 200,000 or fewer. Sponsors could receive an orphan designation for products intended for larger populations if they provided evidence that estimated development expenses were not likely to be recovered through U.S. sales.

The law emphasized the creation of two major market incentives and the reduction of regulatory barriers. The first major market incentive was the granting by the FDA of a seven-year exclusive marketing period to a sponsor for a specific orphan indication of a product. Other sponsors can receive approval for a different drug to treat the same rare disease, or certain other sponsors can receive approval to market an identical drug for some other orphan or common indication. Market exclusivity, therefore, only precludes a second sponsor from obtaining approval to provide an identical drug for the identical orphan indication for which the first sponsor received exclusive market approval. Initially under the act, market exclusivity pertained only to unpatented products. But under a 1985 amendment (Public Law 99–91), exclusive approval was allowed for all orphan products, whether patented or not. This amendment was designed to provide incentives for sponsors of rare-disease products whose patents would expire before or soon after approval, or in cases where prior publication by an academic or government scientist had precluded issuance of a patent.

The second market incentive provided for sponsors to be eligible to receive a tax credit for human clinical testing costs. This originally amounted to 73 cents on the dollar and is now 50 cents. The provision did not pertain to preclinical development costs, since it would be difficult at that early stage to determine that the product was exclusively intended for a rare disease or condition. Finally, the law also provided for FDA grants to support clinical trials of promising orphan products.

Regulatory provisions included a requirement that the FDA communicate with sponsors early in the process, provide written recommendations if requested, and create an open-protocol process to enable physicians to obtain experimental orphan products for patients not involved in clinical trials. These requirements became formulated into a general FDA rewrite of review and protocol procedures for all drugs and biologicals. Tracking of FDA responsiveness specifically to sponsors of orphan products has, therefore, not been required. Nonetheless, an Office of Orphan Products Development within the FDA monitors the review process for all orphan products [40].

Prior to enactment of the law, several private-sector initiatives had been undertaken. These included efforts by the PMA to seek sponsors for promising orphan therapeutics, by the Generic Pharmaceutical Industry Association to seek sponsors for more fully developed products, and by the National Organization for Rare Disorders, representing up to 20 million members, to link patients to researchers and monitor public- and private-sector orphan product activities.

Orphan Drug Activities Since Passage of the Act

In 1983, the first two designated orphan products were approved. According to the FDA, during the first decade of the act (until early 1993), a total of 87 designated orphan products were approved, and 512 products under active development received orphan designations. Six of the approved orphan products had received FDA grants for drug development (the FDA has provided $46 million for a total of 190 grants). As had occurred prior to the act, most of the orphan indications (65%) are for populations of fewer than 50,000 sufferers and about 17% are for populations of more than 100,000 in the United States. Of the 512 orphan product designations, according to the FDA, 50% are for pediatric indications. Of the 87 approved products, 20% are for the treatment of children. There have been 58 drug designations and eight approvals of cancer drugs. Products intended for people aged 65 and older comprise 71 designations. Finally, 24 of the 28 approved "treatment INDs" are for orphan indications [41]. Treatment INDs are made available to physicians for patients with life-threatening or serious conditions (where no products are available on the market).

Tables 1 and 2 provide information on designated and approved orphan products and on the major disease categories involved [42]. Table 3 lists the 93 orphan products approved as of August 1993 [43]. The FDA has changed its system of ranking the therapeutic significance of products to "standard" or "priority" after 1991. Previously, products were ranked as providing "important, moderate, or little" therapeutic gain. Under that system, 38% of the orphan NMEs were ranked as providing important therapeutic gains, and 48% had been ranked as providing moderate gains. Of 32 biologicals deemed "important" by FDA between 1986 and 1990, 22% were for orphan indications [44].

TABLE 1 Designated and Approved Orphan Drug Products[a]

	1989	1991	1992[b]
Total active orphan designations	299	422	488
Total orphan products in development	133	176	189
Cumulative total approved orphan products	36	54	64
Cumulative total orphan product sponsors	85	120	132

[a]From *Orphan Drugs in Development, 1992 Annual Survey*, Pharmaceutical Manufacturers Association, Washington, 1993.
[b]As of March 6, 1992.

TABLE 2 Orphan Drug Disease Categories[a]

Major Categories (N = 6)	Number of Drugs under Development, 1992[b] (N = 195)
AIDS, AIDS-Related conditions	20
Various cancers	58
Childhood diseases	50
Conditions specific to women	17
Genetic disorders	35
Neuromuscular disorders	15

[a]From *Orphan Drugs in Development, 1992 Annual Survey*, Pharmaceutical Manufacturers Association, Washington, 1993.
[b]As of March 6, 1992

Until 1992, FDA approval times for orphan products were 6 to 7 months shorter than those for other products. In 1992, the average time for all drug approvals was 32.6 months, whereas that for orphan drugs was only 17.6 months. This difference could be due to the distribution among FDA divisions (which differ in average review times required) or to other factors, and no trends can be reliably inferred from this single year's experience.

Sales

United States sales data have been collected for 41 of the approved orphan products which have been on the market for one year or more. Mean U.S. sales in the first year of marketing were $19.3 million, median sales $1.6 million. In the first year of marketing, 30 of these 41 orphan products (75%) each earned less than $10 million, three earned between $10 and $25 million, six between $26 and $100 million, and two products more than $100 million. Of the 11 drugs with relatively high sales, four are biotechnology products, which highlights the controversy surrounding the market exclusivity provision of the act. There is no doubt that biotechnology firms are seeking market protection for unpatentable products. They are interested in the protection afforded under the Orphan Drug Act as a vital means of attracting and securing venture capital to survive until they can establish a track record of approved and profitable products. For instance, between 1988 and 1992, the number of biotechnology product designations increased 12%, from 20 products out of 254 in 1988 to 198 products out of 508 designations in 1992 [45].

Remaining Issues

At the time of the passage of the act, the importance of biotechnology was just beginning to be recognized. At present, a few biotechnology products are generating intense controversy over whether the market exclusivity provision is creating an unnecessary monopoly, keeping prices artificially high for products that industry would have developed without the act's protection.

The first example is recombinant human erythropoietin (r-EPO), intended for patients with chronic renal failure-related anemia. It eliminates the need for frequent blood transfusions by patients with end-stage renal disease (ESRD) who are undergoing kidney dialysis. These dialysis patients are covered under the federally financed Medicare program (primarily designed to provide hospital coverage for those over 65 and those who receive Social Security Disability Insurance). When the decision to provide Medicare coverage for these patients was made, the expectation was that the need for dialysis would be replaced by improved therapies, and that coverage for dialysis would enable patients to remain alive until new therapies became available. However, this expectation has not been fulfilled and patients depend on life-long dialysis treatment. Both Amgen Inc. and Genetics Institute applied to the FDA for market exclusivity for their r-EPO products. Amgen was the first to receive FDA approval and market exclusivity, but Genetics Institute was the first to receive a patent. On appeal, the court ruled that Amgen had exclusive marketing rights. Sales of r-EPO exceeded $100 million in the first 6 months of marketing, with reimbursement provided by Medicare. Sales for 1991 totalled $400 million.

The second example is recombinant human growth hormone (r-hGH), intended to treat about 12,000 U.S. children who lack endogenous pituitary hormone, resulting in retarded growth. Two companies provide r-hGH and the shared market has not affected price. Each company receives up to $20,000 annually per child, depending upon the dosage needed. Genetech received FDA market exclusivity in 1985, whereas Eli Lilly received market approval two years later, based on the FDA determination that the two products differed. The Lilly product has one amino acid less, which makes it identical to the natural compound made by the human pituitary. The total market, shared by the two companies, was $150 million in 1991.

The third example, aerosol pentamidine, helps to prevent Pneumocystis carinii pneumonia associated with the human immunodeficiency virus (HIV). In 1991, it derived sales of $130 million; the annual cost per patient is $2400. The number of users will increase with the AIDS epidemic, and for that reason some argue that the product should not enjoy the protection of the act but should be open to price competition by other producers [46–48].

These three examples have intensified the effort to seek a legislative remedy to instances where a small market alone does not make the product unprofitable. A series of amendments dealing with perceived abuses of the act were offered and passed in 1990 (HR 4638), but were vetoed by the President. The amendments would have eliminated orphan status for products used in epidemics where the prevalence exceeds 200,000 and would have allowed shared market access for simultaneously developed identical products intended for the same orphan indication, provided certain stipulations were met.

The three examples of highly profitable orphan products, and the continued attempts to refine the law in response, emphasize the continued importance of the interrelated patent and innovation factors for the pharmaceutical industry. Biotechnology firms are testing the limits of the orphan drug law to deal with patent issues that go far beyond drugs for rare diseases, and the solutions are not yet evident. Nonetheless, despite these controversies yet to be resolved, orphan products have become a new therapeutic resource.

TABLE 3 Approved Orphan Products, January 1983 to August 15, 1993

Generic and Trade Names[a]	Indication Designated	Sponsor, DD = Date Designated, MA = Marketing Approval	Prevalence, Population
Aldesleukin TN = Proleukin	Metastatic renal cell carcinoma	Chiron Corporation DD, 09/14/88; MA, 05/05/92	75,000
Alglucerase injection TN = Ceredase	Replacement therapy in patients with Gaucher's disease Type I	Genzyme Corporation DD, 03/11/85; MA, 04/05/91	20,000
Alpha-1-proteinase inhibitor TN = Prolastin	Replacement therapy in the alpha-1-proteinase inhibitor congenital deficiency state	Cutter Biological DD, 12/07/84; MA, 12/02/87	30,000
Altretamine TN = Hexalen	Advanced adenocarcinoma of the ovary	U.S. Bioscience, Inc. DD, 02/09/84; MA, 12/26/90	11,000
Antihemophilic factor (recombinant) TN = Kogenate	Prophylaxis and treatment of bleeding in individuals with hemophilia A or when surgery is required in individuals with hemophilia A	Miles, Inc. DD, 09/25/89; MA, 02/25/93	16,000
Antithrombin III (human) TN = Thrombate III[b]	Replacement therapy in congenital deficiency of AT-III for prevention and treatment of thrombosis and pulmonary emboli	Miles, Inc. DD, 11/26/84; MA, 12/30/91	24,000
Antithrombin III (human) TN = Atnativ	For the treatment of patients with hereditary AT-III deficiency in connection with surgical or obstetrical procedures or thromboembolism	Kabivitrum, Inc. DD, 02/08/89; MA, 12/13/89	2,500
Atovaquone TN = Mepron	AIDS-1 associated Pneumocystis carinii pneumonia (PCP)	Burroughs Wellcome Company DD, 09/10/90; MA, 11/25/92	45,000

TABLE 3 Continued

Generic and Trade Names[a]	Indication Designated	Sponsor, DD = Date Designated, MA = Marketing Approval	Prevalence, Population
Baclofen TN = Lioresal intrathecal	Intractable spasticity caused by spinal cord injury, multiple sclerosis, and other spinal diseases (including spinal ischemia, spinal tumor, transverse myelitis, cervical spondylosis, and degenerative myelopathy)	Medtronic, Inc. DD, 11/10/87; MA, 06/25/92	40,000
Benzoate and phenylacetate TN = Ucephan	Adjunctive therapy in the prevention and treatment of hyperammonemia in patients with urea cycle enzymopathy (UCE) due to carbamylphosphate synthetase, ornithine, transcarbamylase, or arginosuccinate synthetase deficiency	Kendall McGaw Laboratories DD, 01/21/86; MA, 12/23/87	100
Beractant TN = Survanta intratracheal suspension	Neonatal respiratory distress syndrome (RDS)	Ross Laboratories DD, 02/05/86; MA, 07/01/91	50,000
Beractant TN = Survanta intratracheal suspension	Prevention of neonatal respiratory distress syndrome (RDS)	Ross Laboratories DD, 02/05/86; MA, 07/01/91	35,000
Botulinum toxin Type A TN = Oculinum	Blepharospasm associated with dystonia in adults (patients 12 years of age and older)	Allergan, Inc. DD, 03/22/84; MA, 12/29/89	1,500
Botulinum toxin Type A TN = Oculinum	Strabismus associated with dystonia in adults (patients 12 years of age and older)	Allergan, Inc. DD, 03/22/84; MA, 12/29/89	14,700

TABLE 3 Continued

Generic and Trade Names[a]	Indication Designated	Sponsor, DD = Date Designated, MA = Marketing Approval	Prevalence, Population
Calcitonin, human for injection TN = Cibacalcin	Symptomatic Paget's disease of bone (osteitis deformans)	Ciba-Geigy Corporation DD, 01/20/87; MA, 10/31/86	160,000
Calcium acetate TN = Phos-lo	Hyperphosphotemia in end stage renal failure	Braintree Laboratories DD, 12/22/88; MA, 12/10/90	90,000
Chenodiol TN = Chenix[b]	For patients with radiolucent stones in well opacifying gallbladders, in whom elective surgery would be undertaken except for the presence of increased surgical risk due to systemic disease or age	Reid-Rowell, Inc. DD, 09/21/84; MA, 07/28/83	150,000
Citric Acid, glucono-delta-lactone, and magnesium carbonate TN = Renacidin irrigation	Renal and bladder calculi of the apatite or struvite variety	United-Guardian, Inc. DD, 08/28/89; MA, 10/02/90	72,000
Cladribine TN = Leustatin injection	Hairy cell leukemia	R.W. Johnson Research Institute DD, 11/15/90; MA, 02/26/93	33,000
Clofazimine TN = Lamprene	Lepromatous leprosy, including dapsone-resistant lepromatous leprosy and lepromatous leprosy complicated by erythema nodosum leprosum	Ciba-Geigy Corporation DD, 06/11/84; MA, 12/15/86	4,000
Coagulation factor IX TN = Mononine	Replacement treatment and prophylaxis of the hemorrhagic complications of hemophilia B	Armour Pharmaceutical Company DD, 06/27/89; MA, 08/20/92	4,000

TABLE 3 Continued

Generic and Trade Names[a]	Indication Designated	Sponsor, DD = Date Designated, MA = Marketing Approval	Prevalence, Population
Coagulation factor IX (human) TN = Alphanine	Replacement therapy in patients with hemophilia B for the prevention and control of bleeding episodes, and during surgery to correct defective hemostasis	Alpha Therapeutic Corporation DD, 07/05/90; MA, 12/31/90	4,000
Colfosceril palmitate TN = Exosurf neonatal for intratracheal suspension	Prevention of hyaline membrane disease (HMD); also known as respiratory distress syndrome (RDS), in infants born at 32 weeks gestation or less	Burroughs Wellcome Company DD, 10/20/89; MA, 08/02/90	75,000
Colfosceril palmitate TN = Exosurf neonatal for intratracheal suspension	Established hyaline membrane disease (HMD) at all gestational ages	Burroughs Wellcome Company DD, 10/20/89; MA, 08/02/90	75,000
Cromolyn Sodium TN = Gastrocrom	Mastocytosis	Fisons Corporation DD, 03/08/84; MA, 12/22/89	1,000
Cromolyn Sodium 4% ophthalmic solution TN = Opticrom 4% ophthalmic solution[b]	Vernal keratoconjunctivitis (VKC)	Fisons Corporation DD, 07/24/85; MA, 10/03/84	15,850
Cytomegalovirus immune globulin (human)	Prevention of attenuation of primary cytomegalovirus disease in immunosuppressed recipients of organ transplants	Mass. Pub. Health. Bio. Labs. DD, 08/03/87; MA, 04/17/90	2,000

TABLE 3 Continued

Generic and Trade Names[a]	Indication Designated	Sponsor, DD = Date Designated, MA = Marketing Approval	Prevalence, Population
Digoxin immune fab (Ovine) TN = Digibind[b]	Potentially life-threatening digitalis intoxication in patients who are refractory to management by conventional therapy	Burroughs Wellcome Company DD, 11/01/84; MA, 03/21/86	4,000
Dronabinol TN = Marinol	Apetite stimulation in patients with a confirmed diagnosis of acquired immunodeficiency syndrome (AIDS)	Unimed, Inc DD, 01/15/91; MA, 12/22/92	95,000
Eflornithine HCl TN = Ornidyl	Trypanosoma brucei gambiense infection (sleeping sickness)	Marion Merrell Dow, Inc. DD, 04/23/86; MA, 11/28/90	1
Epoetin Alfa TN = Epogen	Anemia associated with end stage renal disease (ESRD)	Amgen, Inc. DD, 04/10/86; MA, 06/01/89	78,000
Epoetin Alfa TN = Epogen	Anemia associated with HIV infection or HIV treatment	Amgen, Inc. DD, 07/01/91; MA, 12/31/90	28,000
Ethanolamine oleate TN = Ethamolin	To prevent rebleeding of patients with esophageal varices that have recently bled	Block Drug Company, Inc. DD, 03/22/84; MA, 12/12/88	17,300
Etidronate disodium TN = Didronel	Hypercalcemia of a malignancy inadequately managed by dietary modification and/or oral hydration	MGI Pharma, Inc. DD, 03/21/86; MA, 04/21/87	71,000
Felbamate TN = Felbatol	Lennox-Gastaut syndrome	Wallace Laboratories DD, 01/24/89; MA, 07/29/93	125,000

TABLE 3 Continued

Generic and Trade Names[a]	Indication Designated	Sponsor, DD = Date Designated, MA = Marketing Approval	Prevalence, Population
Fludarabine phosphate TN = Fludara	Chronic lymphocytic leukemia (CLL), including refractory CLL	Berlex Laboratories, Inc. DD, 04/18/89; MA, 04/18/91	35,000
Gallium nitrate injection TN = Ganite	Hypercalcemia of malignancy	Fujisawa Pharmaceutical Co. DD, 12/05/88; MA, 01/17/91	121,407
Gonadorelin acetate TN = Lutrepulse	Induction of ovulation in women with hypothalamic amenorrhea due to a deficiency or absence in the quantity or pulse pattern of endogenous GNRH secretion	R.W. Johnson Research Institute DD, 04/22/87; MA, 10/10/89	29,000
Halofantrine TN = Halfan	Mild to moderate acute malaria caused by susceptible strains of *P. Falciparum* and *P. Vivax*	Smithkline Beecham DD, 11/04/91; MA, 07/24/92	5,000
Hemin TN = Panhematin[b]	Amelioration of recurrent attacks of acute intermittent porphyria (AIP) temporarily related to the menstrual cycle in susceptible women and similar symptoms which occur in other patients with AIP, *Porphyria variegata*, and *Heredita Coproporphyria*	Abbott Laboratories DD, 03/16/84; MA, 07/20/83	100
Histrelin acetate TN = Supprelin Injection	Central precocious puberty	Roberts Pharmaceutical Corp. DD, 08/10/88; MA, 12/24/91	5,000

TABLE 3 Continued

Generic and Trade Names[a]	Indication Designated	Sponsor, DD = Date Designated, MA = Marketing Approval	Prevalence, Population
Idarubicin HCl for injection TN = Idamycin	Acute myelogenous leukemia (AML), also referred to as acute nonlymphocytic leukemia (ANLL)	Adria Laboratories, Inc. DD, 07/25/88; MA, 09/27/90	30,000
Ifosfamide TN = Ifex	In combination with certain other approved antineoplastic agents, for third-line chemotherapy germ-cell testicular cancer	Bristol-Myers Squibb DD, 01/20/87; MA, 12/30/88	10,000
Interferon Alfa-2A (recombinant) TN = Roferon-A	AIDS-related Kaposi's sarcoma	Hoffmann-La Roche, Inc. DD, 12/14/87; MA, 11/21/88	10,000
Interferon Alfa-2B (recombinant) TN = Intron A	AIDS-related Kaposi's sarcoma	Schering Corporation DD, 06/24/87; MA, 11/21/88	10,000
Interferon Beta (recombinant human) TN = Betaseron	Multiple sclerosis	Chiron Corporation DD, 11/17/88; MA, 07/23/93	145,000
Interferon Gamma 1-B TN = Actimmune	Chronic granulomatous disease	Genentech, Inc. DD, 09/30/88; MA, 12/20/90	300
Leucovorin TN = Leucovorin Calcium	In combination with 5-fluorouracil for metastatic colorectal cancer	Lederle Laboratories Division DD, 12/08/86; MA, 12/12/91	110,000
Leucovorin TN = Leucovorin Calcium	For rescue use after high dose methotrexate therapy in the treatment of osteosarcoma	Lederle Laboratories Division DD, 08/17/88; MA, 08/31/88	5,000
Leuprolide acetate TN = Lupron injection	Central precocious puberty	TAP Pharmaceuticals, Inc. DD, 07/25/88; MA, 04/16/93	6,000

TABLE 3 Continued

Generic and Trade Names[a]	Indication Designated	Sponsor, DD = Date Designated, MA = Marketing Approval	Prevalence, Population
Levocarnitine TN = Vita Carn[b]	Genetic carnitine deficiency	Sigma-Tau Pharmaceuticals, Inc. DD, 02/28/84; MA, 04/10/86	100
Levocarnitine TN = Carnitor[b]	Primary carnitine deficiency of genetic origin	Sigma-Tau Pharmaceuticals, Inc. DD, 07/26/84; MA, 12/27/85	100
Levocarnitine TN = Carnitor	Secondary carnitine deficiency of genetic origin	Sigma-Tau Pharmaceuticals, Inc. DD, 07/26/84; MA, 12/16/92	100
Levomethadyl acetate hydrochloride TN = Orlaam	Heroin addiction suitable for maintenance on opiate agonists	Biodevelopment Corporation DD, 01/24/84; MA 07/09/93	100,000
Liothyronine sodium injection TN = Triostat	Myxedema coma/precoma	Smithkline Beecham DD, 07/30/90; MA, 12/31/91	14,000
Mefloquine HCl TN = Lariam	Acute malaria due to *Plasmodium falciparum* and *P. vivax*	Hoffmann-La Roche, Inc. DD, 04/13/88; MA, 05/02/89	1,000
Mefloquine HCl TN = Lariam	Prophylaxis of *Plasmodium falciparum* falciparum malaria which is resistant to other available drugs	Hoffmann—La Roche, Inc. DD, 04/13/88; MA, 05/02/89	150,000
Melphalan TN = Alkeran for injection	Multiple myeloma where oral therapy is inappropriate	Burroughs Wellcome Company DD, 02/24/92; MA, 11/18/92	60,000
Mesna TN = Mesnex	Prophylactic agent in reducing the incidence of ifosfamide-induced hemorrhagic cystitis	Degussa Corporation DD, 11/14/85; MA, 12/30/88	40,000

ROYAL PHARMACEUTICAL SOCIETY [illegible]
1, LAMBETH HIGH STREET, LONDON SE1 7JN

TABLE 3 Continued

Generic and Trade Names[a]	Indication Designated	Sponsor, DD = Date Designated, MA = Marketing Approval	Prevalence, Population
Methotrexate sodium TN = Methotrexate	Osteogenic sarcoma	Lederle Laboratories Division DD, 10/21/85; MA, 04/07/88	1,900
Metronidazole (topical) TN = Metrogel	Acne rosacea	Curatek Pharmaceuticals DD, 10/22/87; MA, 11/22/88	136,000
Mitoxantrone HCl TN = Novantrone	Acute myelogenous leukemia (AML), also referred to as acute nonlymphocytic leukemia (ANLL)	Lederle Laboratories Division DD, 07/13/87; MA, 12/23/87	30,000
Monooctanoin TN = Moctanin[b]	Dissolution of cholesterol gallstones retained in the common bile duct	Ethitek Pharmaceuticals, Inc. DD, 05/30/84; MA, 10/31/85	4,500
Morphine suflate concentrate (preservative free) TN = Infumorph	For microinfusion devices for intraspinal administration in the treatment of intractable chronic pain	Elkins-Sinn, Inc. DD, 07/12/90; MA, 07/19/91	25,000
Nafarelin acetate TN = Synarel nasal solution (waived exclusivity)	Central precocious puberty	Syntex (USA), Inc. DD, 07/20/88; MA, 02/26/92	6,000
Naltrexone HCl TN = Trexan[b]	Blockade of the pharmacological effects of exogenously administered opioids as an adjunct to the maintenance of the opioid-free state in detoxified formerly opioid-dependent individuals	Du Pont Pharmaceuticals DD, 03/11/85; MA, 11/30/84	40,000

TABLE 3 Continued

Generic and Trade Names[a]	Indication Designated	Sponsor, DD = Date Designated, MA = Marketing Approval	Prevalence, Population
Pegademase bovine TN = Adagen	Enzyme replacement therapy for ADA deficiency in patients with severe combined immunodeficiency (SCID)	Enzon, Inc. DD, 05/29/84; MA, 03/21/90	40
Pentamidine isethionate TN = Pentam 300[b]	Pneumocystis carinii pneumonia	Fujisawa Pharmaceutical Co. DD, 02/28/84; MA, 10/16/84	3,000
Pentamidine isethionate TN = Nebupent	Prevention of pneumocystis carinii pneumonia in patients at high risk of developing this disease	Fujisawa Pharmaceutical Co. DD, 01/12/88; MA, 06/15/89	17,000
Pentastarch TN = Pentaspan	Adjunct in leukapheresis to improve the harvesting and increase the yield of leukocytes by centrifugal means	Du Pont Pharmaceuticals DD, 08/28/85; MA, 05/19/87	50,000
Pentostatin for injection TN = Nipent	Hairy cell leukemia	Warner-Lambert Co. DD, 09/10/87; MA, 10/11/91	10,000
Potassium citrate TN = Urocit-K[b]	Prevention of uric acid nephrolithiasis	Univ. of Texas Health Sciences DD, 11/01/84; MA, 08/30/85	184,000
Potassium citrate TN = Urocit-K[b]	Prevention of calcium renal stones in patients with hypocitraturia	Univ. of Texas Health Sciences DD, 09/16/85; MA, 08/30/85	17,000
Potassium citrate TN = Urocit K[b]	Avoidance of the complication of calcium stone formation in patients with uric lithiasis	Univ. of Texas Health Sciences DD, 05/29/84; MA, 08/30/85	17,000

TABLE 3 Continued

Generic and Trade Names[a]	Indication Designated	Sponsor, DD = Date Designated, MA = Marketing Approval	Prevalence, Population
Rifabutin TN = Mycobutin	Prevention of disseminated mycobacterium avium complex (MAC) disease in patients with advanced HIV infection	Adria Laboratories, Inc.	100,000
Rifampin TN = Rifadin I.V.	Antituberculosis treatment where use of the oral form of the drug is not feasible	Marion Merrell Dow, Inc. DD, 12/09/85; MA, 05/25/89	40,000
Sargramostim TN = Leukine	Neutropenia associated with bone marrow transplant in patients with non-Hodgkin's lymphoma, Hodgkin's disease, and acute lymphoblastic leukemia	Immunex Corporation DD, 05/03/90; MA, 03/05/91	3,000
Sargramostim TN = Leukine	Treatment of patients who have undergone allogeneic or autologous bone marrow transplantation and in whom engraftment is delayed or in whom engraftment fails	Immunex Corporation DD, 05/03/90; MA, 12/31/91	3,000
Satumomab Pendetide TN = Oncoscint CR/OV	Detection of ovarian carcinoma	Cytogen Corporation DD, 09/25/89; MA, 12/29/92	65,000
Selegiline HCl TN = Eldepryl	Adjuvant to levodopa and carbidopa treatment of idiopathic Parkinson's disease (paralysis agitans), postencephalitic Parkinsonism, and symtomatic Parkinsonism	Somerset Pharmaceuticals, Inc. DD, 11/07/84; MA, 06/05/89	30,000

TABLE 3 Continued

Generic and Trade Names[a]	Indication Designated	Sponsor, DD = Date Designated, MA = Marketing Approval	Prevalence, Population
Somatrem for injection TN = Protropin[b]	Growth failure due to a lack of adequate endogenous growth hormone secretion	Genentech, Inc. DD, 12/09/85; MA, 10/17/85	15,000
Somatropin for injection TN = Humatrope	Growth failure due to inadequate secretion of normal endogenous growth hormone	Eli Lilly DD, 06/12/86; MA, 03/08/87	10,000
Sotalol HCl TN = Betapace	Life-threatening ventricular tachyarrhythmias	Bristol-Myers Squibb DD, 09/23/88; MA, 10/30/92	110,000
Succimer TN = Chemet capsules	Lead poisoning in children	McNeil Consumer Products Co. DD, 05/09/84; MA, 01/30/91	17,000
Teniposide TN = Vumon for injection	Refractory childhood acute lymphocytic leukemia (ALL)	Bristol-Myers Squibb DD, 11/01/84; MA, 07/14/92	1,000
Teriparatide TN = Parathar	Diagnostic agent to assist in establishing the diagnosis in patients presenting with clinical and laboratory evidence of hypocalcemia due to hypoparathyroidism or pseudohypoparathroidism	Rhone-Poulenc Rorer Pharm. DD, 01/09/87; MA, 12/23/87	5,000
Tiopronin TN = Thiola	Prevention of cystine nephrolithiasis in patients with homozygous cystinuria	Pak, Charles Y.C., M.D. DD, 01/17/86; MA, 08/11/88	33,700
Tranexamic acid TN = Cyklokapron	Treatment of patients with congenital coagulopathies who are undergoing surgical procedures, e.g., dental extractions	Kabivitrum, Inc.	20,000

TABLE 3 Continued

Generic and Trade Names[a]	Indication Designated	Sponsor, DD = Date Designated, MA = Marketing Approval	Prevalence, Population
Trientine HCl TN = Cuprid[b]	Patients with Wilson's disease who are intolerant or inadequately responsive to penicillamine	Merck Sharp & Dohme Research DD, 12/24/84; MA, 11/08/85	700
Urofollitropin TN = Metrodin	Induction of ovulation in patients with polycystic ovarian disease who have an elevated LH/FSH ratio and have failed to respond to adequate clomiphene citrate therapy	Serono Laboratories, Inc. DD, 11/25/87; MA, 09/18/86	118,000
Zalcitabine TN = Hivid	Acquired Immunodeficiency Syndrome (AIDS)	Hoffmann-La Roche, Inc. DD, 06/28/88; MA, 06/19/92	30,000
Zidovudine TN = Retrovir	Acquired Immunodeficiency Syndrome (AIDS)	Burroughs Wellcome Company DD, 07/17/85; MA, 03/19/87	10,000
Zidovudine TN = Retrovir	Aids-related complex (ARC)	Burroughs Wellcome Company DD, 05/12/87; MA, 03/19/87	100,000
			Total: 2,815,793

[a]TN = trade name.
[b]Exclusivity expired.

References

1. Asbury, C. H., Medical drugs of limited commercial interest: Profit alone is a bitter pill, *Intern. J. Health Serv.*, 11(3):451–462 (1981).
2. Kemp, B., *Appendix to the Interim Report of the Committee on Drugs of Limited Commercial Value*, FDA (unpublished), Washington, 1975.
3. Woert, M. V., Profitable and non-profitable drugs, *New Engl. J. Med.*, 298(16):903–906 (1978).
4. Rawlins, M., No utopia yet, *Br. Med. J.*, 2(1076) (1977).
5. Rawlins, M., Editorial, *Lancet*, 2(7970):835–836 (1976).

6. Karch, F., *Orphan Drugs*, Marcel Dekker, Inc., New York, 1982, pp. 1–205.
7. Goldberg, L., and Zaroslinski, J., Development of Dopamine. In: *Orphan Drugs* (F. Karch, ed.), Marcel Dekker, Inc., 1982, pp. 118–137.
8. DeFelice, S., The Carnitine Story. In: *Orphan Drugs* (F. Karch, ed.), Marcel Dekker, Inc., 1982, pp. 34–35.
9. Stubbins, J., Alkylating Local Anesthetics. In: *Orphan Drugs* (F. Karch, ed.), Marcel Dekker, Inc., 1982, pp. 74–87.
10. Walshe, J. M., Treatment of Wilson's disease with trientine (triethylene tetramine) dihydrochloride, *Lancet*, 1:643–647 (1982).
11. Food and Drug Administration, Interagency Task Force Report to the Secretary of DHEW, Washington, 1979, pp. 1–82.
12. Finkel, M., Drugs of limited commercial value, *New Engl. J. Med.*, 302:643–644 (1980).
13. Lasagna, L., Who will adopt the orphan drugs? *Regulation*, 3(6):27–32 (1979).
14. Provost, G. P., Homeless or orphan drugs, *Am. J. Hosp. Pharm.*, 25:609 (1968).
15. Schon, D., *Beyond the Stable Stare*, Basic Books, New York, 1981, pp. 120–125.
16. Young, J. H., *The Toadstool Millionaires*, Princeton University Press, Princeton, N.J., 1961.
17. Silverman, M., and Lee, P. R., *Pills, Profits and Politics*, University of California Press, Berkeley, 1974, p. 2.
18. Harris, R., *The Real Voice*, Macmillan, New York, 1964, pp. 21–25.
19. Temin, P., Technology, regulation and market structure in the modern pharmaceutical industry, *Bell J. Econ.*, 10(2):427–446 (1979).
20. U.S. Government Printing Office, *Report of the Panel on Chemicals and Health of the President's Science Advisory Committee*, NSF: 73–500 (1973).
21. Schwartzmann, D., *Innovation in the Pharmaceutical Industry*, Johns Hopkins University Press, Baltimore, 1976, pp. 106–107.
22. Hansen, R. W., The Pharmaceutical Development Process: Estimates of Development Costs and Times and Effects of Proposed Regulatory Changes. In: *Issues in Pharmaceutical Economics* (R. Chien, ed.), Lexington Books, Lexington, MA, 1980, pp. 151–181.
23. DiMasi, J., Hason, R., Grabowski, H., and Lasagna, L., The cost of innovation in the pharmaceutical industry and health economics, *J. Health Econ.*, 10:107–142 (1991).
24. Devita, V., Oliverio, V. T., Muggia, F. M., Wiernik, P. W., Ziegler, J., Goldin, A., Rubin, D., Henney, J., and Schepartz, S., The Drug Development and Clinical Trials Programs of the Division of Cancer Treatment, National Cancer Institute, *Cancer Clin. Trials*, 2:195–216 (1979).
25. Zubrod, C. G., Schepartz, S., Leiten, J., Endicott, K. M., Carrese, L. M., and Baker, C. E., *Cancer Chemotherapy Reports*, October 1966, 50(7), U.S. DHEW, Bethesda, 1968.
26. Final Report for the National Cancer Institute, *Rate of Development of Anticancer Drugs by the National Cancer Institute and the U.S. Pharmaceutical Industry and the Impact of Regulation*, University of Rochester Medical Center, New York, 1981, pp. ii, 40.
27. Krall, R. A., Anti-epileptic drug development. I. History and a program for progress, *Epilepsia*, 19(4):398–408 (1978).
28. National Institute of Neurological and Communicative Disorders and Stroke Antiepileptic Drug Development Program, *Program Performance Summary*, Washington, 1982.
29. Asbury, C. H., *Medical Drugs of Limited Commercial Interest: The Development of Federal Policy*, Johns Hopkins School of Hygiene and Public Health, Baltimore, 1981, pp. 157–175.
30. NIH, *Report of the Commission to Combat Huntingtons Disease and its Consequences*, Bethesda, 1976, pp. 1501–1510.
31. Asbury, C. H., and Stolley, P., Orphan Drugs: Creating a Policy, *Ann. Int. Med.*, 95(2):221–224 (1981).
32. Woert, M. V., L-5-Hydroxytryptophan. In: *Orphan Drugs* (F. Karch, ed.), Marcel Dekker, Inc., 1982, pp. 14–31.
33. Holtzman, E., Rep., H.R. 7089, 96th Congress, 2nd Session, Washington, April 17, 1980.

34. Klugman, J., and Seligman, A., U.S. Government Printing Office, Serial No. 97–17:10–16, Washington, 1981.
35. Leave of reality, Editorial, *Wall Street Journal*, March 12, 1981.
36. Waxman, H. A., The history and development of the Orphan Drug Act. In: *Orphan Diseases and Orphan Drugs* (I. H. Scheinberg and J. Walshe, eds.), Manchester University Press, Manchester, U.K., 1986, pp. 135–145.
37. Waxman, H. A., H.R. 5328, 97th Congress, 1st Session, Washington, 1981.
38. Orphan Drug Act Report, 97th Congress, 2nd Session, September 17, Washington, 1982.
39. Asbury, C. H., Collaborative efforts on behalf of orphan diseases. In: *Orphan Diseases and Orphan Drugs* (I. H. Scheinberg and J. Walshe, eds.), Manchester University Press, Manchester, U.K., 1986, pp. 106–118.
40. Asbury, C. H., *Orphan Drugs: Medical vs. Market Value*, Lexington Books, Lexington, MA, 1985.
41. Haffner, M. E., Tenth Anniversary of the Orphan Drug Act, FDCI/FDA Seminar, Washington, February 23, 1993.
42. Orphan Drugs in Development, *1992 Annual Survey*, Pharmaceutical Manufacturers Association, Washington, 1992.
43. Food and Drug Administration, *Approved Orphan Products, January 1983 to August 15, 1993*, Rockville, MD, 1993.
44. Asbury, C. H., The Orphan Drug Act: The first 7 years, *JAMA*, 265:893–897 (1991).
45. Schuman, S. R., et al., Implementation of the Orphan Drug Act, *Food Drug Law J.*, 47(4):363–403 (1992).
46. Hilts, P. J., Seeking limits to a drug monopoly, *New York Times*, D1,7, May 14, 1992.
47. Asbury, C. H., Evolution and current status of the Orphan Drug Act, *Intern. J. Technol. Assess. Health Care*, 8(4):573–582 (1992).
48. Coster, J. M., Recombinant erythropoietin: orphan product with a silver spoon, *Intern. J. Technol. Assess. Health Care*, 8(4):635–646 (1992).

CAROLYN H. ASBURY

Otic Preparations

Introduction

Otic preparations are commonly used to treat diseases of the external ear and occasionally of the middle ear. Problems include cerumen impaction, dermatitis of the external ear canal, and infectious processes. External otitis and chronic otitis media constitute the majority of infectious diseases of the ear. This article gives an overview of otic preparations, their uses, current availability, and the areas of future development.

Anatomy and Physiology of the Ear

Figure 1 is a diagram of the normal ear comprised of the external ear canal, middle ear space, and hearing canal, or cochlea. The outer two-thirds of the external ear canal is formed by a cartilage framework; it has a thick soft tissue lining containing the apopilosebaceous unit.

External sounds travel through the external ear canal to reach the tympanic membrane. Vibration of the tympanic membrane transmits a sound wave to the three middle ear ossicles. These, in turn, send the sound wave to the inner ear (cochlea), where it is transformed into a nerve impulse. This impulse is sent to the brain, where the perception of hearing occurs.

The normal external auditory canal has several mechanisms that protect it from infections. The S-shaped anatomy of the external auditory canal provides protection from foreign bodies under normal circumstances. The tragus provides protection anteriorly, and hair from follicles found just inside the meatus prevent airborne debris from entering.

The external auditory canal skin is acidic with a pH between 4 and 5. Keratin, which consists of desquamated epithelial cells, is produced by the epithelial lining of the external ear canal; it has an isoelectric point of pH 5. Any increase above this value causes hydration of the keratin layer, increasing susceptibility to pathogenic organisms. As most organisms responsible for otitis externa and chronic superlative otitis grow best at an alkaline pH of 7.2 to 7.6, the acidic pH of the external ear canal is bactericidal or bacteriostatic to many of these pathogenic organisms.

Enzymes produced by sweat and sebaceous glands provide antimicrobial activity. Muramidase, a lysozyme excreted by the sweat glands, may be effective in lysing *Staphylococcus epidermidis* and other gram-positive organisms found on the surface of the ear canal skin. Unsaturated fatty acids, resulting from the breakdown of lipids secreted from sebaceous glands, exert antimicrobial activity against gram-negative organisms and fungi [1].

An intact tympanic membrane protects the normal sterile middle ear space from bacterial pathogens. A ruptured tympanic membrane or tympanostomy tube allows external bacteria access to the middle ear space.

Cerumen, or earwax, is produced in the outer one-third of the external ear canal. It exerts a protective role by forming an oily, mechanical barrier, considered bacteriostatic and fungistatic, over the skin of the external ear canal. A cerumen plug consists mainly

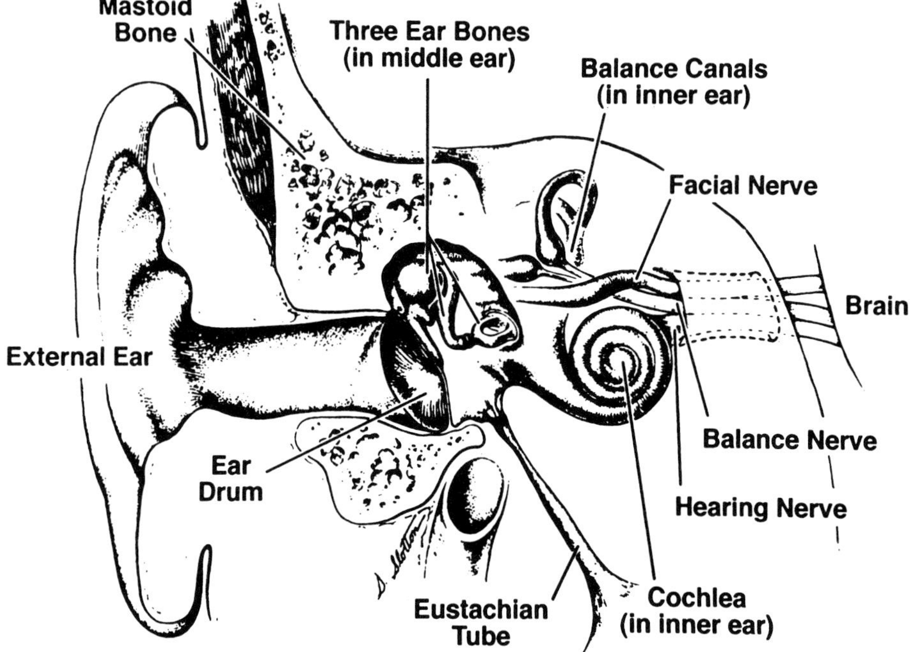

FIG. 1. A diagram of the normal ear. (Courtesy of the House Ear Institute, Los Angeles, CA).

of sheets of keratin. It also contains hair and the secretions of both the sebaceous and ceruminous glands of the external ear canal. Contained within these secretions are glycopeptides, lipids, hyaluronic acid, sialic acid, heparin sulfate, lysosomal enzymes, and immunoglobulin [2]. The overall chemical composition of cerumen consists of saturated and unsaturated long chain fatty acids, alcohols, squalene, and cholesterol [3].

Pathology and Bacteriology of Otitis

To develop new drugs and devices to treat diseases of the external ear requires an understanding of its pathophysiology and a knowledge about the most common organisms responsible for ear inflammation and infections.

Acute otitis externa is an inflammatory condition of the external auditory canal, most commonly precipitated by local trauma, that is, Q-tips, fingernails, or other foreign objects that abrade the external ear canal skin. Other predisposing factors include [4]:

- Maceration of epithelial tissue in the ear canal from prolonged exposure to water or moisture,
- Plugging of sebaceous gland ducts which lowers resistance to infection,
- Moisture absorption by the stratum corneum layer of the epithelium at humidity levels above 80%,
- Elevated ambient temperature against a background of high relative humidity,

- Invasion of exogenous organisms through breaches in a damaged epithelial surface,
- An absence of cerumen, and
- the presence of an alkaline secretion.

Clinical manifestations of the pre-inflammatory stage of external otitis include itching of the external ear canal and congestion of the apopilosebaceous unit. These are thought to result from the loss of lipids in the external auditory canal which, in turn, results in an increase in the aqueous content of the stratum corneum, causing intracellular edema. The acute inflammatory stage is seen with trauma induced by scratching. By this means, bacteria are allowed access to the dermis. A spectrum of clinical manifestations occurs, ranging from mild edema of the ear canal skin with a clear serous discharge to a severe form characterized by intense pain, a grossly edematous ear canal, and a purulent discharge. A chronic inflammatory stage has also been described. It is characterized by thickening of the skin, eczematization, lichenification, and superficial skin ulceration [4].

Otomycosis is the result of a superficial fungal infection in the external auditory canal. This is most commonly the result of an underlying bacterial infection. Fungi initially implant into the stratum corneum, where they lie dormant for several days to weeks. Then they grow in the superficial layer of the skin causing inflammation. Initially the patient usually complains of itching. In the earliest stages, mild edema may be the only clinical symptom. Later, the patient may present with a fungal mass consisting of waxy debris surrounded by a velvety gray membrane with small black spores [5].

Chronic suppurative otitis media is an inflammatory condition of the middle ear. The presence of a tympanic membrane perforation or a tympanotomy tube allows drainage into the external ear canal. Increased vascularity of the mucosa and submucosa combined with acute and chronic inflammatory cells are its hallmark. Granulation tissue, fibrosis, and osteoneogenesis are also commonly present. The granulation tissue contains neutrophils and plasma cells associated with small blood vessels and fibroblasts [6].

Pseudomonas aeruginosa and *Staphylococcus aureus* are the most common organisms responsible for acute otitis externa. *Proteus* species are thought to be responsible for the chronic inflammatory stage associated with it. *Aspergillus niger* and *Candida albicans* are the most common organisms responsible for otomycosis. *Mucormycosis*, yeast-like fungi, dermatophytes, and *Actinomyces* may also be seen [5].

Cultures from patients with chronic suppurative otitis media demonstrate that the most common organisms are *Pseudomonas aeruginosa* and *Staphylococcus aureus*. These are usually mixed infections with a variety of organisms present [7,8]; they exhibit a higher resistance to antibiotics.

Papastavros [9], in a study of 119 cases of chronic suppurative otitis media, noted a large number (81%) of gentamicin-resistant organisms in patients previously treated with topical gentamicin. Brook [7] cultured drainage from 54 children with chronic suppurative otitis media and showed that 70% of these patients harbored beta-lactamase-producing bacteria. Of 37 patients with beta-lactamase-producing bacteria, 32 had previously been treated with an oral penicillin or cephalosporin. No child in this study had received prior ototopical drops. In 39% of the children with bilateral-draining ears, a different organism predominated on each side. Both of these studies demonstrate the potential for encountering resistant organisms in chronic otitis media after prior oral or topical antibiotic therapy.

Cerumen Preparations

Normal desquamation of the epithelial layer of the external ear canal results in migration of cerumen toward the meatus. Any interference with this normal self-cleaning mechanism results in cerumen impaction. An in vitro study has demonstrated that cerumenolysis occurs as the keratin cells, the major constituents of a cerumen plug, are hydrated, resulting in lysis of these cells [2]. Consistent with this finding, aqueous preparations have been demonstrated to be better cerumenolytic products than organic, nonaqueous preparations [2,10,11]. Before using any cerumenolytic agent, the presence of an intact tympanic membrane must be confirmed in order to prevent two possible complications. Introduction of these compounds into the middle ear is often painful, and furthermore the irrigation of cerumen with its keratin cells into the middle ear space may result in a cholesteatoma, a benign but destructive skin growth which requires surgery.

Impacted cerumen can be simply removed by instillation of mineral oil or glycerin into the ear canal. These solutions soften the cerumen, facilitating the separation of the keratin plug from the epithelium, and thus assist the normal migration of cerumen toward the external meatus. Irrigation of the ear canal with hydrogen peroxide is another simple method. The release of oxygen provides a mechanical means for both softening the cerumen and separating it from the canal skin.

Unfortunately, these simple methods are not always successful, and cerumenolytics have been developed to help dissolve cerumen and facilitate its removal. In most cases, however, flushing the ear canal with a rinsing solution or physical extraction is still required.

Over the years, numerous cerumenolytic agents composed of aqueous solutions or organic solvents have been tested (Table 1) [12]. Currently, the most common over-the-counter products consist of carbamide peroxide in glycerin. The latter softens the wax, whereas the oxygen released from the peroxide helps to loosen tissue debris. Usually, this agent may need to be applied repeatedly over several days for the wax to soften. The softened wax may be removed with gentle irrigation or by blowing air into the external canal.

Triethanolamine polypeptide oleate condensate in propylene glycol, Cerumenex, requires a prescription. Its mechanism of action is thought to result from softening of the cerumen plug and lubrication of the ear canal [2], which is usually achieved in 15–20 min; however, mechanical removal of the cerumen plug may still be necessary. Application of this agent is best confined to a physician's office, as severe allergic skin reactions occur occasionally.

TABLE 1 Cerumenolytic Products

Product	Cerumenolytic Agent	Other Ingredients
Cerumenex	Triethanolamine polypeptide oleate condensate	Propylene glycol Chlorbutanol (0.5%)
Debrox drops	Carbamide peroxide (6.5%)	Glycerin Propylene glycol Citric acid
Murine ear drops	Carbamide peroxide (6.5%)	Alcohol (6.3%) Glycerin

Although not marketed as a cerumenolytic, docusate sodium has been found to be a very effective agent [13]. Most commonly used as an aqueous fecal softener, its action on cerumen results in keratin cell expansion and lysis. The preparation is alkaline and in solution releases free hydroxyl ions [2]. Drops placed in the ear canal for 10–15 min usually result in cerumen disimpaction. The plug may then be easily rinsed out of the ear canal or mechanically removed.

The ideal cerumenolytic preparation (a hypo-osmolar, alkaline, aqueous solution) has not yet been developed. It will be able to lyse the keratin cells of cerumen and allow for easy disimpaction [2].

In contrast to the use of cerumenolytic agents, some patients occasionally require cerumen replacement products for conditions such as dry skin, eczema, psoriasis, and chronic otitis of the external ear canal. Unfortunately, there is no product available currently to meet this need.

Antiseptics

Antiseptics agents are often used for the treatment of external ear canal disease. As with cerumenolytics, the presence of an intact tympanic membrane must be confirmed prior to their use. Some antiseptics are commonly used for otologic surgical prophylaxis. Antiseptic otologic preparations are marketed only as the acetic acid solutions.

Acetic acid preparations (usually 2–5% solutions) have both antibacterial and antifungal activity. They are particularly useful against *Pseudomonas aeruginosa*, *Staphylococci*, beta-hemolytic *Streptococci*, *Candida* species, and *Aspergillus*. No organisms are resistant to these preparations [14]. Acetic acid solutions placed in the external ear are generally well tolerated and nonsensitizing; however, instillation into the middle ear cavity is associated with pain. The main drawback of these agents is the vinegar-like smell associated with the instillation. Acetic acid solutions may be combined with aluminum acetate or a steroid compound for anti-inflammatory and antipruritic properties [15].

General antiseptics such as povidine iodine (Betadine), chlorhexidine gluconate (Hibiclens), and hexachlorophene (pHisohex) may be used ototopically for surgical prophylaxis. Povidine iodine is the most commonly employed because of its broad spectrum of activity against microflora, microzoa, and viruses. It is not allowed to enter the middle ear during surgical prophylaxis as it inhibits fibroblast migration during the healing process. However, both chlorhexidine or hexachlorophene may be used for surgical prophylaxis in patients who are allergic to iodine. Chlorhexidine is preferred, because it has a broad spectrum of antimicrobial activity against both gram-positive and gram-negative organisms. The bacteriostat hexachlorophen is more effective against gram-positive than gram-negative organisms; suppuration decreases its activity [15,16].

Isopropyl alcohol is used to rinse the ear canal in patients prone to the development of external otitis. It is commonly applied after swimming as a prophylactic measure. Although isopropyl alcohol has broad bactericidal activity, it is widely used as a drying agent for the external ear canal. Application into the middle ear space causes severe pain, and it should not be used in the presence of an perforated tympanic membrane.

Gentian violet and thimerosal (Merthiolate) are used for the treatment of fungal infections and are discussed below.

Antifungal Preparations

Most otomycotic infections are the consequence of treatment with antibiotics. Simple cleaning of the external ear canal and discontinuation of the medication usually suffice to clear up the infection. However, primary and persistent infections require ototopical antifungal medications (Table 2).

Clotrimazole, as a 1% solution, is the most effective topical fungicide for the treatment of otomycosis. It is active against *Aspergillus* and *Candida* species, the most common pathogens responsible for these infections. It acts by interfering with the biosynthesis of ergosterol and is very effective for refractory or chronic cases caused by the dermatophytes or *Candida* species [17].

Amphotericin B is also an effective ototopical preparation. It may be used as a lotion or in a powder form (see below). Its spectrum of activity covers a variety of fungi, including those responsible for otomycosis. Topical therapy is well tolerated with only rare minor side effects of local skin irritation reported. It is poorly absorbed through the skin [18].

Nystatin and miconazole have a similar spectrum of activity as amphotericin B against the common yeast and fungi responsible for otomycosis [17]. Nystatin is occasionally used in solution as an ototopic drop. Miconazole is rarely used because it is readily available only as a cream. Application into the ear canal is difficult without impairing the hearing.

m-Cresyl acetate (Cresylate), a derivative of cresol, is marketed as a ototopical antifungal preparation. It is highly active against *Candida* and *Aspergillus*. The ear canal may be painted with *m*-cresyl acetate on a cotton-tipped applicator or the compound may be used in solution as an ototopical drop. It is considered the antiseptic of choice for the treatment of otomycosis because it is easily used in the outpatient setting and, in contrast

TABLE 2 Otomycotic Preparations

Product	Antifungal Agent	Other Ingredients
Otic domeboro solution	Acetic acid (2%)	Aluminum sulfate Boric acid
VoSol Otic solution	Acetic acid (2%)	Propylene glycol (3%) Benzethonium chloride
Vosol HC Otic solution	Acetic acid (2%)	Hydrocortisone (1%) Propylene glycol (3%) Benzethonium chloride
Fungizone lotion	Amphotericin B (3%) Thimerosal	Propylene glycol
Lotrimin solution	Clotrimazole	Polyethylene glycol
Mycelex solution	Clotrimazole	Polyethylene glycol
Cresylate solution	*m*-Cresyl acetate (25%)	Propylene glycol Isopropanol (25%)
Gentian violet solution	Gentian violet (1%)	Ethanol (10%)
Merthiolate	Thimerosal 1:1000	
Monistat-Derm lotion	Miconazole (2%)	Pegoxol 7 stearate Mineral oil Benxoic acid
Nystatin suspension	Nystatin, 100,000 units/mL	None

to gentian violet and thimerosal, no staining is associated with its use. However, eczematization may occur if applied to the concha, and therefore its application should be limited to the external ear canal [16,19].

Gentian violet is regularly used in the office setting for the treatment of fungal infections. It also has bacteriostatic and bactericidal activity against most gram-positive organisms. The external ear canal is painted with the gentian violet on a cotton-tipped applicator under direct vision using an operating microscope. This compound is a strong dye and blind application into the external ear canal is difficult without staining. For this reason, it is rarely applied on an outpatient basis [16].

Thimerosal (Merthiolate) may also be used topically for the treatment of otomycosis. Considered a bacteriostat, it is an excellent antiseptic agent in vitro against the common yeast and fungi responsible for otomycosis [16,17].

Fungal cultures are used in refractory or persistent cases of otomycosis, where less common fungi may be responsible, and the appropriate ototopical agent may be selected. Systemic antifungal medications are rarely indicated for the treatment of otomycosis, unless associated with systemic fungal infections.

Topical preparations for the treatment of otomycosis should not be used in the presence of a perforated tympanic membrane.

Antimicrobial Drops

As a group, antimicrobial otic drops are the most commonly prescribed ototopical medication (Table 3). Most of the preparations listed in Table 3 contain a mixture of antibiotics in combination with a steroid agent. Acetic acid or an alcohol may be added for bactericidal activity. Some of these preparations contain acetic acid as the main antibacterial agent. Most of these compounds have a low pH, between 3 and 5, similar to that of the normal external ear canal.

Antimicrobial otic drops should be used with caution in the presence of a tympanic membrane perforation because of the potential for ototoxicity. In the case of suppuration, the ear canal should be cleaned prior to drop instillation.

Neomycin and Polymyxin B are the two most common antibiotic agents found in these preparations. Neomycin is bactericidal to many gram-positive and gram-negative organisms, including those responsible for external and chronic otitis such as *S. aureus*, *C. diphtheriae*, *E. coli*, *Proteus*, *Enterobacter*, *Klebsiella*, and *H. influenzae*. It has no activity against anaerobes, and many strains of *Pseudomonas* are resistant. Cutaneous hypersensitivity is estimated to occur in 6–8 % of patients who receive topical treatment [20].

Polymyxin B and Colistin (polymyxin E), first discovered in 1947, have similar antibiotic spectrums limited to gram-negative organisms. *Pseudomonas aeruginosa* is particularly sensitive to these medications. Other sensitive gram-negative organisms include *Enterobacter*, *E. coli*, *Klebsiella*, and *Haemophilus*. These agents interact with the cell-membrane phospholipids to disrupt the bacterial cells; hypersensitivity is very rare. They are poorly absorbed, even when applied to denuded skin [21].

Chloramphenicol may be used ototopically for selective cases of chronic otitis. Despite its relative lack of activity against *Pseudomonas aeruginosa*, it is bacteriostatic

TABLE 3 Otic Antimicrobial Preparations

Product	Ingredients				
	Antimicrobial	Anti-inflammatory	Acid	Antiseptic	Others
Chloromycetin Otic	Chloramphenicol				Propylene glycol
Coly-Mycin S Otic	Colistin Neomycin	Hydrocortisone (1%)	Acetic	Thiomerosal[a]	Thonzonium Polysorbate 80 Sodium acetate
Cortisporin Otic solution	Polymyxin B Neomycin	Hydrocortisone (1%)	Hydrochloric		Glycerin Propylene glycol
Cortisporin Otic suspension	Polymyxin B Neomycin	Hydrocortisone (1%)	Sulfuric[b]	Alcohol Thiomerosal[a]	Propylene glycol Polysorbate 80
Lazersporin-C solution	Polymyxin B Neomycin	Hydrocortisone (1%)			
Otic Domeboro solution			Acetic Boric		Aluminum sulfate Calcium carbonate
Otobiotic	Polymyxin B	Hydrocortisone (0.5%)	Sulfuric[b]		Propylene glycol Glycerin
Pedi-Otic suspension	Polymyxin B Neomycin	Hydrocortisone (1%)	Sulfuric[b]	Alcohol Thiomerosal[a]	Glyceryl monostearate Mineral oil Polyoxyl 40 stearate Propylene glycol
Pyocidin-Otic	Polymyxin B	Hydrocortisone (0.5%)	Hydrochloric[b]		Propylene glycol
Star-Otic solution			Acetic Boric		Propylene glycol
Tridesilon Otic solution		Desonide (0.05%)	Acetic Citric		Propylene glycol Sodium acetate
VoSol Otic solution			Acetic		Propylene glycol Benzethonium chloride
Vosol HC Otic solution		Hydrocortisone (1%)	Acetic		Propylene glycol Benzethonium chloride

[a]Preservative.
[b]To adjust pH.

against the other common organisms responsible for chronic otitis, including *E. coli*, *Clostridium* species, *Staphylococcus aureus*, *Hemophilus influenzae*, *Bacteroides fragilis*, *Klebsiella* species, and certain strains of *Proteus* [15,22]. However, blood dyscrasias and death have been reported following local application, and local skin hypersensitivity may occur with topical therapy [12]. Although rarely for primary therapy, it is used for refractory chronic otitis, especially when a susceptible organism is cultured.

Despite similar antibacterial composition, these preparations may differ in delivery vehicle and pH. Cortisporin Otic Solution is the most acidic, whereas Coly-Mycin S Otic has a pH of 5, the highest of the group [12,23]. The low pH of these compounds and the alcohol used as an antiseptic agent, cause a burning sensation when in contact with the middle ear.

Otobiotic and Pyocidin-Otic contain only the antibiotic polymyxin B. These compounds are useful for the patient allergic to neomycin but should be used only in certain cases inasmuch as polymyxin B does not act against gram-positive organisms such as *Staphylococcus* and the gram-negative organisms, *Proteus* and *Bacteroides fragilis*.

The ototopical antimicrobial preparations discussed above suffice for most cases of otitis externa and selected cases of chronic suppurative otitis. However, these compounds have a limited effect in certain patients with resistant strains of bacteria, drug-induced allergies, or a tympanic membrane perforation that requires administration into the middle ear space. In the last case, ototopical preparations may cause pain because of the acidic pH or the presence of alcohol. Ototoxicity of neomycin, polymyxin B, and colistin is also of concern, and many otolaryngologists prefer topical ophthalmic preparations [23]. Ophthalmic preparations are discussed in the article Ocular Drug Formulation and Delivery earlier in this volume. This is certainly an important area for pharmacological research in the future.

Ophthalmic compounds that may be used as ototopical remedies are given in Table 4 [12]. Generally, these products differ from the otic preparations in a neutral pH and the absence of alcohol. For example, in contrast to its otic counterpart, Chloromycetin Ophthalmic has a buffered pH and offers a preparation with hydrocortisone. Likewise, the main difference between Cortisporin Ophthalmic and the otic preparation is in the neutral pH.

Compared to the otic antimicrobial preparations, ophthalmologic antimicrobial preparations offer the physician a broader range of antibiotics with which to treat the difficult ear infection. Gentamicin, tobramycin, sulfonamides, and ciprofloxacin are the most common antibiotics used.

Gentamicin and tobramycin ophthalmic preparations are commonly used to treat difficult ear infections. The latter is less toxic than gentamicin and its activity against *Pseudomonas* is higher. These antibacterial agents also have a wide spectrum of activity including *Proteus*, *Klebsiella*, *E. coli*, and *Staphylococcus* [20]. As discussed earlier, resistance to gentamicin develops following topical use [9]. Although both of these drugs are known to be ototoxic, the clinical significance is thought to be minimal.

Sulfonamides are bacteriostatic against a wide range of gram-positive and gram-negative organisms. In chronic otitis, ophthalmic preparations are used for their activity against *Pseudomonas aeruginosa*, *Proteus* species, *Streptococcus*, *Corynebacterium diphteriae*, and *Haemophilus influenzae*.

Ciprofloxacin is well known for its wide range of bactericidal activity, especially against *Staphylococcus aureus*, *Staphylococcus epidermidis*, and *Pseudomonas aeruginosa* [24]. This preparation has the ideal antimicrobial spectrum for refractory otitis, but

TABLE 4 Ophthalmologic Antimicrobial Preparations Commonly Used Ototopically

Product	Ingredients				
	Antimicrobial	Anti-inflammatory	Acid	Antiseptic	Others
Chloromycetin ophthalmic solution	Chloramphenicol		Boric		Buffer
Chloromycetin hydrocortisone	Chloramphenicol	Hydrocortisone (2.5%)	Boric		Buffer Cholesterol Methylcellulose Benzethonium chloride[b]
Ciloxan	Ciprofloxacin		Acetic Hydrochloric[a]		Benzethonium chloride[b] Sodium acetate Mannitol Edetate disodium
Cortisporin ophthalmic solution	Polymyxin B Neomycin	Hydrocortisone (1%)	Sulfuric[a]	Cetyl alcohol	Mineral oil Propylene glycol Polyoxyl 40 stearate Glyceryl monostearate
Gantrisin ophthalmic solution	Sulfisoxazole				Phenylmercuric nitrate
Garamycin ophthalmic solution	Gentamycin				Disodium phosphate Monosodium phosphate Benzalkonium chloride[b]
Metimyd ophthalmic solution	Sulfacetamide	Prednisolone		Thiosulfate Alcohol	Sodium phosphate Tyloxapol Edetate disodium Benzalkonium chloride[b]

Neosporin ophthalmic solution	Polymyxin B Neomycin Gramicidin			Alcohol Thimerosal[b]	Propylene glycol Polyoxyethylene–polyoxypropylene compound
Polytrim ophthalmic solution	Trimethoprim sulfate Polymyxin B		Sulfuric[a]		Benzalkonium chloride[b] Sodium hydoxide
Sulamyd ophthalmic solution	Sulfacetamide			Thiosulfate	Methylcellulose Methylparaben Propylparaben
Terra-Cortril ophthalmic solution	Oxytetracycline	Hydrocortisone (1.5%)			Mineral oil Aluminum tristearate
Tobradex ophthalmic suspension	Tobramycin	Dexamethasone	Sulfuric[a]		Benzalkonium chloride[b] Tyloxapol Edetate disodium Hydroxyethyl cellulose
Tobrex ophthalmic solution	Tobramycin		Boric Sulfuric[a]		Benzalkonium chloride[b] Sodium sulfate Tyloxapol

[a]Preservative.
[b]To adjust pH.

TABLE 5 Ototopical Powder Preparations[a]

Ingredients	Amount per dosage (mg)
1. Chloromycetin	50
Sulfanilamide	50
Fungizone	5
2. Chloromycetin	50
Sulfanilamide	50
Fungizone	5
Hydrocortisone	1

[a]For patients who are allergic to sufanilamide these preparations are available without sulfanilamide.

should not be considered as first-line therapy for more serious infections, such as those with underlying osteomyelitis.

The ophthalmic preparations should only be used in refractory cases of otitis because organism resistance may develop with widespread use.

Powder Preparations

Powdered preparations have been used for many years in otology. These were originally applied as dusting powders for chronic otitis and were especially useful for a mastoid cavity. Prior to the advent of antibiotics, antiseptic and acid powders were insufflated into mastoid cavities. Unlike many other otic preparations, powders do not cause pain upon administration.

A powder insufflator can be used for the instillation of antimicrobial agents into the external ear canal or a mastoid cavity [25]. Current antibiotic preparations suitable for the insufflator device are shown in Table 5 [26]. They are packaged into capsules that fit into the insufflator. The patient can easily blow the powder into the ear canal without spreading it around. Other common antibiotics or antiseptics may be applied in powder form in an otolaryngologist office, boric acid is the most common example.

Anesthetic Preparations

Anesthetic agents (Table 6) are used to eliminate the pain associated with infections such as external otitis, otitis media, and bullous myringitis. They may also be used locally prior to surgical manipulation, most commonly during myringotomy. These agents are only recommended for patients with an intact tympanic membrane.

Most local anesthetic preparations contain benzocaine. As benzocaine is poorly absorbed through the skin, it remains localized for a long time, but its effectiveness is unpredictable. Benzocaine has also been known to produce local hypersensitivity reactions [15].

EMLA is a new anesthetic ointment that anesthetizes the external ear canal and eardrum. After keeping the ointment in the external ear canal for 15–20 min, it is removed;

TABLE 6 Otic Anesthetic Preparations

Product	Anesthetic Agent	Other Ingredients
Americaine Otic	Benzocaine (20%)	Glycerin Polyethylene glycol Benzethonium chloride
Auralgan Otic Solution	Benzocaine Antipyrine	Glycerin
EMLA	Lidocaine Prilocaine	Polyoxyethylene Carboxypolyethylene Sodium hydroxide
Phenol	Carbolic acid	

the surgical procedure may then be completed. This product has been used for myringotomy under local anesthesia [27].

Phenol is the common topical anesthetic for myringotomies. It is applied over the specific area of the tympanic membrane where the myringotomy is to be performed. It acts by causing instant epidermal destruction. The section of the tympanic membrane that is in contact with the phenol turns white due to precipitated proteins, indicating an anesthetic effect. Healing occurs by hyperplasia of the epithelium and connective tissue, but may take some time after application [16].

Other Preparations

Propylene glycol is a good base for many of the combination antibiotic drops. It acts as a dehydrating agent to fungi and enhances the effectiveness of other antifungal medications. Occasionally a patient may develop a contact dermatitis.

Corticosteroids are added to many ototopical combination drops to reduce the inflammation and puritis associated with the acutely infected ear. Corticosteroids may also be used primarily to treat dermatoses found in the external ear canal, mainly psoriasis and seborrheic dermatitis. These compounds may reduce the scaling, itching, and inflammation.

Silver nitrate, as a solution or as a powder on a stick applicator, is occasionally used in the external ear canal as a cauterizing agent. It may be applied to granulation tissue or to the site of a superficial infection. Generally it is well tolerated; however, if it is excessively applied and bone is exposed, the area does not heal and surgical correction may be required.

Ototoxicity

The subject of ototoxicity must be addressed whenever discussing the development of new ototopical preparations. It is an important topic from a clinical standpoint and a medico-legal point of view.

TABLE 7 Ototoxic Otic Preparations

Solvent	Antifungal
Propylene glycol	Cresylate
Antiseptics	VoSol
Acetic acid	Antimicrobial
Alcohol	Chloramphenicol
Benzalkonium chloride	Colistin
Iodochlorhydroxyquinolone	Gentamycin
Chlorhexidene acetate	Neomycin
Povidone-iodine	Polymyxin B
	Anti-inflammatory
	Hydrocortisone

In the presence of an intact tympanic membrane, ototoxicity is less important, inasmuch as the preparation has to be systemically absorbed for an ototoxic effect to occur. The issue is most relevant in cases of chronic suppurative otitis media with a perforated tympanic membrane, where the ototopical medication has the potential to reach the inner ear via the middle ear. Placed within the middle ear, ototopical medications may diffuse across the oval or round window, resulting in inner ear absorption. These windows consist of a thin membrane separating the middle ear space from the inner ear fluids. There is controversy regarding the clinical relevance of ototoxicity in cases of chronic suppurative otitis media.

A comprehensive review of the ototoxicity of the various ototopical preparations has recently been published [28]. Table 7 lists the agents in which ototoxicity has been demonstrated in animal models. There is no antiseptic that is thought to be free of ototoxicity. The antifungal medications nystatin, amphotericin B, clotrimazole, and tolnaftate have been tested in animal models and found to be free of ototoxicity. All four antibiotics found in current otic compounds have demonstrated ototoxicity. The antibiotics sulfacetamide and ciprofloxacin present in ophthalmic preparations have not demonstrated ototoxicity. No evaluation of the ototoxic effects of topical tobramycin has been published; it is thought to be similar to gentamicin in this regard. Although hydrocortisone has demonstrated ototoxicity in animal models, other corticosteroids such as triamcinolone and dexamethasone have not. Desonide has not been tested.

Numerous animal studies have been undertaken to evaluate the ototoxic effects of these different medications but the results must be examined with caution because of the differences between the animal models and the human temporal bone. The small mammals used in these studies, usually chinchillas or guinea pigs, have a round window that is easily exposed and very thin compared to the human ear. The human round window is more deeply recessed in bone and is six times thicker than that in the chinchilla. Some human temporal bones may actually demonstrate a thin shelf of bone covering the round window. Further studies must be completed to determine the significance of these differences with respect to ototoxicity and ototopical preparations.

A 1992 survey of otolaryngologists revealed that 80% believed that the risk of sensorineural hearing loss due to otitis media was higher than that from using an ototopical agent known to be ototoxic [29]. As McCabe pointed out in his editorial comment [30]:

In 30 years of practice, I have not recognized a single ear damaged in hearing from any antibiotic ear drop, however long term. This total experience has not changed since then. This comment is important not only for patient care but for medicolegal reasons.

Summary

A variety of otic preparations have been reviewed here, including indications, side effects, and limitations. The ideal cermenolytic compound has not yet been developed, nor has a cerumen replacement product. Antiseptics enjoy wide application but are limited when used in the presence of a perforated tympanic membrane. Available antifungal medications appear to be adequate for the treatment of otomycosis, although none have been approved as otic preparations. The limitations of the otic antimicrobial drops have been discussed, including the potential for organism resistance and for ototoxicity. Powder preparations are not widely available and must be specifically prepared by a pharmacist each time they are dispensed.

The current practice of some otolaryngologists using medications that have not been approved by the FDA for ototopical use, demonstrates the need for new otic preparations. It is hoped that this article will lay the foundation that will enable the development of these new products.

References

1. Cassisi, N., Cohn, A., Davidson, T., and Witten, B., Diffuse otitis externa, clinical and microbiologic findings in the course of a multicenter study on a new otic solution, *Ann. Otolaryngol. Rhinol. Laryngol.*, 86(Suppl. 39):–b (1977).
2. Robinson, A. C., Hawke, M., Mackay, A., Ekem, J. K., and Stratis, M., The mechanism of cerumenolysis, *J. Otolaryngol.*, 18(6):268–273 (1989).
3. Okuda, I., Bingham, B., Stoney, P., and Hawke, M., The organic composition of earwax, *J. Otolaryngol.*, 20(3):212–215 (1991).
4. Senturia, B. H., Marcus, M. D., and Lucente, F. E., *Disease of the External Ear*, Grune & Stratton, Orlando, FL, 1980, pp. 31–56.
5. Lucente, F. E., Smith, P. G., and Thomas, J. R., Disease of the External Ear. In: *Otologic Medicine and Surgery* (P. W. Alberti and R. J. Ruben, eds.), Churchill Livingstone, New York, 1988, pp. 1073–1092.
6. Meyerhoff, W. L., Pathology of chronic suppurative otitis media, *Ann. Otolaryngol. Rhinol. Laryngol.*, 97(Suppl. 131):21 (1988).
7. Brook, I., and Yocum, P., Quantitative bacterial cultures and beta-lactamase activity in chronic suppurative otitis media, *Ann. Otolaryngol. Rhinol. Laryngol.*, 98:293–297 (1989).
8. Kenna, M. A., Rosane, B. A., and Bluestone, C. D., Medical management of chronic suppurative otitis media without cholesteatoma in children—update 1992, *Am J. Otolaringol.*, 14(5):469–473 (1993).
9. Papastavros, T., Giamarellou, H., and Varlejides, S., Role of aerobic and anaerobic microorganisms in chronic otitis media, *Laryngoscope*, 96(April):438–442 (1986).
10. Robinson, A. C., and Hawke, M., The efficacy of ceruminolytics: Everything old is new again, *J. Otolaryngol.*, 18(6):263–267 (1989).
11. Bellini, M. J., Terry, R. M., and Lewis, F. A., An evaluation of common cerumenolytis agents: An in-vitro study, *Clin. Otolaryngol.*, 14:23–25 (1989).

12. *Physicians Desk Reference*, Medical Economics Company, Oradell, NJ, 1993.
13. Chen, D. A., and Caparosa, R. J., A nonprescription cerumenolytic, *Am. J. Otolarynol.*, 12(6):475–476 (1991).
14. Jones, E. H., *External Otitis. Diagnosis and Treatment*, Charles C Thomas, Publisher, Springfield, IL, 1965.
15. *Drug Evaluations Annual 1992*, American Medical Association, Washington, 1992, pp. 1479–1515.
16. Harvey, S. C., Antiseptic and Disinfectants: Fungicides; Ectoparasiticides. In: *The Pharmacological Basis of Therapeutics*, 5th ed. (L. S. Goodman and A. Gilman, eds.), Macmillan Publishing Co., New York, 1975, pp. 987–1017.
17. Stern, J. C., Shah, M. K., and Lucente, F. E., In vitro effectiveness of 13 agents in otomycosis and review of the literature, *Laryngoscope*, 98:1173–1177 (1988).
18. Lopez, L., and Evens, R. P., Drug therapy of aspergillus otitis externa, *Otolaryngol. Head Neck Surg.*, 88:649–651 (1980).
19. Personal communication, The Recsei Laboratories, Goleta, CA, 1991.
20. Sande, M. A., and Mandell, G. L., Antimicrobial Aents: The Aminoglycosides. In: *Goodman and Gilman's The Pharmacological Basis of Therapeutics*, 8th ed. (A. G. Gilman, T. W. Rall, A. S. Nies, and P. Taylor, eds.), Pergamon Press, New York, 1991, pp. 1098–1116.
21. Sande, M. A., and Mandell, G. L., Antimicrobial Agents: Tetracyline, Chloramphenicol, Erythromycin, and Miscellaneous Antibacterial Agents. In: *Goodman and Gilman's The Pharmacological Basis of Therapeutics*, 8th ed. (A. G. Gilman, T. W. Rall, A. S. Nies, and P. Taylor, eds.), Pergamon Press, New York, 1991, pp. 1117–1145.
22. Fairbanks, D. N. F., Otic topical agents, *Otolaryngol. Head Neck Surg.*, 88:327–331 (1980).
23. Hoffman, R. A., and Goldofsky, E., Topical ophthalmologics in otology, *Ear Nose Throat J.*, 70(4):201–205 (1991).
24. Mandell, G. L., and Sande, M. A., Antimicrobial Agents: Sulfonamides, Trimethoprim, Sulfamethoxazole, Quinolones, and Agents for Urinary Tract Infections. In: *Goodman and Gilman's The Pharmacological Basis of Therapeutics*, 8th ed. (A. G. Gilman, T. W. Rall, A. S. Nies, and P. Taylor, eds.), Pergamon Press, New York, 1991, pp. 1047–1064.
25. House, J. W., and Sheehy, J. L., Powder insufflator for the ear, *Otolaryngol. Head Neck Surg.*, 91(4):461–462 (1983).
26. Personal communication, Medical Square Pharmacy, Los Angeles, CA, 1992.
27. Hickey, S. A., Buckley, J. G., and O'Connon, A. F. F., Ventilation tube insertion under local anesthesia, *Am. J. Otolaryngol.*, 12(2):142–143 (1991).
28. Rohn, G. N., Meyerhoff, W. L., and Wright, C. G., Ototoxicity of topical agents, *Otolaryngol. Clinic North Am.*, 26(4):747–758 (1993).
29. Lundy, L. B., and Graham, M. D., *Ototoxicity and Ototopical Medications: A Survey of Otolaryngologist*. Presented at the Ninth Shambaugh-Shea Weekend of Otology, Chicago, IL, March 6–8, 1992.
30. McCabe, B. F., Editorial Comment, *Ann. Otolaryngol. Rhinol. Laryngol.*, 99:41 (1990).

WILLIAM H. SLATTERY III
RICHARD E. BROWNLEE, JR.

Parenterals: Large Volume

Large-volume intravenous solutions refer to injections intended for intravenous use. They are packaged in containers holding 100 mL or more. Other sterile large-volume solutions include those used for irrigation or dialysis. These may be packaged in containers designed to empty rapidly, containing a volume of more than 1000 mL. They are packaged in single-dose units in suitable glass or plastic containers and, in addition to being sterile, are nonpyrogenic and free of particulate matter. Because of the large volumes administered, bacteriostatic agents are never included, since toxicity may result from administering large quantities of bacteriostatic agent.

Large-Volume Solutions for Intravenous Use

Large-volume parenterals (LVPs) intended to be administered intravenously are frequently called, "intravenous" (iv) fluids or "infusion" fluids (Fig. 1). Their most common applications include the correction of serious disturbances in electrolyte and fluid balances in the body and a means of providing basic nutrition. In recent years, they have been used as vehicles for other drugs and as a method of providing parenteral nutrition. Infusion or intravenous fluids are packaged in containers with a capacity of 150 to 1000 mL. Mini-type infusion containers of 250-mL capacity are available, with 50 and 100 mL fills for the dilution of drugs when used in the "piggyback" technique (Fig. 2).

Solutions to be administered intravenously or by infusion (venoclysis) must be clear and contain substances that can be assimilated and utilized by the circulatory system, such as sodium chloride, amino acids, dextrose, electrolytes, and vitamins. Many different kinds and combinations of intravenous solutions are commercially available. The most commonly used are listed in Table 1. Examples of intravenous admixture systems and equipment are shown throughout this article.

Although it is desirable that intravenous fluids be isotonic to minimize trauma to the blood vessels, hypertonic or hypotonic solutions can be administered successfully. Highly concentrated hypertonic nutrient solutions are being used in parenteral nutrition. To minimize vessel irritation, these solutions are administered slowly with a catheter inserted in a large vein such as the subclavian.

On rare occasions, intravenous fluids are administered into the subcutaneous tissues. This type of administration is called "hypodermoclysis" and is used for infants or obese patients, with inaccessible veins.

With few exceptions (e.g., urea, pentothal), LVPs are available in clear liquid form (usually aqueous) and as clear liquids for direct iv injection. The only LVP nonsolutions injected iv are parenteral "iv fat." Parenteral emulsions contain particle sizes of approximately 0.5 μm and, with appropriate precaution, can be administered iv.

All LVPs are required to be:

- Sterile
- Non-pyrogenic
- Free of particulate matter
- Packaged as single-dose containers

A primary iv container is utilized for fluids, nutrition electrolyte replacement, and drug therapy by the continuous method. It may also be used for KVO (keep vein open) for future therapy. Drugs can be added to the LVP and infused over a period of 4-8 hours. This method achieves continuous blood levels of drug once steady state has been reached.

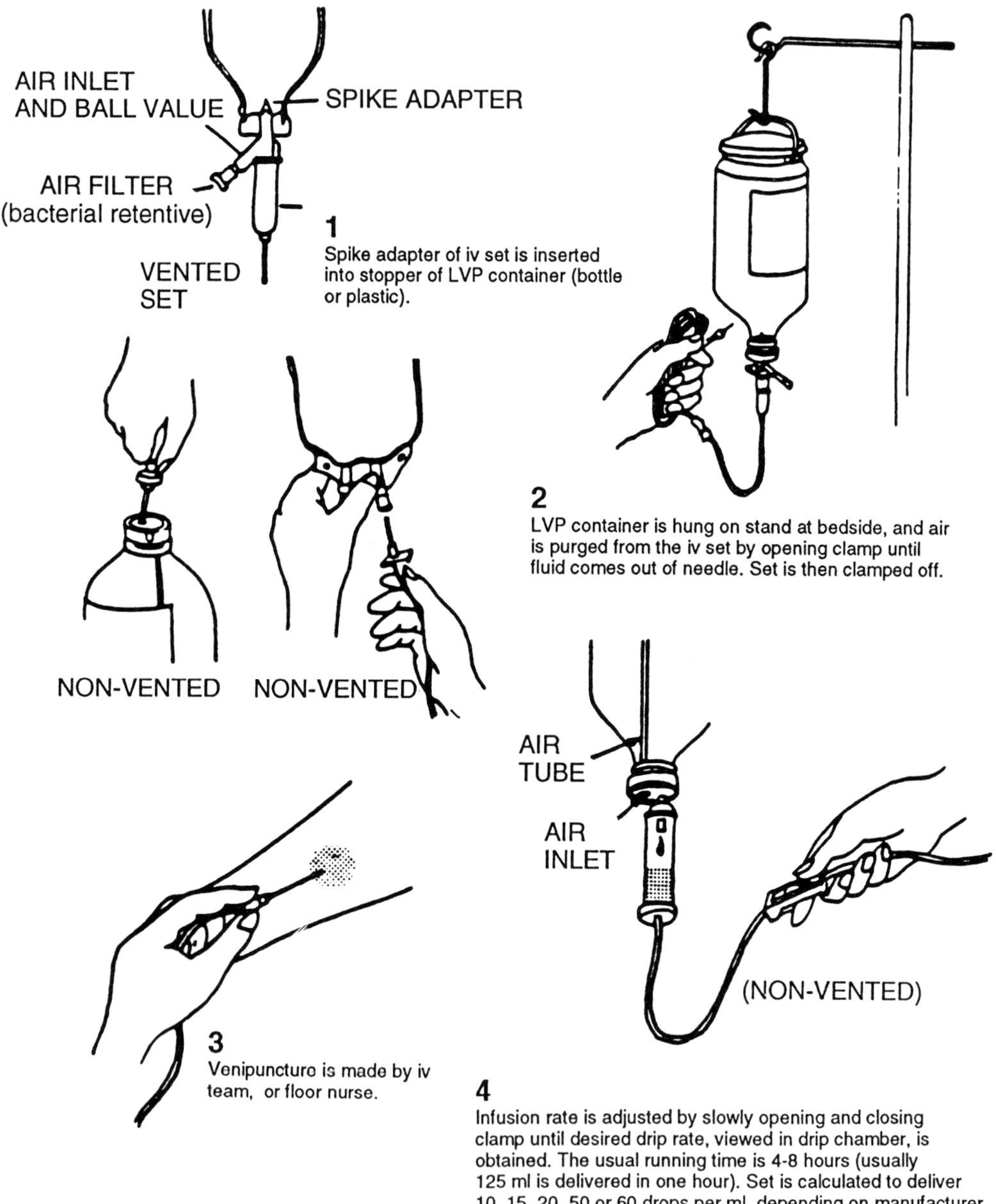

FIG. 1. Starting an LVP infusion continuous therapy.

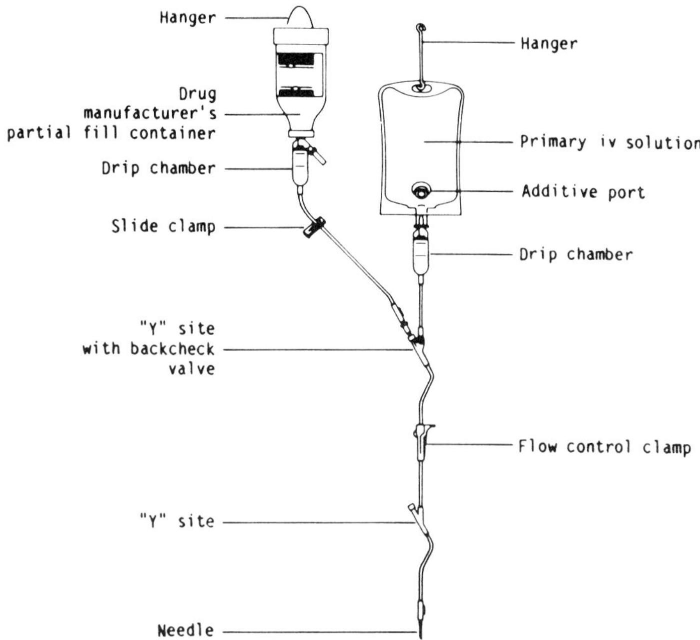

FIG. 2. Drug manufacturer's partial-fill piggyback (DMP).

- Free of preservatives, and
- The volume must not exceed 1000mL (except for irrigation solutions)

Sterility

All LVPs must meet the requirement of sterility without compromise. This is ensured by initially subjecting the product to a valid sterilization process and packaging the product in a form that ensures sterility for shelf life.

Non-Pyrogenic

Pyrogens or bacterial endotoxins are metabolic by-products of microbial growth. These water-soluble, heat-resistant lipopolysaccharides cannot be destroyed by steam sterilization or filtration.

Pyrogen contamination in parenteral products usually eminates from three main sources: the water used as the solvent; the containers with which the solution has come into contact during its preparation, packaging, storage, or administration; or the chemicals used in the preparation of the product.

The injection of pharmaceuticals containing pyrogens is more significant when given in large volumes by the iv route as compared to other routes of injection and volumes. The labels of iv fluids describe the contents as nonpyrogenic, which indicates that pyrogen tests gave negative findings. However, minute quantities of pyrogens may be present which have not been detected by testing, and therefore these fluids are labeled ''Non-pyrogenic'' and not ''Pyrogen free.''

TABLE 1 Large Volume Solutions for Intravenous Use

Injection[a]	Common Name[a]	Concentration (%)	pH	Therapeutic Value
Dextrose	Glucose	2.5	3.5–6.5	Hydration, calories
	5% D/W	5		Hydration, calories
		10		Insulin shock, calories
		20		Insulin shock, calories
		50		Insulin shock, calories
		70		Calories
Sodium chloride	Normal saline	0.9	4.5–7.0	Extracellular fluid replacement
	N.S.S. 1/2	0.45		Dehydration
	Normal saline	3		Hyponatremia
		5		Hyponatremia
Ringer's	Ringer's		5.0–7.5	
NaCl		0.86		Fluid and electrolyte replacement
KCl		0.03		
$CaCl_2$		0.033		
Lactated Ringer's	Hartmann's		6.0–7.5	
NaCl		0.6		Fluid and electrolyte replacement
KCl		0.03		
$CaCl_2$		0.02		
Na lactate		0.3		
Sodium bicarbonate		1.4	8	Metabolic acidosis
		5		Metabolic acidosis
Ammonium chloride		2.14	4.5–6.0	Metabolic alkalosis, hypochloremia
Sodium lactate	M/6 Sodium lactate	1/6 molar	6.0–7.3	Metabolic acidosis
Mannitol		5	5.0–7.0	Osmotic diuresis
		10		
		15		
		20		
Alcohol			4.5	
with 5% D/W		5		Sedative, analgesic, calories
with 5% D/W in N.S.S.		5		Sedative, analgesic, calories
Dextran 40 in N.S.S.		10	5	Priming fluid for extracorporeal circulation
in 5% D/W		10	4	Priming fluid for extracorporeal circulation
Dextran 70 in N.S.S.		6	5	Plasma volume expander
		6	4	Plasma volume expander
Multiple electrolyte solutions[b]			5.5	Fluid and electrolyte replacement

[a]5% D/W = 5% dextrose in water; N.S.S. = normal saline solution.
[b]Varying combinations of electrolytes, dextrose, fructose, and invert sugar.

Particulate Matter (PM)

"Particulate matter consists of extraneous, mobile, undissolved substances, other than gas bubbles, unintentionally present in parenteral solutions" according to *USP XXII*. The composition of unwanted particulate matter varies. In some instances, the composition is due to many sources, whereas in others it eminates from one specific source. Extraneous materials found in parenterals include cellulose, cotton fibers, rubber, metal, plastic particles, undissolved chemicals, rust, and dandruff. The theoretical possibilities include any environmental material to which the product is exposed. Although the biologic effects of particulate matter are not well defined, the quality control ramifications are clear.

Particulate matter is undesirable, unwanted, and clinically not necessary for therapy. Constant efforts must be made to eliminate its sources and occurrence. Particulate matter in a parenteral product can be due to many sources and activities:

1. The solution itself and the chemicals comprising it;
2. The manufacturing process and its variables, such as the environment, equipment, and personnel;
3. The packaging components with which the product is in contact;
4. The sets and devices used in administering the product; and
5. The manipulations involved in the preparation of the product as well as the environment in which it is prepared.

During the manufacture and packaging of the solution, the environment, personnel, and filling equipment can contribute to particulate matter. The environment and equipment are more easily monitored than the personnel. Identification of the particulate matter may be helpful in locating the sources and eliminating them. Particles of 50 μm or larger diameter can be detected by visual inspection.

For smaller particles special instrumental techniques must be used. All the techniques require scrupulously clean equipment and environment for satisfactory performance, even though they may be based on different physical principles. Packaging components, such as glass or plastic containers or the rubber closure, can generate particulate matter if they are not washed and handled properly. Touching administration devices such as syringes or infusing fluid can also generate particulate matter. During storage, particulate matter can be generated by chemical reactions among components of the solution, reaction of the chemical components with the packaging materials, or degradation of the solution. Control and detection of particulate matter have long been of concern to the pharmaceutical industry.

Packaging

All LVPs are required to be packaged as single-use containers (one-time use). All multiple-dose parenteral containers are required to contain a preservative system (bacteriostatic agent). Bacteriostats in significant quantities, that is, in concentrations necessary for microbial effectiveness, can have detrimental effects because of the large volumes administered with LVPs. The containers are usually made of glass, or flexible and semi-rigid plastic.

Volume Requirement

All LVPs for iv use must be packaged in containers having a minimum volume of 100 mL and a maximum volume of 1000 mL, except for irrigation solutions (not given iv) which are permitted to be packaged in volumes over 1000 mL.

Excess Fills

All parenteral containers must contain an excess in the fill volume to ensure complete administration. Loss results from clearing of air in the administration set and volume retained after completed infusion, and LVPs are no exception. The excess suggested is based on the volume contained in the parenteral (Table 2). The excess volume or contents in a parenteral package allows the user to remove the volume stated on the label. The excess amounts are not stated on the label.

Tonicity

Large-volume parenterals are not required to be isotonic, although many are. However, hypertonicity or hypotonicity are frequently a requirement for therapeutic effectiveness. If a hypotonic solution is injected into biological cells, water from the product permeates the cell membrane in an effort to equalize the osmotic pressure on both sides of the membrane, causing the cell membrane to swell and possibly burst; this swelling produces a hemolytic effect termed "hemolysis." If hypertonic solution is injected into biological cells, water from the cell permeates the membrane in an effort to dilute the hypertonic solution and produces a shrinkage of the cell termed "crenation." A wide range of osmotic pressure can be tolerated (250–350 mOsm). The tolerance of osmotic pressure is related to the volume administered. Since LVPs deliver larger volume than small volume parenterals (SVPs), the issue of tonicity becomes more meaningful with LVP iv administration.

In order to achieve therapeutic effectiveness, some LVPs are not isotonic (e.g., 0.45% sodium chloride injection and 10% dextose injection).

Packaging Systems

Abbott, Baxter, and McGaw supply LVP fluids in plastic and glass containers (Table 3). The plastics used are polyvinyl chloride (PVC), polyolefin, copolyester, or laminates of

TABLE 2 Recommended Excess Volume for LVPs

Labeled Size (mL)	For Mobile Liquids (mL)[a]	For Viscous Liquids (mL)[a]
0.5	0.10	0.12
1.0	0.10	0.15
2.0	0.15	0.25
5.0	0.30	0.50
10.0	0.50	0.70
20.0	0.60	0.90
30.0	0.80	1.20
50.0 or more	2%	3%

[a]Except where otherwise stated.

TABLE 3 Intravenous Fluid Systems

Manufacturer	Container	Characteristics
Abbott	Glass	Vacum Air filter
Abbott	Plastic	Polyvinyl chloride Flexible Non-vented
Abbott	Plastic	Copolyester Flexible Non-vented
McGaw	Glass	Vacuum Air Tube
McGaw	Plastic	Copolymer Flexible Non-vented
Baxter	Glass	Vacuum Air Tube
Baxter	Plastic	Polyvinyl chloride Flexible Non-vented
Baxter	Plastic	Laminate

these. The glass is classified as Type I or Type II glass. Type I glass (borosilicate glass) is the highest quality available for commercial use. It is more expensive than Type II glass (soda-lime glass) which is mostly used for LVP packaging. Drug absorption is a consideration with some drugs and some plastics. Nitroglycerin, for example, is significantly absorbed by PVC but not by glass. For examples of current containers and administration options see Figures 3–8.

Clinical Utilization of LVPs

Basic Nutrition

In addition to maintaining normal body functions, hospitalized patients require adequate caloric intake to survive the insults of illness or operation. This is a requirement for wound healing. For those patients who are not able to satisfy their food requirements orally, nutrition must be supplied by the intravenous route, and proteins, carbohydrates, and vitamins can be administered in this way.

Amino Acids

Various commercial solutions containing amino acids are available. They are used to supply the body's nitrogen requirements. Recommended daily allowances of protein are ap proximately 0.9 g/kg of body weight for a healthy adult and 1.4–2.2 g/kg for healthy growing children and infants. Protein requirements may be higher for traumatized or malnourished patients. To supply adequate protein parenterally, various kinds of solutions and combinations of synthetic essential and nonessential amino acids are available in 5,

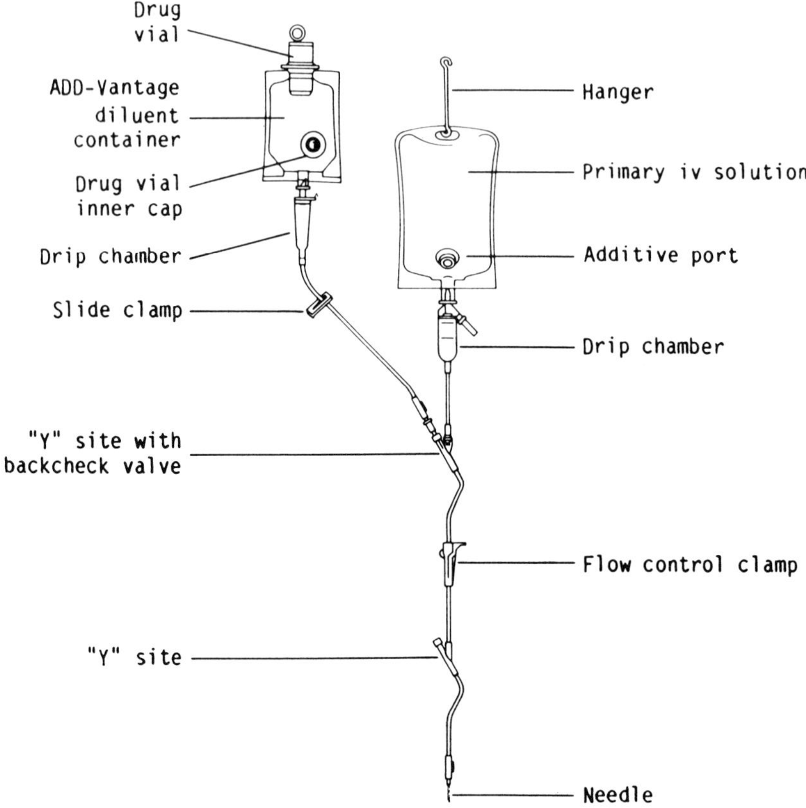

FIG. 3. Add Vantage™ LVP setup and intermittent drug-delivery system.

10, and 15% concentrations as well as others. Amino acids are used when oral feeding is not possible or gastrointestinal absorption is impaired.

Carbohydrates

Dextrose is an important nutrient, with 1 g providing 3.4 cal (14.2 J). Thus, a 1000 mL Dextrose Injection, 5%, contains 50 g dextrose and supplies 170 cal (711.5 J). Traditionally, 1 g of dextrose has been calculated to provide 3.75 cal (15.7 J). Commercial dextrose is in the monohydrate form and a 0.91 correction factor is required (3.75 cal $\times$ 0.91 $=$ 3.4 cal or 14.2 J). The body utilizes dextrose at a rate of 0.5 g/kg of body weight per hour. Therefore, 1000 mL of Dextrose Injection, 5%, requires 1½ h for assimilation. The pH range for Dextrose Injection, 5%, is given as 3.5 to 6.5 in *USP XXII*. The low pH is due to the sugar acids present. Some practitioners believe that the acidity of dextrose solutions and other acid intravenous solutions may cause vein irritation and phlebitis. A few investigators have advocated the addition of sodium bicarbonate to neutralize the acid pH of intravenous solutions. A 1% sodium bicarbonate solution packaged in 20-mL containers is available for this purpose (Neut, Abbott). An acid pH is essential to ensure stability of the dextrose solution during sterilization and storage. As the pH increases, caramelization occurs and the dextrose solution darkens.

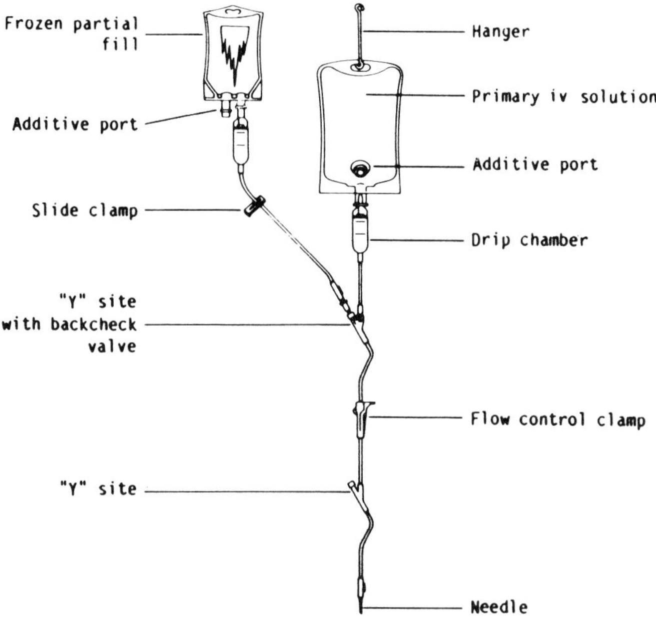

FIG. 4. Frozen partial fill.

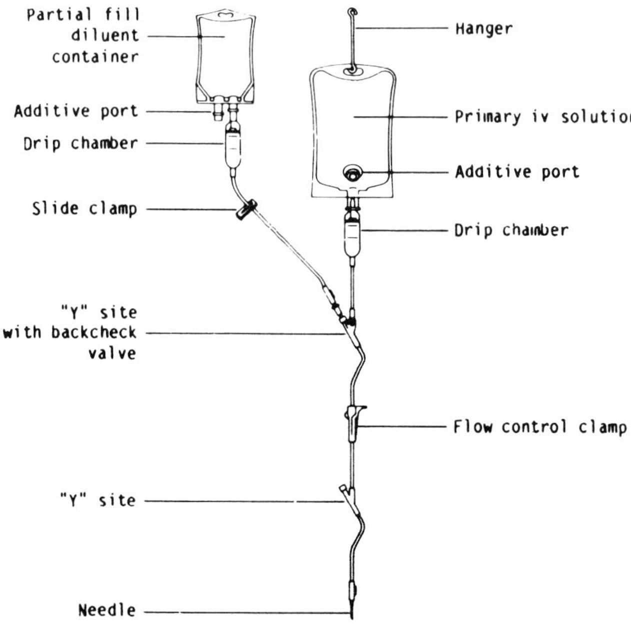

FIG. 5. Partial-fill diluent container.

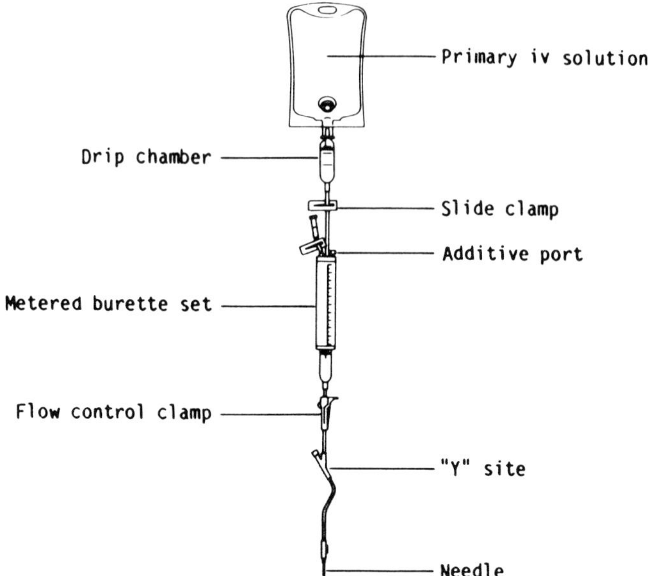

FIG. 6. Burette set.

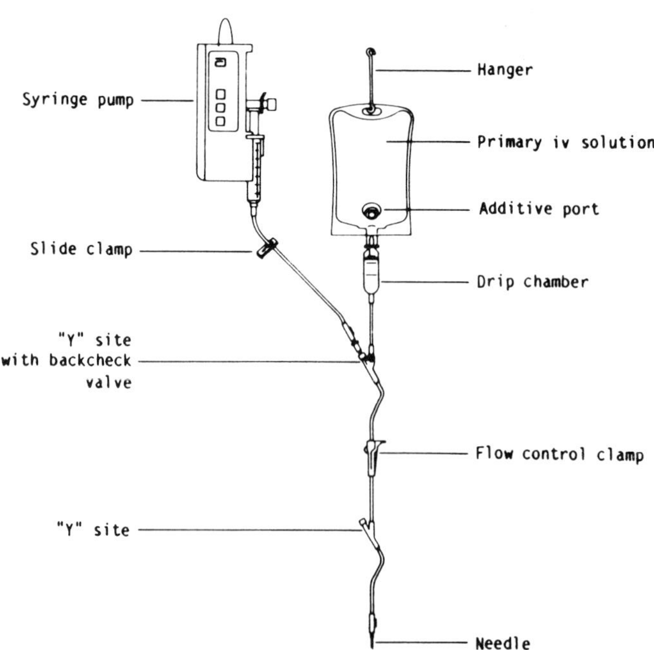

FIG. 7. Syringe pump.

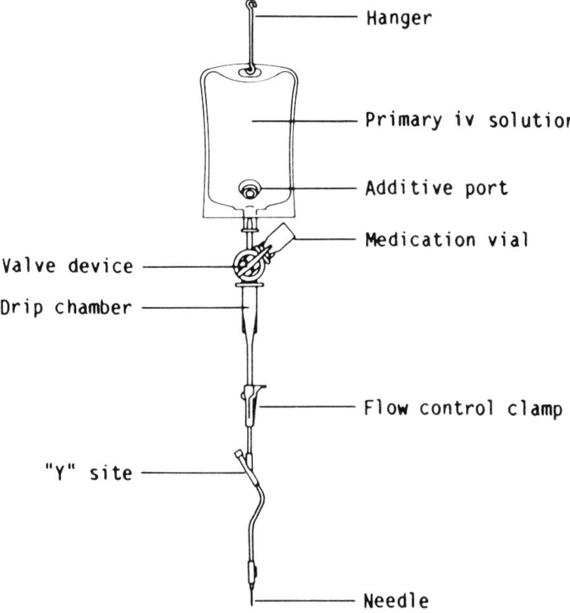

FIG. 8. Cris™ infusion system.

Alcohol

Other sources of energy include ethanol solutions supplying about 7 cal (29.3 J)/g ethyl alcohol. When administered too rapidly, ethanol solutions have a depressant effect on the central nervous system (CNS).

IV Fat

For intravenous feeding, fat must be in a suitable form, usually emulsions. In the past, difficulty with fat emulsions was related to untoward reactions believed to have been caused by the emulsifier. Fat emulsions for intravenous administration are being used both in Europe and in the United States.

Given intravenously, fat droplets are distributed in the blood and metabolized in the same pathways as are chylomicrons. Most of this lipid or lipoprotein is hydrolyzed by lipoprotein lipase, and the hydrolytic products (free fatty acids and monoglycerides) are taken up by the cells and metabolized. The metabolism of 1 g of fat provides 9.1 kcal (38 kJ) of energy, compared to 3.4 kcal (14.2 J) provided by the metabolism of 1 g of glucose. The diameter of lipid particles ranges from 0.1 to 0.5 μm, which is comparable to the size of physiologic blood chylomicrons.

Intralipid

Intralipid contains 10 or 20% wt/v of purified soybean oil, 1.2% egg yolk phospholipid, the emulsifier, and 2.25% glycerin, making the emulsion isotonic. Sodium hydroxide is added to adjust the pH between 5.5 and 9.0. Soybean oil comprises a number of neutral triglycerides, most of which are largely unsaturated fatty acids, such as linoleic (54%), oleic (26%), palmitic (9%), and linolenic (8%). These, together with the glycerin and egg lecithin, provide 1.1 kcal/mL (4.6 J/mL) of emulsion. The osmolality of Intralipid 10% is 280 mOsm, comparable to that of blood.

Liposyn (Abbott)

Liposyn II is supplied in 10 and 20% concentrations, containing 5 and 10% soybean oil and 5 and 10% safflower oil, respectively; each also contain 1.2% egg phospholipids and 2% glyerol. Liposyn III is supplied in 10 and 20% concentrations of soybean oil.

Parenteral Nutrition

Total parenteral nutrition (TPN) is the long-term intravenous feeding of amino acid solutions containing high concentrations of dextrose (approximately 20%), electrolytes, vitamins, and in some instance insulin. The need to maintain adequate caloric intake while keeping the volume of solution required to a minimum necessitates the use of this hypertonic solution. The basic solution can be prepared by the combination of commercially available dextrose and amino acids. These solutions are usually combinations of 50–70% dextrose and 5% amino acid solutions. After mixing, they supply approximately 1 cal (4.2 J) per mL of solution. Required supplements such as electrolytes and vitamins are frequently added to the basic solution. Many manufacturers provide the solutions in ready-to-mix units. The solutions are administered via a large vein, such as the subclavian, over 8 to 24 h. The purpose of using this vein and slow administration is to minimize adverse effects. The subclavian vein is large and close to the heart; therefore, the solution is diluted rapidly by the large volume of blood in this vessel. Numerous references in the literature fully describe the methods of preparation and parenteral implications.

Peripheral-vein total parenteral nutrition (PV-TPN) utilizes glucose, amino acids, and lipids as the energy sources and appropriate electrolytes and micronutrients. PV-TPN is designed to deliver approximately 70–100 g protein and 1200–2000 kcal/day (5000–8400 kJ/day) to patients with mild to moderate nutritional deficits. PV-TPN avoids the complications associated with CNS catheters. Solutions of amino acids containing 3.5, 5 and 7% solutions are available for PV-TPN.

In addition to its value as a partial source of energy in a balanced program of total parenteral nutrition (TPN), including amino acids, dextrose, minerals, vitamins, and electrolytes, a lipid emusion is useful in treating or preventing essential fatty acid deficiency (EFAD).

Other Applications

Restoration of Electrolyte Balance

Electrolyte disturbances can be caused by a variety of clinical conditions, such as trauma, injury, burns, shock, diarrhea, vomiting, and electrolytic shifts in body compartments. If the oral route cannot be used to correct the difficulty, electrolytes are administered intravenously. The condition of the kidneys must be considered before electrolyte replacement is initiated. Urinary depression may be the result of decreased fluid volume or renal impairment. A hydrating solution such as 5% D/W in 0.2% sodium chloride are administered. Urinary flow is restricted if the retention is functional. The most frequently used solution is Sodium Chloride Injection, 0.9%, an isotonic solution containing 154 mEq each of sodium and chloride ions. Ringer's Injection and Lactated Ringer's Injection contain small quantities of calcium and potassium ions. Deficits of these ions require additional supplementations. Lactated Ringer's Injection contains sodium lactate, which is used for metabolic acidosis. Solutions with multiple electrolytes are available commercially to simplify therapy (Normosol, Abbott). These solutions closely resemble the composition of plasma electrolytes.

Fluid Replacement

Dehydration requires fluid replacement. Sodium chloride and dextrose injections can be used as basic solutions for fluid replacement. Excessive use of large volume solutions can cause edema and water intoxication.

Blood and Blood Products

Blood and blood products can only be administered intravenously. They are used in cases of shock, hemorrhage, or blood protein loss. No drug should be mixed with blood prior to administration.

Drug Carriers

Because of convenience, the irritation potential of the drug, and the desire for continuous drug therapy, intravenous fluids are frequently used as vehicles for the intravenous administration of drugs. In some instances, the combination of one or more drugs in an intravenous fluid impairs drug stability and may promote parenteral imcompatibilities. In addition, the drug or the LVP may contribute to infusion phlebitis.

Arginine Hydrochloride Injection

This amino acid is believed to be effective in stimulating the utilization of ammonia by the body. Elevated levels of ammonia correlate with cerebral dysfunction and result in liver damage. Elevated ammonia levels may be due to high protein feedings and excessive intake of ammonium chloride, and cause intestinal tract bleeding. Arginine enhances the formation of urea and thus reduces the ammonia level; however, clinical results are poor. The product R-Gene was removed from the market, but was subsequently reintroduced as R-Gene 10(KabiVitrum). The official indications for this product are as an iv stimulant to the pituitary and as a diagnostic test for human growth hormone (HGH).

Urea, Lyophilized Form

Solutions of urea are administered intravenously to reduce edema associated with trauma, and especially to reduce intracranial and intraocular pressure. Urea is not metabolized by the body. The administration of this concentrated solution causes osmotic diuresis, reducing the fluid present in tissue.

Mannitol

The intravenous administration of mannitol solutions results in osmotic diuresis. The solution is eliminated by the body almost entirely unmetabolized. Mannitol is of value in the prophylaxis of oliguria from tubular necrosis, the treatment of cerebral edema, and the promotion of diuresis; dosages contain 50 to 200 g as 5, 10, or 20% solution. The 20% solutions are saturated, and a reduction in temperature may cause crystallization. If this occurs, the injection should be warmed prior to administration in order to dissolve the mannitol. Administration of the 20% injection requires a blood filter to ensure against infusion of mannitol crystals.

Dextrans

Dextrans are polymolecular polysaccharides composed of glucose units. The average molecular weight of Dextran 70 is 70,000, and the average molecular weight of Dextran 40 is 40,000. When given intravenously, Dextran 70 is an effective plasma volume expander. It is used in the treatment of trauma, hemorrhage, burns, and surgical shock. Because of its lower molecular weight, Dextran 40 is less effective as a plasma volume expander than Dextran 70. It is used as a priming fluid in pump oxygenators during extracorporeal circulation. Dextran 40 has also value as a prophylactic agent against thrombus formation. The drug prevents rouleau formation of red blood cells.

Sodium Bicarbonate

In addition to its availability in ampuls, vials, and prefilled syringes, sodium bicarbonate, 5% injection, is also packaged in 500-mL bottles as 1.4%, 1/6 molar, and 5% solutions. This infusion fluid is packaged in a Type I glass container sealed with a rubber closure; it requires a vented administration set. It is used to combat acidosis by supplying a ready source of bicarbonate ion and can be administered as an intravenous fluid. The pH of sodium bicarbonate solutions is approximately 8. Although a simple compound, sodium bicarbonate presents problems in manufacture and administration; for example, it decomposes to sodium carbonate with the liberation of carbon dioxide.

Sodium Lactate Injection (1/6 molar)

This injection contains 167 mEq sodium and lactate ions per liter, and provides a source of sodium for the elevation of bicarbonate levels in severe acidosis. The lactate portion is metabolized by the liver into glycogen. This solution is used in the emergency treatment of metabolic acidosis.

Ammonium Chloride Injection (2.14%)

Solutions containing 400 mEq of ammonium and chloride ions per liter are used in the treatment of metabolic alkalosis and hypochloremia.

Lactated Ringer's Injection (LRI) (Hartmann's Solution)

This product contains small amounts of sodium, potassium, and calcium chlorides and low amounts of sodium lactate, and approximates the extracellular fluid composition. It is utilized in the initial treatment of hypovolemic shock in adults; 1–2 L may be infused in the initial treatment. LRI is also utilized as a source of fluid and electrolytes.

Hetastarch

Hetastarch is composed primarly of amylopectin treated with sodium hydroxide and ethylene oxide. It is utilized as a substitute for serum ablumin for plasma volume expansion. Hetastarch molecules range from 10^4 to 10^6 Daltons. These large molecules are slowly metabolized and, administered iv, are capable of maintaining intravascular volume for a longer period of time than crystalloids. Hetastarch is used for the treatment of hypovolemia.

Large-Volume Solutions Not Administered Intravenously

Although solutions for irrigation and dialysis resemble intravenous fluids in many respects, they are not administered directly into the venous system. Their manufacture is subject to the same stringent controls as that for intravenous fluids, but they may be packaged in containers that are larger than 1000-mL capacity and that are designed to empty rapidly.

Surgical Irrigating Solutions (Splash Solutions)

Surgical irrigating solutions are used to bath and moisten body tissue. They may be used topically for moistening dressings, for wound irrigation, or as soaking or washing fluids for instruments. Sodium Chloride for Irrigation and Sterile Water for Irrigation are commonly used for these purposes, in addition to Lactated Ringer's Injection. Solutions for irrigation are available in flexible and semirigid plastic containers.

Urologic Irrigation Solutions

Surgeons performing urologic procedures generally use a large amount of irrigation solutions during procedures. The solutions help to maintain the integrity of the tissue, remove blood, and provide a clear field of view for the surgeon. Urologic solutions require an administration set and are used with Foley catheters by connection to a cystoscope. Sterile Water for Irrigation and Sterile Glycine Solution are commonly used. Antibiotics are sometimes added, as in the case of Neosporin G.U. Irrigant.

Sorbital solution 3% is a nonhemolytic urologic irrigant used for transurethral resection.

Glycine Solution

Glycine, a nontoxic amino acid, is commonly used to eliminate the risk of intravascular hemolysis during transurethral resection. It is supplied as a 1.5% solution in Water for Injection and packaged in 1000- 15000-, and 3000-mL pour bottles; 15% solution concentrates are available for dilution. The 1.5% solution is slightly hypotonic. Glycine solution is nonconducting and does not cause dispersion of high frequency current and loss of electrosurgical cutting efficiency.

Peritoneal Dialysis Solutions

Peritoneal dialysis solutions (Inpersol, Abbott) are not administered directly into the circulatory system, but rather into the peritoneal cavity. Peritoneal dialysis is used to remove toxic substances normally excreted by the functioning kidney. In cases of poisoning or renal shutdown, or in patients awaiting renal transplants, dialysis is a lifesaving measure used to remove toxic substances, excessive body waste, and serum electrolytes. The composition of these commercially available solutions resembles that of potassium-free extracellular fluid. Solutions are available containing 1.5 and 4.25% dextrose and electrolytes. Solutions are made hypertonic to plasma with dextrose to prevent absorption of water into the intravascular compartment. By osmosis and diffusion the peritoneal cavity behaves as a semipermable membrane. Catabolities and other substances may be removed from the body. An incision is made on the linea alba (midline), and a trocar connected to a catheter attached to the container of the dialysis solution is inserted. The solution is permitted to flow into the abdominal cavity where it remains for 30 to 90 min and drained by a siphon action. The procedure is repeated many times and may require 30 to 50 L of solution for daily treatment. Common additives to peritoneal dialysis solutions include heparin and potassium chloride.

Solutions for peritoneal dialysis containing various concentrations of dextrose (1.5, 2.5, 4.25%), and sodium, calcium, and magnesium chloride and lactate are commercially available in containers as large as 3000 mL.

Bibliography

Boylan, J. C., and Fites, A., *Parenteral Products, Modern Pharmaceutics*, 2nd ed., Marcel Dekker, Inc., New York, 1990.

Gennaro, A. J., ed., *Remington's Pharmaceutical Sciences*, 18th ed., Mack Publishing Co., Easton, PA, 1990.

Mehta, R. C., et al., Fat emulsion partical size distribution in total nutrient admixture, *Am. J. Hosp. Pharm.*, 49:2749 (1992).

Parenteral Drug Association, *Depyrogenation*, Technical Report No. 7, Philadelphia, 1985.

Avis, K. E., ed. *Pharmaceutical Dosage Forms, Parenteral Medications*, 2nd ed., Vol. 1, Marcel Dekker, Inc., New York, 1992.

Practical Aspects of PV-TPN, a Clinician's Guide to Peripheral Vein Total Parenteral Nutrition, Abbott Lab., HPD North Chicago, 1984.

Turco, S., *Sterile Dosage Forms*, 4th ed., Lea & Febiger, Philadelphia, 1994.

United States Pharmacopeia XXII, The United States Pharmacopeial Convention, Inc. Rockville, MD, 1989.

SALVATORE J. TURCO

Parenterals: Small Volume

Introduction

The *United States Pharmacopeia XXII* [1] defines a small volume parenteral (SVP) (actually the USP replaces ''parenteral'' with ''injection'') as ''. . . . an injection that is packaged in containers labeled as containing 100 mL or less.'' Therefore, all sterile products packaged in vials, ampuls, syringes, cartridges, bottles, or any other container that is 100 mL or less fall under this classification. Ophthalmic products packaged in squeezable plastic containers, although topically applied to the eye rather than administered by injection, also fall under the classification of small volume injections as long as the container size is 100 mL or less. (See the article Ocular Drug Formulation and Delivery in this volume.) Large volume parenterals (LVPs) have to be terminally sterilized, whereas SVPs can be sterilized terminally or by aseptic filtration and processing. Large volume parenterals usually involve intravenous infusion, dialysis, or irrigation fluids containing electrolyes, sugar, amino acids, blood and blood products, and fats [2]. The LVPs must be administered by intravenous routes; in fact, any injection volume greater than 10 mL must be administered by intravenous administration. Small volume injection or parenterals involve all other types of parenteral products for topical ophthalmic application or injection by various routes.

- Primary routes
  - Intramuscular
  - Intravenous
  - Subcutaneous
- Secondary routes
  - Hypodermoclysis
  - Intra-abdominal (Intraperitoneal)
  - Intra-arterial
  - Intra-articular
  - Intracardiac
  - Intracisternal
  - Intradermal
  - Intralesional
  - Intraocular
  - Intrapleural
  - Intrathecal
  - Intrauterine
  - Intraventricular

The formulations are relatively simple, involving the drug, possibly ingredients added for various reasons (to be described), a solvent system (preferably aqueous), and the appropriate container and closure packaging system.

This article will introduce the reader to the basic aspects of small volume parenteral products, including their use, types and primary characteristics of dosage forms, formulation ingredients, and packaging systems. Several excellent references are available for

ROYAL PHARMACEUTICAL SOCIETY LIBRARY
1, LAMBETH HIGH STREET, LONDON SE1 7JN

additional information [2–6]. Harwood et al. [7] recently published an extensive article on processing aspects of small volume parenterals which are not covered here. Large volume parenterals are covered in a complementary article in this volume by Turco.

Primary Uses of SVPs

Small volume parenterals can be therapeutic injections, ophthalmics, diagnostics, radiopharmaceuticals, or allergenic extracts.

Therapeutic Injections

Therapeutic injections include anti-infectives, steroids, hormones, vitamins, cardiovascular agents, barbiturates, central nervous system agents, proteins, and many other types of drugs. There are over 400 injection products listed in the USP. The injections are usually solutions containing the active ingredient and other substances. Alternatively, the solution contains only the drug, or the drug is suspended in a suitable medium or formulated as a sterile emulsion. Injections are ready-to-use (e.g., Amobarbital Sodium for Injection) or need to be reconstituted from solids to a solution or suspension prior to injection (e.g., Amoxicillin for Injectable Suspension). Injections can also be commercially available concentrated liquids (e.g., Potassium Chloride for Injection Concentrate) which must be diluted prior to application. Injectable products are available in single or multiple dosages. Multiple-dose injections must contain an antimicrobial preservative system; usually, the volume of injection cannot exceed 30 mL [8].

Ophthalmic Products

Ophthalmic drug products include drugs in solution, suspension, gel, or ointment, administered topically to the corneal surface of the eye. Ophthalmic products also include irrigating solutions in SVP sizes. There are many different types of ophthalmic drug products to treat glaucoma, infection, inflammation, and other diseases of the eye. Ophthalmic products must be sterile, but since they are topically applied, are not required to be pyrogen-free. Ophthalmic solutions and suspensions are usually packaged in squeezable low-density polyethylene containers for easy administration. Ophthalmic ointments also are sterile and must be free from metallic particles; they are packaged in ointment tubes. Since ophthalmic products are multiple-dose products, they must contain antimicrobial preservative agents. A thorough reference on ophthalmic dosage forms has been contributed by Hecht et al. [9].

Diagnostic Agents Including Diagnostic Radiopharmaceuticals

There are many SVP diagnostic agents available, including solutions containing radioactive iodine, chromium, technetium, iron, and other radioactive elements. These products are used primarily to evaluate organ functions. Most of these are produced to be used within hours of preparation because of extremely short half-lives of the radiopharmaceutical agent. Although usually not tested because of almost-immediate use, these products are required to be sterile and pyrogen-free. For more information the reader is referred to the excellent article on sterile diagnostic dosage forms written by Olsen [10].

Allergenic Extracts

Allergenic extracts are sterile concentrates (solutions or suspensions) of the substances (allergens) responsible for unusual sensitivities in humans. These products can be used for therapeutic or diagnostic purposes. Extracts are aqueous (normal saline is used as the diluent) or glycerinated (50% glycerin is the diluent). Most preparations are buffered at pH 8 and contain phenol (usually 0.4%) as an antimicrobial preservative. They are sterilized by aseptic filtration. For more information on allergenic extracts the reader is referred to the article by Shough [11].

Formulations

Small volume parenterals are usually thought of as small-volume solutions in vials or ampuls, but are available in a variety of dosage forms and packaging systems.

Liquids

Small volume parenteral liquids are primarily aqueous solutions, but some commercial products contain oily solutions or mixtures of water and water-miscible cosolvents.

Aqueous Solutions

Aqueous ready-to-use SVPs contain the active ingredient, additional substances, if necessary, and water as the solvent. Water-for-Injection (WfI), USP, is the solvent of choice for aqueous SVPs. It is prepared by distillation or reverse-osmosis technologies. Of all the USP types of water (Table 1), WfI is the purest form available for parenteral products. An essential requirement is its freedom from pyrogenic contamination. Pyrogens are metabolic by-products of microbial growth which cannot be destroyed by conventional sterilization techniques. Aqueous SVP solutions are prepared either by filling the product into containers and terminally sterilizing the finished product or, for drugs which cannot physically or chemically withstand the high temperatures required for terminal heat sterilization, the drug product in WfI is sterile filtered and aseptically filled into the final container.

Nonaqueous Solutions

A few SVPs are oily solutions (Table 2). The oil is always a vegetable oil (sesame, olive, or cottonseed oil most commonly) because of its safety, relative purity, and biocompatibility. Oils for injection must meet certain USP requirements, such as the solid paraffin test (measurement of oil clarity), a saponification value between 185 and 200, an iodine value between 79 and 128, and tests for unsaponifiable matter and free fatty acids [12]. Oily solutions are prepared by separately sterilizing the solvent (usually by dry heat) and the drug (dry heat or a gas such as ethylene oxide) and combining the drug and solvent aseptically. Terminal sterilization cannot be used for oily solutions because of the lack of moisture within the product necessary to generate a saturated steam under pressure

TABLE 1 Types of Water Described in the *United States Pharmacopeia*

Type	Preparation	Pryogen free	Comments
Purified Water USP	Distillation or ion exchange	No	Pharmaceutical solvent
Water for Injection USP (WfI)	Distillation or reverse osmosis	Yes	Not sterile Must be used within 24 h or stored below 5°C or ≥80°C; used for manuf. of parenteral products to be sterilized
Sterile Water for Injection USP	Distillation or reverse osmosis	Yes	Same as WfI; single-dose containers; also used to reconstitute sterile solids and dilute sterile solutions
Bacteriostatic Water for Injection USP	Distillation or reverse osmosis	Yes	Multiple and single dose
Sterile Water for Irrigation USP	Distillation or reverse osmosis	Yes	1 L or larger, wide mouth, does not meet particulate matter requirements for LVP; labeled "For Irrigation Only"

TABLE 2 Small Volume Parenteral Products Containing Oil(s) as the Solvent System[a]

Product, USP XXII	Oil
Ampicillin (suspension)	Vegetable
Desoxycorticosterone acetate	Sesame
Diethylstilbestrol	Sesame, cottonseed
Dimercaprol (suspension)	Peanut
Epinephrine (suspension)	Sesame
Estradiol benzoate	Sesame
Estradiol cypionate	Cottonseed
Estradiol valerate	Sesame
Estrone	Sesame
Ethiodized iodine	Poppyseed
Fluphenazine enanthate	Sesame
Hydroxyprogesterone caproate	Sesame
Menadione	Sesame
Nandrolone decanoate	Sesame
Penicillin G procaine (suspension)	Vegetable
Propyliodone (suspension)	Peanut
Testosterone cypionate	Cottonseed
Testosterone enanthate	Sesame
Testosterone propionate	Sesame

[a]From Ref. 4, p. 193

to destroy microorganisms. Sims and Worthington [13] and Radd et al. [14] have reported on product development experiences with oily injection formulations.

Cosolvent

A great number of SVPs contain cosolvent systems (Table 3). Cosolvents are used to increase the solubility of the drug in water or minimize or prevent the chemical degradation of the drug by water. Therapeutic protein dosage forms usually require water-miscible cosolvents to enhance water solubility and protein stability in aqueous environments. However, the possible adverse effect on protein conformation must be taken into account.

Water-miscible co-solvents operate on the principle of lowering the dielectric constant of water, thereby increasing the aqueous solubility of poorly water-soluble drugs. Depending on drug stability, products containing cosolvents can be sterilized terminally by saturated steam under pressure or aseptically filtered. A primary concern in using cosolvents in injectable formulations is their potential to cause lysis of red blood cells when administered intravenously [15]. Therefore, any addition of a co-solvent to a formulation intended for parenteral administration must be studied for its safety and potential toxicological effects.

Solids

Small volume parenterals are available as sterile dry solids which must be reconstituted with Sterile Water for Injection, USP, or Bacteriostatic Water for Injection, USP, prior to being administered primarily as a solution, or, in some cases, as a suspension. Sterile dry SVPs are prepared by two methods.

Freeze-Drying

Most commercial sterile dry powders are manufactured by freeze-drying, also called lyophilization. In this process, under strict aseptical conditions, the product is aseptically

TABLE 3 Small Volume Parenteral Products Containing Cosolvents[a]

Trade Name	Manufacturer	Cosolvent Composition
Dramamine	Searle	50% Propylene glycol
Apresoline	Ciba	10% Propylene glycol
MVI	US Vitamins	30% Propylene glycol
Nembutal	Abbott	40% Propylene glycol, 10% ethanol
Luminal	Winthrop	67.8% Propylene glycol
Dilantin	Parke-Davis	40% Propylene glycol, 10% ethanol
DHE 45	Sandoz	15% Glycerin, 6.1% ethanol
Cedilanid	Sandoz	15% Glycerin, 9.8% ethanol
Robaxim	Robbins	50% Polyethylene glycol
Serpasil	Ciba	50% Polyethylene glycol, 10% dimethylamine
Ativan	Wyeth	20% Polyethylene glycol, 80% propylene glycol
Librium	Roche	20% Propylene glycol
Valium	Roche	40% Propylene glycol, 10% ethanol
Lanoxin	Burroughs Wellcome	40% Propylene glycol, 10% ethanol

[a]From S. Yalkowsky and T. Roseman, *Techniques of Solubilization of Drugs*, Marcel Dekker, Inc., New York, 1981, p. 91.

filtered and filled as a solution. Special slotted rubber closures are partially inserted into the vials, which are transferred to a freeze-dryer. Freeze-drying involves three primary operations:

- Freezing of the product,
- Sublimation of the frozen solvent (phase transition from a solid (ice) phase to a gaseous phase), and
- Heating the product to room temperature, resulting in a crystalline or amorphous solute.

The partially inserted rubber closures are then fully seated in the vials, and the finished product contains a white or off-white sterile dry solid.

Freeze-drying is used primarily because of the limited stability of certain drugs in solution, especially therapeutic proteins. Freeze-dried formulations usually contain bulking agents, excipients to enhance physical and sometimes chemical stability of the drug as well as to provide an esthetic dried solid matrix. Freeze-dried vials are usually stable for at least two years at room temperature, except for certain protein products which may be stable for only 18 months under refrigeration. Once the freeze-dried product is reconstituted (usually with Sterile Water for Injection, USP), it has a relatively short usage period at room temperature (12 hours to seven days).

Freeze-drying technology is reviewed by Pikal [16] and Nail and Gatlin [17].

Powder-Filled SVPs

Many SVP antibiotics, particularly the cephalosporins, are manufactured by sterile crystallization of the active ingredient and aseptically filling the sterile powder into the final container. The drug is dissolved in an appropriate solvent before filtering through a 0.22 μm membrane filter. Several techniques can be used for sterile crystallization, including adding sterile seed crystals and adjusting the pH, or adding a sterile antisolvent in which the drug is insoluble. The resultant slurry is usually collected on a Buchner funnel-type of filter and dried, and the resultant crystals are milled and blended. Several variables are critical in controlling the purity and quality of the final crystals, including temperature, rate of addition of antisolvent, adjustment of pH, mixing time, and the quality of the seed crystals.

Compared to freeze drying, sterile crystallization and powder filling is much more economical, but also more subject to process variability and possible microbial and particulate contamination.

Suspensions

In parenteral suspensions (Table 4) the active drug ingredient is suspended in a liquid carrier, either ready to use or reconstituted as a suspension. Drugs are formulated as suspension dosage forms because of poor solubility in aqueous solution or because of the need for a prolonged-acting delivery system. Suspension products are prepared by com-

TABLE 4 Small Volume Parenteral Suspensions

Product	Manufacturer	Suspending Agent
Aristocort	Lederle	Propylene glycol 4000
Bicillin C-R	Wyeth	Lecithin, carboxymethylcellulose
Decadron-LA	Merck	Carboxymethylcellulose
Depo-Medrol	Upjohn	PEG 3350 (polyethylene glycol)
Duracillin	Lilly	Procaine salt
Hydeltra-TBA	Merck	Tebutate salt
Lente Insulins	Lilly, Novo	Polymorphic
NPH Insulins	Lilly, Novo	Protamine
PZI Insulins	Lilly, Novo	Protamine, zinc
Prolixin Decanoate	Princeton	Decanoate salt

bining sterile vehicle and sterile powder aseptically or by combining two sterile solutions, whereby the drug solution is insoluble in the other solution and the drug precipitates out of solution.

Major concerns for SVP suspensions include:

1. Resuspendability of the drug in the vehicle to permit homogeneous filling of the product into the container and homogeneous dosing.
2. Caking or settling of the drug, resulting in a physically unstable product, and
3. Syringeability (the ability to withdraw a homogeneous dose from the vial into a syringe) and injectability (the ability to eject the product through the needle into the patient).

Formulation ingredients include the suspending agent (usually a wetting agent), a buffer, and an antimicrobial preservative. Akers et al. [18] have published a comprehensive review of the formulation development and manufacturing methodology involved in parenteral suspension products.

Emulsions

Emulsions are mixtures of oil- and water-based vehicles with an appropriate surface-active agent to facilitate and maintain the miscibility of the oil-in-water phase. The only emulsified SVP product to date commercially available is Alpha-Tocopherol, a sustained-release intramuscularly injected vitamin E product. Diazepam has also been formulated as an injectable emulsion; its stability assessment has been described by Levy and Benita [19]. Emulsified dosage forms have been studied for sustaining the release of drugs administered intramuscularly. LVP emulsions are widely used as nutrient sources given intravenously.

Basic Characteristics of SVPs

Like any sterile dosage form, SVPs must be sterile and free of pyrogens and foreign particulate matter. These three characteristics distinguish sterile dosage forms from any other type of pharmaceutical product. They are treated in significant detail in a recently revised book on parenteral quality control [20].

Sterility

Sterility is the state of absolute freedom from microbial contamination. Interestingly, "Sterile" on the label of a SVP means literally that a sample of the lot of the product has passed the USP test for sterility [21]. Needless to say, much more is done to ensure product sterility than simply testing a sample of a lot prior to its release. Achievement of sterility involves the combination and coordination of a host of activities and processes, among them cleaning and disinfection of the facility; cleaning and sterilization of equipment, packaging, and all other articles potentially in contact with the product; aseptic filtration of the product itself and terminal sterilization of the product; installation and certification of laminar air-flow areas where sterile air is provided by high efficiency particulate air (HEPA) filters; environmental monitoring of the facility, equipment, water, and personnel for strict microbiological and particulate control; appropriate gowning and training of personnel in aseptic techniques, validation of sterilization processes, integrity testing of the container-closure system to maintain a sterile product, and conducting the sterility test itself, not only prior to release of the product, but also, at least, at the end of the shelf life (expiration date) of the product.

The end-product sterility test suffers from at least three serious limitations, and therefore one cannot depend solely on this test to be assured of sterility.

1. Concern that the small sample (usually 20 containers per batch) truly represents the entire batch. Probability statistics reveal that with such a small sample size the extent of contamination must be significant (on the order of 1% of the batch) for the sample to fail the sterility test.

2. Concern that the culture media used for the sterility test can support the growth of any microbial life (bacteria, fungi, mold), possibly contaminating the product.

3. Concern that no accidental contamination was introduced during the performance of the sterility test. There is always a finite probability (although usually below 1.0%) that personnel, testing environment, testing materials, etc., may introduce contamination, resulting in a false positive sterility test. This concern is being addressed with the help of isolation sterility test chambers (e.g., LaCalhene, Amsco) which remove direct human contact with the product samples.

Freedom from Pyrogens

Pyrogens are metabolic by-products of microbial growth. Injected in sufficient amounts in humans, pyrogens can react with the hypothalamus of the brain to raise the body temperature. In addition, they can cause a number of other adverse physiological effects, including, at sufficiently high doses, death. Pyrogens are minute, water-soluble, heat-resistant lipopolysaccharides which cannot be destroyed by steam sterilization or removed by 0.2-μm membrane filters. Prevention rather than elimination is the key for pyrogen removal. The primary source of pyrogenic contamination in parenteral products is water. Fortunately, pyrogens are destroyed by distillation. Water used to clean containers and closures can also be a source of pyrogens. However, glass is sterilized by dry heat at temperatures (>200º C) hot enough to destroy pyrogens. Rubber closures are steam sterilized which does not destroy pyrogens, and therefore the water used to clean rubber closures much be pyrogen free. Chemical raw materials used in parenteral formulations must be crystallized using pyrogen-free water or other solvents. The only other possible, although usually impractical way to remove pyrogenic contamination from parenteral products is to use ultrafilters (<0.1 μm) to remove the smallest unit of lipopolysaccharide.

Pyrogenic contamination is detected by two tests. In the older method, rabbits are injected with the products and the rectal temperature is measured. The more recent method involves a relatively simple in vitro method, the Limulus amebocyte lysate (LAL) test. It is based on the fact that the amebocytes of the horseshoe crab (Limulus) are highly sensitive to the lipopolysaccharide contained in endotoxins from gram-negative bacteria. The LAL test is the USP method of choice, and endotoxin limits have been established for most SVPs [22].

Freedom from Particulate Matter

Particulate matter, as contaminant in SVPs, creates problems in product quality and possibly clinical hazards although direct evidence of adverse effects has never been found. The primary source of particulate matter is the container–closure system (glass and rubber), although particulates can originate from a variety of sources including the environment, processing equipment, undissolved raw materials, drug degradation product(s), and personnel. At present, the United States is the only country whose compendia require tests and set limits for particulate matter in SVPs.

Stability

Drugs in SVPs are generally unstable. Many drugs are so unstable that they cannot be marketed as ready-to-use solutions. Drugs with sufficient solution stability require various formulation, packaging, and storage conditions to maintain stability during shelf-life. The primary path of drug degradation involves oxidation and hydrolytic reactions. Drugs can also react with packaging and formulation components, resulting in physical and chemical degradation. Oxidation attacks functional groups (e.g., phenolic or sulfhydryl) that form free radicals under certain conditions which react with molecular oxygen. Free-radical formation is catalyzed by a variety of factors, including light, heat, metal ions, pH, peroxides, and, of course, oxygen itself. For this reason, many SVP products are packaged in light-protective packaging, require storage at controlled room or lower (refrigeration) temperatures, are formulated at low pH, contain antioxidants and/or chelating agents, and are processed where, prior to sealing the container, the product is overlayed with an inert gas (usually nitrogen) to remove oxygen from the container.

The other primary mechanism of drug degradation in liquid SVPs is by reaction with water. Hydrolysis and decomposition occur with pH changes and are catalyzed by resulting hydrogen or hydroxide ions. For this reason, buffers are needed in certain liquid parenteral products to achieve tight control of solution pH.

Hydrolysis of solid SVPs is caused by moisture in the atmosphere or trace moisture in packaging (primarily rubber closures) or the dry powder itself. Thus, control of residual moisture during and after processing and effective container–closure systems to prevent atmospheric moisture from entering the product are of utmost importance.

Isotonicity

Small volume parenterals should be isotonic with blood, tears, and other biological fluids in muscle, tissue, and spinal fluid, wherever the product is injected. This means that the biological cell contains the same number of solute "particles" (in solution) from the injected solution as the number of particles within the cell itself. If a product is injected (or instilled in the eye) containing fewer solute particles (a hypotonic solution) than those contained in biological cells, water from the product permeates the cell membrane to equalize osmotic pressure on both sides of the membrane, causing it to swell and possibly burst. In blood this is called hemolysis. If an injected or instilled product contains more solute particles (a hypertonic solution) than those contained in the cell, water from the cell permeates the membrane to dilute the hypertonic solution and the cell shrinks (crenation). In either case, cellular damage potentially can occur causing pain and tissue irritation. Blood, muscle, and subcutaneous tissue cells can withstand a fairly wide range of osmotic pressure from injected solutions (250–350 mOsm/kg), whereas tear and spinal fluids are much more sensitive to even slight differences in osmotic pressure of instilled or injected solutions. However, in practice, wide osmolarity ranges of SVPs can be tolerated when injected into the body (other than intrathecally) without any serious problems.

Formulation Ingredients

Small volume parenterals are simple formulations compared to other pharmaceutical dosage forms. Solution SVPs contain water, the active ingredient, and up to three to five inactive ingredients. Solid SVPs contain the active ingredient and up to one or two inactive ingredients. Formulators are severely restricted in the choice of inactive ingredients because of safety considerations. For example, only eight antimicrobial preservative agents are generally acceptable for SVP administration. If none of these are compatible or efficacious with a particular new drug SVP, the formulator has no other choices available.

Solvent

The most widely used SVP solvent is Water for Injection (WfI), USP. As a solvent, WfI is used in formulation compounding and must be terminally sterilized in the final package. It is prepared by distillation or reverse osmosis and is highly purified water without endotoxin contamination. Sterile Water for Injection (SWfI), USP, is used for reconstitution of solid SVPs prior to administration. It is terminally sterilized prior to commercial distribution. Bacteriostatic Water for Injection is commercially available as a reconstitution vehicle for certain products which require a preservative for multiple usage. The most common bacteriostatic agent is benzyl alcohol. Sesame oil or cottonseed oil are used as vehicles for water-insoluble drugs such as corticosteroids and certain vitamins.

Solubilizers

Solubilizers for drugs that are poorly soluble in water include a wide variety of agents, shown below, with different mechanisms of increasing water solubility.

- Cosolvents
  - Glycerin
  - Polyethylene glycol 300 and 400 (PEG)
  - Propylene glycol
  - Ethanol
- Surface active agents
  - Polyoxyethylene sorbitan monooleate (0.1–0.5%, Polysorbate 80)
  - Polyoxyethylene polyoxypropylene ethers (0.05–0.25%, Pluronic 68)
- Complexing agents
  - Beta-cyclodextrins
  - Polyvinylpyrrolidone

Liquid solubilizers include primarily water-miscible cosolvents such as ethanol, propylene glycol, polyethylene glycol 400, and glycerin. These solvents act simply to reduce the dielectric constant of water (its high capability to conduct electricity) in order to increase solubility of hydrophobic or slightly hydrophilic drugs. For example, Lanoxin (Digoxin Injection, Burroughs-Wellcome), Valium (Diazepam Injection, Roche), and Nembutal (Pentobarbital Sodium Injection, Abbott) each contain 40% propylene glycol and 10% ethanol in order to solubilize drugs of low water solubility for intravenous injection. Gibson et al. [23] studied the use of PEG solutions as solubility and stability enhancers of a new cytotoxic agent. Interestingly, they included information on the effects of PEG on sterile filtration, lyophilization, and reconstitution of the drug and found that a 50% PEG 3400 aqueous vehicle yielded the best overall results. Other pertinent references are available describing various liquid solubilizers enhancing aqueous solubility of poorly soluble active ingredients [24–27].

Surface active agents increase the dispersability and water solubility of poorly soluble drugs due to their unique chemical properties of possessing both hydrophilic and hydrophobic functional groups in the same molecule. The hydrophobic functional groups adsorb to surface molecules of the drug, while the hydrophilic functional groups interact with water molecules. Therefore, the poorly soluble molecules of the drug locate in the core of the surface active agent (the so-called micelle), while the polar molecules of the surface active agent associate with polar substances such as water. Pluronics (polyoxyethylene-polyoxypropylene-polyoxyethylene) block copolymers and polysorbate 80 are the most widely used surface active agents in enhancing water solubility or aqueous dispersibility of poorly soluble drugs.

Solid solubilizers include the cyclodextrins which act by forming soluble inclusion complexes in aqueous solutions. These molecules, like surface active agents, are amphiphillic, that is, they contain hydrophobic interior functional groups and hydrophilic hydroxy functional groups at the exterior. Brewster et al. [28] reviewed the application of cyclodextrins in parenteral formulations, particularly for the solubilization and stabilization of various proteins and peptides. Simpkins [29] reported on the solubilization of ovine growth hormone using 2-hydroxypropyl-β-cyclodextrin.

Antimicrobial Preservative Agents

These agents serve to maintain sterility of the product during its shelf life and use. They are required in preparations intended for multiple dosing from the same container be-

TABLE 5 Antimicrobial Preservative Agents in Small Volume Parenterals

Agent	Concentration Range (%)	Products
Phenol	0.065–0.5	Humulin N, Zantac, Tensilon, Tagamet, Phenergan, Imferon
m-Cresol	0.16–0.3	Humulin N, Humulin R, Humatrope, Demerol
Methylparaben	0.05–0.18	Decadron, Elavil, Prostigmin
Propylparaben	0.011–0.035	Garamycin, Prolixin, Bicillin
Chlorobutanol	0.5–0.55	Epitrate, Bentyl, Dopram
Benzyl alcohol	0.75–2.0	Valium, Protropin, Geopen, Compazine, Pronestyl, Cleocin
Benzalkonium chloride	0.01–0.025	Most ophthalmic products
Thimerosal	0.0075–0.01	Neosporin, Rhogam, Wydase

cause of the finite probability of accidental contamination during use. They are also included, although this is controversial, in single-dose products that are aseptically manufactured to provide additional sterility assurance. This is acceptable as long as it is shown that the antimicrobial agent is not used to ''cover-up'' for inadequate aseptic processing. The combination of antimicrobial preservative agents and adjunctive heat sterilization (at temperatures below 121° C) is widely employed for drug products sensitive to high temperatures. Only eight agents (Table 5) are used for SVP formulations. Most substances with antimicrobial activity are irritating and toxic at relatively low concentrations, and usually have stability problems. They can be incompatible with the drug and formulation ingredients as well as with the packaging components. For example, the most commonly used antimicrobial preservative agents are alcoholic or phenolic chemicals. Alcohols and phenols are highly toxic even at low concentrations, and are extremely volatile and can thus permeate certain rubber closure and plastic formulations. In addition, phenols are readily oxidized and lose their antimicrobial activity.

Buffers

Buffers are used to maintain the pH of the solution in the range that provides maximum stability to the drug against hydrolytic degradation. Buffer systems used in SVPs contain simple weak acids and their corresponding sodium salts (Table 6). The appropriate choice of buffer depends on the pH range where the drug in question is most stable. The concentration of buffer depends on the strength of buffer capacity (an indication of the resistance of the buffer system to changes in pH when acidic or basic substances are added) required to maintain the pH within the range of maximum drug stability throughout the intended shelf life.

TABLE 6 Common Buffer Systems Used in Small Volume Parenteral Products

pH	Buffer System	Concentration (%)
3.5–5.7	Acetic acid–acetate	1–2
2.5–6.0	Citric acid–citrate	1–5
6.0–8.2	Phosphoric acid–phosphate	0.8–2
8.2–10.2	Glutamic acid–glutamate	1–2

Antioxidants

Antioxidants function by preferentially reacting, rather than the drug, with molecular oxygen, thus minimizing or terminating the oxidation reaction. Oxidation reactions involve the formation of free radicals (e.g., from sulfhydryl or phenolic groups) catalyzed by environmental factors such as light, heat, heavy metals, peroxides, hydroxide ions, and air. Many drugs used in SVP products are sensitive to oxygen and degrade rapidly in the absence of protection. In addition to antioxidants, other precautions must also be taken, such as protection from light, heat, heavy metals, and peroxides; formulating the product at low pH is another safety measure. Common SVP antioxidants are shown in Table 7. The most widely used agent is sodium bisulfite because its oxidation-reduction potential lies in the range where it does not preferentially oxidize too slowly or too rapidly. Sometimes combinations of antioxidation agents strengthen oxidative drug protection as well as combining an antioxidant and a chelating agent such as ethylenediaminetetraacetic acid (where the chelating agent removes heavy metal contaminants). See also the article Autoxidation and Antioxidants in Vol. 1 of this encyclopedia [30].

Protein Stabilizers

Therapeutic proteins and peptides have become important in SVP formulations. They are very reactive with water, other formulation components, packaging components, and air

TABLE 7 Antioxidants Commonly Used in Small Volume Parenterals

Antioxidant	Concentration Range (%)
Water soluble	
Sulfurous acid salts	
Sodium bisulfite	0.05–1.0
Sodium sulfite	0.01–0.2
Sodium metabisulfite	0.025–0.1
Sodium thiosulfate	0.1–0.5
Sodium formaldehyde sulfoxylate	0.005–0.15
Ascorbic acid isomers	
L- and D-ascorbic acid	0.02–1.0
Thiol derivatives	
Acetylcysteine	0.1–0.5
Cysteine	0.1–0.5
Thioglycerol	0.1–0.5
Thioglycolic acid	
Thiolactic acid	
Thiourea	0.001–0.05
Dithiothreitol	
Glutathione	
Oil soluble	
Propyl gallate	0.05–0.1
Butylated hydroxyanisole	0.005–0.02
Butylated hydroxytoluene	0.005–0.02
Ascorbyl palmitate	0.01–0.02
Nordihydroguaiaretic acid	0.01–0.05
α-Tocopherol 9	0.05–0.075

in the package, and highly sensitive to changes in environmental conditions such as temperature, pH, light, moisture, and mechanical manipulations. Degradation reactions are both chemical and physical. Proteins are well known to aggregate at excessive temperature (hot and cold) or by shaking and handling. Protein aggregation not only potentially affects chemical potency, but also physical appearance and quality. Various ingredients have been used to minimize protein degradation in SVPs. The most prominent stabilizers include serum albumin; amino acids such as glycine, lysine, and glutamine; surface active agents, primarily poloxamer 188 (Pluronic 68) and polysorbate 80; polyhydric alcohols such as sorbitol, glycerol, and polyethylene glycol; carbohydrates such as sucrose, lactose, and maltose; and antioxidants, chelating agents, polyvinylpyrrolidone, polyvinyl alcohol, dextran, and gelatin. Protein stabilization is reviewed in Refs. 31 to 33.

Tonicity Adjusters

A wide variety of agents are used to adjust SVP tonicity. Most common are simple electrolyes, such as sodium chloride and other sodium salts, and nonelectrolytes such as glycerin and lactose. Normally, the SVP formulator first considers the drug concentration and other ingredients necessary for solubility, stability, or other purposes. Once these have been formulated, osmolarity is measured and, if hypotonic, the tonicity-adjusting agents are added. If the formulation is hypertonic but at a level not acceptable for the intended administration, the formulation needs to be diluted or ingredients reduced.

Other Ingredients

Bulking agents are used in freeze-dried preparations to increase the solid content of the plug resulting from the lyophilization process to help inspecting the quality of the final product. Cryo- or lyoprotectants are used in freeze-dried preparations, particularly for proteins that are sensitive to freezing and drying procedures. These agents stabilize and prevent degradation of a protein during freeze drying and storage [34]. Suspending agents keep the drug suspended in the solvent after shaking and resuspending. Emulsifying agents lower the interfacial tension to allow the mixing of oil and water solvents in the formulation. Semisolid agents aid in the dispersability of the drug in ophthalmic ointments and provide the ointment base. Examples of these agents are give below

- Bulking agents for freeze-dried preparations
  - Mannitol
  - Lactose
  - Sucrose
  - Dextran
- Suspending agents
  - Carboxymethylcellulose (CMC) sodium
  - Gelatin
  - Sorbitol
- Cryo- and lyoprotectants
  - Sucrose
  - Polyvinylpyrrolidone

Methylcellulose
Gelatin
- Ophthalmic ointment bases
  Petrolatum

Packaging

The packaging system is an essential part of the parenteral formulation, providing long-term protection and maintenance of physical and chemical stability. Packaging is a major source of particulate contamination and can contribute to physical and chemical degradation of the product due to leaching of packaging constituents or adsorption of product constituents onto the surface of the container and closure. Packaging systems provide unique opportunities for convenient SVP deliver (e.g., cartridges, syringes). The main types of packaging systems, are glass, rubber, and plastic. Metal tubes used for packaging of sterile ophthalmic ointments are not discussed here.

Glass

Glass used for parenteral products is classified as Type I, Type II, and Type III (Table 8). Type I is the highest quality grade, composed almost exclusively of borosilicate (silicon dioxide), making it chemically resistant to extreme acidic and alkaline conditions. Type I glass, although the most expensive, is preferred for most parenteral products, especially ready-to-use solution products. It can be used for any parenteral packaging. Type II glass is soda-lime glass (treated with sodium sulfite or sulfide to neutralize surface alkaline oxides), whereas Type III glass is untreated soda-lime glass. Types II and III glasses are used for dry powder and oily solution parenteral products. Type II can be used for solution products with a pH below 7.0 as well as for acidic and neutral preparations. The *USP XXII* gives tests for the different types of glass [35].

The formulator must be aware that within each type of glass there are different types and levels of additives (boron, sodium, potassium, calcium, iron, and magnesium) which affect chemical and physical properties. Therefore, the formulator should have all the necessary information from the glass manufacturer(s) to ensure that the glass formulation is consistent from batch to batch and that additive specifications are consistently met.

TABLE 8 Glass Used for Small Volume Parenterals

			Limits	
Type	General Description	USP Test	Size (mL)	mL of 0.02 N Acid
I	Highly resistant, borosilicate glass	Powdered glass	All	1.0
II	Treated soda-lime glass	Water attact	100 or less	0.7
			Over 100	0.2
III	Soda-lime glass	Powdered glass	All	8.5
NP[a]	General-purpose soda-lime glass	Powdered glass	All	15.0

[a]For nonparenteral articles.

Amber glass containers are used for light sensitive products. The amber color is produced by the addition of iron and manganese oxides to the glass formulation. These, however, can leach into the formulation and catalyze oxidative reactions. See also the article Glass as Packaging Material for Pharmaceuticals in Vol. 7 of this encyclopedia [36].

Rubber

Rubber formulations are used in SVPs for closures for vials and cartridges and plungers for syringes. These formulations are extremely complex. Not only do they contain the basic rubber polymer, but also many additives such as plasticizers, fillers, vulcanizing agents, pigments, activators and accelerants, and antioxidants. Many of these additives are not fully characterized for content or purity and can be sources of physical and chemical degradation problems in parenteral products. Like with glass, the formulator must work closely with the rubber manufacturer to choose the correct rubber formulation with consistent specifications and characteristics to maintain product stability.

The most common rubber polymers used in SVP closures are natural and butyl rubber, with silicone and neoprene rubber used less frequently (Table 9). Butyl rubber is preferred because it requires fewer additives, has low water vapor permeation characteristics (therefore, excellent for sterile dry powders sensitive to moisture), and moderate characteristics with respect to gaseous permeation and reactivity with the pharmaceutical product.

Problems with rubber closures include leaching of constituents into the product, adsorption of active ingredients or antimicrobial preservatives by the elastomer, and coring of the rubber by repeated insertion of a needle. Coring produces rubber particulates which affect the quality and potentially the safety of the product.

Siliconization of rubber closures is a common practice to facilitate the movement of rubber through equipment during processing and seating into vials. However silicone is incompatible with hydrophilic drugs, especially proteins. Excessive contact with siliconized rubber can result in protein aggregation. Elastomer manufacturers have developed formulations which do not require application of silicone to function in high speed production operations. See also the article Elastomeric Parenteral Closures in Vol. 5 of this encyclopedia [37].

Plastic

Plastic packaging is very important for ophthalmic dosage forms administered by flexible plastic bottles, involving squeezing to emit droplets of sterile solutions, suspensions, or gels. Plastic SVP containers for other than ophthalmic products are becoming more

TABLE 9 Autoclavable Rubber Compounds Used in Small Volume Parenterals

Type	Additives	Water-Vapor Permeation	Potential Reactivity with Product
Butyl	Moderate	Low	Moderate
Natural	High	Moderate	High
Neoprene	High	Moderate	High
Polyisoprene	High	Moderate	Moderate
Silicone	Moderate	Very high	Low

widely accepted because of cost savings, elimination of glass breakage, and convenience of use. Like rubber formulations, plastic formulations can interact with the product, causing physical and chemical problems. Plastic formulations are less complex than rubber and tend to have a lower potential for leachability of its constituents. The most commonly used plastic polymer for ophthalmic products is low density polyethylene. For other SVPs, polyolefin formulations are widely used as well as polyvinyl chloride, polypropylene, polyamide (nylon), polycarbonate, and copolymers (e.g., ethylene–vinyl acetate).

Containers

The most common container type for SVPs is a glass or polyethylene vial with a rubber closure and a metal seal. Glass ampules used to be the most popular type of SVP packaging systems, but are used less today because of the problem of glass particles when the neck of the ampule is broken. Both syringe (prefilled) and cartridge containers have increased in popularity and use because of their convenience compared to vials and ampules. Vials and ampules require withdrawal of the product from the package prior to injection, whereas the product in syringes and cartridges is ready for administration. Bottles are used for large volume parenterals (LVPs).

Plastic containers are used for instillation of ophthalmic products. Metal ointment tubes are used to package sterile ophthalmic ointments.

Storage

Proper storage of SVPs is critical to the safety and potency of the active ingredient contained in the packaging system. Long-term stability studies are necessary for the appropriate storage conditions, involving temperature, light protection, relative humidity, and protection from excessive mechanical stress during transportation and handling. Studies on storage conditions are becoming even more important as products are exported globally and exposed to a wide range of environmental conditions. Protein dosage forms are especially sensitive to extremes in temperatures and handling. In addition to concerns regarding maintenance of chemical and physical stability of the drug product during storage, there is also concern that the container and closure systems are adequate to maintain the sterility and other microbiological quality attributes of the sterile product. Container and closure integrity studies are of great importance and are being scrutinized in great detail by regulatory bodies such as the Food and Drug Administration. An excellent review of container and closure integrity issues and methods is given by Guazzo [38].

References

1. *United States Pharmacopeia, XXII National Formulary XVII*, The United States Pharmacopeial Convention, Inc., Rockville, MD, 1989, p. 1470.
2. Turco, S., and King, R. E., *Sterile Dosage Forms*, 3rd ed., Lea & Febiger, Philadelphia, 1987, pp. 116–127.

3. Avis, K. E., Sterile Products. In: *The Theory and Practice of Industrial Pharmacy*, 3rd ed. (L. Lachman, H. A. Lieberman, and J. L. Kanig, eds.), Lea & Febiger, Philadelphia, 1986, pp. 639–677.
4. DeLuca, P. P., and Boylan, J. C., Formulation of Small Volume Parenterals. In: *Pharmaceutical Dosage Forms: Parenteral Medications*, 2nd ed., Vol. 1 (K. E. Avis, H. A. Lieberman, and L. Lachman, eds.), Marcel Dekker, Inc., New York, 1992, pp. 173–248.
5. Boylan, J. C., and Fites, A. L., Parenteral Products. In: *Modern Pharmaceutics*, 2nd ed. (G. S. Banker and C. T. Rhodes, eds.), Marcel Dekker, Inc., New York, 1989, pp. 491–538.
6. Avis, K. E., Parenteral Preparations. In: *Remington's Pharmaceutical Sciences*, 18th ed. (A. R. Gennaro, ed.), Mack Publishing Company, Easton, PA, 1990, pp. 1545–1569.
7. Harwood, R. J., Portnoff, J. B., and Sunbery, E. W., The Processing of Small Volume Parenterals and Related Sterile Products. In: *Pharmaceutical Dosage Forms: Parenteral Medications*, 2nd ed., Vol. 2 (K. E. Avis, H. A. Lieberman, and L. Lachman, eds.), Marcel Dekker, Inc., New York, 1993, pp. 1–92.
8. *United States Pharmacopeia, XXII, National Formulary XVII*, The United States Pharmacopeial Convention, Inc., Rockville, MD, 1989, p. 1472.
9. Hecht, G., Roehrs, R. R., Cooper, E. R., Hiddemen, J. W., and Van Duzee, B. F., Design and Evaluation of Ophthalmic Pharmaceutical Products. In: *Modern Pharmaceutics*, 2nd ed. (G. S. Banker, and C. T. Rhodes, eds.), Marcel Dekker, Inc., New York, 1989, pp. 539–603.
10. Olsen, L. E., Sterile Diagnostics. In: *Pharmaceutical Dosage Forms: Parenteral Medications*, 2nd ed., Vol. 1 (K. E. Avis, H. A. Lieberman, and L. Lachman, eds.), Marcel Dekker, Inc., New York, 1992, pp. 321–359.
11. Shough, H. R., Allergenic Extracts. In: *Remington's Pharmaceutical Sciences*, 18th ed. (A. R. Gennaro, ed.), Mack Publishing Company, Easton, PA, 1990, pp. 1405–1415.
12. *United States Pharmacopeia, XXII, National Formulary XVII*, The United States Pharmacopeial Convention, Inc., Rockville, MD, 1989, p. 1471.
13. Sims, E. E., and Worthington, H. E. C., Formulation studies on certain oily injection products, *Int. J. Pharm.*, 24:287–296 (1985).
14. Radd, B. L., Newman, A. C., Fegely, B. J., Chrzanowski, F. Lichten, J. L., and Walkling, W. J., Development of haloperidol in oil injection formulations, *J. Parenter. Sci. Tech.*, 39:48–53 (1985).
15. Reed, R. W., and Yalkowsky, S. H., Lysis of human red blood cells in the presence of various cosolvents, *J. Parenter. Sci. Tech.*, 39:64 (1985).
16. Pikal, M. J., Freeze Drying. In: *Encyclopedia of Pharmaceutical Technology*, Vol. 6 (J. Swarbrick and J. C. Boylan, eds.), Marcel Dekker, Inc., New York, 1992, pp. 275–303.
17. Nail, S. L., and Gatlin, L. A., Freeze Drying: Principles and Practice. In: *Pharmaceutical Dosage Forms: Parenteral Medications*, 2nd ed., Vol. 2 (K. E. Avis, H. A. Lieberman, and L. Lachman, eds.), Marcel Dekker, Inc., New York, 1993, pp. 163–233.
18. Akers, M. J., Fites, A. L., and Robison, R. L. Formulation development of parenteral suspensions, *J. Parenter. Sci. Tech.*, 41:88–96 (1987).
19. Levy, M. Y., and Benita, S., Short- and long-term stability assessment of a new injectable diazepam submicron emulsion, *J. Parenter. Sci. Tech.*, 45:101–107 (1991).
20. Akers, M. J., *Parenteral Quality Control: Sterility, Pyrogen, Particulate, and Package Integrity Testing*, 2nd ed., Marcel Dekker, Inc., New York, 1994.
21. *United States Pharmacopeia, XXII, National Formulary XVII*, The United States Pharmacopeial Convention, Inc., Rockville, MD, 1989, Sterility Tests, pp. 1483–1488.
22. *United States Pharmacopeia, XXII, National Formulary XVII*, The United States Pharmacopeial Convention, Inc., Rockville, MD, 1989, 5th Supplement, 1992.
23. Gibson, M., Denham, A. J., Taylor, P. M., and Payne, N. I., Development of a parenteral formulation of trimelamol, a synthetic S-triazine carbinolamine-containing cytotoxic agent, *J. Parenter. Sci. Tech.*, 44:306–313 (1990).
24. Chien, Y. W., Solubilization of metronidazole by water-miscible multi-cosolvents and water-soluble vitamins, *J. Parenter. Sci. Tech.*, 38:32–36 (1984).

25. Howard, J. R., and Gould, P. L., The use of co-solvents in parenteral formulation of low-solubility drugs, *Int. J. Pharm.*, 25:359–362 (1985).
26. Tarr, B. D., and Yalkowsky, S. H., A new parenteral vehicle for the administration of some poorly water soluble anti-cancer drugs, *J. Parenter. Sci. Tech.*, 41:31–33 (1987).
27. Rajagopalan, N., Dicken, C. M., Ravin, L. J., and Sternson, L. A., A study of the solubility of amphotericin B in nonaqueous solvent systems, *J. Parenter. Sci. Tech.*, 42:97–102 (1988).
28. Brewster, M. E., Simpkins, J. W., Hora, M. S., Stern, W. C., and Bodor, N., The potential use of cyclodextrins in parenteral formulations, *J. Parenter. Sci. Tech.*, 43:231–240 (1989).
29. Simpkins, J. W., Solubilization of ovine growth hormone with 2-hydroxypropyl-β-cyclodextrin, *J. Parenter. Sci. Tech.*, 45:266–269 (1991).
30. Johnson, D. M., and Gu, L. C., Autoxidation and Antioxidants. In: *Encyclopedia of Pharmaceutical Technology*, Vol. 1 (J. Swarbrick and J. C. Boylan, eds.), Marcel Dekker, Inc., 1988, pp. 415–449.
31. Wang, Y. J., and Hanson, M. J., Parenteral formulations of proteins and peptides: stability and stabilizers, *J. Parenter. Sci. Tech.*, 42 Suppl. (1988).
32. *Stability and Characterization of Protein and Peptide Drugs* (Y. J. Wang, and R. Pearlman, eds.), Plenum Publishing Corp., New York, 1993.
33. *Stability of Protein Pharmaceuticals* (T. J. Ahern, and M. C. Manning, eds.), Plenum Publishing Corp., New York, 1992.
34. Townsend, M. W., and DeLuca, P. P., Use of lyoprotectants in the freeze-drying of a model protein, ribonuclease A, *J. Parenter. Sci. Tech.*, 42:190–199 (1988).
35. *United States Pharmacopeia, XXII, National Formulary XVII*, The United States Pharmacopeial Convention, Inc., Rockville, MD, 1989, p. 1571.
36. Abendroth, R. P., Glass as a Packaging Material for Pharmaceuticals. In: *Encyclopedia of Pharmaceutical Technology*, Vol. 7 (J. Swarbrick, and J. C. Boylan, eds.), Marcel Dekker, Inc., New York, 1993, pp. 79–99.
37. Avis, K. E., and Smith, E. J., Elastomeric Parenteral Closures. In: *Encyclopedia of Pharmaceutical Technology*, Vol. 5 (J. Swarbrick, and J. C. Boylan, eds.), Marcel Dekker, Inc., New York, 1992, pp. 73–88.
38. Guazzo, D. M., Container/Closure Integrity. In: *Parenteral Quality Control: Sterility, Pyrogen, Particulate, and Package Integrity Testing*, 2nd ed. (M. J. Akers, ed.), Marcel Dekker, Inc., New York, 1994. Chap. 4.

MICHAEL J. AKERS

Particle-Size Characterization

Sampling Procedures

It should be a self-obvious truth that any size-characterization procedure must be preceded by an efficient sampling procedure to obtain a representative sample. Unfortunately, in many companies, the group requesting a fine-particle characterization forward the sample from a remote location within an industrial plant, and the scientists charged with the size characterization procedure never inquire as to the sampling procedures. It is usually assumed that the sample is a representative sample when, in fact, a process worker may have simply removed it, at random. The worker may not have received any guidance as to the necessity of obtaining a representative sample. The problems of obtaining a representative sample of a fine-particle system are often very complex and require expensive procedures. The subject of powder sampling has been discussed extensively in standard reference books. Several companies sell sampling equipment for installation in industrial systems [1–7].

Even when the sample received by the laboratory is a representative sample, the analyst still faces the difficult task of taking a small subsample from the powder supplied. It has been shown that one of the most efficient devices for taking a subsample of the powder is to use a device known as the spinning riffler shown in Fig. 1(a). It consists of a ring of containers which rotate under the powder supply. The total powder supply is processed by this instrument. It has been shown that to obtain a representative sample, the time of powder flow through the apparatus divided by the time of rotation of the ring of containers should be a large number [5–7]. Difficulties arise using such devices with very fine powders because air currents caused by the rotation of the system can blow the fines away. Furthermore, if the powder is cohesive (sticky), the powder flow through the funnel can be impeded. In some situations, the flow properties of the powder can be modified by adding a silica flow agent, provided that this does not interfere with the size characterization procedures employed subsequent to the sampling procedure [8].

Recently, a new approach to the sampling of powders has been developed by Kaye and co-workers. In this procedure, the powder is thoroughly mixed in such a way that any sample taken at random is a representative sample [9,10]. The equipment used in this technique is shown in Fig. 1(b). The mixing chamber is placed in a slowly rotating drum lined with dimpled foam. The foam serves two purposes, first of all, it promotes gentle and quiet tumbling of the chamber. Secondly, it accentuates the lifting power of the slowly rotating cylinder which lifts the partially filled chamber up the wall of the rotation cylinder until it tumbles randomly down to a new position of equilibrium before it is again lifted up prior to the next tumble. The chaotic tumbling of the mixing chamber creates ideal conditions for powder mixing, and short mixing times have proved to be efficient in mixing the ingredients [11]. At the cessation of the tumbling procedure, a small sampling cup attached to the lid of the mixing chamber is used to retrieve a representative sample. The tumbling chamber can have various geometric shapes, and provided that dimpled foam is used, even the classical 225-g laboratory jar can be tumbled on laboratory-scale equipment. Efficiency of mixing falls off if the jar is more than half filled, because this imposes restrictions on the free random movement of the powder in the chamber. It is recommended that this type of device be used to homogenize any powder sample before

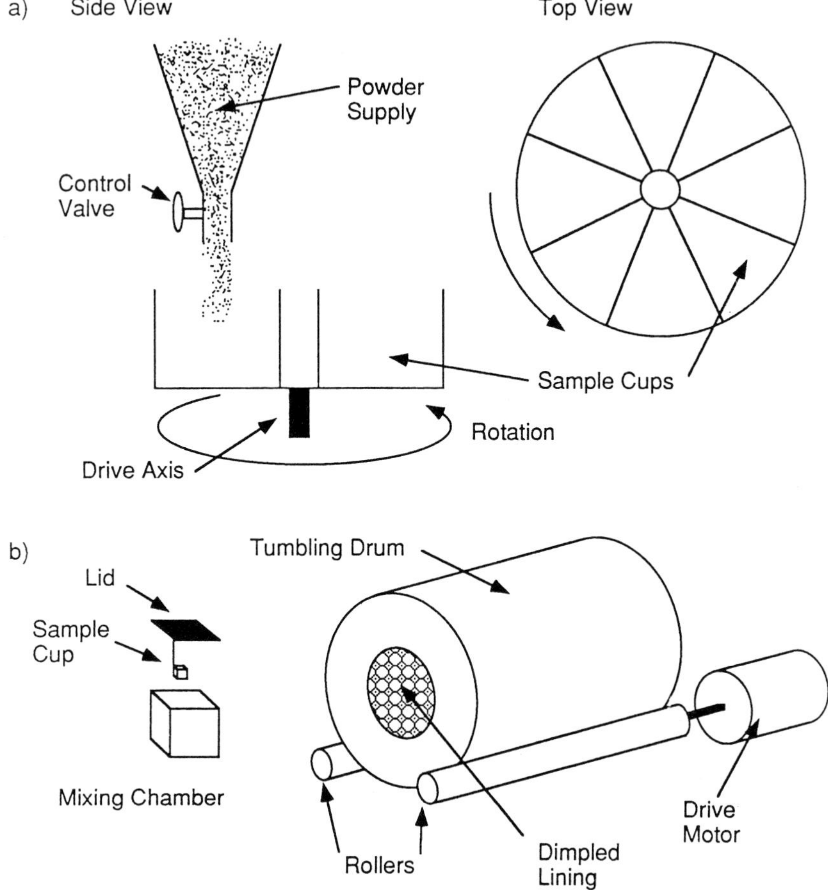

FIG. 1. Systematic representative sampling of a powder can be achieved with the spinning riffler. Chaos-generating devices can be used to generate representative samples taken at random. (a) Spinning riffler [7]. (b) Free-fall tumbling powder mixer used for powder homogenization and sampling [10].

using a subsample in any experimental investigation if the sample had been kept for some time or been poured in a laboratory environment. Powder segregation mechanisms are far more widespread in the laboratory than generally known [12]. For taking a sample of a suspension from a slurry process line the Isolock sampler is a useful piece of equipment [13].

The study of the size distributions of therapeutic aerosols creates a very difficult sampling task for the specialist. Wherever possible, size characterization of an aerosol system should be carried out in situ, using the diffractometers discussed later. For sampling an aerosol system, a cascade impactor is used to fractionate the aerosol into various size groups. (A full discussion of these instruments is given in Ref. 1.) Aerosols can also be sampled through various filter systems for subsequent examination by image analysis procedures. If the aim of the sampling process is to generate a deposit which can be examined through a microscope with an imaging system, surface filters such as the Nuclepore filter of Fig. 2 can be used [14–16]. The traditional paper filter is described

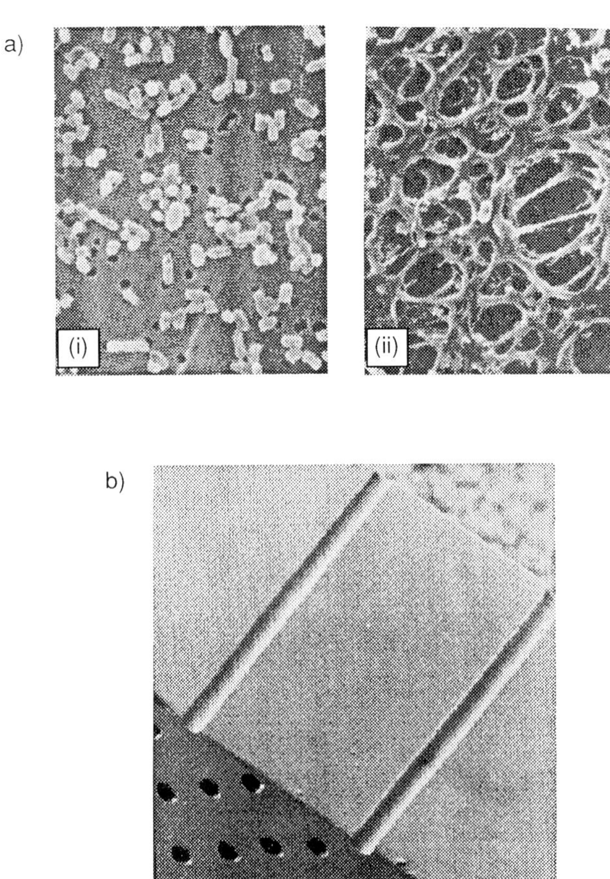

FIG. 2. Various types of filters for sampling aerosols to generate fields of view useful in characterization by image analysis. (a) Nuclepore surface filter (i) and cellulosic depth filter (ii). (b) Oblique view of a 25 μm "collimated hole" sieve [17].

technically as a depth filter. Although depth filters can sometimes be rendered transparent by using immersion oil, it is normally difficult to view the fine particles on depth filters because they penetrate into the pore structure of the filter. The Nuclepore filter of Fig. 2(a) and similar polycarbonate filters are called surface filters. They are available in various pore sizes for filtering aerosols of a given size [14–16].

The most recent innovation in the preparation of fine-particle fields of view for image analysis are the glass filter sieves shown in Fig. 2(b). They are made by a process in which a fiberoptic array is assembled, and the cores are dissolved to generate orthogonal holes of closely controlled dimensions in the filtering-sieving surface [17]. These glass sieves are proving to be useful in the concentration of fine particles contaminating parenteral fluids prior to their characterization [18].

Sample Preparation

In many situations, a powder sample to be characterized has to be prepared in a specified format for the characterization procedure. Thus, the powder may have to be spread out on a glass slide prior to microscopic examination or a suspension of the material may have to be prepared in an appropriate liquid or gas. The act of dispersing the powder can radically change the size distribution of the powder to be studied and the procedure used to prepare the sample for characterization should respect what is known as the operational integrity of the fine particles. Thus, if the fine particle is to be dispersed in water, the use of ultrasonics to disperse the powder in the liquid can result in the shattering of fine-particle agglomerates which normally would persist throughout the treatment that the powder receives in the manufacturing and usage operation.

In general, the technology used to disperse a powder prior to a characterization study should match the severity of dispersion forces that the powder will experience in use. Alternatively, if ultrasonics are used to generate a well-dispersed powder, the analytical procedure protocol should be defined rigorously in order to avoid variations from operator to operator. A dispersing agent is used frequently and great caution should be exercised since it can alter the structure of the system in a fundamental manner [19].

Size Characterization of Fine Particles and Powders

Direct Examination with Microscopes and Other Imagining Devices

Extensive pioneering studies of fine-particle characterization by examining their images through the microscope and other imaging devices were carried out by Heywood as well as Hausner [20,21]. In this early work, the areas or dimensions of profiles were measured by direct comparison of the profile images with sets of reference circles engraved on what was known as an eye piece reticule [1]. More recently, several sophisticated systems have been developed for computer-aided image analysis [22,23]. These devices often have built-in logic procedures to process the image before characterization experiments to avoid problems associated with deep convolutions in the profile. Thus, in Fig. 3 the modification of the image of an agglomerate by two processes known as image erosion (a) and image dilation (b) is shown. It can be seen that in some cases, the break down of a complex profile during image erosion allows the investigation of the possibility that subunits have joined together, resulting in the overall structure of an aerosol agglomerate. Redilation of an image to its original size after several erosions removes convolutions from the profile. This can create problems when intercept logic is used to measure the perimeter and area of the profiles [25,26].

The increased power of processing logic available in modern computer-aided analysis systems makes it possible to characterize the shape of fine-particle profiles, using Fourier analysis techniques and to describe structures by means of fractal dimensions. The Fourier analysis techniques can be carried out in one or two dimensions [24]. When exploring the structure of a profile in one-dimensional space by means of Fourier analysis, a reference point is located within the profile and a geometric signature wave form is generated by rotating a vector at uniform angular velocity around the perimeter of the profile. The magnitude of the vector plotted against the angle of the vector generates a wave form-type function. This wave form is subjected to Fourier analysis to generate a power

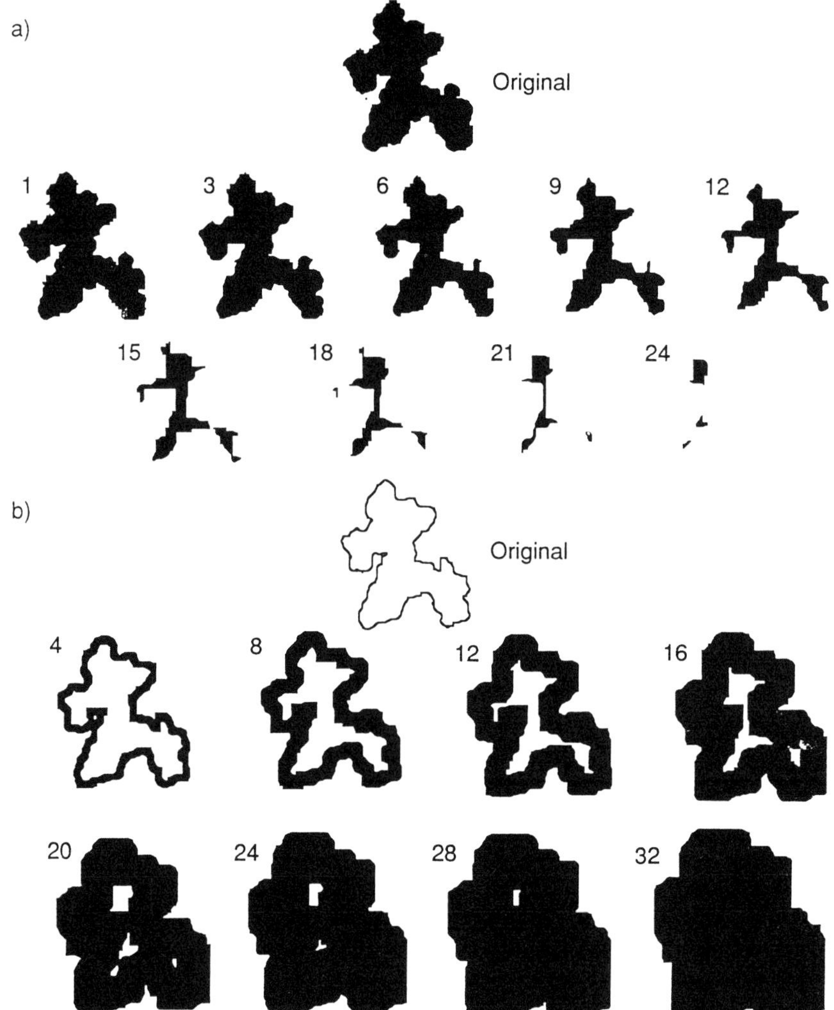

FIG. 3. Computer-aided image profile characterization logic enables routine characterization of convoluted profiles. (a) Repeated erosion of an aerosol agglomerate profile suggests that the cluster was formed by the collision of several subunits. (b) Dilation logic can be used to fill in internal holes and deep fissures in an image to be evaluated.

spectrum of the various harmonics contributing to the structure of the wave form. This technique is useful for round objects but generates complex information if there are deep convolutions or sharp edges on the profile. For such profiles, two-dimensional Fourier transform can be generated by computer. Any sharp edges or deep crevices of the profile show up as high frequencies in the two-dimensional Fourier transform. These high frequencies are probably related to the dissolution rates and bioavailability of any drug particles. In general, powder-flow problems are more complex the more high frequencies are present in the two-dimensional Fourier transform [28].

A different procedure for describing the structure of rugged profiles has been developed from the theorems of a new subject known as fractal geometry [26–29]. The basic

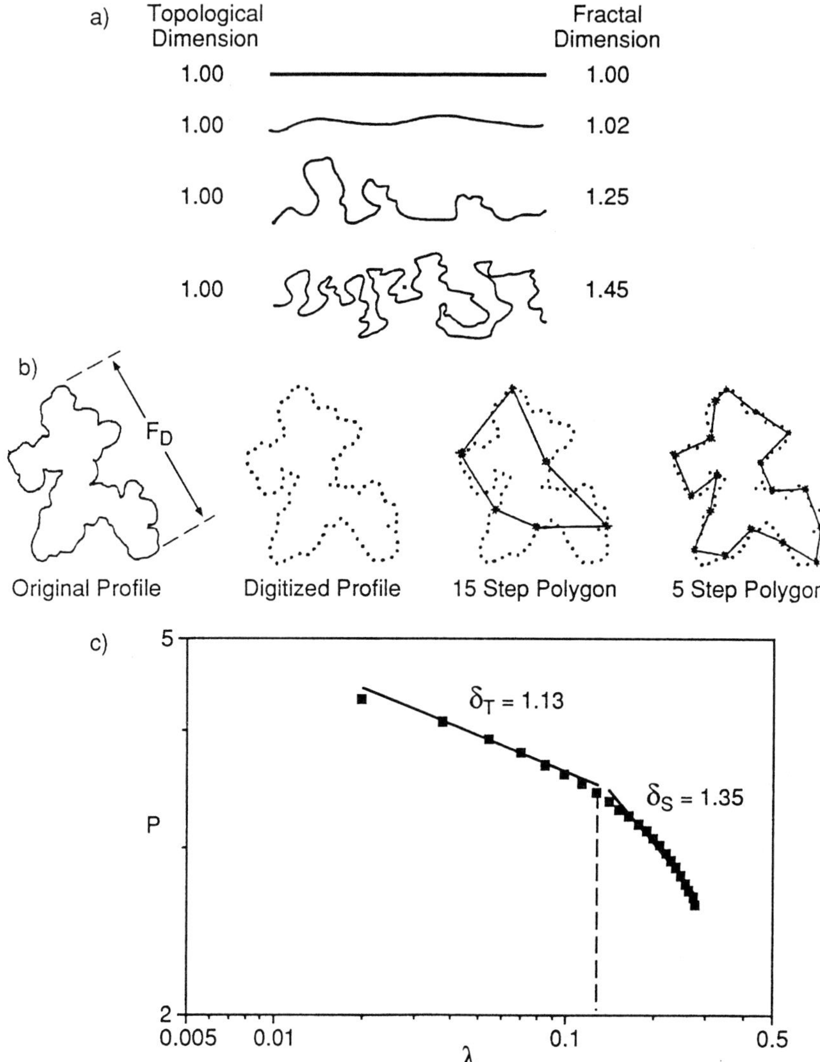

FIG. 4. Fractal dimensions can be used to evaluate the rugged structure of fine particles. (a) Fractal dimensions describe the ruggedness of various rugged lines. (b) Physical basis of the equipaced exploration technique for evaluating the fractal dimensions of rugged boundaries. (c) Data generated by the equipaced exploration technique for the profile of (b).

concept employed in fractal geometry is to add a fractional number to the topological dimension of a system to describe the space-filling ability of the system being described. Thus, in Fig. 4(a) all the lines have a topological dimension of one. The fractional number added to this dimension creates the boundary fractal dimension of the line, a parameter that describes the ruggedness of the line. In Fig. 4(b) the basic logic used to evaluate the fractal dimension of a profile of a powder grain is shown. Polygons are constructed on a digitized form of the profile by pacing out a given number of steps around the profile. Polygons constructed in this way become the perimeter estimate at the inspection resolution represented by the distance paced out along the profile. The perimeter estimate and the distance between exploratory steps taken around the perimeter are normalized with respect to the maximum projected length of the profile. To estimate the magnitude of the fractal dimension of the profile, the perimeter estimates are plotted against the exploration steps, as indicated in Fig. 4(c). This plot is known as a Richardson plot in honor of one of the pioneers of the detailed studies of convoluted profiles such as these of islands [1]. The slope of the data lines on the Richardson plot represents the fractional number that has to be added to the topological dimension to describe a structure of the boundary. As in the case of the profile studied in Fig. 4(b), some fine-particle profiles exhibit different fractal dimensions at different levels of inspection. Thus, in this profile, what is known as the structural boundary fractal dimension is revealed by the course-resolution data, and what is known as the textural boundary fractal dimension is revealed at high resolution inspection. The structural fractal dimension probably governs the packing and flow properties of a powder, whereas the texture governs the dissolution rate, adsorptive capacity, and chemical activity.

Because of the large amount of visual information imparted by an image of a fine particle, there has been a tendency to regard image-analysis inspection as a fundamental method against which all others should be measured. Recently it has been shown that the methodology normally used in the image analysis of profiles is vulnerable to coincidence errors of the type discussed later when stream methods of characterization are described. In essence, the principal problem involved in the inspection of a system by image analysis is the difficulty of deciding what constitutes a separate and operationally functional fine particle. A failure to record the density of coverage of the surface used in a microscopic study of a powder is a major source of uncertainty in the value of the reported data [30].

Sieve Fractionation

Sieving is a widely used method for characterizing the range of grain sizes present in a powder. In this technique, a quantity of powder is separated into two fractions on a surface containing holes of a specified uniform size. The two main problems associated with sieve characterization are the difficulty of determining the completion of the fractionation process and secondly, coping with the variation in sieve apertures present in new and worn sieves. (See discussion of sieve characterization in Refs. 1 and 23.) The photomicrograph of a woven wire sieve surface in Fig. 5(a) illustrates the problems associated with the variations in sieve apertures. In Fig. 5(b) the data on the variation of the sieve apertures as characterized by various studies are plotted [31]. First of all, the minimum midpoint diameter of the trapezium created by the projected image of the wire-woven surface provides the operational diameter of the sieve. Then the size distribution of the apertures can be measured with the help of image-analysis techniques. The size distribution determined in this way is then normalized by the nominal aperture of the sieve. It can be seen from the data in Fig. 5(b) that the aperture distribution is Gaussian.

In an alternative technique, some near mesh-sized glass beads are separated on the sieve and the beads trapped in the mesh are sized. If sand is used in such an experiment, a typical set of grains trapped in the opening of the sieve allows to determine the shape of the profiles, as illustrated by the data of Fig. 6. Electroformed sieves have a much narrower distribution of aperture sizes but are more fragile and expensive than wire-woven sieves [1]. Recently glass sieves with very exact holes have been developed (see Fig. 2); this type of device is very accurate but they have to be handled with great care.

a)

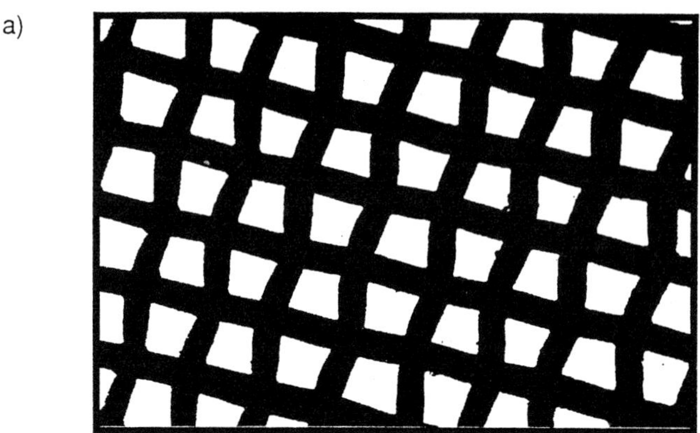

b)

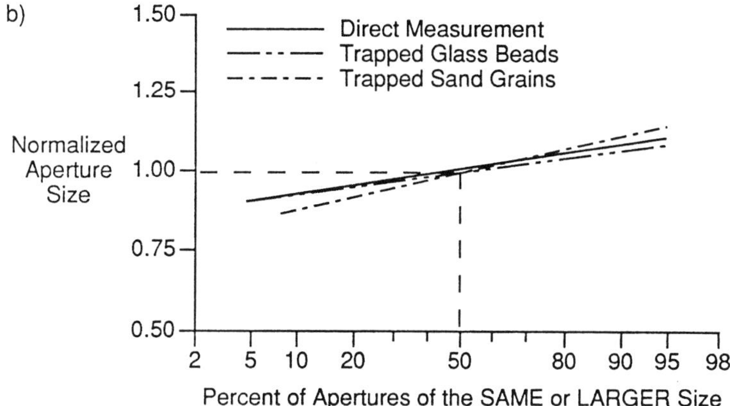

FIG. 5. Variations in mesh apertures; aperture sizes increase with sieve usage. (a) Photograph of a wire-woven sieve. (b) The variations in sieve apertures can be determined either by direct inspection of the aperture or by examining near mesh sizes of fine particles trapped in the apertures during a sieving experiment.

Sedimentation Techniques

Sedimentation procedures to evaluate particle size in terms of the equivalent spheres, which have the same settling speed in laminar flow conditions, are the basis of many techniques used to characterize fine particles. A suspension of fine particles is prepared and their falling speed is determined with an immersed balanced pan or by monitoring the settlement of the fine particles with the help of light beams or x-ray beams (Fig. 7). The measured falling speeds of the fine particles are inserted, along with the other appropriate parameters of the suspension, into Stokes' law, as shown in Eq. (1).

$$d_s = \sqrt{\frac{18\eta t}{(\rho_p - \rho_L)gh}} \tag{1}$$

where d_S = Stokes diameter of the fine particle
η = viscosity of the suspension

g = acceleration due to gravity
h = distance through which the fall is timed
t = time required to fall the distance h
ρ_P = density of the powder
ρ_L = density of the liquid

The configuration of the actual instrument used to measure the Stokes diameters of fine particles varies between instrument manufacturers [1,23]. In some devices the fine-particle sedimentation is monitoned with a light beam; these instruments are known as photosedimentometers. Because of the difficulties of interpreting the concentration measurement of fine particles with diameters close to that of the wavelength of the light being

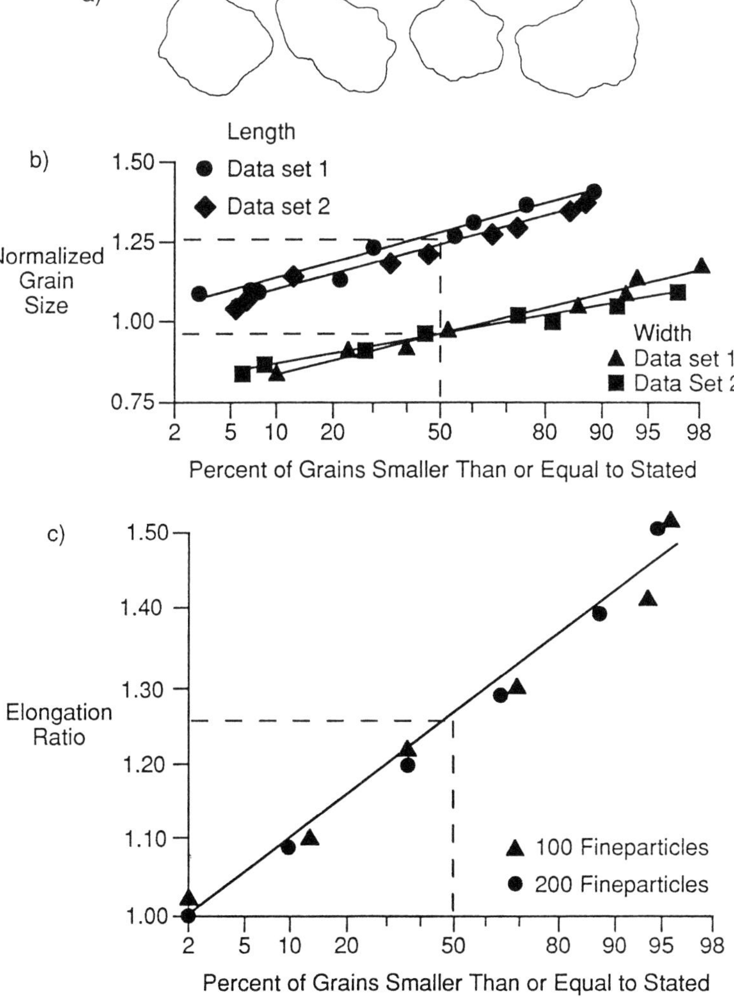

FIG. 6. When calibrating a sieve mesh with trapped irregularly shaped grains, a subset of powder grains is obtained which can be used to generate a shape description of the powder grains [31]. (a) Typical sand grain profiles. (b) Length and width distributions of sand grains trapped in a sieve mesh. (c) Elongation ratio distribution for sand grains trapped in a sieve mesh.

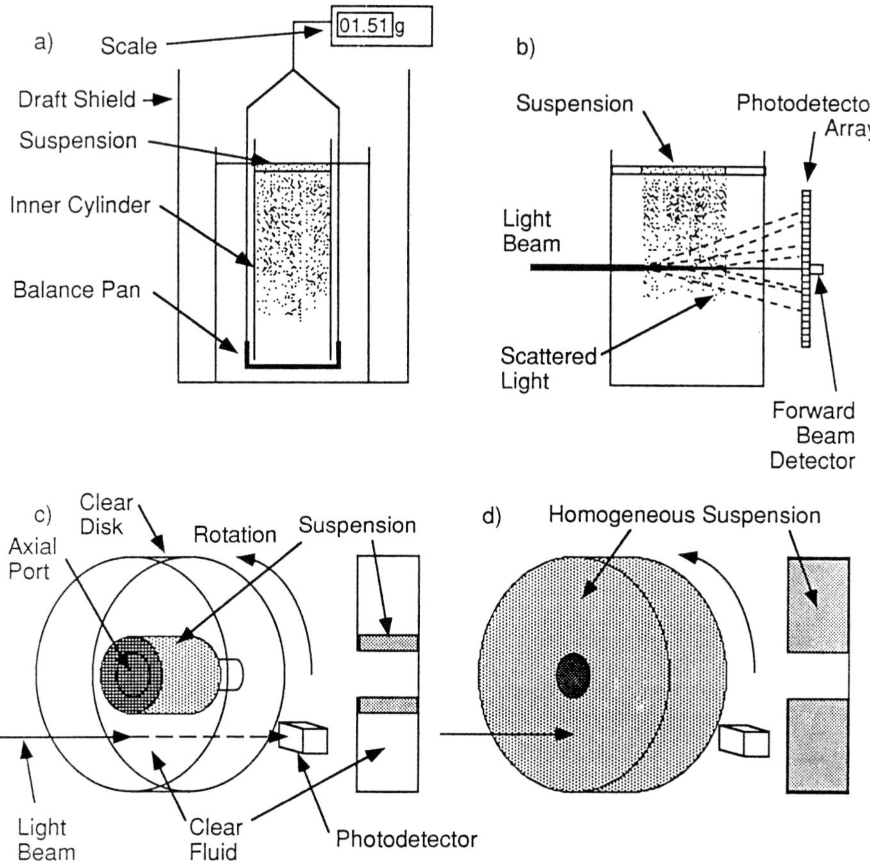

FIG. 7. Sedimentation methods for characterizing the sizes of powder grains. The settling speeds of fine particles in a suspension are measured and interpreted as equivalent spheres using Stokes' law. (a) In a sedimentation balance, the sedimenting fine particles are weighed as they arrive at the base of the sedimentation column. (b) In a photosedimentometer the movement of fine particles is monitored and recorded by means of light beams. In some cases x-rays are used rather than visible light. (c) In a line-start centrifugal method all the fine particles to be studied start at the same distance from the centre of rotation. (d) The homogeneous-start centrifugal method.

used to monitor the dynamics of the suspension, some instruments employ x-ray beams to monitor the fine-particle movements. Other instruments use centrifugal force to accelerate the settling dynamics of the suspended fine particles.

Sedimentation methods were the dominant size-characterization procedures in the 1950s and 1960s. In recent years, they have been displaced from the powder laboratory by the diffractometers described below. Diffractometers have the advantage of speed, but problems occur in the interpretation of the diffracted light signals. The x-ray-based sedimentometer manufactured by the Micromeretics Corporation, called the Sedigraph, is still widely employed, partly because its use is written into some industrial standards governing size-characterization procedures [23].

Recent years have seen a revival of disk centrifuges to characterize fine particles smaller than one micron, basically because of the work carried out by Provder and co-workers in cooperation with Brookhaven Laboratories Ltd. [32,33]. Extensive reviews of the classical sedimentation methods are presented in Refs. 1 and 23; see also Ref. 34.

Diffractometers

The advent of the laser has made the generation of diffraction patterns by a suspension of fine particles a relatively easy task. At the same time, the rapid development of computer processing equipment and specialized photocells has made it possible to process the information in a group diffraction pattern to generate the particle size distribution of the fine particles in suspension. One of the first commercially available equipment for generating size-distribution information from a group diffraction patterns of a randomly dispersed array of fine particles was the CILAS equipment developed in France to measure the size distribution of cement [34]. The basic system of the CILAS laser diffractometer equipment is shown in Fig. 8, where the information from the photodiode array is sent to a computer. The companies that have developed diffractometers do not divulge the structure of their software. The user of this equipment should be careful to gain information on the data-processing protocol followed in any specific instrument to change the diffraction information into a size-distribution function. Some of the instruments assume a given distribution function and curve fit to accelerate the data processing. Sometimes such curve fitting can distort the data generated. Several manufacturers of these instruments provide extensive technical data on their performance, and the International Standard Organization is currently preparing a standard procedure for diffractometers [35–38]. The laser diffractometers are particularly useful for studying the size distributions of sprays and aerosol clouds [38–41].

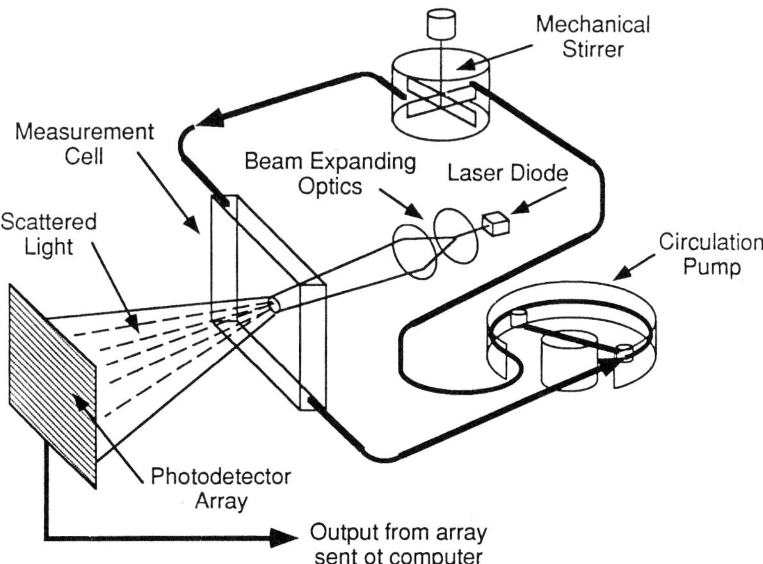

FIG. 8. In a laser diffractometer size analyzer the size distribution of a random array of fine particles is deduced from their group diffraction pattern. (From the commercial literature of the CILAS Corp. [34], by permission.)

Time-of-Flight Instruments

Another type of instrument which has been made possible by the availability of lasers is known as time-of-flight instrument. Here a narrow focused beam of laser light explores an area of a suspension. The size of the particles in suspension is measured by the time it takes for a laser beam to pass across the profile of the fine particle. Sophisticated optical recording devices and electronic editors are used to generate the size distribution data from the information generated by the device.

In Fig. 9 the basic system is shown of the instrument developed and marketed by Galai instruments of Israel [42]. (It was sold in the United States for several years by the Brinkmann organization, but it is now marketed by Galai Instruments.) A useful feature of this instrument is that, as the fine particles are being characterized by the scanning laser beam, they are also imaged on a television screen in such a way that any agglomeration can be detected during the analysis. The logic of the Galai system allows the fine-particle shape to be measured concurrently with size.

Another time-of-flight size analyzer is known as the LASENTECH. This system is portable and has been suggested for use as an online monitor for fine particles moving in a system as well as in the laboratory [43]. A different type of time-of-flight instrument, based on different physical principles, is manufactured by Amherst Instruments Limited [44]. Here the stream of aerosol fine particles is accelerated across a gap defined by two laser beams. The time of flight across this gap is measured from the light signals scattered from the two light beams, and an electronic editor ensures single occupancy for the measurement series. The larger fine particles are slow to accelerate across the gap, whereas the smallest move with the speed of the feed air jet. The system is calibrated using standard fine particles.

A similar instrument is manufactured by the TSI Corporation [45]. The basic system for measuring the aerodynamic diameter of aerosol fine particles is shown in Fig. 10. In this instrument the velocity of a moving fine particle being accelerated across the inspection zone is measured by the Doppler shift in two beams which have a different directional reference to the moving airstream. From one perspective, the two lasers beams

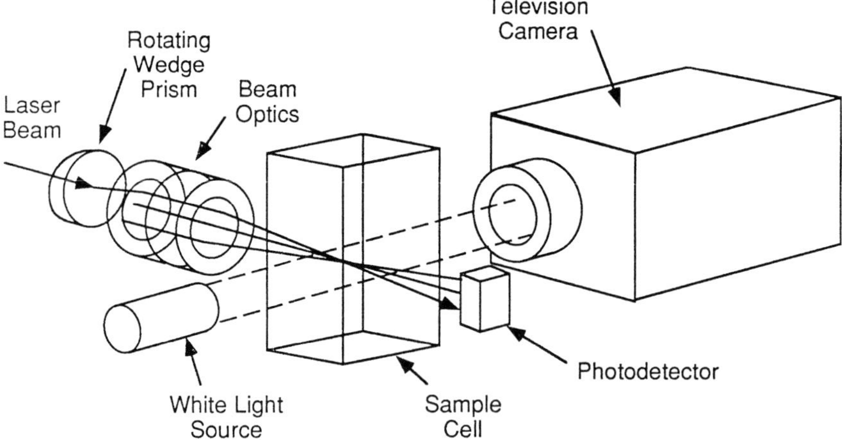

FIG. 9. The Galai time-of-flight laser-based system for characterizing fine particles. (By permission of Galai Instruments.)

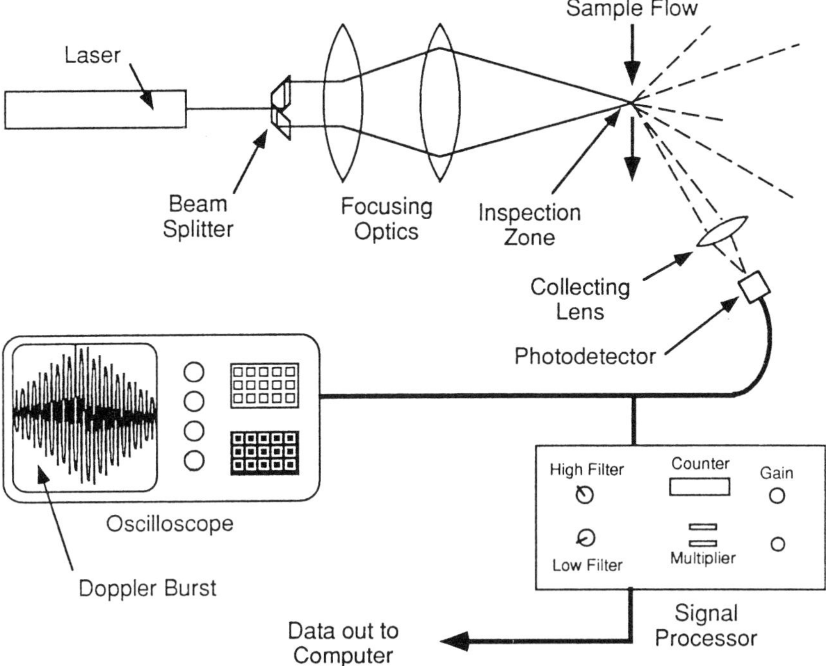

FIG. 10. A Doppler-shift procedure for measuring the aerodynamic size of aerosol fine particles [1].

can be regarded as creating interference fringes, whereas the aerosol fine particle moving across the fringe system creates an oscillating signal which can be related to the fine-particle size via calibration measurements. Several instruments based on this principle are available from different manufacturers [40,45,46]. The fact that the instruments in which aerodynamic sizes are measured by the movement of the fine particles across crossed laser beams involves laser Doppler shifts is not immediately obvious from reading the trade literature of companies marketing this type of instrument. Indeed, in this class of instrument the interpretive theory is complex and the user is generally provided with a calibrated instrument to carry out the characterization studies of interest.

Photon-Correlation Spectroscopy

Another instrument, where the physics of the measurements are not immediately obvious to the outside observer, is in a group of instruments variously referred to as photon-correlation, dynamic light scattering, or quasi-elastic light scattering spectroscopes (often referred to as PCS, DLS, or QUELS). In this discussion, the term photon-correlation spectroscopy is used [47]. Its physical basis is the monitoring of the Doppler shifts in reflected laser light created by the Brownian motion of submicron fine particles. In some cases, the technique can also be applied to fine particles of several microns in diameter. The equipment for actually measuring the Doppler shifts is relatively simple, but the overall expense is increased by the data-processing computer which is usually included. This instrument is useful for studying relatively simple size distributions such as latex suspensions. However, interpreting a wide range of sizes in suspension with this technique can involve complex data processing which, if carried out incorrectly, can generate confusing data [47–49].

Thus far, in this article, several instruments have been discussed in which a stream of aerosol fine particles are characterized by the rate at which they are accelerated across an inspection zone. In an instrument known as the E-SPART analyzer the aerosol fine particles are oscillated in an inspection zone by means of an acoustic wave. The inspection zone is the location of an optical fringe system created by crossed laser beams. The movement across this fringe system of oscillated fine particles is used to characterize the aerodynamic diameter of the fine particles. The aerodynamic size of a fine particle is the size of a sphere of unit density that has the same dynamic behavior as the fine particle being studied. This system can measure the aerodynamic size distribution in real time of aerosols which are breathable hazards for industrial workers. It is also used for studying household products, and asthma therapy and other respiratory problems [50].

Stream Counters

Another size-characterization instrument group is known as stream counters, where a stream of fine particles is passed through an inspection zone. The physical properties of the inspection zone are changed by the presence of the fine particles. The size of the fine particle is deduced from this change. In the Coulter counter (Fig. 11), the fine particles to be characterized are placed in an electrolyte and a stream of suspension is passed through an orifice between two electrodes. The size of the fine particle is deduced from the measured resistance change between the electrodes [51]. A major problem with stream counters is the single occupancy of the fine particles in the inspection zone. Should there be inadvertently two fine particles in the orifice, they register as one large fine particle and the counting of the smaller-sized particles has a deficit of two. This type of error is referred to as primary count loss (the undercounting of the smaller fine particles) and secondary count gain (the false registering of larger fine particles due to multiple occupancy of the zone). Normally the analysis with this type of instrument is carried out in a series of increasing dilutions until further dilution does not affect the measured size distribution. A difficulty sometime encountered with this method is the availability of a conducting fluid which does not interact with the fine particles to be inspected. Over the years, various sophisticated data-processing techniques have been used to allow for problems associated with the Coulter counter, for example, when the fine particles are too close to the walls of the orifice or have extreme shape [1,23]. Another counter working on the same general principles is known as the Electrozone counter [52].

In another group of stream counters, the fine particles in the inspection zone are monitored with a light beam. Various models of this type of instrument have been developed to count fine particles in liquids; others are specialized for the counting of dust fine particles in the air [1,23,53–55].

Elutriators for Size Characterization Studies and Fine Powder Fractionation

Elutriators are a class of instruments which fractionate fine particles according to their size by manipulating them in a moving fluid. They are among the first devices used for measuring size distributions of powders by fractionating them into various size groups

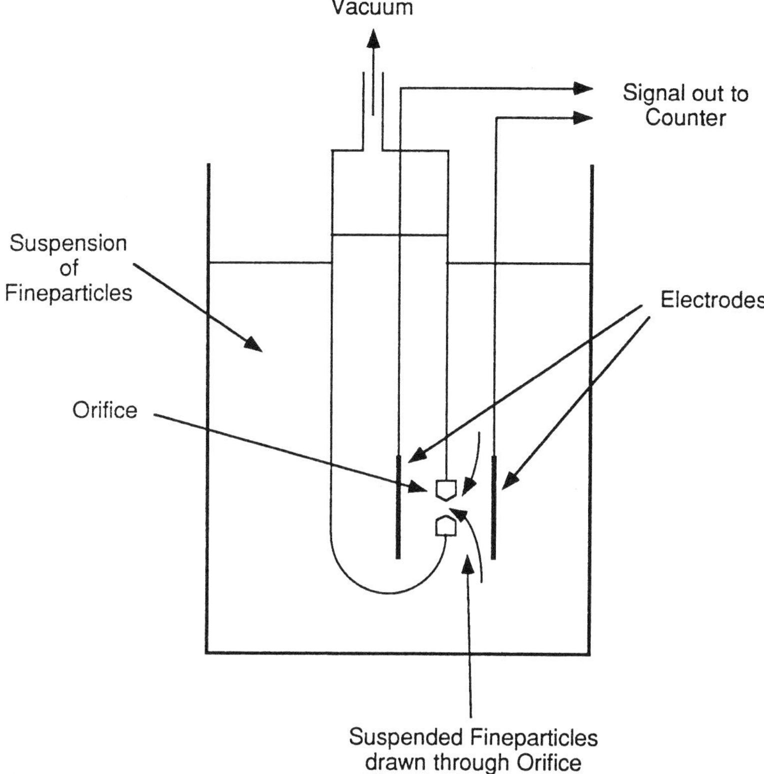

FIG. 11. Schematic diagram of the Coulter counter.

and weighing the amount of powder in each group. The Roller elutriator was widely used in the powder metals industry [1]. In recent years, elutriators have tended to be displaced from common use by diffractometers and other optically based instruments. They are still extremely useful, however, for fractionating powders into different size to study the physical variations of properties with size. Thus, a drug powder can be fractionated into various sizes to study the dependence of the bioavailability of a drug on its particle size. Fig. 12 shows three basic types of elutriators for fractionating powders and studying aerosol fine particles. In the gravity elutriator shown in Fig. 12(a), air or another suitable fluid is passed upward through powder placed on a filter. As the air moves up through the column, the velocity of the moving fluid can be adjusted to move all fine particles below a certain size from the elutriator body to a fines collector which may be a filter or a cyclone. The size limit defining the size of the fine particles remaining in the elutriator is called the cut size of the elutriator. Because it is difficult to control the movement of the fluid and because of turbulence, the cut size and the fractionating power of an elutriator are not precise. A microscope or other suitable device is needed to investigate the actual fractionation of the powder in a given elutriator.

Cyclones are widely used in industry to fractionate powders. The operation of a cyclone, which is in fact a centrifugal elutriator, is shown in Fig. 12(b) [56]. The stream of fluid suspension containing the fine particles to be fractionated enters the top of the cy-

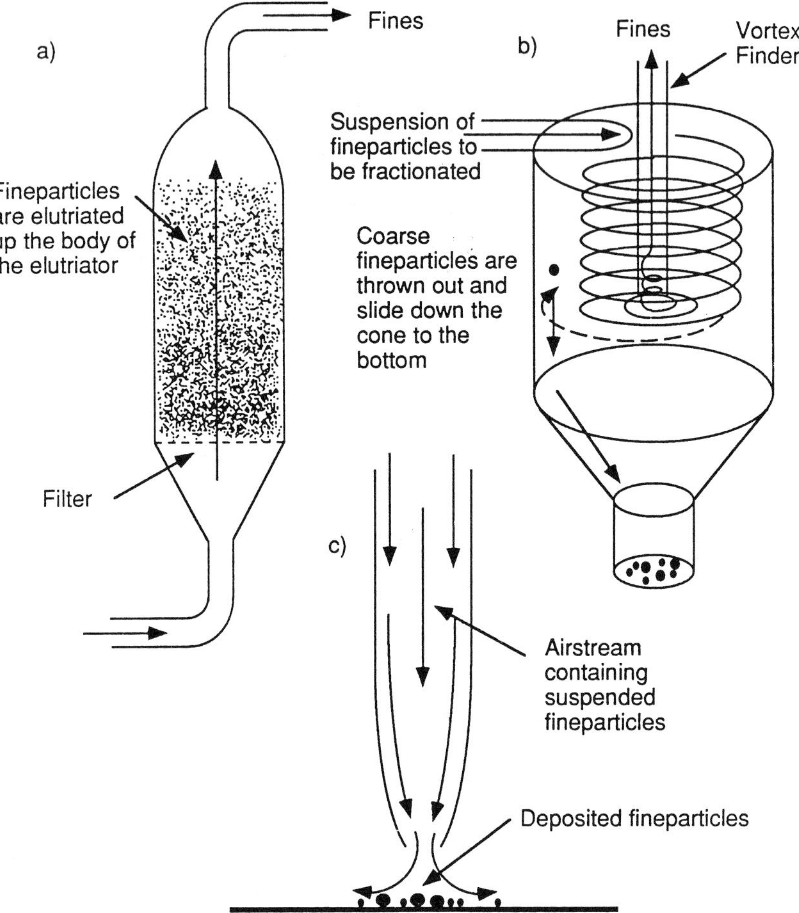

FIG. 12. Elutriators. (a) Gravity elutriator. (b) Cyclone (centrifugal elutriator). (c) Impactor. (From Ref. 1.)

lindrical body tangentially. The fluid stream is made to spiral downward through the body of the cyclone until it can reverse its flow and leave through a pipe known as the vortex finder. As the feed stream spins around the body of the cyclone, the fine particles in suspension are thrown to the wall by centrifugal force. At the wall, the coarser particles fall down into the conical bottom of the cyclone. The cut size of the cyclone, which determines how small the fine particles leaving through the vortex finder are, is determined by the dimensions of the cyclone and the velocity of the fluid stream. Small cyclones are widely used in occupational hygiene studies.

Another device for depositing fine particles from an airstream is the jet impactor, shown in Fig. 12(c). The airstream containing the suspended particles is impinged onto a glass slide. As the airstream is forced to turn because of the slide under the jet, a centrifugal force pushes the suspended fine particles onto the slide. The smallest fine particle, which is just deposited on the slide, is determined by the jet-slide configuration and the speed of the airstream moving through the equipment [1].

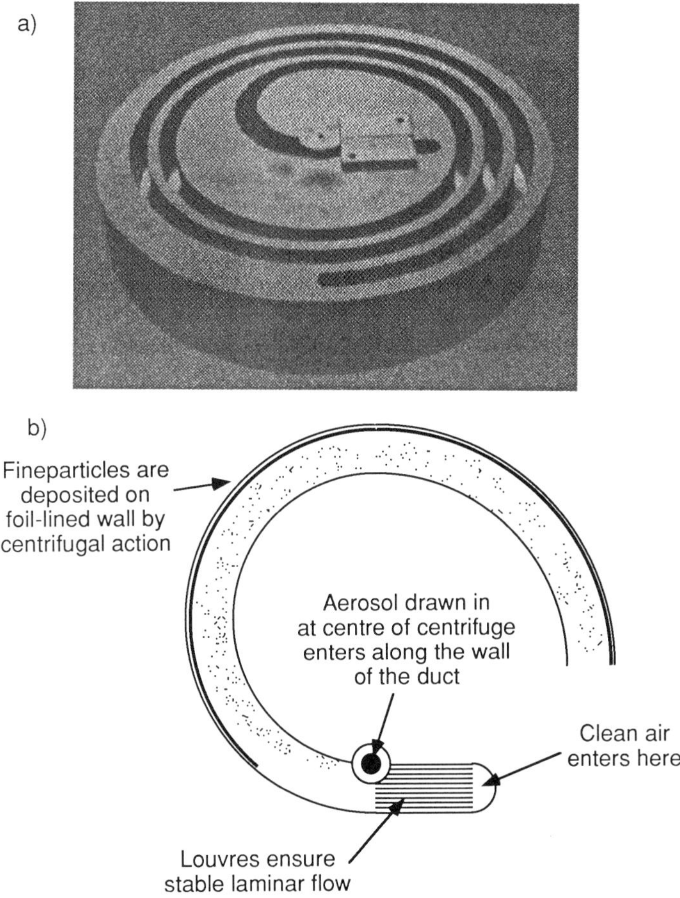

FIG. 13. Cross-flow classifier (elutriator). (a) Fractionation chamber of the spiral duct centrifuge aerosol spectrometer. (b) Schematic diagram of the operating principles of the spiral duct centrifuge developed by Stöber and co-workers. (From Ref. 57.)

In a another type of elutriator, the cross-flow classifier, the particles are made to pass across a moving stream of fluid. In Fig. 13, the equipment for the study of aerosol fine particles, such as those used in therapeutic sprays, is shown. The rotor in Fig. 13(a) is made to spin at high speed. A spray, generated across the central hole (seen in the disk at the center of the rotor), results in a thin stream of aerosol entering along the wall of the spiral duct. The opposite side of the duct is lined with foil, and under the centrifugal action of the rotating disk the fine particles in the airstream move along and across the duct. The rate at which they move across is determined by their size and the centrifugal forces generated by the spinning rotor. Consequently, when the foil is removed from the spiral duct, the aerosol particles have been deposited along the foil in order of their size. The spiral duct centrifuge of Fig. 13 was developed by Stöber and Flachsbart [57]. In an advanced version of the spiral disk centrifuge, piezoelectric devices are placed on the walls of the duct opposite the entry stream and connected to transmitters in the lid of the centrifuge. With this equipment, the rate of particle deposition at certain locations along the duct wall can be telemetered to a distant recording device [1].

Giddings and co-workers have developed a series of cross-flow classifiers known as field-flow fractionation devices [58]. The procedures, often referred to as FFF, are defined by Giddings [58] as:

> . . . a family of high resolution techniques capable of separating and characterizing materials in the macromolecular and colloidal range and beyond. Applications of FFF span a ten- to fifteen-fold mass range, extending from molecules under 1000 molecular weight to particles 100 microns in diameter. Particles as diverse as cells, subcellular particles, viruses, liposomes, protein aggregates, fly ash, waterborne colloids, and industrial latexes and pigments have been separated.

Characterization of Powder Surface Areas

In powder studies, the surface area of the powder is an important parameter. It can be measured directly by means of gas adsorption studies, where the amount of gas or another molecular item, such as dye molecules adsorbed onto the powder to form a monolayer, is determined. Several books have been written describing the theory and procedures for gas adsorption studies. Prior to 1977, it was believed that one of the basic problems with surface area estimates by gas adsorption was that uncertainties in the knowledge of the cross-sectional area of the absorbed molecules made the estimates depend upon the gas being used [59]. In recent years, the gas adsorption studies of surface areas have been reinterpreted from the viewpoint of fractal geometry. It is now recognized that the surface area measured, using a given gas, depends upon the accessibility of the rough surface to the adsorbed molecules as illustrated by Fig. 14(a). In a study of a series of absorbent molecules of increasing size, Avnir and co-workers have shown that the surface area estimates can be plotted against the molecular size to obtain a Richardson plot from which the fractal roughness of the powder surface can be deduced [60,61]; a graph generated by Avnir and co-workers is shown in Fig. 14(b). The slope of its data line can be used to deduce a fractal dimension of the rough surface. The fractal description of powder roughness is an important parameter for the bioavailability of a drug or the chemical reactivity of powder. Neimark has recently described a method for calculating the surface area and roughness of a powder by studying capillary condensation of a liquid on a powder [62].

The fineness of a powder can be studied with the help of permeability techniques, where the resistance to fluid flow of a powder plug is measured, and the fineness of the powder deduced from this measured resistance using various equations such as the Kozeny-Carmen equation. The interpretive equations used to calculate the surface area from permeability measurements make several assumptions concerning the pore structure of the packed powder bed, and the measured surface area from permeability studies should be regarded only as a measure of fineness and not as an absolute measure of surface. Instruments such as the Fisher subsieve sizer and the Blaine fineness tests are permeability-based methods which, in the past, have been widely used in industry and are still often used for quality control by industry. A major advantage of permeability methods is the fact that they use large amounts of powder which minimizes the problems of surface-area measurement [63,64].

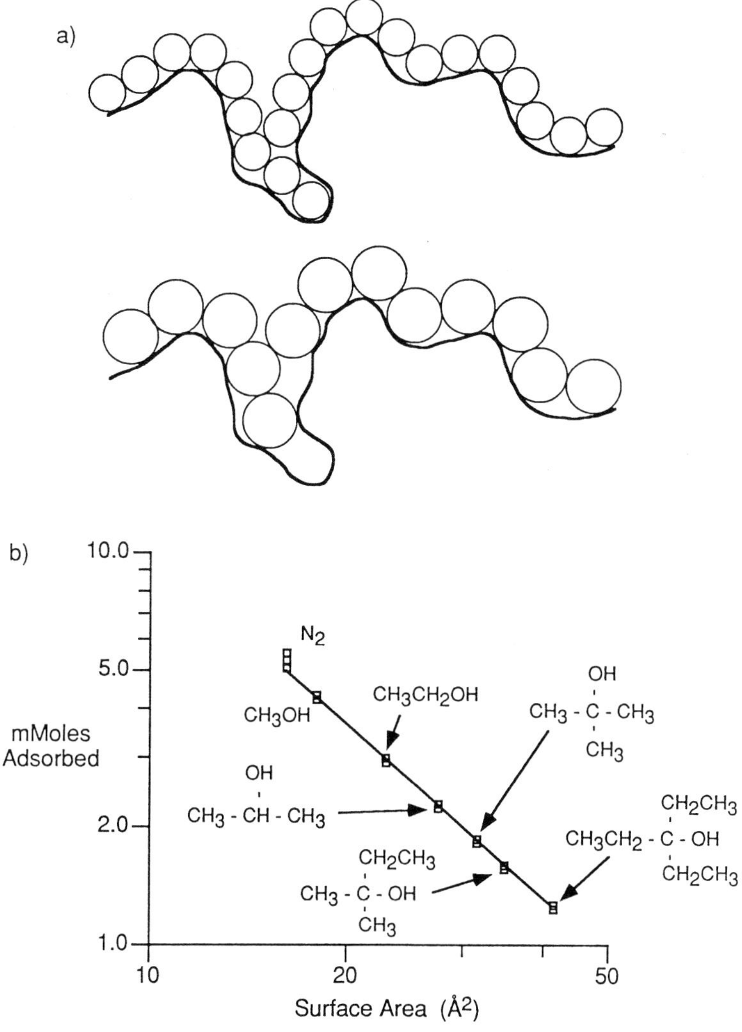

FIG. 14. Gas adsorption data permit the determination of the fractal dimension of a rough surface. (a) The surface is estimated from the number of gas molecules which cover the surface. The estimate depends on the size of the gas molecule. (b) The fractal dimension of a surface is derived from the results of gas adsorption with several differently sized molecules. (From Ref. 60 by permission of Dr. D. Avnir.)

Pore Size-Distribution Measurements

When the pore size of a packed powder bed or of the structure of porous powder grains is of interest, mercury-intrusion studies can be used to investigate the pore structure. Figure 15 shows data of a study using the mercury-intrusion technique to examine the structure of a powder bed of porous grains [65]. The amount of mercury entering a bed at different pressures is used to generate the data. Using the known contact angle of mercury

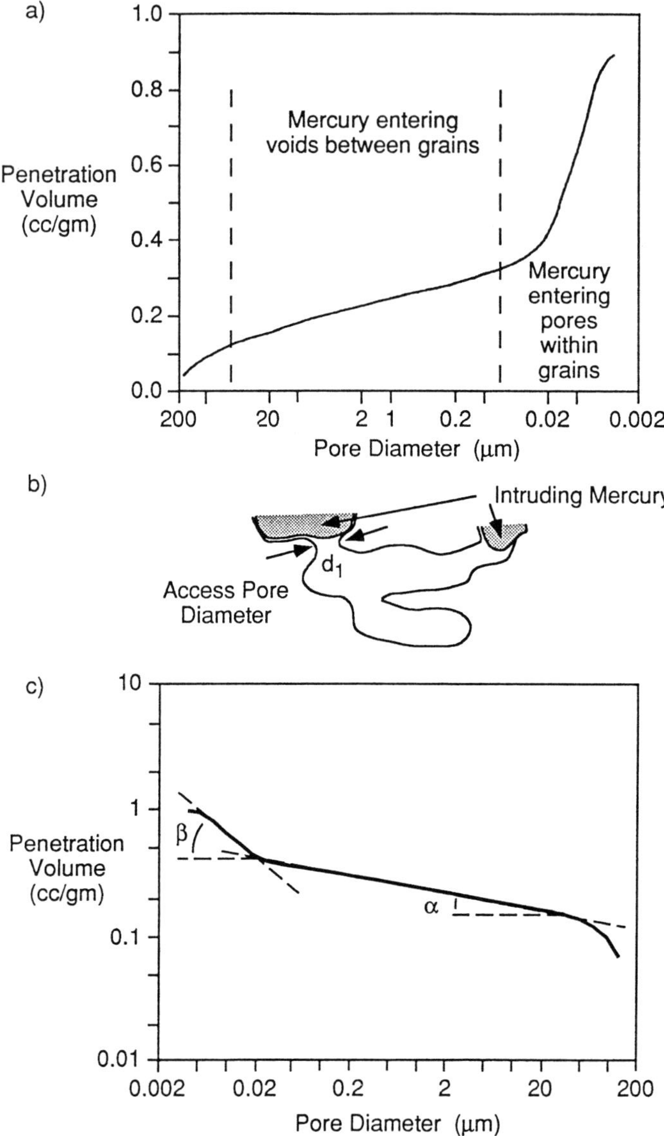

FIG. 15. Mercury intrusion porosimetry. (a) Traditional representation of mercury intrusion data. (b) The physical significance of "bottleneck" theories of mercury intrusion have always been the subject of debate. (c) A possible reinterpretation of the data of (a) as fractal data.

with the material of the powder, the applied pressure can be interpreted in terms of the capillary tube through which mercury moves at that pressure. However, there has always been some controversy as to the physical significance of mercury-intrusion data since it only measures access pore diameter not the size of the pore behind the pore neck. (Theories interpreting mercury-intrusion data in terms of pore diameter are often referred to as ink-bottle interpretive models, the idea being that the pore is the bottle behind the neck

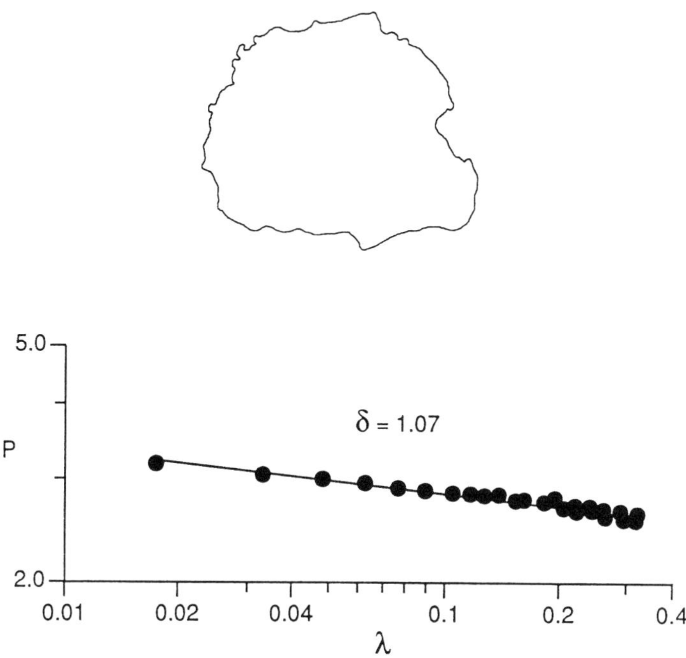

FIG. 16. (a) The fractally structured boundary of a spreading drop. (b) Richardson plot of the boundary of a fluid drop on a tablet of acetaminophen.

of the ink bottle which represents the penetration diameter.) For the data in Fig. 15(a), the mercury is entering the voids between the grains of the powder at low pressures, whereas when a pressure of approximately 13.8 MPa (2,000 psi) is reached, the mercury starts to intrude into pores within the powder grains having access diameters of the order of 0.1 μm. It has recently been shown that the traditional way of presenting mercury-intrusion data can be revised to generate a fractal dimension in data space. The revised data of Fig. 15(a) are shown in Fig. 15(c). The slopes α and β of these diagrams are fractal dimensions in data space [67].

In Fig. 16 a recently suggested technique for studying the pore structure of articles such as drug tablets is illustrated. In this technique, a drop of a suitably colored fluid is placed on a porous pharmaceutical tablet. As the fluid moves outward through the pore structure, a fractal boundary is created which is related to the pore structure of the tablet (Fig. 16(a)). Studies are underway to link the fractal structure of a boundary to the measured pore size distribution of the tablet [66]. The Richardson plot (Fig. 16(b)) of the boundary of the fluid drop on a tablet of commercial acetaminophen shows that the fractal dimension of the boundary of fluid is 1.07.

Standard Reference Powders

Some makers of instruments for characterizing fine particles claim that their instruments are perfect and do not need calibration. Such claims should be treated with skepticism, and in practice many sizing instruments have to be calibrated using standard powders available from several vendors [68,69]. Because the various methods of exploring the size distribution of a powder evaluate different physical parameters, the size distributions of a powder generated by different methods do not always agree. The relationship between distribution functions, as evaluated by different methods, should be explored experimentally. In Fig. 17(a) the empirically established correlation is shown between Blaine

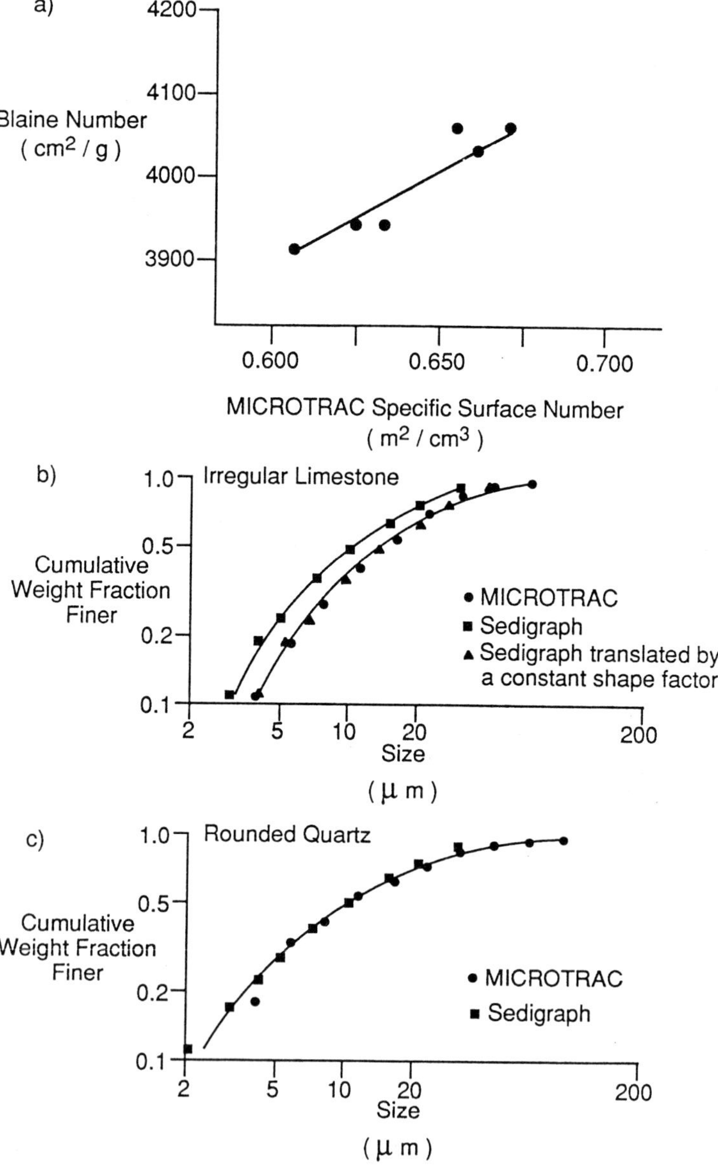

FIG. 17. The size distribution function of a powder measured by different instruments. (a) Empirically established correlation between Blaine fineness number and surface area deduced from diffractometer data. (b) Sometimes a simple correlation factor can link two distribution functions deduced from different size characterization methods. (c) For sperical powder grains, the data generated by different methods usually agree with one another.

numbers (measured in square centimeters per gram and based on permeability methods of characterization) and the surface area of the cement powder, based on data generated by a diffractometer (specifically the Leeds and Northrop MICROTRAC) [41]. Sometimes the correlation can be interpreted as a shape factor. Thus the size characterization of an irregular-shaped limestone powder by the Sedigraph (a Stokes' law-based procedure) and diffractometer data from the MICROTRAC instrument can be correlated (Fig. 17(b)) by a simple factor which is probably related to the shape characteristics of the powder. This interpretation is strengthened by the fact that when the two methods are used to study a powder with basically spherical grains, the two deduced size-distribution functions correlate to a substantial degree [41].

References and Footnotes

1. Kaye, B. H., *Direct Characterization of Fineparticles*, Wiley, New York, 1981. A revised version of this book entitled *Characterizing Powders, Mists, and Fineparticles Systems* is in preparation to be published by VCH in Spring 1995.
2. Kaye, B. H., Efficient sample reduction of powders by means of a riffler sampler, *Soc. Chem. Ind. Monographs.*, 18:159–163 (1964).
3. *British Standards Methods for the Determination of Particle Size Powders*, Part 1, Subdivision of gross sample down to 0.2 mL, BS3406, Part 1, London, 1961.
4. Kaye, B. H., An investigation into the relative efficiency of different sampling procedures, *Powder Met.*, 9:213–234 (1962).
5. Sampling equipment literature is available from Gustafson, 6340 LBJ Freeway, Suite 180, Dallas, TX 75240.
6. Sampling equipment literature is available from Gilson Screen Company, P.O. Box 99, Malinta, OH 43535.
7. Information on the spinning riffler system is available from Microscal Ltd., 20 Mattock Lane, Ealing, London, W5 5BH.
8. For a discussion of the effect of flow agents on the rheology of powders, see Chap. 3, Kaye, B. H., *Powder Mixing*, Chapman & Hall, London (anticipated publication, spring 1995).
9. See discussion of Poisson trackers in Kaye, B. H., *Chaos and Complexity*, VCH Publishers, Weinheim, Germany, 1993. See also appropriate sections in Ref. 8.
10. Plessis, P., and Kaye, B. H., *Powder Sampling from Mixing Chambers*, Rosemont Conference 1991, Cahners Exposition Group, Des Plaines, IL 60018.
11. Kaye, B. H., and Clark, G. G., Evaluating the Performance of Chaotic Powder and Aerosol Sampling Devices Using Tracker Fineparticles, *Nürnberg Conference on Particle Size, May, 1989*. Proceedings published by Nürnberg Messer Centrum.
12. See discussion of powder segregation mechanics in Ref. 8.
13. Isolock samplers are available from Bristol Engineering Company, 204 South Bridge St., Box 696, Yorkville, IL 60560.
14. Nuclepore is the registered trademark of the Costar Corporation, 7035 Commerce Circle, Pleasanton, CA 94566. Comprehensive literature on the structure and properties of Nuclepore filters is available from the manufacturer who kindly provided the photograph reproduced in Fig. 2(a).
15. Gelman Science., Ann Arbor, MI.
16. The Poretics Corporation, 151 Lindbergh Avenue, Livermore, CA.
17. Collimated Holes Incorporated, 460 Division St., Campbell, CA 95008.
18. Allen, T., Application of precision transparent sieves to the determination of low number concentrations of oversized particles in powders, *Part. Part. Syst. Charact.*, 9:252–258 (1992).

19. Parfitt, G. D., *Dispersion of Powders in Liquids*, 2nd ed., Wiley, New York, 1973.
20. Heywood, H. H., Size and Shape Distribution of Lunar Fines, Sample, 12057, 72. In: *Proceedings of Second Lunar Science Conference*, Vol. 13, 1971, pp. 1989–2001; see also Ref. 1.
21. Hausner, H. H., Characterization of the Powder Particle Shape. In: *Proceedings of the Symposium on Particle Size Analysis, Loughborough, England, 1967*. Published by the Society for Analytical Chemistry, London, 1967, pp. 20–27; see also discussion in Ref. 1.
22. See discussion in Refs. 1 and 23.
23. Allen, T., *Particle Size Analysis*, 4th ed., Chapman and Hall, London, 1992.
24. See discussion of the use of Fourier techniques to characterize the shape of profiles in Chap. 15 of Ref. 25.
25. Kaye, B. H., *Chaos and Complexity, Discovering the Surprising Patterns of Science and Technology*, VCH, Weinheim Germany, 1993.
26. Kaye, B. H., *A Randomwalk through Fractal Dimensions*, VCH, Weinheim, Germany, 1989.
27. Mandelbrot, B. B., *Fractals: Form, Chance, and Dimension*, Freeman, San Francisco, 1977.
28. See Chap. 15 of Ref. 25, Kaye, B. H., Applied fractal geometry and the fineparticle specialist, Part 1, *Part. Part. Syst. Charact.*, 10 (3):99–110 (1993).
29. Schaeffer, D. W., Fractal models and the structure of materials matter, *Res. Soc. Bull.*, 13: 22–27 (1988).
30. Kaye, B. H., Multi-fractal description of a rugged fineparticle profile, *Part. Part. Syst. Charact.*, 1:14–21 (1984).
31. Kaye, B. H., and Yousufzai, M. A. K., Calibrating and monitoring woven wire sieving surfaces, *Powder Bulk Solids*, 1992 (Jan.):29–34.
32. Provder, T. ed., *Particle Size Analysis*, ACS Symposium Series 332, American Chemical Society, Washington, 1987.
33. *Sieves Sieving and other Sizing Methods*. Draft of standard *Determination of Particle Size Distribution, Laser Diffraction Methods*. Some of the classical sedimentation equipment as well as other sizing equipment is available from Gilson Company Inc., P.O. Box 677, Worthington, OH 43085-0677.
34. CILAS U.S.A. Agents Denver Autometrics, Inc., 6235 Lookout Road, Bolder, CO 80301. Company headquarters in France, Osi 47, Rue de Javel, 75015 Paris.
35. Sympatec Inc. Princeton Service Center, 34890 U.S. Route 1, Princeton, NJ 08540-5706.
36. Kaye, B. H., Dangers of curve fitting in the deduction of size distribution from diffraction data, *Proceedings of the Powder and Bulk Solids Conference, Rosemont, IL, May 6–9, 1991*.
37. See trade literature of Shimatzu Scientific Instruments Incorporated, 7102 Riverwood Drive, Columbia, MD 21046.
38. Holve, D. J., Using ensemble diffraction to measure particle size distribution, *Powder Bulk Eng.*, 1991 (June):15–19; see also trade literature of INSITEC, 2110 Omega Road, Suite D, San Ramon, CA 94583.
39. See trade literature of Coulter Counter Electronics, 590 West 20th St., Hialeah, FL 33010.
40. Malvern Instruments Incorporated, 10 Southview Rd., Southborough, MA 01772.
41. MICROTRAC System manufactured by Leeds and Northrop Instruments, 3000 Old Roosevelt Blvd., St. Petersburg, FL 33702.
42. Technical literature available from Galai Production Limited, Industrial zone, 10500 Migdal, Haemek, Israel.
43. LASENTECH is available from Laser Sensor Technology Inc., P.O. Box 3912, Belleview, WA 98009.
44. Amherst Process Instruments Inc., Mountain Farms Mall, Hadley, MA 01035.
45. TSI Inc., 2500 Cleveland Avenue, N, St. Paul, MI 55113.
46. Dantech Corporation, 777 Corporate Drive, Mahwah, NJ 07430.
47. Weiner, B. B. In: *Modern Methods of Particle Sizing* (H. Barth, ed.), Wiley-Interscience, New York, 1984, Chap. 3. See also Ref. 32.
48. See technical literature of Brookhaven Instruments Corporation, Brookhaven Corporate Park, 750 Bluepoint Road, Holtsville, NY 11742.

49. Nicoli, D. F., Wu, J. S., Chang, Y. J., McKenzie, D. C., and Hasapidis, K., Automatic high resolution particle size analysis by single particle optical sensing, *Am. Lab.*, 1992, (July):39.

50. Halbert, M. K., Mazumder, M. K., and Baum, R. L., Respirable particulates in household aerosols, *Environ. Res.*, 1981: 105–109. See also review article in KONA, 1993. KONA is produced by the Hosokawa Micron Corporation which market the SPART analyzer; literature is available from Micron Powder Systems (a member of the Hosokawa group), 10 Chatham Rd., Summit, NJ 07901. (The term SPART analyzer stands for single particle aerodynamic relaxation time analyzer.)

51. Information on the Coulter counter is available from Coulter Electronics, Inc., 590 West 20th St., Hialeah, FL 33010.

52. Information on the Electrozone counter is available from Particle Data, Inc., P.O. Box 265, Elmhurst, IL 60126.

53. An optical stream counter is available from the Climet Corporation, 1320 Colton Avenue, Redlands, CA 92373.

54. Royco instruments for studying aerosols and fineparticles in liquids are available from Royco Instruments, Inc., 141 Jefferson Drive, Menlo Park, CA 94025.

55. The widely used stream counter for fineparticles in fluid is the HIAC counter, HIAC Instruments Division, P.O. Box 3007, 4719 West Brooke St., Monte Claire, CA 91763.

56. Humann, W. L., Cyclone separators, a family affair, *Chem. Eng.*, 1991 (June):118–123.

57. Stöber, W., and Flachsbart, H., *Environ. Sci. Technol.*, 3:1280 (1969).

58. Giddings, J., Field flow fractionation, *Chem.* & *Eng.* News, 1988 (Oct. 10): 34. See also review in KONA 1991 (Ref. 50). For information on field flow fractionation reserach development and industrial applications, contact Field Flow Fractionation Research Center, Department of Chemistry, University of Utah, Salt Lake City, UT 84112.

59. See discussion of gas adsorption methods in Ref. 23.

60. See review of Avnir's work in Takayasu, H., *Fractals in the Physical Sciences*, John Wiley & Sons, New York, 1990.

61. The reinterpretation of gas absorption data from a fractal geometry perspective is discussed extensively in D. Avnir, ed., *Fractal Approach to Heterogeneous Chemistry*, John Wiley & Sons, London, 1989.

62. Neimark, A. V. Calculating surface fractal dimensions of absorbents, *Adsorp. Sci. Technol.* 7(4): 210–216 (1990); Neimark, A. V., Percolation theory of capillary hysteresis phenomena and its application for characterization of porous solids. *Characterization of Solids, II* In: (F. Rodrigues - Reinoso, et al., eds.), Elsevier Science Publishers, Amsterdam, 1991, pp. 67–75.

63. Kaye, B. H., Permeability techniques for characterizing fine powders, *Powder Technol.*, 1: 11–22 (1967).

64. Kaye, B. H., and Legault, P. E., Real-time permeability for the monitoring of fineparticle systems, *Powder Technol.*, 23:179–186 (1973).

65. Orr, C., Application of mercury penetration in material analysis, *Powder Technol.*, 3: 117–123 (1969–1970).

66. Kaye, B. H., Applied fractal geometry and the fineparticle specialist: Part 1, Rugged boundaries and rough surfaces, *Part. Part. Syst. Charact.*, 10 (3):99–110 (1993).

67. Kaye, B. H., Fractal dimensions in data space; new descriptors for fineparticle systems, *Part. Part. Syst. Charact.*, 101:191–200 (1994).

68. Standard powders are available from Duke Scientific Corporation, 135D San Antonio Rd. Palo Alto, CA 94303.

69. Calibration fineparticles are available from Dyno Particles A. S., P.O. Box 160N-2001, Lillestrom, Norway.

BRIAN H. KAYE

Particulate Matter in Parenteral Products

Introduction

Over the past 30 years, foreign particulate matter introduced into the body through a pharmaceutical product has been the subject of a great deal of debate, much of it emotional and, frankly, some of it ill informed. More recently, two books have appeared on the subject that provide some objectivity to the debate [1,2]. Nevertheless, like so many other controversies, opinions differ according to the individual standpoint. A medical practitioner, for example, might take the view that foreign particulate matter is unacceptable contamination in a product used to save, not complicate, a patient's life. A producer, on the other hand, will point out that it is impossible to remove every vestige of foreign matter, and that there is no objective evidence about the hazard to the patient, at levels currently accepted in the industry as being realistic, without significantly increasing the cost of the product. Caught in between these two extremes is the individual in the regulatory area who knows (or should know) that to demand no particulate "contamination" is unrealistic in the sense that no product could be made to this degree of perfection, but who also appreciates that the industry does need to make products that are suitable for use by current standards. It might be pointed out that the consumer, unaware of this debate for the most part, demands to have a product that is of the highest quality at the lowest cost possible.

The purpose of this article is to draw attention to some of the issues in this ongoing debate and to attempt to provide some objectivity to a subject that has occasionally provided "more heat than light." See also the articles Parenterals: Large Volume and Parenterals: Small Volume in this volume of this encyclopedia.

Definitions

Particulate Matter is defined in Chapter ⟨788⟩ of the *United States Pharmacopeia XXIII* (USP), as " . . . extraneous, mobile, undissolved substances, other than gas bubbles, unintentionally present in parenteral solutions." In addition, injectable solutions are required to be " . . . essentially free from particles that can be observed on visual inspection."

These definitions, important for understanding the compendial language, actually provide some problems of their own. For example, extraneous simply means that the undissolved substance is a foreign material, presumably not declared on the label of the product, which does not belong in the product. This has allowed some authors to use the loaded term contamination which, as demonstrated later, is inappropriate in the context of most pharmaceutical products. The word mobile infers that the particles are capable of moving around inside the product. Unfortunately, there are examples that are not difficult to find in which the particles are capable of sticking to the container surface or, in the case of plasticizer droplets, actually become resorbed by the plastic container wall, only to become mobile again when the container is agitated or flexed.

The USP mentions that gas bubbles are excluded from consideration. Since there are only three states of matter, this infers that the remaining substances are comprised of either solid or liquid, without exception. Some authors, again, have attempted to suggest that oily plasticizer droplets are not "particulate matter," which, of course, is not true.

Of some importance is also the term unintentionally since it should be evident that a manufacturer would not intentionally add material to a products without declaring it on the label. The USP does not, however, infer that such material is inevitably present although, as observed earlier, this is the situation in a real world.

A definition of particulate matter was suggested [1] as: unwanted, mobile, insoluble matter, inevitably and inadvertently present in the product. Here "unwanted" carries the same implication as "unintentionally," whereas "inevitably and inadvertently" emphasizes the point that it is virtually impossible to eliminate all foreign particles from a product.

The real issues become evident when the USP phrase "essentially free from particles that can be observed on visual inspection" is examined. There is a fundamental problem in deciding what "essentially free" means and this has not been satisfactorily resolved to date. Visual inspection, as discussed later, is a probalistic procedure in which the observer stands a chance of detecting the particle or not. The other question, related to this one, is the definition of particle. Common dictionary definitions of the term are different [3] but seem to infer, overall, that a particle is just visible to the naked or unaided eye. This leads to the other question of what is just visible to the eye. Again, there is a literature on this subject but, for the sake of discussion at this point, it may be assumed that a single discrete particulate entity with a diameter of between 50 to 100 μm is just about at the edge of visual acuity. Thus, in a discussion of particulate matter, it has to be presumed that there are two basic regions based on a consideration of their particle size or diameter: one region in which the particles are larger than those detected at the edge of visual acuity, and the other where the particles are so small as to require instrumental detection and quantitation. Characteristically, the particles larger than, say, 100 μm, are relatively few in number when considered in terms of the volume of the container as a whole; they only stand a chance of being detected visually. The smaller particles increase in number per unit volume as the particle size decreases, and it is possible to measure a particle size distribution if the analyst uses an appropriate instrument to detect and, more to the point, count the particles as a function of size.

Origins

Particulate matter found in injection solutions can be categorized as intrinsic or extrinsic. Intrinsic materials are due to inherent properties of the solution or its container, such as precipitates formed between components of the ingredients of the formulation or between interactions of the materials constituting the container wall and the solution. An example of the former type of reaction would be the formation of insoluble sodium or magnesium acid phosphates from phosphate buffer solutions. The second type of reaction is exemplified by the formation of glass spicules from soda-glass containers holding citrates. A newer type of intrinsic particulate matter has recently appeared with some of the biotechnological products. Some proteins, such as somatotropins, are exquisitely sensitive to shear produced by shaking. A reconstituted somatotropin solution therefore precipitates out when a vial containing it is shaken too vigorously.

Extrinsic particulate matter can be thought of as matter that drops into the solution from various sources during its preparation, processing, or filling. In the main, this material comes from various surfaces with which the solution comes into contact. Here examples would be iron oxides formed in stainless steel tubing, glands, or packing materials that shed during pumping operations, and lubricating oils. The container components probably represent the principal source of particulate matter under the control of the manufacturer. Inadequately cleaned containers are an obvious source of insoluble materials but the elastomeric stoppers are commonly associated with significant levels of particulate matter. Elastomers are usually filled with insoluble materials to obtain the necessary physical properties required to perform their function as a sealant. Surface abrasion during cleaning and transport often generates particles of the elastomer itself or of the filler. Some additives, such as antioxidants incorporated in elastomers in order to enhance chemical stability, may produce insoluble reaction products with solution components. Phosphates are a source of intrinsic particulate matter, and phosphate buffers can precipitate aluminum, magnesium, or calcium salts, reacting with otherwise soluble ions extracted on storage from the glass wall or even the stopper. Plastic containers have their own formulation problems. For example, polyvinyl chloride (PVC) sheets used to prepare plastic bags widely employed for intravenous solutions contain as much as 30% by weight of plasticizers, such as dioctylphthalate, which are insoluble oils. These oils can be liberated into the bag contents as droplets which constitute particulate matter that is introduced into the veins of the patient. As noted earlier, an aqueous solution presents the possibility that the hydrophobic oil used as a plasticizer for PVC sheeting is present in the product in the form of droplets that can be resorbed into the PVC wall. However, when used to store blood or blood products, the oil tends to remain within the bag, and the plasticizer itself is administered to the patient in relatively large quantities associated with some of the more hydrophobic elements in the blood.

Another source of oily droplets is silicone oil used as lubricant to help the insertion of closures into the container. Technically these oils are extremely effective but if used incorrectly, the excess oil can become emulsified in the product and is undoubtably administered to the patient. If the product itself is lyophilized the oil can become closely associated with the particles or aggregates in the dried powder, making them hydrophobic and difficult to redissolve on reconstitution.

Since the sources of insoluble particulate matter are various, the chemical and physical nature of the particles themselves is widely different. Table 1 gives sizes of extraneous particulate matter found in parenteral solutions.

Among the best "hands-on" account of particulate matter sources is the review by Borchert et al. from Upjohn [4]. They observe that the volume and depth of the literature on particulate matter in parenteral products attest to the commitment of the pharmaceutical industry to address this complex issue. From an outsider's perspective, this point must be considered to be basically correct, although there is a certain self-congratulatory element about it. Another point made by these authors is the importance of applying a scientific approach to the resolution of problems in this area, and this is also true from a number of perspectives. However, without concerns being expressed by consumers, compendia, and regulatory authorities at various times, it is doubtful if the demonstrable progress made over the past 30 years would have been so evident. Formerly, the attitude

TABLE 1 Approximate Sizes of Extraneous Particulate Matter Found in Parenteral Solutions[a]

Material	Approximate Diameter (μm)
Clay	<1
Kaolin	<1
Mineral oil	<1
Talc	<1
Titanium dioxide	<1
Viruses	<1
Ultramarine	1
Carbon black	>1
Crystalline materials[b]	>1
Glass fragments	>1
Metal fragments	>1
Iron oxide	>1
Starch	<2
Stearic acid	<5
Diatoms	1–5
Asbestos fibrils	1–10
Barium sulfate	<10
Magnesium oxide	<10
Magnesium stearate	<10
Phthalates	<10
Silicone oils	<10
Sulfur	<10
Vegetable oils	<10
Whiting (chalk)	<10
Zinc oxide	<10
Trichomes	>10
Bacteria, bacterial spores	2–20
Fungi and fungal spores	20–50
Cellulose fibers and fragments	1–100
Bentonite	10–100
Paraffin wax	10–100
Sand	>100
Plastic fragments	1–500
Rubber fragments	1–500
Human skin flakes	10–10,000
Miscellaneous biological debris	10–10,000
Insect parts	20–10,000

[a]Reported by various authors.
[b]Antioxidants, additives.

among producers seemed to be "if you cannot see it, it does not exist!" There has indeed been considerable progress in the intervening years.

Detection

The detection and subsequent counting or measurement of subvisible (<100 μm) or visible particles suspended in a drug solution are two separate processes.

Visual Inspection

If a solution has been passed through a sequence of filters in a properly controlled production process, very few particles per unit volume of solution are left in the product visible to the unaided eye. Any particles remaining in the product that are larger than the pore size of the filters could be considered to be inadvertent particulate, even contamination, since they probably originated in the atmosphere or surrounding environment before the container was sealed. In addition, some particles may have been detached from the filling or pumping equipment used in the processing. There is only a slim chance of the particles being detected on inspection because this whole process is, by its very nature, a chance or random process, usually termed probalistic. Clearly, the chance of detecting a particle increases or decreases with its size. The laws of chance have been explored carefully for much of the past century, but the relationship between detection and particle size has received serious attention only over the past few decades. As noted later, the compendia tended not to recognize this fact, since most simply state that the product passes or fails the inspection process, apparently not realizing that in this area, as in so many others, there are gradations.

The problem is partly due to the fallability of human inspectors. These are for the most part filling-line operators who have been chosen for their visual acuity and are often poorly qualified, although careful selection and training are required for their task [1]. However, even under optimal conditions, human factors that influence the inspection process include [5] actual visual acuity, aptitude, fatigue, environment, intensity of illumination, and inspection speed.

Visual acuity is of utmost importance, with the operator or inspector wearing any visual aid necessary.

Aptitude for inspection can be determined by appropriate tests during the selection process. Godding [6] suggested that a simple test of behavior while reading two long paragraphs of small print was adequate to determine if the candidate had the appropriate psychological profile for the task. In a developing country this test may not be entirely appropriate since it is unlikely that the candidate would have sufficient reading skills.

The major issue appears to be fatigue. It is essential that the inspectors be able to concentrate on their task which becomes very difficult after a while. For young girls to be on inspection duty for a complete 8-h shift is unacceptable, and happens today only rarely. It is far better for operators to rotate from inspection duties to some other task for periods under an hour, with at least another 2 h in between sessions in the inspection booth. No matter how dedicated the personnel is to the task, it is inevitable that detection levels vary over any given time frame. It is therefore important to minimize the variability of the results by improving the working conditions for the inspectors. This includes lighting levels both inside and outside of the inspection booth, low background noise, and controlled environmental temperature and humidity. Disturbances in the familiar work routine can cause loss of concentration. Therefore visitors to the immediate area should be discouraged or only allowed to observe through a glass window or, better, a one-way mirror. Individual factors such as mood, boredom induced by fatigue, or lack of interest also need to be considered in the management of the inspection system.

Another issue is the rate at which products are passed to the inspector. Rates of 5 pieces per minute for 20 mL ampules and three pieces per minute for 50 mL ampules have been suggested as optimal [7], but higher rates have been used in some plants, which would put their effectiveness in serious doubt. The Parenteral Drug Association's

(PDA) guidelines for visual inspection procedures [7] are helpful but do not pay sufficient attention to the human factors involved.

From a manufacturer's perspective, the final inspection process becomes a final safety product check and is therefore critical to the whole production process. There is a need to appreciate that inspectors are, above all, human and frail. They need to be treated with respect, and all precautions have to be taken in order to optimize their performance.

Improving the Chances of Visual Detection

The chances of detecting visible particulate matter can be improved by close attention to the conditions under which the inspection process is carried out. The PDA guidelines [7] are helpful in this respect. Saylor [8] suggested that individual inspectors must be seated and provided with their own inspection booth or work station, minimizing the opportunity to disturb them. Perhaps the best and most detailed description of the inspection process is given in *USP XIII* (1947). It still provides an excellent basis for a standard operating procedure designed today, and is worth quoting in full:

> A suitable device for observing the clarity of parenteral solutions may be provided by placing a ''gooseneck'' desk lamp in front of a vertical screen. The screen, covered with a black or white surface fore the detection of light or dark-colored particles, has a dull or ''flat'' finish, to reduce reflection to a minimum. The desk lamp is provided with a parabolic hemispherical shade, preferably lined in frosted white to prevent reflection of images. The front of the reflector is tilted downward slightly to protect the observer's eyes from direct illumination. With such a lamp the source of light is a 100-Watt, inside-frosted, incandescent bulb operated at rated voltage. Approximately the same intensity of illumination is given by three 15-Watt fluorescent lamps. The intensity of illumination, determined with a light meter, at a distance of 10 in. [25 cm] from the source, is not less than 100 and not more than 350 foot candles [3.76 Mlux].
>
> For examination the surface of the ampoule or other container of a parenteral solution shall be free from attached labels and thoroughly cleaned. Holding the container by the neck, slowly invert it to prevent the formation of fine air bubbles and twirl it slightly to rotate the liquid therein. Then hold the container horizontally about 4 in. [10 cm] below the front edge of the light source and examine the contents against the white and against the black backgrounds. Preferably make the examination in subdued light or in a dark room to eliminate extraneous light from the walls of the container.

Knapp [9] reviewed the literature on the subject of particle detection and summarized the essential elements of the process as

- The capability of the viewer
- The size of the target
- The total background illumination, and
- The contrast of the target or particle against the viewing background

Viewing condition can be improved by utilizing the appropriate design of the inspection booth, according to Knapp's concepts, shown in Figs. 1 and 2. Essentially based on the earlier USP XIII description, this design is more modern, and two 20-Watt fluores-

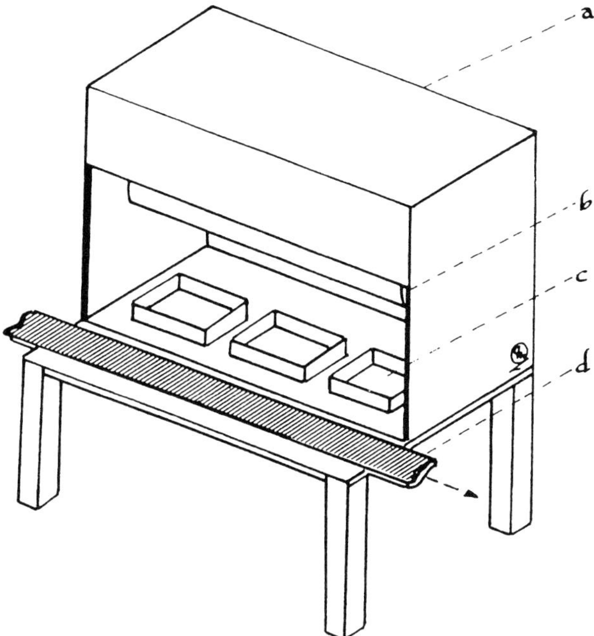

FIG. 1. Inspection booth. Key: a = backboard of booth painted half black and half white (vertically); b = two-tube strip light; c = baskets or boxes to collect rejects, organized according to white floaters, black floaters, bad seals, etc.; d = conveyor belt, foot activated by the operator to bring material into and out of the inspection area (moves in opposite direction for left-handed operators who would be located at the back of this booth, in a mirror-image). (According to concepts advocated by Knapp [9].)

cent lamps are used together to suppress the inherent flicking of a single tube which can be a source of operator fatigue. In addition, automatic or semi-automatic product feeding can be incorporated into the system.

Devices to Enhance Viewing

The inspection booth in its present manifestation is probably optimally designed and located in the plant. Nevertheless, issues of detection certainty remain, and furthermore the speed of operation is reduced. Devices, ranging from very simple to extremely complex, have been proposed to improve the inspection process. Perhaps the simplest of these was the bottle-inspection device [6], shown in Fig. 3. It is likely that it would allow for the detection of colloidal particles and turbidities due to precipitates. Unfortunately, since it is loaded manually, it would be slow to operate. However, a device like this could still be helpful at the patients' bedside, where it could be used to inspect a parenteral solution prior to administration. A modern device, the Allen Viewer is probably more convenient for this purpose [1,2]. It consists of a magnifying lens covered by a polarizing material. The container is held behind the lens against a polarizing screen in front of a light source. Effectively the bottle is viewed in polarized light which allows anisotropic materials such as cellulose particles, at one time a common contaminant in parenteral solutions, to be readily detected against a black background.

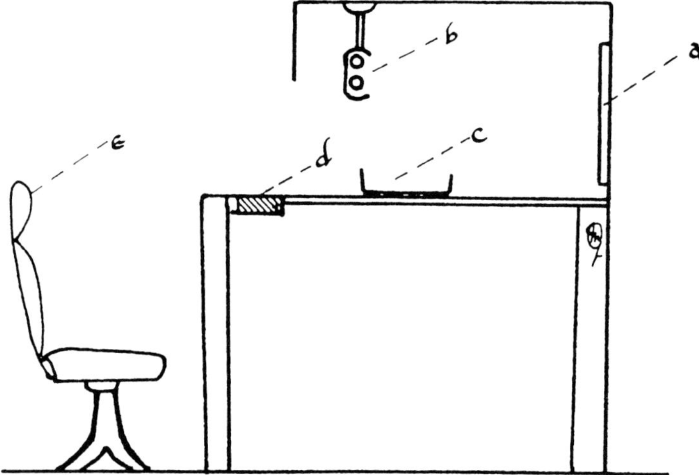

FIG. 2. Cross-section of inspection booth. Key: a = black and white backboard; b = two-tube strip light; c = collection baskets or boxes for rejects; d = conveyor belt, e = laboratory chair (must be comfortable and adjustable).

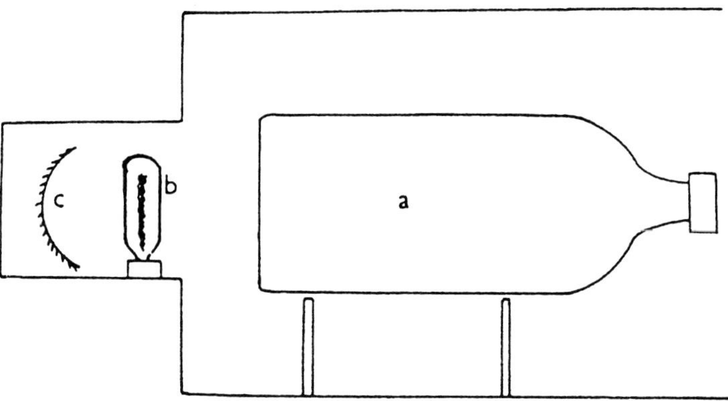

FIG. 3. Bottle-inspection device. Key: a = bottle being viewed normally to beam of light; b = lamp; c = parabolic focusing mirror. The background is painted matte black and the viewer is shielded from direct light by screens.

Manufacturers of equipment used to fill, seal, and inspect parenteral products have made various attempts to automate the inspection process. In one version, the container passes the inspector who makes a decision about whether or not to pass it. Although appreciably faster, this device still depends critically upon the human inspector for a decision, with all of the attendant concerns about accuracy and sensitivity noted above. A serious attempt to overcome these problems can be seen in the various automatic inspection machines (AIMs) marketed by the Eisai Company (Figs. 4–6). These machines take advantage of the latest advances in computers and light-detection systems. Fiber optics are used to bring light to the spinning ampules, and light scattered by any particles in the system is collected by fiber optic bundles and carried to charged coupling devices or sil-

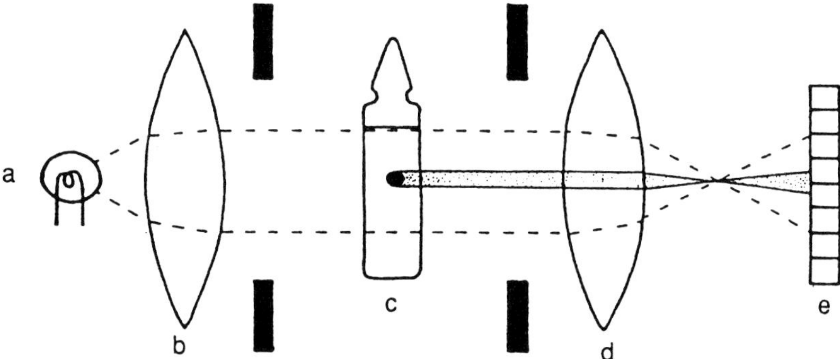

FIG. 4. Eisai Automatic Inspection Machine (AIM). Key: a = lamp; b = focusing lens; c = ampule after spinning; d = collecting lens onto fiber optic array; e = diode array.

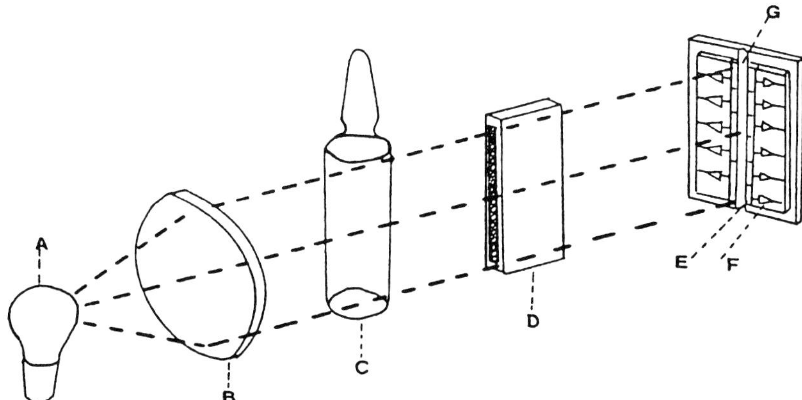

FIG. 5. Detection system of the Eisai Automatic Inspection Machine. Key: A = white light lamp; B = focusing lens; C = spinning ampule held in beam and locked in position so that only solution spins; D = collimating lens (a parallel fiber optic array); E = silicon photodiodes, detecting moving shadow of particles; F = amplifier; G = slit to fixed width of light beam. (Adapted from Eisai promotional material, with permission.)

icon photodiodes. Effectively the moving shadows due to particles are digitized. In one device these can be used to examine the profile of the ampule for imperfect seals, flattened edges, bulges, or other imperfections and the presence of carbonized fragments, all at an amazing rate of up to 18,000 ampules per hour. Inspection devices for particles are similar, with a consistency and a speed that could not be matched by human operators. These devices have the advantage that they provide objective evidence of the particulate matter levels in a batch which otherwise is not feasible. In part because of their sophistication, these devices require expensive capital investment not justified for the small product runs that are a general feature of the pharmaceutical industry (obviously, there are some exceptions). The devices have been validated using ampules repeatedly inspected by human inspectors [10], but some questions about what is actually detected remain unanswered at present. There is little information on the limits of size detection in terms of the particle size threshold and the numbers of particles at those thresholds.

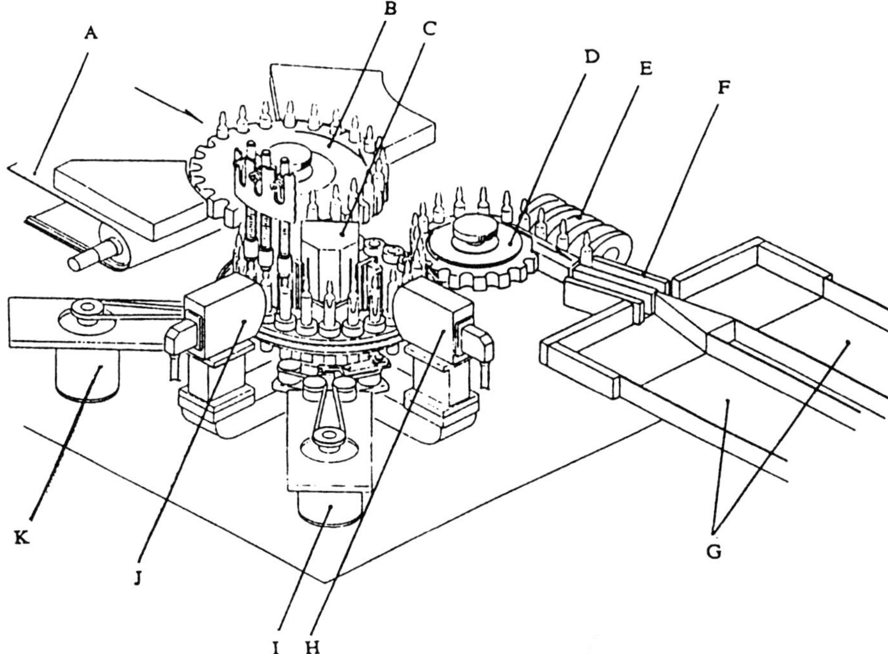

FIG. 6. The conveyance mechanism for the Eisai Automatic Inspection Machine. The ampules (or other containers) are moved by the starwheel onto the slowly rotating inspection table and spun three times before inspecting twice for foreign particulate matter and once for fill volume. Key: A = feed belt; B = infeed starwheel; C = SD head containing the photodiode detectors; D = discharge starwheel; E = screw conveyor; F = sorting pendulum; G = collection hopper; H = light projector; I = spinning motor; J = light projector; K = spinning motor. (Adapted from Eisai promotional material, with permission.)

The devices are therefore being used in a comparative fashion: ''is this lot as good as the standard lot?'' In terms of quality, this is a legitimate question and a valid way of carrying out inspections.

Instrumental Detection and Measurement of Particulate Matter

The basic problem of detecting random particulate matter in injection solutions is due to the fact that the quantities involved are very small and that the chances of detection vary for many of the reasons noted above. When the particle size decreases to the point where they are difficult to see with the unaided eye ($<100\ \mu m$), the numbers per unit volume are increasing to the point where they are detectable by instruments. Scientifically, if an instrument can detect a particle, it should be capable of determining the count per unit volume. It is the measurement of the number of particles in a system that remains the key issue. Various instrumental methods have been available to the analyst for the past 30 years. However, not all instruments are equally sensitive or useful, and not all instruments are capable of making accurate measurements in a system where there are only a few particles per unit volume. As the particles in a parenteral system decrease in size from the visible region ($>100\ \mu m$) to the colloidal region ($<1\ \mu m$), the numbers per unit volume increase exponentially. There is a questionable interim size range, in which a tran-

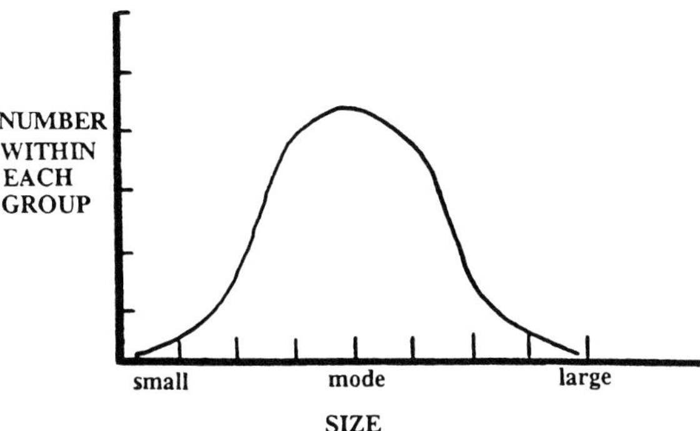

FIG. 7. Gaussian distribution relating number of particles and their size from the smallest to the largest.

sition exists from a probalistic detection principle to a point where there is a reasonable certainty that the instrument will, indeed, detect and count particles with the required accuracy and precision. Under the latter circumstances, an instrument can be used to determine if there is a relationship between the size and number of particles per unit volume. If there is, this relationship can be used to make other measurements and predictions about the nature of the distribution.

Size distribution of a particulate suspension consisting of just one species of particles implies that there are small and large particles in the system, with a continuum between the two extremes of size that is frequently represented by the familiar Gaussian distribution (Fig. 7). As it stands, this distribution is a differential which, by integrating, can be converted into an integral or cumulative distribution (Fig. 8). As shown in Fig. 8, the differential distribution is asymmetric or skewed to the left, suggesting many more small particles in the system than large ones. This, in fact, is the situation in a parenteral solution since, as noted earlier, there is an exponential increase in the number of particles as the size is decreased. This implies a logarithmic relationship between the size and number and, generally, if the differential distribution shown in Fig. 8 is plotted as the logarithm of size, there is a tendency for this skewdness to be straightened out, and the plot resembles the one in Fig. 7, a Poisson distribution. As it happens with the particulate matter found in injection solutions, in order to obtain a symmetrical distribution, the numbers have become so vast at the lower end of the counting range that it is usually necessary to take logarithms of both the size axis and the number axis, a so-called log–log plot.

In a mixed system, containing a number of different materials, each with its own characteristic size distribution, an instrument attempting to measure the properties of the system is only be able to measure the resultant size distribution obtained by adding the individual distributions. The effect this has on the particle size distribution between limits is illustrated in Fig. 9. In a real system, there would be random numbers of random identities. The integral between limits (or the sum between the two extremes) is a direct measurement of the total number of particles present of that component. In reality, of course, these would not all be the same, as suggested in Fig. 9, but would vary, as shown in Fig. 10. Summing the resultant distribution, measured by an instrument, usually results in a reasonably straight log–log plot too. This discussion assumes random identities of particles; if there were only one species, or one that dominates the rest, the instrument

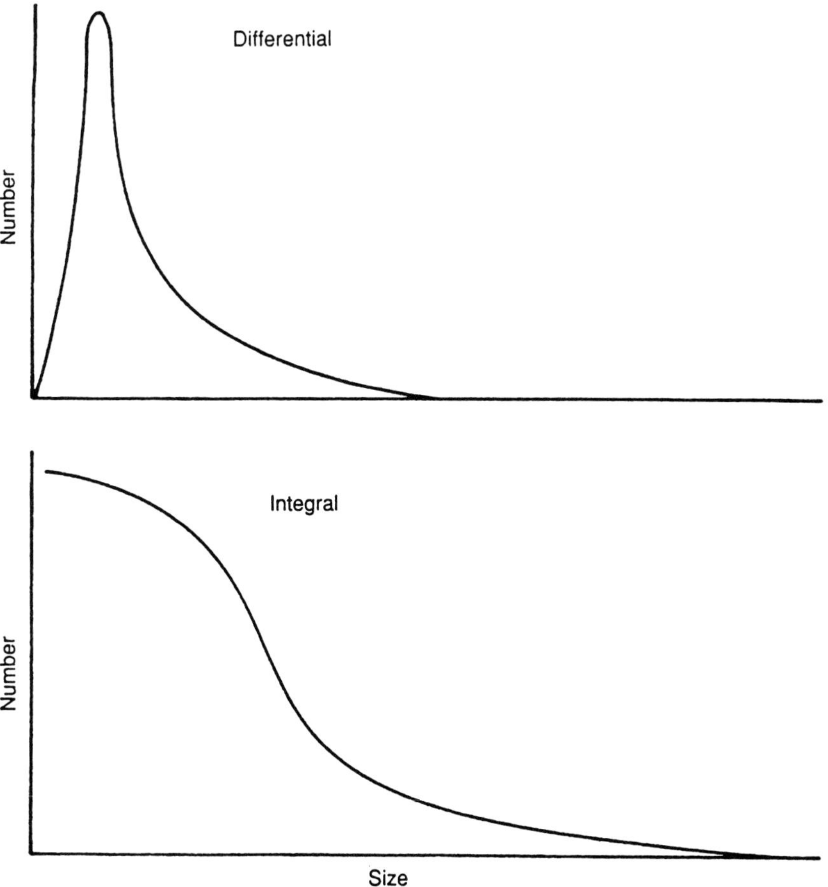

FIG. 8. Differential and integral size-distribution plots.

would measure the size distribution of this dominant. This is an important point, since it should be emphasized that if, indeed, a parenteral product contains a dominant species, it could be said that product is contaminated and probably not suitable for its stated purpose.

The linear log–log plot for particulate matter in injection solutions has been frequently found in parenteral products over the past 30 years [1], and has proved to be a very convenient approximation in practice. However, filtration results in much cleaner solutions (Fig. 11), as particle groups are removed sequentially. Modern filtration procedures give solutions containing so few particles that significant problems are encountered in detecting an accurate and precise count by instrument at the thresholds employed for compendial testing. This has resulted in some, as yet unpublished, observations that the log–log plot is not necessarily valid (Barber, private communication). This is partly due to a much higher degree of sophistication associated with current computers, which are capable of fitting data into some linear format based on various mathematical models, even with severely limited numbers in the original data set. The main advantage of

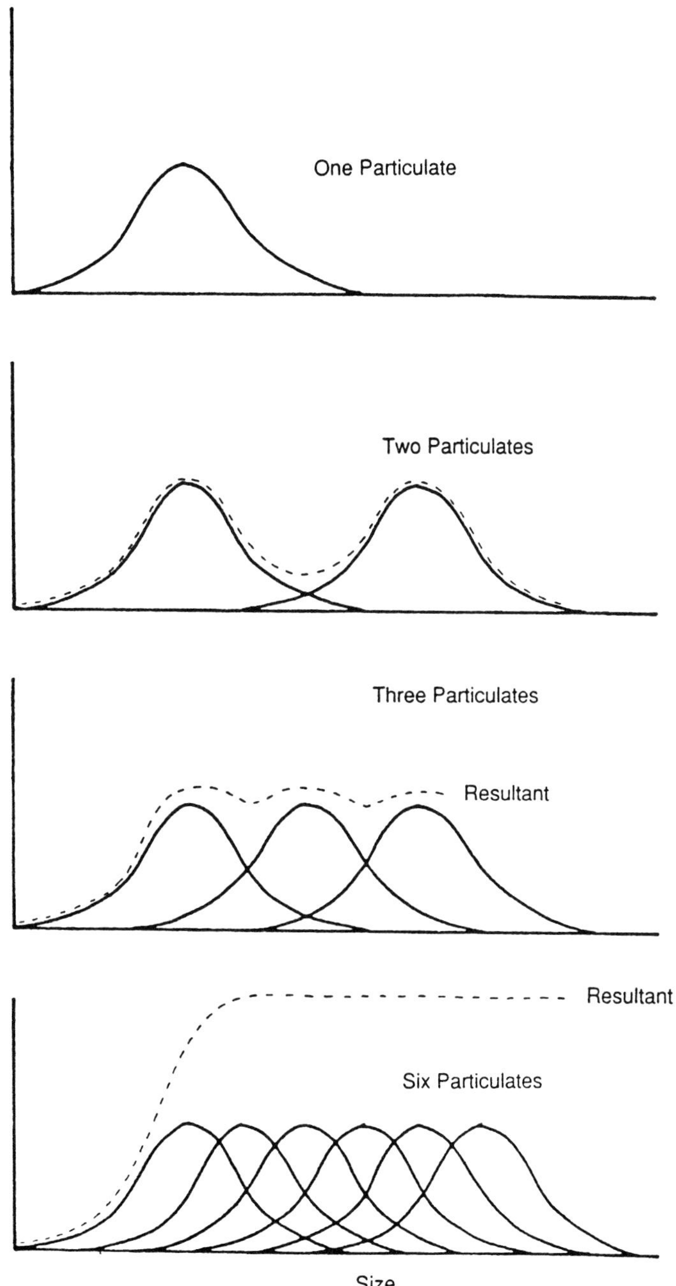

FIG. 9. The effect of increasing random numbers on the particle size distribution between limits.

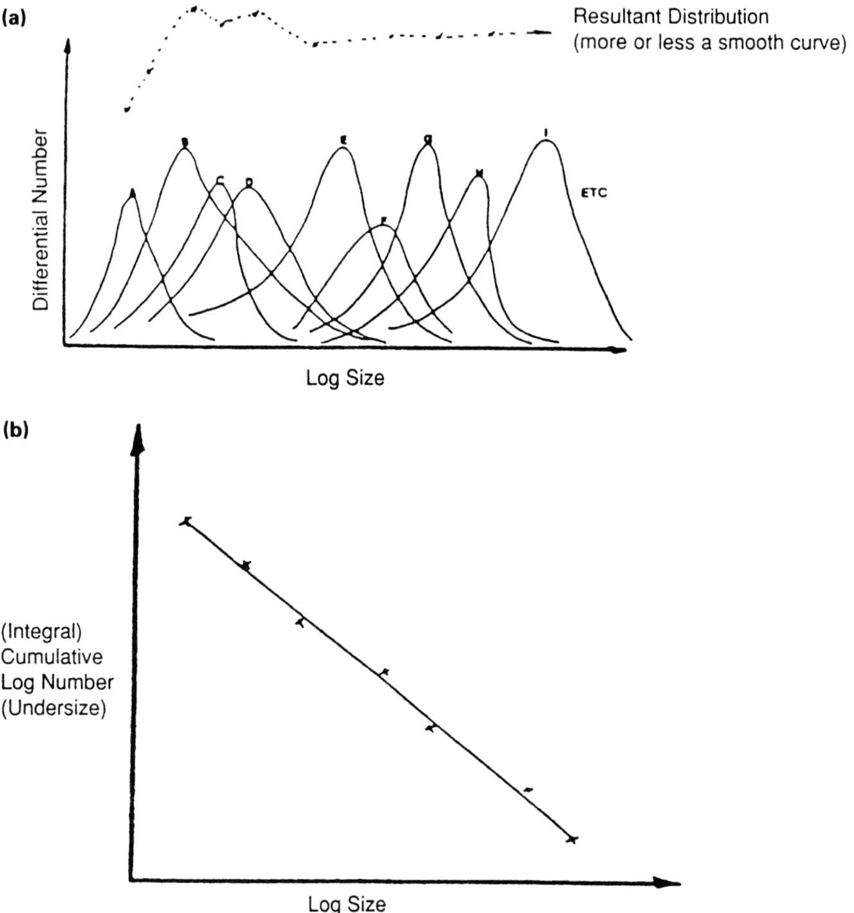

FIG. 10. The effect of a range of (random) size distributions on (a) the differential size distribution and (b) the integral size distribution, shown as a cumulative number undersize curve against size.

the log–log plot is precisely that it is unsophisticated and insensitive over a very wide range of numbers and sizes.

Instruments for Counting Particles in Parenteral Solutions

The Coulter Principle

The first quantitative determination of particulate matter in an injectable product was carried out in 1964 with a Coulter Counter [10]. This instrument had been devised in the late 1940s as a method of automatically counting blood cells; it is still widely utilized in hospitals for this purpose today. The Coulter Counter consists of two electrodes at either side of an orifice in a tube immersed in the sample under examination (Fig. 12). As a particle is passed through the orifice, it causes a momentary increase in the resistance between the two electrodes. This can be displayed as a pulse, the size of which is directly proportional to the volume of the particle (or, more accurately, the volume of the electrolyte displaced by the particle). The instrument can therefore both count and size par-

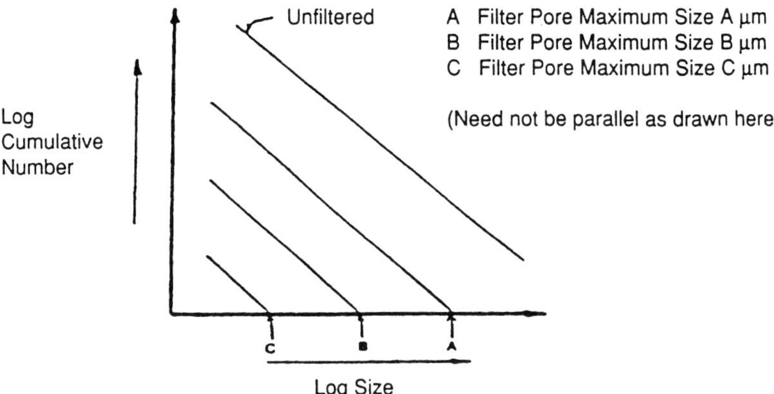

FIG. 11. The effect of filtration producing a truncation of the size distribution.

ticles in a suspension. This principle has been repeatedly demonstrated to be both accurate and precise under a wide variety of experimental conditions. However, there are some limitations which have become more evident as the quality of parenteral solutions has improved [1]. The main problem is that electrolyte is needed to carry the current between the two electrodes. If a solution such as Dextrose Injection is to be inspected, it requires the addition of electrolyte and any manipulation of the test solution carries with it the risk of the procedure adding extraneous particles to the system. A main limitation of the method is simply that it is difficult to carry out sufficient analyses in a reasonable time frame. This is a major issue in industry where the analyst may be presented with samples from a number of batches each day which cannot be analyzed in a timely fashion. Nevertheless, the device has proved valuable for hospital pharmacists who have access to instruments in their own hospital pathology laboratories. For this reason the Coulter Counter was described in the British Pharmacopoeia (BP) as being suitable for the Limit Test for Particulate Matter. However, in the current (1993) BP this device has been dropped from the monograph.

Light-Obscuration Instruments

Light blockage or, more accurately, light-obscuration instruments were introduced in the late 1950s as an automatic method for measuring suspended particulate matter in hydraulic oils used to control aircraft surfaces. Over the years, the principle and application of these instruments have become better understood and it is now the USP method to measure particulate matter in all injectable solutions.

The principle is simple: in a cell the solution is carried through a zone separating a light source and a light detector. Unencumbered, the light sensor, usually a silicon photodiode (otherwise a transistor) emits a constant current, but as a particle is carried between it and the light source, a shadow is cast on the surface and the current is diminished in proportion to the area of the sensing surface that is blocked out or obscured (Figs. 13 and 14). Initially the light source was a white light lamp, but recent developments using monochromatic solid-state lasers, which have a much longer life, have probably im-

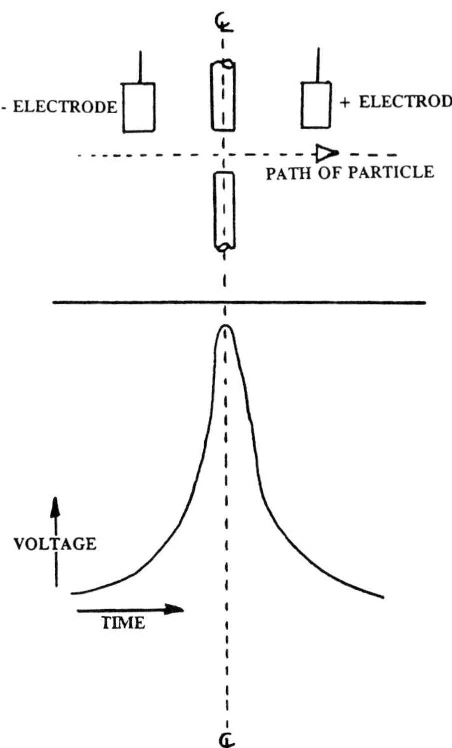

FIG. 12. The Coulter principle. The orifice is in a tube inserted into an electrolyte solution. The two electrodes are inside and outside of the orifice tube; the polarity reverses each time the machine is switched on. Distorted curves arise if the particle approaches the orifice at an angle, but normally this is not evident because the curve is compressed into a spike. The area under the curve is a function of the particle volume and, as a spike, the height of the spike is also a measure of particle volume.

proved the sensitivity of these devices. The advantages and disadvantages of the numerous current instruments are described in detail in Refs. 1 and 2. The main advantages are that they are generally accurate and precise, do not require electrolyte, and are rapid in operation, allowing large numbers of samples to be processed each day. The disadvantages are a sensitivity to shape since the instrument only "sees" the size as a function of the shadow cast. If a particle is flaky, for example, the "size" detected will vary according to the orientation of the particle as it passes through the sensing zone. If a particle is transparent, allowing some light to pass through it, it will appear to be slightly smaller than it would appear in, for example, a Coulter instrument. There is some evidence that the color and refractive index of the carrying fluid, if not the particle itself, may also affect the sensitivity of the resulting data. Some authors have commented on the possibility of count loss occurring because the instrument does not have time to respond as the particles are carried through the sensing zone if the flow rate of the carrying liquid is too high. Others have suggested, without sufficient evidence, that subthreshold particles detected by the instrument produce spurious counts at the measuring threshold. This effect, if indeed it occurs, is most unlikely to contribute any significant numbers of particles to the threshold count [1].

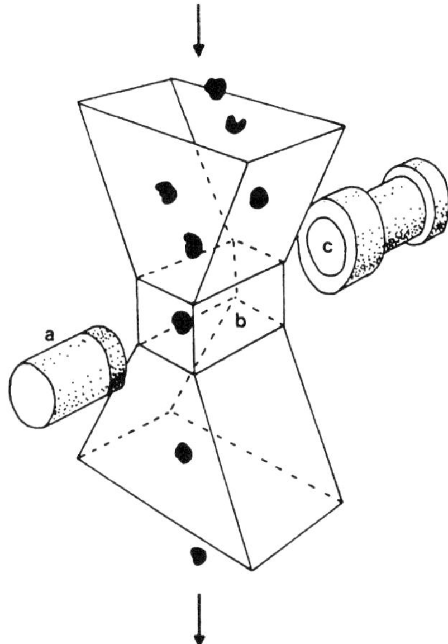

FIG. 13. Light-obscuration sensor. Key: a = light source; b = sensing zone; c = detector.

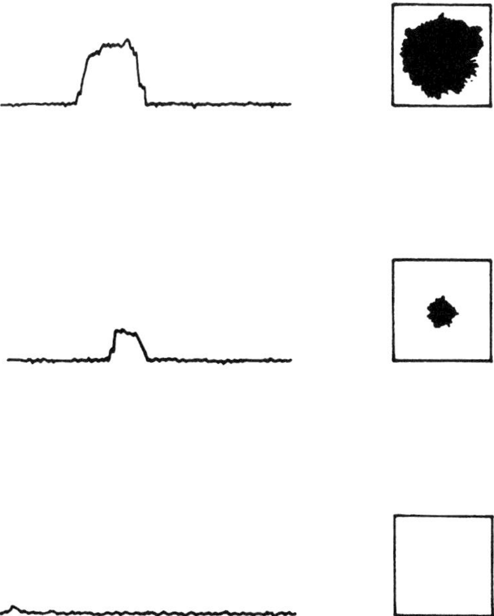

FIG. 14. The change in base-line signal from a light-obscuration counter as a function of the cross-sectional area of the particle in the beam.

Optical Microscope

In this procedure the solution under examination is passed through a filter, the surface of which is examined under the microscope. The method was published first in 1960 in a paper describing this procedure as applied to injectable solutions [11]. However, following a growing concern in the United States about particulate matter in parenteral products, the Millipore Company advocated a filtration procedure based on the standardized technique developed by the American Society of Automotive Engineers, Aeronautical Recommended Practice (ARP) No. 599. After the method was improved by cleaning the collecting filters prior to the sampling procedure, it was published by the Millipore Company as a pharmaceutical procedure and was eventually adopted by the United States Pharmacopeia (*USP XIX*) in 1975. In this format it was only applied to the evaluation of large-volume parenterals (LVP). The method gives good service and has been substantially retained as a compendial procedure for over 20 years.

The procedure involves filtering a 25 mL sample of the injection solution through a gridded filter that has been carefully rinsed with filtered particle-free water. After drying in the air, the collected particles are examined with surface or side illumination under low magnification. Trasen claimed that the procedure has certain advantages [12]:

1. Particles are measured directly by the analyst and can be characterized morphologically if required (although not by the USP).
2. Particles are measured directly by the analyst.
3. Particles are sampled from the container in the same way a patient would receive its content.
4. Sampling can be carried out in a closed system, thereby avoiding external contamination.
5. Results are unaffected by bubbles.
6. The container is penetrated only once.
7. No periodic calibration is required.
8. Agglomerated particles are recognized and can be sized individually.
9. The entire container can be sampled, if required.
10. Ultraclean equipment is used.
11. The membrane can be retained by the laboratory for subsequent evaluation as part of the batch record.

In his enthusiasm Trasen may have overstated the case and some claims were soon found to be misleading. For example, claims 4 and 10 become superfluous since it is obvious that the manufacturer would not wish to add particles to the product during the analysis and would take every precaution accordingly.

As experience with the method developed, workers in the area realized that the method, as published, suffered from a number of disadvantages. Barber and his colleagues improved the procedure, which is described at some length in his book [2]. This procedure has been substantially adopted by the *USP XXIII*, which will be published in 1994 and becomes official on January 1, 1995.

In the new procedure the entire content of a container is examined, and the filter is viewed by incident oblique illumination and by episcopic bright-field illumination internal to the microscope. Particles are judged or measured by reference to an improved design of a circular-diameter graticule.

Nevertheless, the optical microscopic procedure has inherent disadvantages that are not removed by the new procedure.

1. The filter absorbs oily materials such as silicone lubricants and some preservatives which are then not seen as particles.
2. Some amorphous and gelatinous materials are only seen with difficulty against the matrix of the filter and are therefore difficult to measure.
3. Using white light illumination the discrimination of a typical optical microscope is around 1.0 μm [1], and hence there is a built-in error at the lower-size threshold at 10.0 μm of around ±10 %.
4. Although, nominally, the method only requires a microscope, a filtering apparatus, a few filter membranes, and a technician, it is not an inexpensive procedure. The analytical environment must be protected from external contamination, which requires a clean room and laminar-flow hoods. The principal cost element is the time for analysis and the careful training of dedicated technicians.

In addition, Draftz, himself a professional microscopist, noted that the method is slow, boring, and labor intensive [13]. It is imprecise by its very nature and gave poor reproducibility between and within laboratories and, as a sizing procedure, is generally inaccurate. Some of these problems are eliminated with the help of an automatic scanning optical microscope [2]. These instruments are relatively expensive and not every organization is willing to devote resources to the installation, validation, and continued operation of this type of instrument. Furthermore, although some of the human factors are removed, the question of discriminating between amorphous and oily materials remains.

A major advantage of the method is that the operator sees and in some cases can identify the particulate matter collected on the filter. The identification procedures can be improved with the help of *The Particle Atlas* [34] and made more certain by examination under a scanning electron microscope fitted with an energy dispersive x-ray detector [2]. Although this is now a required procedure under the Good Manufacturing Practices (GMPs) that control the manufacture of parenteral products, no pharmacopeia requires the identification of particulate matter.

In summary, the use of a relatively simple filtration and microscope system has some advantages for determining the relative amount of particulate matter in injectable solutions. The accuracy and precision of the method are both poor, and the fact that oily materials cannot be visualized is a major drawback. The possibility of being able to archive or store the collected particulate with the batch records offers a considerable advantage. Provided there is no attempt to correlate the microscopic procedure with other methods of particle counting and sizing, the method itself is useful in a comparative sense in order to compare material lots. Other pharmacopeias use the method for the evaluation of large-volume parenterals, but the USP has recently stated that the improved method will provide an essential element in the examination of both large- and small-volume parenterals in the future.

Current Compendial Limits

In the now famous preface to the first edition of the *United States Pharmacopoeia* (the spelling changed in 1955), published in 1820, it was noted that its value depended on the fidelity with which it conformed to the best state of medical knowledge of the day. Traditionally the various compendia worldwide have always been slow to follow technical developments in pharmacy. For example, injectable products were first used around the time of the American Civil War, but the first compendial monograph was published in the *British Pharmacopoeia* (BP) of 1874. No method of sterilization was indicated until 1923 when the BP monograph also indicated that the intravenous injections should be "free from solid particles." By 1926, the *USP X*, the *DAB VI* (Deutsches Arzneibuch) and the *Dutch Pharmacopoeia VIII* all included an autoclaving procedure for the preparation of a sterile product. The *British Pharmacopoeia* of 1932 went even further by offering autoclaving, sterile filtration, aseptic manipulation, and an intermittent heating process.

The first injectable product to be included in the USP was the Diphtheria Antitoxin in the *USP VIII* of 1905. In 1915, two more products were included, but particulate matter was not mentioned until the *National Formulary VI* added a heading "Clearness" that required an aqueous ampuled product to be clear, and, when viewed under a bright light, to be substantially free of precipitate, cloudiness or turbidity, speck or flecks, fibers or cotton hair or any undissolved material. An issue that remains unresolved today is the use of the words "substantially free from" (particulate). This issue was addressed in the subsequent edition of the NF by the following statement:

> Substantially free shall be construed to mean a preparation which is free from foreign bodies that can be readily discernible by the unaided eye when viewed through a light reflected from a 100-W Mazda lamp, using as a medium a ground glass and a background of black and white.

The *USP XII*, which appeared in 1942 when considerable amounts of injectable solutions were required by the military, went one step further and omitted the essential word substantially. The problem came to a head when one manufacturer objected to material being rejected by the FDA because it contained excessive quantities of particulate matter. Complaining that the pharmacopeial test was unrealistic (a common complaint still heard today), the matter went to court. The FDA inspector was unable to demonstrate that he could unequivocally decide which product was "contaminated" and which was not. As a result, the court decided that the test described in the *USP XII* was too arbitrary and unreliable and therefore unsuitable for legal purposes. Consequently, the *USP XIII* was more cautious in its approach and simply required individual visual inspection of each ampule.

Dissatisfaction with the official tests for clarity were being expressed on the other side of the Atlantic at about the same time. Godding [6] ventured so far as to actually propose that a standard should be adopted that was as close as possible to the ideal of a complete freedom from particulate matter, an ideal that still remains unattainable and unrealistic today.

Some 20 years later, the situation started to change following two incidents on both sides of the Atlantic in which patients died following the administration of a contaminated intravenous product. It is true that, in both cases, the particulate matter just happened to be visable, but they served to point to the fact that particulate matter of all types provide a clue as to the conditions under which they were manufactured. Following an FDA symposium organized in Washington in 1966, the *USP XIX* introduced the microscopic procedure for the evaluation of large-volume parenterals in 1975. In the United Kingdom, following a governmental inquiry, an instrumental procedure based on the Coulter Counter was featured in the 1973 *British Pharmacopoeia*.

Since that time the various compendia have reacted to the advance of technology, some more rapidly than others. For example, the BP introduced the HIAC (high accuracy counter) as an alternative to the Coulter in 1978. However, it was rapidly realized that the two instruments, operating on different principles of particle detection, gave different results, which meant that the same limits on particulate matter could not apply. This was corrected in the 1983 edition and there have been no changes since then.

Based on the principle of being in the forefront of technical development, the USP has become a leader in this area. After a prolonged period of debate, the filtration procedure was introduced in 1975 (*USP XIX*), but with only two size thresholds being specified (Table 2) in an attempt to characterize the log–log size distribution intrinsic to most parenteral solutions. The limiting particle numbers allowed at each size threshold were somewhat loosely based on the standards suggested a decade earlier by Kendall in Australia [1] and have remained in force since that time. As noted earlier, the 1995 edition of the USP (XXIII) will feature the improved microscopic procedure which in practice is more sensitive to solid particles. In order to reflect improvements in the industrial quality of large-volume parenterals that have taken place over the past two decades, the allowable limiting particle numbers have been lowered to about one quarter of the previous limits (Table 2).

A significant change occurred, however, in the philosophy of the USP in the 1985, *USP XXI*, edition. For the first time, a limit test was introduced for the allowable particulate matter in small-volume injection solutions. The method was based on the HIAC or light-obscuration procedure. The numbers of producers of these materials are both larger and more sophisticated in their degree of appreciation of the technical issues involved. In addition, the products themselves were much more varied in composition than the relatively simple salt and sugar solutions of large-volume parenteral products. The net effect of this diversity was a brief period of confusion, and the implementation of the new standards was delayed for a year until 1986. The new standards were based on the observation that the average large-volume parenteral was administered to a patient who had been treated with at least five additional small-volume injections, and it was intended that the small-volume limits should not be more than five times those of the large-volume injections. The allowable numbers are shown in Table 3 and are given in terms of the total numbers of particles in each individual container.

An even more significant change is to occur in *USP XXIII*. In principle, the methods of analysis are to remain the same, but the test is conducted in two stages which are applicable to both large- and small-volume parenteral solutions alike. The product will be tested by a light-obscuration procedure first, and the new limiting numbers have been

TABLE 2 Quality Improvement of Large-Volume Parenteral Solutions: Allowable Limits of Particulate Matter per mL

Size Threshold (μm)	*USP XIX*, 1975	*USP XXIII*, 1995
10	50	12
25	5	2

TABLE 3 Allowable Limits for Particulate Matter per Container in Small-Volume Parenteral Solutions Detected by a Light-Obscuration Procedure

Size Threshold (μm)	*USP XIX*, 1985	*USP XXIII*, 1995
10	10,000	6,000
25	1,000	600

TABLE 4 The 1995 *USP XXIII* Limit Test for Particulate Matter in Injections

Size Threshold (μm)	Stage 1, Light Obscuration	Stage 2, Microscope
Small-volume parenterals		
10	6,000 per container	3,000 per container
25	600 per container	300 per container
Large-volume parenterals		
10	25 per mL	12 per mL
25	3 per mL	2 per mL

selected to allow about 90% of product to pass at this stage. However, should the product fail this test, it can then proceed to a filtration and microscopic procedure. The basic intention of having a two-stage procedure is to limit the amount of silicone and other oily particulate materials present in injectables. The original intention was to have an additional chemical limit test for silicones but this has proved to be difficult to implement, given the present state of knowledge in this area. Although it cannot be directly calculated because the two tests measure the particles by different instrumental principles, the implication is that the light-obscuration procedure counts all particles above 10 μm in diameter in the system under examination, whereas the microscope sees only solid particles since the oils will have been absorbed into the filtration matrix. The difference, therefore, may be assumed to be silicone or other oily particles.

To demonstrate the sensitivity of this method, it can be assumed for the sake of this discussion, that the oil has an average density of 0.8 g/mL. If there are (6000−3000 = 3000) particles of silicone oil of particle size 10 μm (a low level for the sake of illustrating a point), the mass of silicone per container is:

$$0.8 \cdot 4/3 \cdot \pi \cdot 3000 \cdot (10/2)^3 \cdot 10^{-12}\ \text{ng} = 40\ \text{ng}$$

This corresponds to 40 ppm in a 1-mL ampule which, in any discussion about purity, must be regarded with some satisfaction. The same type of calculation, applied to a 500-mL large-volume parenteral, shows that the "contamination level" has dropped to about 0.5 ng silicone oil or about 1 ppb, well below current methods of detection using chemical or other physical principles.

The new light-obscuration limits are shown in Table 3 for comparative purposes, and the allowable limits for the two stages of *USP XXIII* are shown in Table 4.

Physiological Effects

The physiological effects produced by particulate matter when introduced into the human or animal body remain an area of considerable dispute, perhaps best summarized by the

Scottish legal verdict of "not proven." This is especially true today since there can be little objective doubt that the quality, and therefore the particle burden, of commercial injectable products is far better than it was 20 years ago. The chance, therefore, of injecting harmful particulate matter into a patient must have decreased significantly. Nevertheless, it might be assumed that some effects might be produced if a particle, for example, blocked a blood vessel or induced a foreign-body reaction, ultimately resulting in a tumorous response.

Passive Blockage

The mammalian blood system effectively consists of two sections connected together. The high pressure (arterial) side is connected to the low pressure (venous) system through the capillaries at one end and the heart at the other. It is unlikely that a particle, introduced into the venous system by an injection into the radial vein in the upper arm, would lodge in the veins as they are carried forward, since the veins enlarge as they approach the heart. Once through the heart, however, the particle would enter the pulmonary artery and, from that point onward, the arteries decrease in size as they approach the capillary beds. This is demonstrated in Table 5. The net effect is that particles could lodge in the system according to their diameter (Table 6). This is a theoretical concept, however, since the blood itself is particulate and is equipped with an extremely effective system for collecting and destroying foreign particulate matter, especially if it is an invasive microorganism. This is the reticuloendothelial system (RES), which attempts to remove

TABLE 5 Subdivision of the Arterial Blood Supply in the Canine Lung[a]

Tissue	Number	Diameter (μm)
Pulmonary artery	1	15,500
Right and left branches	2	11,500
Lesser arteries	8	5,960
First-order arteries	24	3,960
Second-order arteries	164	2,260
Third-order arteries	1121	1,000
Lobular arteries	1.6×11^4	300
Atrial arteries	6.4×11^4	165
Sac arteries	1.28×11^5	165
Capillaries	6×11^8	7

[a]From Ref. 38.

TABLE 6 Site of Particle Lodgement According to Size

Diameter (μm)	Site
>50	Large veins and arteries
25	Smaller veins and arteries
15	Lungs
10	Upper limit of RES interaction
5	Capillaries
1	Lower limit of RES interaction
0.1	Seepage through capillary fenestrations

foreign particles by phagocytosis or ingestion, following a process in which the surface of the particle is coated with a protein that enables it to be recognized by cells associated with the RES. This process, termed opsonization, does not occur with all particles and the RES appears to capable of removing only particles between 1 and 10 μm in diameter. Outside this range it is conceivable that large particles, for example, between 20 and 50 μm in diameter, could block blood vessels as has been demonstrated in experimental animals. The body contains an extensive system of collateral circulation pathways. If one blood vessel is blocked for any reason, there are many alternative pathways to carry blood to essential organs. Problems obviously arise if there are so many large particles introduced into the body that all of the collateral pathways are blocked. This has apparently led to fatalities due to intravenous administration of narcotics derived from tableted material. However, this situation is hardly relevant to the deliberate administration of an intravenous drug product manufactured under good manufacturing conditions.

Physiologically, most injected particulate matter between about 5 to 15 μm tends to be trapped in the capillary beds of the lung and, to a lesser extent, in the spleen and liver. Once trapped in the lung, there appears to be a mechanism for the particles to pass through the capillary walls and be ultimately excreted in the sputum. There is some evidence [14,15] that there are large arteriovenous shunts which allow particles to pass around the natural collection system associated with the lung. However, Schroeder et al. [16] demonstrated that the removal of particles from the blood stream is directly related to size, the larger particles being removed more rapidly.

It has been only rarely demonstrated that the presence of particulate matter is harmful. An example is the work by Hearse and co-workers [17] who noted hemodynamic changes in isolated rat heart preparations following the infusion of unfiltered intravenous solutions. The heart recovered when washed through with filtered solutions, but the exact cause of the effect does not appear to have been determined. In addition, the effect has not been detected in humans, and therefore the overall significance of the observation is less than certain.

Physiological Interactions with Particles

Although the passive interaction of the body with injected particles is possible, the fact that the body is a very interactive system must not be forgotten, and other possible interactions should be looked for. To a certain degree, the fate of an injected particle depends on its chemical nature and its shape. It is possible to block the RES by injecting quantities of small particles such as heat-denatured albumin microparticles. The coating of foreign particles with protein prior to ingestion by phagocytes of the RES system has been mentioned, but this reaction depends on the chemical nature of the particles themselves. As discussed by Davis et al. [18], it is possible to frustrate the normal physiological system by coating the particles with appropriate polymers, and this has been used to target particulate systems containing drugs to sites such as lung, liver, and spleen. In recent years various particulate systems have been delivered to the body such as sterile phospholipid-stabilized oil emulsions, liposomes, and nanoparticles. Studies of the fate of these systems have helped to understand what happens when relatively large numbers of particles are deliberately injected into the body. This work has never provided any reason to be concerned about effects produced by the very small numbers of particles that may be inadvertently introduced from an injection of, for example, a drug solution. This subject appears to be irrelevant to the main problem of defining the desirable degree of quality that should be built into the product.

Opsonization due to the coating process mentioned earlier may, however, result in the particle being coated with phagocytes that ultimately form a large mass of cells or granulomata. This would have the effect of increasing the size of the contaminating particle, potentially blocking blood vessels. In addition, some granulomata could be the focus of a tumorous or cancerous response, perhaps because of some interaction, necrosis, or anaerobic reaction at the center of the cellular mass. This is not an inevitable response to the formation of granulomas but a significant proportion are likely to form cysts or some similar reaction. Pulmonary-artery granulomata associated with particles in intravenous fluids and emulsions have been blamed for the death of children on parenteral feeding regimens [35].

An effect due to shape of the particles has been reported, especially if the particles are fibers. It appears that fibers may form sites of attachment for fibroblasts if they have an appropriate length-to-breadth ratio or, perhaps, diameter. This area is controversial but may provide an explanation for why asbestos fibrils appear to produce cancerous reactions [19,20] and why glass or cellulose fibers may be intrinsically undesirable as injectable contaminants [21,22].

The chemical nature of the particulate may be unlikely to produce an immediate effect, and acute physiological responses are unlikely to be evident except in extreme situations. On the other hand, chronic effects over time are more possible. Concern about injection of glass spicules and fragments following the routine breaking of an all-glass ampule prior to administration of the contents was expressed at least half a century ago, and the first examination of the pathology of glass particles can be traced back to the classical investigations of Gardner and Cummings in 1931 [23]. Numerous investigations since that time have failed to demonstrate any foreign body reaction, granuloma formation, or pyrogenic response to glass.

This is different, however, for the natural cellulose particles commonly found in injections up until fairly recently. Various authors have shown that cellulose does prompt a severe physiological response [22,24–30,36] and therefore cellulose fibers must be excluded from injection solutions. This is also true for talc, although the main sources of this material are surgeons rubber gloves [31,32]. Unfortunately, until recently talc was used as a mold-release agent for pharmaceutical-grade rubber stoppers and was therefore inevitably present in injections solutions until this was recognized and the material rigorously removed from contact with the product.

Silicone oil is currently a source of controversy since it too is inevitably present in injectable products from a variety of sources, but mainly as a lubricant for the insertion of stoppers. Initially regarded as inert, the problems found with massive quantities of silicone released into the body from leaking silicone oil-filled prosthetic devices such as breast implants has prompted a reevaluation of the situation. There is a possibility that chronic effects on the immune system or other physiological functions due to relatively small amounts of silicone oil from contaminated parenteral products may eventually be discovered [37].

Glaser [33] has recently reviewed the physiological problems associated with particulate matter, bubbles, and aerosols related to the use and reuse of medical and dental devices. He concluded that particulate matter in injectables is dealt with by the RES. However, potential issues are associated with inhalation of aerosols from devices such as dental drills. At this stage of development the significance of the inhalation issue is not clear and is probably irrelevant to the injected product.

A recent FDA safety alert (April 18, 1994) has drawn attention to an incident in which a hospital pharmacist added calcium gluconate and potassium phosphate to a Total Parenteral Nutritional formulation containing amino acids, a lipid emulsion, and dextrose. Not surprisingly, a precipitate of calcium phosphate formed which was obscured by the presence of the emulsion. Unfortunately, two patients died and two others suffered respiratory distress, apparently as a result of diffuse microvascular pulmonary emboli containing calcium phosphate. This incident serves to emphasize that inappropriate procedures outside of the general control of the product manufacturer may result in the formation of insoluble particles from interactions between mixture components. Massive doses of insoluble particulate matter are, indeed, hazardous to the patient, although, as emphasized in this review, levels of particulate material present in current commercial products are too small to be considered an issue.

GMP and Contamination

Mainly originating from the United States, and, in particular, from the FDA during the 1960s, GMPs have been broadly accepted around the world. Quality should be built into a product and not only tested for at the end of the production process. Unfortunately, in some quarters, GMPs have acquired excessive importance. It seems to be difficult to define the simple (and key) word "quality." Statements by the FDA (from the Rockville Vatican, as the headquarters are variously called) have defined quality as a fitness for a defined purpose. This is considered to include the fact that the product is not "contaminated," which would render it unfit for use. The real issue here is that particulate matter in a pharmaceutical parenteral product is regarded by some as "contamination" but in reality it is physically impossible to make a product without some insoluble particulate matter present, albeit a small amount [1].

Pragmatically, therefore, it has to be decided quite arbitrarily, what is acceptable and what is not. The stigma associated with "contamination" must be removed and the inevitability of the presence of small amounts of inadvertently present material must be accepted; it could be termed particle burden. Then, and only then, can it be accepted that, by applying GMPs, the "quality" of the product can be improved, no matter how the word is defined. The word contamination is too emotive and, with one very important exception, is unacceptable. The exception is contamination with living microorganisms in a supposedly sterile product when the word assumes its correct connotation and meaning. If the product is truly sterile and conforms to the compendial requirements for particulate matter, that product is not contaminated in any sense.

Facilities and Equipment

The detailed GMPs make it obligatory that sterile products be made in dedicated facilities, using specialized equipment which is chosen and designed to ensure that cleanliness is maintained throughout the process. Materials of construction are carefully selected to make certain that integrity is maintained and that the product coming into contact with the system is not contaminated, thereby increasing the particle burden. The particle burden originally present can be significantly reduced by repeated filtration. The object of any subsequent stage in the process is to ensure that the particle burden remains low and is not increased by material falling into the product prior to the filling and sealing process.

Procedures and Personnel

The GMPs are based on written procedures for every stage of the production process. This serves to draw attention to the fact that production and manipulation of every pharmaceutical product involves people. Not all pharmaceutical organizations recognize that product quality critically depends on personnel. Even in a totally automated plant a few individuals are needed for maintenance and adjustment, although the size of most pharmaceutical lines does not justify the significant cost of installing an automatic operation. Operator training is an essential element in any GMP facility and recent events suggest that some managements may have lost sight of the importance of a dedicated work force. This issue, at a time of considerable cutback in the industry, will become relevant when the industry realizes fully that without the appropriately trained work force product quality cannot be maintained.

Conclusions

In some sense, the jury can be regarded as being still out and likely to come up with a verdict of ''not proven.'' Indeed, it is not very likely that a clear opinion will ever result since very few people would wish to volunteer for the type of clinical trial that would be needed to provide definite information on the subject. This is even assuming that there could be a medical and pharmaceutical consensus as to the basic requirements of any clinical protocol for a trial of this nature. In a 1965 *Lancet* editorial Sir Harold Dodd, concludes that: ''Running the risk of injecting fungal spores, mycelia, and debris causing granulomata of the lungs, brain and other organs is unwarrantable.'' This opinion remains reasonable today, especially when it can be pointed out that materials thought to provide problems such as talc or asbestos can be eliminated and, by monitoring overall particulate found in parenteral solutions, the levels found in commercial products today are significantly lower than they were in Sir Harolds' day. The issue is one of pharmaceutical quality, not of physiological significance and danger. By reducing the levels of particulate matter to the very low levels implied in the application of GMPs, the product quality is always maintained and the patient is safeguarded.

Acknowlegment

I am grateful to Michael Anisfeld and Interpharm Press for the permission to publish Tables 1, 5, and 6 and Figs. 1–14 from my earlier book [1].

References

1. Groves, M.J., *Particulate Matter: Sources and Resources for Healthcare Manufacturers*, Interpharm Press, Buffalo Grove, IL, 1993.

2. Barber, T.A., *Pharmaceutical Particulate Matter: Analysis and Control*, Interpharm Press, Buffalo Grove, IL, 1993.
3. Groves, M.J., Defining parenteral particulates, *Proc. PDA Int. Conf. on Particle Detection, Metrology and Control, Washington*, Parenteral Drug Association, Arlington, VA, 1990, pp. 82–102.
4. Borchert, S.J., Abe, A., Aldrich, S.D., Fox, L.E., Freeman, J.E., and White, R.D., Particulate matter in parenteral products, *J. Parent. Sci. Technol.*, 40: 212–239 (1986).
5. Hodgson, I., Current trends in ampoule inspection, *Manuf. Chem.*, 56(2): 29–31 (1985).
6. Godding, E.W., Foreign matter in solutions for injection, *Pharm. J.*, 154: 124–125 (1945).
7. Hamlins, W.E., General guidelines for the visual inspection of parenteral products in final containers and in-line inspection of container components, *J. Parent. Drug Assoc.*, 32: 63–66 (1978).
8. Saylor, H.M., Particulate matter. II. Visual inspection, *Bull. Parent. Drug Assoc.*, 20: 31–44 (1966).
9. Knapp, J.Z., Detection and Measurement of Particles in Sealed Containers. In: *Filtration in the Pharmaceutical Industry* (T.H. Meltzer, ed.), Marcel Dekker, Inc., New York, 1987, pp. 587–706.
10. Groves, M.J., and Major, J.F.G., Assessment of particulate material in normal saline solution for injection B.P. by means of the Coulter Counter, *Pharm. J.*, 193: 227–228 (1964).
11. Termansen, J.B., Filtration testing of injections and eyedrops, *Arch. Pharm. Chem.*, 67: 1155–1162 (1960).
12. Trasen, B., Membrane filtration technique in analysis for particulate matter, *Bull. Parent. Drug Assoc.*, 22: 1–8 (1968).
13. Draftz, R.G., Microscopical counting, sizing and statistical strategies for LVP contaminants. In: *Proc. PDA Int. Conf. on Particle Detection, Metrology and Control, Washington*, Parenteral Drug Association, Arlington, VA, 1990, pp. 458–466.
14. Prinzmetal, M., Ornitz, E.M., Smukin, B., and Bergman, H.C., Arterio-venous anastomoses in liver, spleen and lung, *Am. J. Physiol.*, 152: 478–502 (1948).
15. Haley, T.C., Asbestos—a reassessment of the overall problem, *J. Pharm. Sci.*, 64(9): 1435–1449 (1975).
16. Schroeder, H.G., and Simmons, G.H., and DeLuca, P.P., Distribution of radiolabelled subvisible microspheres after intravenous administration to beagle dogs, *J. Pharm. Sci.*, 67(4): 504–507 (1978).
17. Hearse, D.J., Erol, C., Robinson, L.A., Maxwell, M.P., and Braimbridge, M.V., Particle-induced coronary vasoconstriction during cardioplegic infusion, *J. Thorac. Cardiovasc. Surg.*, 89: 428–438 (1985).
18. Davis, S.S., Illum, L., McVie, J.M., and Tomlinson, E., *Microspheres and Drug Therapy: Pharmaceutical, Immunological and Medical Aspects*, Elsevier, Amsterdam, 1984.
19. Stanton, M.F., Some Etiological Considerations of Fibre Carcinogenesis. In: *Biological Effects of Asbestos* (P. Bogovski, V. Timbreli, J.C. Gibson, et al., eds.), WHO, Int. Agency for Research on Cancer, Publication No. 8, Lyon, France, 1973, pp. 289–294.
20. Wagner, J.C., Experimental production of mesothelial tumors in the pleura by implantation of dusts in laboratory animals, *Nature*, 196: 180–181 (1962).
21. Maroudas, N.G., O'Neill, C.H., and Stanton, M.F., Fibroblast anchorage in carcinogenesis by fibres, *Lancet*, 1: 807–809 (1973).
22. Garvan, J.M., and Gunner, B.W., Intravenous fluids: A solution containing such particles must not be used, *Med. J. Austral.*, 2: 140–145 (1963).
23. Gardner, L.V., and Cummings, D.E., Studies of experimental pneumonokoniosis. VI. Inhalation of asbestos dust, *J. Ind. Hyg.*, 13: 112–120 (1931).
24. Von Glahn, W.C., and Hall, J.W., The reaction produced in the pulmonary arteries by emboli of cotton fibers, *Am. J. Pathol.*, 25: 575–595 (1949).

25. Jaques, W.E., and Mariscal, G.G., A study of the incidence of cotton emboli, *Bull. Inst. Assoc. Med. Museums*, 32: 63–72 (1951).
26. Garvan, J.M., and Gunner, B.W., Particulate contamination of intravenous fluids, *Brit. J. Clin. Pract.*, 25: 119–121 (1971).
27. Garvan, J.M., and Gunner, B.W., The harmful effects of particles in intravenous fluids, *Med. J. Austral.*, 2: 1–6 (1964).
28. Purkiss, R., Effects of distribution of intravenously administered cellulose particles in mice, *J. Pharm. Pharmacol.*, 27: 290–292 (1975).
29. Brüning, E.J., Origin and significance of intra-arterial foreign body emboli in the lungs of children, *Virch. Arch. Pathol. Anat. Physiol. Clin. Med.*, 327: 460–470 (1955).
30. Sarrut, S., and Nezelof, C., A complication of intravenous therapy, *Pract. Med.*, 68: 375–380 (1960).
31. Antopol, W., Lycopodium granuloma: Its clinical and pathological significance, together with a note on granuloma produced by talc, *Arch. Pathol.*, 16: 326–331 (1933).
32. Roberts, G.B.S., Granuloma of the fallopian tube due to surgical glove talc: silicious granulomata, *Brit. J. Surg.*, 34: 417–419 (1946).
33. Glaser, Z.R., Some health and safety aspects involving *in vivo* particulates, bubbles and aerosols related to the use or reuse of medical and dental devices, *Pharmacopeial Forum*, 20(1): 6949–6955 (1994).
34. McCrone, W.C., et al., eds., *The Particle Atlas*, Vols. 1–6, Ann Arbor Scientific Publisher, Ann Arbor, 1973 to present.
35. Puntis, J.W.L., Wilkins, K.N., Ball, P.A., Rushton, D.I., and Booth, I.W., Hazards of parenteral treatment: Do particles count? *Arch. Dis. Childr.*, 76:1475–1477 (1992).
36. Bavikatte, K., Hilliard, J., Scheiner, R.L., Merkin, D., Williams, B., Lemons, J.A., and Gresham, E.L., Systemic vascular cotton emboli in the neonate, *J. Pediatr.*, 95(4): 614–616 (1979).
37. Hunt, J., Farthing, M.J.G., Baker, L.R.I., Crocker, P.R., and Levison, E.A., Silicone in the liver: Possible late effects, *Gut*, 30:239–242 (1989).
38. Gross, M.A., and Carter, C.J., Pathogenic hazard of particulate matter in solutions for parenteral use, *Proc. Symp. on Safety of Large-Volume Parenteral Solutions*, Food and Drug Administration, Rockville, MD, 1966, pp. 31–35.

MICHAEL J. GROVES

Partition Coefficients

Historical Background

The first observation that the ratio of concentrations of a solute (e.g., I_2 or Br_2) when distributed between an organic solvent (e.g., CS_2 or ether) and water, remained constant even when the volume ratio of the immiscible solvents changed widely, was first reported by Berthelot and Jungfleisch [1] in 1872, as illustrated by Eq. (1).

$$P = \frac{C_o}{C_{aq}} = \text{equilibrium constant K} \tag{1}$$

Smith [2] in 1921 suggested that partition coefficient P can be converted from one solvent system to another. Collander [3–5] 30 years later, presented the standard linear free energy relationship, shown in Eq. (2), using water and different alkanols.

$$\log P_2 = a \log P_1 + b \tag{2}$$

where a is a coefficient and b a constant.

Meyer [6,7] and Overton [8–10], at the turn of the century, discovered that most organic compounds (except nutrients) penetrate tissue cells as a lipid barrier and that their narcotic action [10,11] parallels the oil–water partition coefficients of the compounds. In the early 1950s, Collander [12] demonstrated that the penetration rate of plant cell membranes by various organic compounds was related to their oil–water partition coefficient. Cohen and Edsal [13] studied the ratios of alcohol solubility to water solubility to define the relative lipophilic character of amino acids. The limited additivity of the partition coefficients of organic compounds was observed by Collander, Cohen, and Edsal in their studies. In the early 1960s, Salame and Pinsky [14,15] derived the permachor method, given in Eq. (3), for calculation of the P factor for the prediction of chemicals permeation through a plastic membrane.

$$\log P_f = 16.55 - \frac{3700}{T} - 0.22\pi \tag{3}$$

where π is the permachor constant, and T is the absolute temperature. A general equation was presented by these authors as in Eq. (4).

$$\log P_f = K - R\pi \tag{4}$$

where K is a temperature correction constant and R is a polymer (e.g., plastic) correction term. Interestingly, about the same time Hansch, Fujita, and co-workers [16,17] made the most significant contributions toward the understanding and application of partition coefficients (log P and π) and greatly extended the linear free-energy-related (LFER) approach from organic chemistry to medicinal chemistry and biology. This renewed interest in the application of partition coefficients has stimulated many excellent reviews, books, and monographs (see Bibliography and Refs. 18–22).

Theory and Experimental Methods of Measurements

Why log *P*?

Since the partition coefficient is measured when an equilibrium is reached, it is characterized by the equality of the chemical potentials, μ_o and μ_{aq}, of the solute in the two phases (organic and aqueous), as shown by Eqs. (5) to (7).

$$\mu_o = \mu^0_o + RT \ln C_o \tag{5}$$

$$\mu_{aq} = \mu^0_{aq} + RT \ln C_{aq} \tag{6}$$

If $\mu_o = \mu_{aq}$, then

$$P = C_o/C_{aq} = e^{-(\mu^0_{aq} - \mu^0_o)/RT} = e^{-\Delta\mu^0/RT} \tag{7}$$

where C_o and C_{aq} are the equilibrium concentrations of the solute in the organic and the aqueous phases, respectively; μ^0_o and μ^0_{aq} are the chemical potentials (in the organic and aqueous phases, respectively) at infinite dilution; and *R* is the gas constant, *T* the temperature (K), and *P* the partition coefficient; *P* is a constant for any compound in a given solvent system at a given temperature, this relationship is known as the Nernst law [23].

Just like any equilibrium constant *K*, *P* is linearly related to the standard free-energy change when it is converted to the logarithmic scale [24], as in Eqs. (8) to (10).

$$\Delta G^0 = -RT \ln K \tag{8}$$

For any equilibrium:

$$\Delta G^0 = -2.303\ RT \log K \tag{9}$$

For partition processes:

$$\Delta G^0 = -2.303\ RT \log P \tag{10}$$

For this reason of linear free-energy relationship (LFER), log *P* is commonly used in most correlation studies instead of *P*.

In the past 30 years or so, 1-octanol–water has been the most commonly used solvent system. It has been shown that for correlation with biological activity, organic solvents (like 1-octanol) capable of forming hydrogen bonds usually give better correlation than those not able (e.g., CCl_4, cyclohexane, and other hydrocarbons). Extensive compilations on 1-octanol–water partition coefficient are available (see Bibliography).

On the other hand, if one is interested in separating out thermodynamic properties like enthalpy change (ΔH) and entropy change (ΔS), a solvent with minimum mutual solubility with water (like cyclohexane or heptane) is preferable.

Apparent vs. true partition coefficient (log *P'* vs. log *P*)

If a solute is ionizable (either acidic or basic), two different species can exist in the aqueous phase, and therefore the apparent partition coefficient (*P*') or the true partition coefficients (*P*) can be measured, as shown below and in Eqs. (11) to (15).

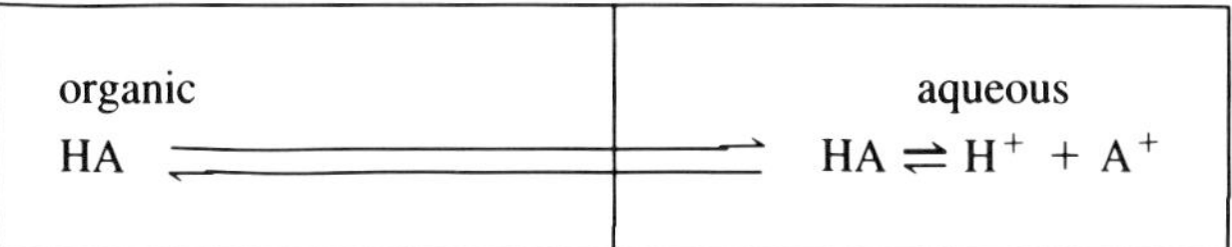

where

$$P = \frac{[HA]_o}{[HA]_{aq}} \tag{11}$$

$$P' = \frac{[HA]_o}{[HA]_{aq} + [A^-]_{aq}} \tag{12}$$

and

$$P = \frac{P'}{1 - \alpha} \tag{13}$$

where α is the degree of ionization, defined in Eqs. (14) and (15).

For acids:
$$\alpha = \frac{1}{1 + \text{antilog}(\text{pKa} - \text{pH})} \tag{14}$$

For bases:
$$\alpha = \frac{1}{1 + \text{antilog}(\text{pH} - \text{pKa})} \tag{15}$$

Since the degree of ionization is a function of the pH of the aqueous phase and the pKa of the solute, the apparent partition coefficient P' fluctuates as the pH of the aqueous phase (usually a buffer solution) is changed, while the true (or corrected) partition coefficient (P) should remain constant. However, in reality the different buffer species may not only affect P' but also P because of different degrees of ion-pair formation and the different polar nature of the counterions used. Among the different buffer species, 1-octanol–phosphate buffer appears to give the most consistent results as compared to octanol–water [25]. In some publications the apparent partition coefficient P' is also described as the distribution coefficient D.

Since the separation of immiscible phases takes place only in the presence of gravity, it would not be possible to measure partition coefficients in outer space where the gravity is zero.

Shake-Flask Method

The shake-flask method is most commonly used in the measurement of partition coefficients. It is also the standard procedure to validate other methods. A solute is simply shaken with two immiscible solvents (organic and aqueous), followed by analyzing the solute concentration in one or both phases. To avoid any volume changes in both phases, one phase is saturated with the other before the partitioning process. It is important to ensure that equilibrium is reached before the analysis. If a solute does not cause emulsification, vigorous shaking can reduce the time required to reach equilibrium, usually in a few minutes. However, if a solute with both polar and nonpolar groups present (like saponin glycosides or surfactant-type compounds), a gentle and slow shaking procedure should be used or even special devices like a Doluisio and Swintosky Y-tube [18,26] or a Schulman-type cell [18,27].

Some true (undissociated, corrected) partition coefficients of representative drug molecules ranging from − 2.26 to + 5.48 are shown in Table 1.

For the quantitative analysis of the solute distributed in one or both phases, the most commonly used analytical methods include uv–visible spectrophotometric analysis for compounds with chromophore groups [28], and gas–liquid chromatography (GLC) [29]. Colorimetric methods have also been used for specific compounds [30,31].

With proper choice of solvent volume and sensitive analytical methods, log P values ranging from − 5 to + 5 can be measured [18]. The temperature dependence of many partitioning systems is on the order of 0.01 log unit per degree in the 25°C range [18]. Adequate temperature control is needed for high accuracy. This is more critical for volatile solvents like ether, choloroform, low-boiling hydrocarbons, and alcohols lower than 1-octanol.

Chromatographic Methods

In recent years the availability of reproducible systems and precision instruments in high-performance liquid chromatography (HPLC) has prompted the application of chromatography in rapid measurement of partition coefficients [32–34]. In general, a linear relationship between log P and log K' from a set of compounds is required for the interpolation or extrapolation of log P values of additional compounds of congeneric nature, as shown in Eq. (16).

$$\log P = a \operatorname{Log} K' + b \tag{16}$$

where the capacity factor K' is determined from the net retention time t_R relative to the nonadsorbed time t_0 as defined by Eq. (17).

$$K' = (t_R - t_0)/t_0 \tag{17}$$

This is similar to the linear relationship R_m measured by thin-layer chromatography (TLC) [35,36], given by Eq. (18).

$$R_m = \log K' = \log\left(\frac{1 - R_f}{R_f}\right) = log \left(\frac{1}{R_f} - 1\right) \tag{18}$$

Because of the limits inherent in the mathematical formula, R_m ranges only from − 1.996 to + 1.996 for all possible compounds. This makes it less sensitive than the direct measurement of log P. Nevertheless, for many compounds it is much easier and more economical to measure log K' or R_m than log P.

Countercurrent and Filter Probe Methods

A countercurrent-based device, known as AKUFVE, is useful when a large amount of information resulting from varying T or pH is required on one or only a few compounds [37,38]. This method suffers the disadvantages of difficulties in cleaning and operation

TABLE 1 Selected True (Corrected) Partition Coefficients of Representative Drug Molecules Measured in 1-Octanol–Water or 1-Octanol–Phosphate Buffer[a]

Drug	log *P*
L-Tyrosine	− 2.26
Citric acid	− 1.72
Phenol red	− 1.45
Streptozotocin	− 1.45
Sulfanilamide	− 0.73
Theobromine	− 0.72
Chlortetracycline	− 0.62
Ethanol	− 0.31
Cimetidine	0.40
Atenolol	0.43
Metiamide	0.50
Procainamide	0.51
Morphine	0.76
Ephedrine	0.87
Aminopyrine	1.00
Colchicine	1.03
Chloramphenicol	1.14
Atropine	1.24
Digoxin	1.26
Nalidic acid	1.41
Phenobarbital	1.47
Hydrocortisone	1.61
Benzoic acid	1.72
Salicylic acid	1.73
Benzylpenicillin	1.83
Chloroform	1.97
Dexamethasone	1.99
Podophyllotoxin	2.01
Metoprolol	2.04
Naloxone	2.09
Mathapyrilene	2.81
Phenformine	2.94
Labetalol	3.18
Benadryl	3.20
Propranolol	3.29
Clobetasol-17-butyrate	3.63
Progesterone	3.87
Propoxyphone	4.18
Mefepristone (Ru 486)	5.48[b]

[a]Adapted from Refs. 21 and 24 and A. Leo Pomona College Medicinal Chemistry Project Data Base (1986).

[b]Calculated from the log *P* of progesterone and the π values of the substituents:

$$\begin{aligned}\log P_{\text{Ru 486}} &= \log P_{\text{progesterone}} - \pi_{CH_3} + \pi_{\text{double bond}} \\ &+ \pi_{(CH_3)2N-} + \pi_{-C_6H_4} - \pi_{-COCH_3} + \pi_{-C\equiv C-} \\ &+ \pi_{CH_3} + \pi_{OH} \\ &= 3.87 - 0.5 - 0.2 + (-0.18) + 1.96 \\ &- (-0.71) + 0.48 + 0.5 + (-1.16) = 5.48\end{aligned}$$

ROYAL PHARMACEUTICAL SOCIETY LIBRARY
1, LAMBETH HIGH STREET, LONDON SE1 7JN

as well as the need of large quantities of materials [39]. Another recently reported method is Tomlinson's filter-probe method [22,40,41], which samples the phase with the larger volume (generally the aqueous phase) and pumps it through a uv detector to monitor the state of equilibrium. A heavy metal probe is attached to the circulating stainless steel tubing with a special filter that prevents entrapment of the unwanted phase. This method is related to the shake-flask method at high phase–volume ratio. It may be useful for unstable compounds and, as a closed system, be used over a wide temperature range [40,41]. Kaufman et al. [42] have reported a microelectrometric titration method for the direct measurement of the pKa and partition and distribution coefficients of narcotics and narcotic antagonists and their pH and temperature dependence. Based on this principle, an automated instrument (PCA 101) is now available for the simultaneous measurement of pKa and log P (Sirius Analytical Instruments Ltd., East Sussex England, RH185AF).

Calculation of Partition Coefficients

Fujita-flask π constant

In 1964 Fujita et al. [43] proposed that log P was an additive-constitutive property and can be calculated by taking the sum of the log P of the parent molecule and the π of the substituent, as in Eqs. (19) to (21).

$$\log P = \Sigma\pi \tag{19}$$

$$\pi_{\text{substituent}} = \log P_{\text{substituted molecule}} - \log P_{\text{parent molecule}} \tag{20}$$

For example:

$$\begin{aligned}\pi_{CH_3} &= \log P_{CH_3C_6H_5} - \log P_{C_6H_6} \\ &= 2.69 - 2.13 = 0.56\end{aligned} \tag{21}$$

$$\begin{aligned}\log P_{Cl(C_6H_4)CH_3} &= \log P_{C_6H_6} + \pi_{Cl} + \pi_{CH_3} \\ &= 2.13 + 0.71 + 0.56 \\ &= 3.40 \text{ (calculated)} \\ &\text{measured value} = 3.33\end{aligned}$$

By definition the π of hydrogen is zero. A scale of the π values of various groups from very hydrophilic to very hydrophobic is shown in Table 2. Extensive compilations of the π constants of various functional groups are available in the literature [18,21].

Rekkers' Fragmental Constant *f*

The fragmental (reductionist) approach of calculating log P was initiated by Rekker and co-workers [20,44,45]. Based on a collection of measured log P values, they applied statistical analysis to determine the average contribution of simple fragments like C, CH, CH_2, CH_3, OH, NH_2, $CONH_2$, OCH_3COOH, etc. (see Table 2). It was found that it was necessary to introduce corrections if two polar groups were separated by only one or two aliphatic carbons. Their postulation is given in Eq. (22).

TABLE 2 The π and *f* Constants for Some Functional Groups[a]

Function *x*	π_x Aromatic System	π_x Aliphatic System	f_x Aromatic System	
			Rekker	Leo-Hansch
H−	0	0	0.18	0.23
F−	0.13	− 0.17	0.42	0.37
Cl−	0.76	0.39	0.93	0.94
Br−	0.94	0.60	1.18	1.09
I−	1.15	1.00	1.47	1.35
CH_3−	0.50	0.50	0.70	0.89
CH≡C−		0.48		
CH_2 = CH−		0.70		
C_2H_5−	1.00	1.00		
$CH_2 = CCH_3$ (with bond ǀ below C)		1.00		
CH_2 = $CHCH_2$−		1.20		
n−C_3H_7−	1.50	1.50		
i−C_3H_7−	1.30	1.30		
n−C_4H_9−	2.00	2.00		
s−C_4H_9−	1.80	1.80		
t−C_4H_9−	1.68	1.68		
cyclo−C_3H_5−		1.21		
cyclo−C_5H_9	2.14	2.14		
cyclo−C_6H_{11}−	2.51	2.51		
Adamantyl	3.30			
C_6H_5−	2.13	2.13	1.89	1.90
−$(CH_2)_3$−	1.04			
−$(CH_2)_4$−	1.39			
−$(CH)_4$−	1.24			
−CF_3	1.07		1.25	1.11
−CH_2OH	− 1.03	− 0.66		
−CH_2COOH	− 0.72	− 0.76		
−COOH	− 0.32	− 1.26	0.00	− 0.03
−COO^-	− 4.36			
−$CONH_2$	− 1.49	− 1.71	− 1.13	− 1.26
−$COOCH_3$	− 0.01	− 0.27		
−$COCH_3$	− 0.55	− 0.71		
−CN	− 0.57	− 0.84	− 0.23	− 0.34
−OH	− 0.67	− 1.16	− 0.36	− 0.44
−OCH_3	− 0.02	− 0.47		
−OCH_2COOH	− 0.86			
−$OCOCH_3$	− 0.64	− 0.91		
−CH=$NNHCONH_2$	− 0.85			
−CH=$NNHCSNH_2$	− 0.27			
−O−β−Glucose	− 2.84			
−NH_2	− 1.23	− 1.19	− 0.90	− 1.00
−$N(CH_3)_2$	− 0.18	− 0.32		
−NO	− 0.12			0.11
−NO_2	− 0.28	− 0.82	− 0.09	− 0.03
−$NHCOCH_3$	− 0.97			
−$NHCOC_6H_5$	0.72			
−N=NC_6H_5	1.69			
−$NHCONH_2$	− 1.01			
−$N(CH_3)_3^+$	− 5.96			

TABLE 2 Continued

Function x	π_x Aromatic System	π_x Aliphatic System	f_x Aromatic System	
			Rekker	Leo-Hansch
$-N_3$	0.46			
$-SH$	0.39	0.28	0.62	0.62
$-SCH_3$	0.62			
$-SCF_3$	1.44			
$-SCCl_3$	1.65			
$-SO_2$				− 2.17
$-SO_2F$				0.30
$-SO_2CH_3$	− 1.26			
$-SO_2CF_3$	0.55			
$-SF_5$	1.55			
$-SO_2NH_2$	− 1.82			− 1.59

[a]Adapted from Refs. 18, 20, 21, and 46.

$$\log P = \Sigma a_n f_n + \Sigma b_m F_m \tag{22}$$

where a = the number of occurrences of fragment f of type n, and
b = the number of occurrences of correction factor F of type m

Leo-Hansch *f* Constant

Hansch and Leo [21] used a constructionist (synthetic) approach by starting with a few carefully measured values of log P of simple structures like H_2 and CH_4 and derived a separate set of fragment constants. The two columns in Table 2 show the slightly different values obtained by the two groups. Different π and f values should be used for an aliphatic system [46].

It is worth noting that although π_H is zero, f_H according to the Rekker's scale is 0.18 and according to the Hansch-Leo scale 0.23. The calculation of log P using the fragment method has been computerized by the Hansch-Leo group [47]. In this CLOGP program all known correction factors have been incorporated. The structure of any compound can be entered by a linear notation called SMILES [48], and by going through a substructure search algorithm GENIE [48] the log P value can be calculated according to Eq. (22). The SMILES program includes all isomerism. For a detailed discussion of this approach, the original references [47,48] should be consulted.

Other Methods

Other published methods [22] of estimating partition coefficients include the use of molecular surface and volume in predicting solubilities and free energies of desolvation, and the application of principal-component analysis based on partition coefficient data. Suzuki and Kudo's CHEMICAL (Combined Handling of Estimation Methods Intended for Completed Automated log P Calculation) [49] as well as a mutidescriptor highly nonlinear regression model proposed by Bodor et al. [50] were applied, where a 10-parameter (15-term) equation was used to correlate with the log P values of 118 compounds of varying complexity. (All the descriptors were derived from AM1 calculation and were related to the surface area, dipole moment value, and charge densities of the molecule.) Some of the terms were raised to 10^4 and 10^2 powers to give the best fit. It is difficult to explain the physical meaning of the highly complex polynomial equation.

Several experts in the field suggest that the ultimate goal of flawless calculation of log *P* has not yet been fully realized [51,52], especially when dealing with a highly complex structure with de novo functional groups.

Physical Factors Contributing to Log *P* or π: Bulk and van der Walls Forces, Dipolar Interactions, and Hydrogen bonding

Over the last two decades, considerable efforts have been devoted to delineate the fundamental nature of partition coefficients (log *P* or π). As a result, many correlations between log *P*(or π) with other structural descriptors or physicochemical parameters have been reported by various investigators. For example, Moriguchi et al. [53,54] dissected log *P* into two intrinsic components, namely molecular volume and polar effect, and showed that the partition coefficient of a nonpolar molecule is a linear function of the volume; for polar molecules, a hydrophilic group effect has to be added as a correction term in the evaluation of log *P*. Kamlet et al. [55,56] correlated log *P* with the solvatochromic parameters π^* and β, which were derived to measure dipolar and hydrogen-bond acceptor strengths of pure bulk solvents as well as the corresponding properties of solutes.

Franke et al. [57] examined the dependence of hydrophobicity on solvent and structure and showed that log *P* values depend on solute bulk and polar and hydrogen-bonding effects. Ou et al. [58] examined the quantitative relationship of log *P* with molecular weight (log *MW*), dipole moment (μ), and hydrogen-bond capability (HB_2) of various compounds. For 222 of 282 compounds, Log *P* values were correlated with these three parameters with a correlation coefficient of 0.938 and standard deviation of 0.492, as shown in Eq. (23).

$$\log P = 5.84 \cdot \log MW - 0.36 \cdot \mu - 0.77 \cdot HB_2 - 8.86 \tag{23}$$
$$n = 222,\ r = 0.938,\ s = 0.492$$

where HB_2 is the sum total of energy decrement in a hydrogen-bond group.

In a similar fashion, Yang et al. [59] reported the general Eq. (24) to be applicable to a wide range of nonpolar and polar substituents (with only a few notable exceptions).

$$\pi = + a \cdot MW \text{ (or } vW) - \text{b} \cdot \text{HB} - \text{C} \cdot \mu + d \tag{24}$$

where vW is the van der Waals volume and HB can be the number of atoms in a group capable of forming H bonds (HB_1), or HB_1 X energy (HB_2).

This general model has been extended to the log *P* of disubstituted aromatic compounds [60] and the solubilities of tetracycline derivatives [61].

Applications

Extraction

In both organic and analytical chemistry laboratories, it is a common procedure to extract a compound from one solvent to another. It is also a common knowledge that it is more efficient to use small volumes and multiple extractions. This is shown by Eqs. (1) and (25) to (27), assuming the two solvents are completely immiscible (e.g., H_2O–CCl_4).

$$P = \frac{C_o}{C_{aq}} = \text{constant } K \tag{1}$$

$$P = \frac{W_o/V_o}{(W - W_o)V_{aq}} \tag{25}$$

or

$$W_o = W\frac{PV_o}{PV_o + V_{aq}} \tag{26}$$

after n extractions

$$W_n = W\left(\frac{PV_o}{PV_o + V_{aq}}\right)n \tag{27}$$

where W is the water phase and V the volume.

If two solvents are partially miscible (e.g., ether–H_2O), the equation provides only approximate values which may still be useful for practical purposes [62].

Preservation of Oil–Water Systems

Many pharmaceutical preparations containing oil–water systems (creams, ointments, or suspensions) are subject to microbial contamination. Bacteria in these heterogenous systems are usually grown in the aqueous phase and at the oil–water interface. To preserve the shelf life of these preparations, benzoic acid or other organic acids are added as preservatives. Since the microbial cell membrane is lipophilic in nature, the bacteriostatic actions of the acidic preservative are due almost entirely to the undissociated acid and not to the ionized form [63]. A good understanding of the partition coefficient and the degree of ionization allows accurate calculation of the free unionized acid in the aqueous phase which provides the bacteriostatic concentration. Specific examples of the calculation can be found in Ref. 62.

Quantitative Structure–Activity Relationships (QSAR)

Since the early work of Hansch et al. [16–18] numerous examples of the quantitative correlation of biological activity with chemical structure have been reported [19,22,24–25,39,43,47,48]. The success of QSAR relies heavily on the use of partition coefficients (log P or π) in extending the linear free-energy relationship (LFER) from homogenous organic chemical systems (i.e., the Hammett-Taft type approach) to compartmentalized heterogenous biological systems.

Further analysis of the physical nature of the partition coefficient reveals that it is a composite property depending on size, shape, dipole moment, and hydrogen-bonding ability. Although many researchers have attempted to replace log P with other simple parameters, only limited success has been achieved for some but not all molecules. It appears that for entirely new complex molecules, it would still be necessary to measure the partition coefficient, preferably validated by the conventional shake-flask method.

Summary

A thorough understanding of partition coefficients is important to all research scientists and product development staff in various branches of the pharmaceutical field. The principle and applications are involved in several different areas of current pharmaceutical interest. These include the techniques of extraction, preservation of oil–water systems, penetration through packaging materials, absorption and distribution of drugs in vivo, protein binding and hemodialysis [64], drug metabolism, enzyme inhibition, drug–receptor interactions, drug-delivery systems, and drug targeting. Since the partition coefficient is a measure of hydrophobic-bonding tendency, and all proteins (enzyme, membrane, plasma, and receptor proteins) [65] contain 20–45% of amino acids with nonpolar groups (e.g., leucine. isoleucine, phenylalanine, tyrosine, tryptophan, etc.) [66], continuing interest in using partition coefficients in correlating biological activity with molecular structure is expected. Other areas of interest in the application of partition coefficient fall beyond the scope of this article. These include analytical chemistry, toxicology, forensic medicine, ecology, and environmental protection [67,68]. Interested readers should consult the biography and references cited.

Since an increasing number of new compounds are being synthesized every day, it is not feasible to have the partition coefficient of every new structure experimentally determined. When a close congener with measured log P value is available, it is easier to use the $\Sigma\pi$ method in calculating the log P of a structurally similar new derivative. On the other hand, for a large number of different structure, the CLOGP method based on the f constant of Hansch and Leo [66] is suitable for obtaining calculated log P values fairly efficiently. Regardless of the method used, it is necessary to measure the log P of a few model compounds for comparison. Many times careful examination of the large deviation between the experimentally measured and the theoretically calculated values can uncover intra- or intermolecular interactions and thus lead to a better understanding of the phenomenon of partitioning of a solute between two immiscible phases saturated with each other.

The initial development of the fragmental constant f by Rekker [44,45] has stimulated that of the systematic CLOGP method. Rekker has further compared the model of partition process with the passage of a ball through a "brick wall," in order to account for a frequently observed "magic number." The model does not take into account the fact that neither 1-octanol nor the aqueous phase consists of homogeneous and ordered "bricks" as depicted in his diagram [20]. At the present time, there is no rigorous theoretical method available for the calculation of log P of a complex de novo structure. Therefore, semi-empirical methods and experimental methods will continue to be employed.

For QSAR analysis, distribution coefficients (D) of ionizable compounds have been used by some investigators [69]. From the mathematical formula of D, it can be demonstrated that it is the same as the apparent partition coefficient (P') and can be easily converted to a true (or corrected) partition coefficient P [70], as shown by Eqs. (28) to (30).

$$D = \frac{[HA]_o}{[HA]_{aq} + [A^-]_{aq}} \tag{28}$$

$$P' = \frac{[HA]_o}{[HA]_{aq} + [A^-]_{aq}} \tag{29}$$

$$\begin{aligned} \frac{D}{(1-\alpha)} &= \frac{[HA]_o}{([HA]_{aq} + [A^-]_{aq})\left(1 - \dfrac{[A^-]_{aq}}{[HA]_{aq} + [A^-]_{aq}}\right)} \\ &= \frac{[HA]_o}{([HA]_{aq} + [A^-]_{aq})\left(\dfrac{[HA]_{aq}}{[HA]_{aq} + [A^-]_{aq}}\right)} \\ &= \frac{[HA]_o}{[HA]_{aq}} = P \end{aligned} \tag{30}$$

If limited data points are available in QSAR analysis, log P' (log D) can be used to account for different degrees of ionization as well as different lipophilicities. If on the other hand, sufficient number of data points are available (more than five data points for each parameter being examined), it will be advantageous to use the log of the [undissociated] vs. [dissociated] ratio log U/D (= pKa − pH for acids, and pH − pKa for bases) as an independent variable as well as log P [71]. This will separate the effect of ionization from that of relative lipophilicity.

Avdeef [72] has recently reported refinement of partition coefficients and ionization constants of multiprotic substances, based on a generalized, weighted, nonlinear least-squares procedure and pH titration curve. This method allows the determination of pKa and log P values of multiprotic substances with fairly close ionization constants.

Bibliography

Dunn, III, W. J., Block, J. H., and Pearlman, R. S., eds. *Partition Coefficient Determination and Estimation*, Pergamon Press, New York, 1987.

Hansch, C., and Leo, A., *Substituent Constants for Correlation Analysis in Chemistry and Biology*, Wiley, New York, 1979.

Leo, A., Hansch, C., and Elkins, D., *Chem. Rev.*, 71:525–616 (1971).

Martin, Y. C., *Quantitative Drug Design*, Marcel Dekker, Inc., New York, 1978.

Mckinney, J. D., ed., Monograph on structure–activity correlation in mechanism studies and predictive toxicology, *Environ. Health Perspec.*, 61 (Sept.):3–349 (1985).

Rekker, R. F., *The Hydrophobic Fragmental Constant*, Elsevier, Amsterdam, 1977.
Rekker, R. F., and Mannhold, R., *Calculation of Drug Lipophilicity*, VCH, Weinheim, Germany 1992.
Rydberg, J., Musikas, C., and Choppin, G. R., eds., *Principles and Practices of Solvent Extraction*, Marcel Dekker, Inc. New York, 1992.

References

1. Berthelot, M., and Jungfleisch, E., *Ann. Chim. Phys.*, 4:26 (1872).
2. Smith, H. W., *J. Phys. Chem.*, 25:204–263 (1921).
3. Collander, R., *Acta Chem. Scand.*, 3:717–747 (1949).
4. Collander, R., *Acta Chem. Scand.*, 4:1085–1098 (1950).
5. Collander, R., *Acta Chem. Scand.*, 5:774–780 (1951).
6. Meyer, H. H., *Arch. Exptl. Pathol. Pharmakol.*, 42:109–118 (1899).
7. Lipnick, R. L., *TIPS*, 10:265–269 (1989).
8. Overton, E., *Z. Physikal. Chem.*, 22:189–209 (1897).
9. Overton, E., *Vierteljahresschr. Naturforsch. Ges. Zürich*, 44:88–135 (1899).
10. Overton, E., *Studien über die Narkose, zugleich ein Beitrag zur allgemeinen Pharmackologie*, Fisher, Jena, Germany, 1901.
11. Lipnick, R. L., *TIPS*, 7:161–164 (1986).
12. Collander, R., *Physiol. Plant*, 7:420 (1954).
13. Cohen, R., and Edsal, J., *Proteins, Amino Acids and Peptides*, Reinhold, New York, 1943, p. 200.
14. Salame, M., *Soc. Plast. Eng. Trans.*, 1:153–163 (1961).
15. Salame, M., and Pinsky, J., *Mod Packag.*, 36:153–156 (1962).
16. Hansch, C., Maloney, P. P., Fujita, T., and Muir R. M., *Nature (London)*, 194:178–180 (1962).
17. Hansch, C., and Fujita, T., *J. Am. Chem. Soc.*, 86:1616–1626 (1964).
18. Leo, A., Hansch, C., and Elkins, D., *Chem. Rev*, 71:525–616 (1971).
19. Purcell, W. P., Bass, G. E., and Clayton, J. M., *Strategy of Drug Design, a Guide to Biological Activity*, Wiley-Interscience, New York, 1973, pp. 1–193.
20. Rekker, R. F., *The Hydrophobic Fragmental Constants*, Elsevier, Amsterdam, 1977, pp. 1–132.
21. Hansch, C., and Leo, A., *Substituent Constants for Correlation Analysis in Chemistry and Biology*, Wiley, New York, 1979, pp. 1–339.
22. Dunn, III, W. J., Block, J. H., and Pearlman, R. S., *Partition Coefficient Determination and Estimation*, Pergamon Press, New York, 1987, pp. 1–154.
23. Nernst, W., *Z. Physical. Chem.*, 8:110–113 (1891).
24. Lien, E. J., *SAR Side Effects and Drug Design*, Marcel Dekker, Inc., New York, 1987, pp. 52–90.
25. Wang, P. H., and Lien, E. J., *J. Pharm. Sci.*, 69:662–668 (1980).
26. Doluisio, J. T., and Swintosky, J. V., *J. Pharm. Sci.*, 53:597–601 (1964).
27. Rosano, H. L., Duby, P., and Schulman, J. H., *J. Phys. Chem.*, 65:1704–1708 (1961).
28. Silverstein, R. M., Bassler, G. C., and Morrill, T. C., *Spectrometric Identification of Organic Compounds*, 5th ed., Wiley, New York, 1991.
29. McNair, H. M., and Borelli, E. J., *Basic Gas Chromatography*, Consolidated Printers, Berkeley, 1968, pp. 1–306.
30. Boltz, D. F., *Chemical Analysis*, Vol. III, *Colorimetric Determinations of Nonmetals*, Interscience Publishers, New York, 1958, pp. 1–372.

31. Bundgaard, H., and Ilver, K., *J. Pharm. Pharmacol.*, 24:790–794 (1972).
32. Carlson, R. M., Carlson, R. E., and Kopperman, H. L., *J. Chromatogr.*, 107:219–223 (1975).
33. Tomlinson, E., Poppe, H., and Kraak, J. C., *Int. J. Pharmaceut.*, 7:225–243 (1981).
34. Unger, S. H., Cheung, P. S., Chiany, G. H., and Cook, J R., RP-HPLC Determination of 1-Octanol Partition and Distribution Coefficients: Experience and Results. In: *Partition Coefficient Determination and Estimation* (W. J. Dunn, III, J. H. Blodker, and R. S. Pearlman, eds.), Pergamon Press, New York, 1987, pp. 69–82.
35. Boyce, C. B. C., and Miborrow, B. V., *Nature*, 208:537–539(1965).
36. Stahl, E., *Thin-layer Chromatography*, Academic Press, London, 1965, pp. 1–510.
37. Reinhardt, H., and Rydberg, J., *Acta Chem. Scand.*, 23:2773–2780 (1969).
38. Davis, S. S., Elson, G., Tomlinson, E., Hanison, G., and Dearden, J. C., *Chem. Ind. (London)*, 1976, pp. 677–683.
39. Taylor, P. J., Hydrophobic Properties of Drugs. In: *Comprehensive Medicinal Chemistry*, Vol. 4 (C. Hansch, P. G. Sammes, and J. B. Taylor, eds.), Pergamon Press, New York, 1991, pp. 272–274.
40. Tomlinson, E., Davis, S. S., Parr, G. D., James, M., Farraj, N., Kinkee, J. M. M., Gaisser, D., and Wynne, H. J., The Filter Probe Extractor: A Versatile Tool for the Rapid Determination of Solute Oil–water Distribution Coefficients. In: *Partition Coefficient Determination and Estimation* (W. J. Dunn, III, J. Block, and R. S. Pearlman, eds.), Pergamon Press, Oxford, 1986, pp. 83–100.
41. Tomlinson, E., *J. Pharm. Sci.*, 71:602–604 (1982).
42. Kaufman, J. J., Semo, N. M., and Koski, W. S., *J. Med. Chem.* 18:647–655 (1975).
43. Fujita, T., Iwasa, J., and Hansch, C., *J. Am. Chem. Soc.*, 86:5175–5180 (1964).
44. Nys, G. G., and Rekker, R. F., *Chim. Thérap.*, 8:521–535 (1973).
45. Rekker, R. F., and Dekort, H. M., *Eur. J. Med. Chim. Ther.*, 14:479–488 (1979).
46. Lien, E. J., Molecular Structure, Properties and States of Matter. In: *Remington's Pharmaceutical Sciences*, 18th ed. (A. R. Gennaro, ed.), Mack Publishing Co., Easton, PA, 1990, pp. 170–171.
47. Leo, A. J., Methods of Calculating Partition Coefficients. In: *Comprehensive Medicinal Chemistry*, Vol. 4 (C. Hansch, P. G. Sammes, and J. B. Taylor, eds.), Pergamon Press, New York, 1990, pp. 295–319.
48. Weininger, D., *J. Chem. Inf. Comput. Sci.*, 28:31 (1988).
49. Suzuki, T., and Kudo, Y. J., *Comput-Aided Mol. Design*, 4:155–198 (1990).
50. Bodor, N., Gabanyi, Z., and Wong, C. K., *J. Am. Chem. Soc.*, 111:3783–3786 (1989).
51. Rekker, R. F., and DeVries, G., A Basic Confrontation of Rekker's Revised Sf-system with HPLC-retention Data Obtained on a Mixed Series of Aliphatic and Aromatic Hydrocarbons. In: *9th Europ. Symp. on SAR:QSAR and Molecular Modelling*, Strasbourg, Sept. 1992, Abs. p. 38.
52. Mannhold, R., Rekker, R. F., and ter Laak, A. M., Calculated Log P Values: Are They Reliable? In: *9th Europ. Symp. on SAR:QSAR and Molecular Modelling*, Strasbourg, Sept, 1992, Abs. p. 44.
53. Moriguchi, I., *Chem. Pharm. Bull.*, 23:247–257 (1975).
54. Moriguchi, I., Kanada, Y., and Komatsu, K., *Chem. Pharm. Bull.*, 24:1799–1806 (1976).
55. Kamlet, M. J., Abraham, M. H., Doherty, R. M., and Taft, R. W., *J. Am. Chem. Soc.*, 106:464–466 (1984).
56. Kamlet, M. J., Abboud, J. L. M., Abraham, M. H., and Taft, R. W., *J. Org. Chem.*, 48:2877–2887 (1983).
57. Franke, R., Kuhne, R., and Dove, S., Dependence of Hydrophobicity on Solvent and Structure. In: *Quantitative Approaches* (J. C. Dearden, ed.), Elsevier, Amsterdam, 1983, pp. 15–32.
58. Ou, X. C., Ouyang, Y., and Lien, E. J., *J. Mol. Sci. (Wuhan, China)*, 4:89–95 (1986).

59. Yang, G. Z., Lien, E. J., and Guo, Z. R., *Quant. Struct.–Act. Relat.*, 5:12–18 (1986).
60. Lien, E. J., Gao, H., Wang, F. Z., and Shinouda, H. G., Partition Behaviors of Solvents, Drugs and Chemicals. In: *9th Europ. Symp. on SAR:QSAR and Molecular Modelling*, Strasbourg, Sept. 1992, Abs. p. 115.
61. Lien, E. J., Banerjee, S., Khan, A., Gao, H., and Wang, F. Z., Dipolar, Hydrogen Bonding and van der Waals Forces and their Contributions to the Partition Coefficients and Solubilities of Chemicals and Drugs. In: *9th Europ. Symp. on SAR:QSAR and Molecular Modelling, Strasbourg*, Sept. 1992, Abs. p. 14.
62. Martin, A., Swarbrick, J., and Cammarata, A., *Physical Pharmacy*, 3rd ed., Lea & Febiger, Philadelphia, 1983, pp. 306–308.
63. Rahn, O., and Conn, J. E., *Ind. Eng. Chem.*, 36:185–187 (1944).
64. Schreiner, G. E., *Drug Intell.*, 5:322–339 (1971).
65. Putnam, F. W., Structure and Function of Plasma Proteins. In: *The Proteins*, 2nd ed., Vol. III (H. Neurath, ed.), Academic Press, New York, 1965, pp. 154–253.
66. Leo, A. J., Hydrophobic Parameter: Measurement and Calculation. In: *Methods in Enzymology*, Vol. 202 (J. J. Langone, ed.), Academic Press, New York, 1991, pp. 544–591.
67. Draber, W., and Fujita, T., eds., *Rational Approaches to Structure, Activity and Ecotoxicology of Agrochemicals*, CRC Press, Boca Raton, FL, 1992.
68. Hermens, J. L. M., and Operhuizen, A., eds., *QSAR in Environmental Toxicology*-IV, Elsevier, Amsterdam, 1991.
69. Scherrer, R. A., and Howard, S. M., *J. Med. Chem.*, 20:53–58 (1977).
70. Alhaider, A. A., Selassie, C. D., Chua, S. O., and Lien, E. J., *J. Pharm. Sci.*, 71:89–94 (1982).
71. Lien, E. J., The Relationship Between Chemical Structure and Drug Absorption, Distribution, and Excretion. In: *Medicinal Chemistry*, IV, *Proceedings of the 4th International Symposium of Medicinal Chemistry* (J. Maas, ed.), Elsevier, Amsterdam, 1974, pp. 319–342.
72. Avdeef, A., *J. Pharm. Sci.*, 82:183–190 (1993).

ERIC J. LIEN

Patents in the Pharmaceutical Industry

The only thing that keeps us alive
is our brilliance.
The only thing protecting
our brilliance
is our patents.
Edwin H. Land, 1976

This statement from the inventor of the instant camera was made at the time Polaroid Corporation instituted patent litigation against Kodak at Kodak's introduction of their instant camera system. Although hidden within this quotation is the metaphor referring to the brilliant colors of their color photographic process, the statement would seem to apply equally well to the pharmaceutical industry. Its success has been based upon the discovery of new products which treat human disease states in new and unique ways. The patent system has provided protection for these innovative products for a period of time, allowing the industry to use the revenues gained to search for the next generation of products which will improve the health of society.

What is a Patent?

A patent is a grant by a government of exclusive rights to an inventor for his invention in exchange for the inventor disclosing his invention to society. This quid pro quo is valuable to society as the disclosure stimulates further innovation and development. The alternative for the inventor is to keep his invention secret and so deprive society of the opportunity for further advancement.

Patent rights are limited in time and are also limited to the sole right of excluding others from making, using, and selling the invention. Since these rights are granted by governments, they are effective only in the area controlled by that government. Thus, a United States patent provides protection only for the United States and its territories, such as Puerto Rico. If the inventor desires protection in Japan, Canada, or any of the European countries, he must apply for a patent in each of these countries as well.

It is important to understand that this right granted by the patent is solely a right to exclude others. It does not carry with it the right to practice the invention by the inventor himself. This right to use by the inventor may be limited by the existence of other patents which would need to be used in order to practice his invention or by laws or regulations having nothing to do with patents. Examples of the latter are the health registration regulations present in the countries where pharmaceutical products are being sold. An inventor not being free to use his invention because of patents owned by others is also a common situation. For example, Party X may have a patent claiming a broad genus of compounds useful to treat hypertension. An inventor discovers a specific compound not disclosed specifically in the patent of Party X but through selection of the appropriate substituents in the defined genus this compound can be found. Its hypertensive properties are far superior to those of the compounds disclosed in Party X's patent. This inventor can obtain a patent for the compound in question but must obtain permission from Party X before marketing because of the patent of Party X.

Patents belong to a class of property referred to as "intellectual property." Included are not only patents but also trade secrets, trademarks, registered designs, and copyrights.

A trade secret is any information unknown to the public but which gives the owner an economic or competitive advantage. Trade secrets have value only as long as they remain secret, which is difficult in this modern day. Within the pharmaceutical industry, it is rare for any invention to be maintained as a trade secret because the most important inventions are those which can be easily "reverse engineered" or identified by competitors in the field. However, occasionally an invention, such as a process improvement, may be held as a trade secret if it is such that it cannot be discovered by analysis or study of the product which is sold. If a patent was obtained, the world would be informed of the improvement; however, the patent owner would be in a very difficult position to determine if anyone was using the patented invention without special permission.

A trademark is a word, name, or symbol which identifies the source of the goods to which it is attached. The same product can be sold by two or more companies but the public can identify each company's goods by the trademark. Pharmaceutical products available from multisources carry the same generic name but also the unique trademark of the specific seller; an example is the Tagamet® brand of cimetidine. Trademarks carry the "good will" developed by the owner and last as long as they are used and protected by owner. Aspirin was a trademark at one time but is now generic.

A copyright protects the creation of artists and authors. Within the pharmaceutical industry copyrights are used to protect advertisements, product literature, and other copy used for product promotion.

The patent system traces its history back to the early days in Venice when the government provided traders with exclusive rights in various fields. Patents for inventions were granted in Venice at least as early as 1460. The Anglo-American systems found their basis in Great Britain where parliament enacted the Statute of Monopolies in 1624. This law provided the basis for the British patent system for many years. From the 1400s to 1700s, inventors were granted patents not only for inventions as known today but also for new articles that were brought into the country for the first time.

The American colonies, before achieving independence, had no power to grant patents for inventions under the British system. The Massachusetts legislature in 1621 did enact a law giving exclusive rights to persons who introduced new industries into the colonies. South Carolina in 1784 enacted a statute providing for protection of inventions for 14 years. The basic U.S. patent system rests on one of the powers given to Congress in the United States Constitution. Article I, Section 8, gives Congress the power "to promote the progress of science and useful arts by securing for limited times to authors and inventors the exclusive right to their respective writings and discoveries." The first patent and copyright act of the United States was enacted on April 10, 1790.

Patents and Pharmaceuticals

Over the years, the patent system, as applied to pharmaceuticals, has been an area of great controversy. Many countries, especially those with few technology-based industries, have held that providing protection for drug products is against society's interest.

Some countries include food within this category as well. Based on this theory, patents for pharmaceutical products have been limited or not allowed at all. The limitation generally provided is that chemical compounds can be claimed only by the process of their preparation. Thus, if someone develops a different process to make the compound, they have avoided the patent to the innovator. Some "process protection" countries further weaken the protection by placing the burden of proving the process used by infringers on the patent owners. Others have what is referred to as "reversal of proof," where, if the product is new, the infringer is assumed to be using the patent owner's process and must prove that he or she is not using it.

As a country becomes more industrialized, it strengthens its patent system by providing protection for compounds per se, often referred to as "product protection." Examples are Germany and Japan which had process protection for pharmaceutical products until 1968 and 1978, respectively, when they amended their laws to provide product protection. China had no patent law until June 1, 1985. At that time, pharmaceuticals were given only process protection. Effective January 1, 1993, China amended its patent laws to allow product protection.

In summary, patent protection for pharmaceutical products has improved significantly over the last ten years. Countries where no patents could be obtained have put patent laws into effect and process-protection-only countries have changed to allow product protection. Countries have lengthened the patent term to 20 years from a shorter term. Some of these changes have been the result of pressure from the U.S. Government on other countries to improve their intellectual properties right or be subject to sanctions under U.S. trade regulations.

New compounds are not the only inventions important to the pharmaceutical industry. Many products have been developed from natural sources, such as extracts from plants or compounds isolated from fermentation broths from various microorganisms. Protecting these inventions has been difficult at times in various countries due to the fact that the materials were present in nature and thus were viewed as natural products and not new or novel. These difficulties can be overcome in certain cases by claiming the compounds in their pure form.

With regard to compounds made by fermentation, these may also be claimed as new compounds or as products made by a certain fermentation process. However, claiming of the microorganism per se has changed in recent years. Prior to the arrival of biotechnology methods, microorganisms were generally not patentable. However, compounds produced by these "factories" were patentable provided the patent application contained a morphological description of the organism and a sample of the organism was deposited with a national depository in order to make samples available to others. The microorganisms themselves were viewed as unpatentable, because they are obtained by random selection from soil or other sources, and the inventor has difficulty describing how to reproduce the invention. This was also true where the organism was made by a random mutation process since it was impossible for another researcher to reproduce the results with predictability.

Patenting of "living matter" changed dramatically with the arrival of biotechnology methods and procedures. In 1980, the famous Diamond vs. Chakrabarty case was decided by the U.S. Supreme Court. In this case, a new strain of bacteria, produced by a reproducible artificial procedure, had the ability to digest oil and thus was useful in dispersing oil slicks. It was important to have patent protection on the bacteria per se because they were used themselves and not in a process to produce another product. Certain groups and individuals in the public sector expressed great concern that this decision would lead to patenting other higher forms of life. Only a few cases of higher life forms exist as of today. One is the "Harvard mouse" which was patented in U.S. Patent No. 4,736,866 (1988). This transgenic mouse has the special property of having an oncogene sequence in the germ and somatic cells which make the mouse useful in testing for carcinogenic materials or for compounds that confer protection against neoplasms.

International Treaties and Systems

As noted earlier, patent protection is obtained on a country-by-country basis and therefore applications must be filed in each country where protection is desired in order to obtain worldwide protection. International treaties and regional conventions have been set up to coordinate worldwide protection and make it convenient and efficient. Several important treaties have been developed and are administered by the international organization known as the World Intellectual Property Organization (WIPO) located in Geneva, Switzerland.

Paris Convention

The Paris Convention for the Protection of Industrial Property was first signed in Paris in 1883 by 11 countries and has been revised several times over the years. Today it is ratified by more than 107 countries. A notable country of concern to the pharmaceutical industry which is not a member of the Paris Convention is Taiwan.

The important feature of the Paris Convention is allowing an applicant to claim priority to his first-filed application in any member country, provided the applicant files a patent application in that country within one year. This is referred to as convention priority and is of great importance in the patent strategies developed within the pharmaceutical industry. These strategies are more clearly described below. If the first application meets the conditions of the Convention, the applications in all member countries are treated as if they were filed on the same day as the first application. The one-year period is a rigid date which must be adhered to with the exception that when the convention year ends on a Saturday, Sunday, or a public holiday, the application may be filed on the next working day.

Budapest Treaty

When an invention involves a microorganism, most countries require that disclosure be completed by the deposition of the biological material. The WIPO established international uniformity under the Budapest Treaty of 1977 which came into force in 1980. This treaty has been ratified by 24 countries plus the European Patent Office. It provides for the establishment of a group of international deposit authorities. When a strain of microorganisms is deposited in any one of these authorities, this single deposit satisfies the necessary requirements for all countries which are a signatory of this treaty. Under this convention, the formal requirements for making the deposit and maintaining the culture are set forth. Included within this is the possibility of a redeposit, should the initial deposit become nonviable. The maintenance of the deposit is for a minimum time of 30 years from the date of deposit.

Patent Cooperation Treaty

An important recent development is the Patent Cooperation Treaty (PCT) which is administered by WIPO. This treaty first came into force in January 1978, and is today an extremely useful convention in the patent-filing strategy for much of the pharmaceutical industry. As of October 1, 1993, it is in effect in 60 countries. Included are the United States, all the countries of the European Patent Convention, Japan, and Canada; China joins on January 1, 1994.

This treaty puts forth a process in which an applicant, through a simplified procedure, can file one application and designate that it be treated as an application in one or up to all of the PCT member countries. This application is filed in one of the official receiving offices in any of the official languages, English, German, French, Japanese, Russian, Spanish and, as of January 1994, Chinese. The PCT is offering a very important mechanism within the pharmaceutical industry in providing an efficient means of obtaining maximum patent protection around the world in the most efficient and cost effective manner.

The PCT application can be filed under the terms of the Paris Convention at the end of the one-year period from the priority filing. The receiving office passes an application on to an international searching authority where a search for the novelty of the invention is carried out. The application, together with the search report, is published 18 months from the priority date. After this publication, the applicant can choose two avenues for the application. First, if he or she wishes to proceed directly to each of the designated countries, the filing can be perfected in each of the designated countries within 20 months of the priority date by submitting the required formal documents and translations which are combined in each local patent office with a copy of the PCT application received from WIPO. Alternatively, by the end of 19 months, a "demand" can be filed that a preliminary examination on patentability be carried out by the Preliminary Examining Authority of the PCT. This examination occurs between the 19th and 30th month from the priority date. During this period, the applicant receives from the Preliminary Examining Authority the results of the examination and has the opportunity to present arguments and/or amend the claims. Before the end of 30 months from the priority date, WIPO sends the application, search report, and results of the preliminary examination to each of the designated National Patent Offices. If the applicant wishes to continue to maintain an application in these countries, all documents and translations required by that country must be submitted by the end of the 30th month to perfect the national filing.

The main advantage of the PCT process is that it allows the applicant time to more clearly determine the commercial viability and importance of his invention. In the pharmaceutical industry, patents are filed on new potential products very early in their development. Many of these fall by the wayside during the development process. The PCT allows for an application to be filed and maintained with minimum expense up to the 30th month before the significant expenses of national filing fees and translations are required. Thus, under a strategy using the PCT, the pharmaceutical company can maintain patent applications for the major economically important countries of the world at minimum cost while having 30 months in which to study the invention and determine its commercial potential.

The treaty has been gaining in popularity and use in recent years. In 1992, the PCT was used to file 25,917 applications as compared to 4,675 in 1982 and 459 in 1978.

European Patent Convention

A regional system is one that arises from a regional treaty entered into by a number of countries within a geographic area. The European Patent Convention (EPC) is the most important of several regional patent systems. It was negotiated by a number of European countries and entered into force on October 7, 1977, with the formation of the European Patent Organization (EPO). This convention was ratified by eight countries by the time the European Patent Office began accepting applications on June 1, 1978; 17 countries have ratified the EPC as of January, 1993.

Under the EPC, an applicant can file one application in the European Patent Office and designate in which of the 17 countries the application should have effect. If, after examination by the European Patent Office, the invention is found patentable, the application is granted. This grant is not as a single patent but as a national patent in each country designated by the applicant at the time of filing. At the time of grant, if the applicant wishes to validate the patent in the designated countries, translations need to be filed in the individual countries as appropriate. Enforcement and challenges to the validity of the patent take place in each country under the national patent laws of that country. Under the EPC, a challenge can be made within nine months of the patent grant. This procedure is referred to as an opposition and is still administered within the European Patent Office.

This convention provides an efficient means of obtaining patent protection in up to 17 countries through the filing and prosecution of only one application. When the EPC first went into effect, there was concern that if the prosecution was unfavorable, the applicant would not have any patent protection, whereas under the national systems, patents would have been granted. With the passage of time, this concern has been greatly diminished and now the convention is used by most, if not all, within the pharmaceutical industry.

Other Regional Systems

There are two regional systems for countries in Africa. They are the African Regional Industrial Property Organization (ARIPO), formed in 1976, and the African Intellectual Property Organization (OAPI), formed in 1962. Each system has 14 member states.

Another regional system, which has, however, not yet gone into effect, is the European Community Patent. This system would cover all members of the European Economic Community (EC). It differs from the EPC in that one application would be filed which would result in one patent covering all EC countries. In order to go into effect, this treaty must be ratified by all the EC members. This has not happened yet and may happen only as the EC moves to a single market economy.

Claimable Inventions in the Pharmaceutical Area

Section 101 of the U.S. Patent Law defines inventions and discoveries for which a patent can be obtained in very broad terms. Specifically, these are processes, machines, articles of manufacture, and compositions of matter, or any new and useful improvements of these. Article 52 of the European Patent Convention states that a patent shall be granted for any invention which meets the three requirements for patentability. It then lists exclusions which include "scientific theories and mathematic methods," in addition to medical treatments as noted below. Many different inventions arising out of research in the pharmaceutical field can be protected under these broad definitions.

Chemical Inventions

Within the pharmaceutical field, chemical inventions have become of primary importance. The traditional inventions for which the pharmaceutical industry has sought patents are shown below.

Potential Chemical Inventions

- Compound per se
- Pharmaceutical compositions of new compounds
- New pharmaceutical compositions of old compounds
- Method of treatment, mechanistically or by disease state or both
- Compound for use (broad first use)
- New medical use for old compound (second use)
- Analogy processes for new compounds
- Process per se (when novel and inventive)
- Intermediates
- Processes for preparing compositions
- Different salt forms, hydrates, or polymorphs

Specifically, new compositions of matter (NCM) (new chemical compounds) prepared by synthetic methods are the primary area of interest. They may be made by synthetic methods or isolated from natural sources such as plant or oceanic material or from fermentation broths. At times a compound is known in an impure state which is unusable as a pharmaceutical product. If it is obtained in a purified state and meets the requirements of patentability, it can be claimed as a compound of a defined purity.

In addition to the compound per se, chemical processes for the preparation of the compound can be claimed. In the United States, proving patentability of a process is difficult when the process is a known chemical reaction which produces an old or new compound or uses new starting materials. These processes, known as analogous processes, have varied standards of patentability in different countries.

Pharmaceutical compositions of new compounds or new improved formulations of old compounds are also patentable. For a new drug-delivery system, patent protection can be very important and useful.

A method of treating a particular disease or physiological condition is another important type of invention in the pharmaceutical field. It may be necessary to claim this type of invention by what is called "Swiss claims" in order to overcome the industrial applicability requirement in Europe. In the United States, the applicant may be required to provide proof to support the treatment claim. This is especially true if the invention is treating a disease which has been difficult or impossible to treat in the past, such as cancer or AIDS. A claim to a method of treating cancer with a certain compound will be challenged during examination. The most likely result will be an amendment of the claim to a method of treating specific cancers for which data can be provided to demonstrate utility.

Biotechnology Inventions

With the blossoming of the biotechnology area, a whole new specialty in patent law has developed since approximately 1980. In general, it is viewed that the principles of chemical patent practice apply equally well to the biotechnology field. The Court of Appeals for the Federal Circuit (the U.S. Federal Court that hears all patent appeals from the patent office and federal district courts) has stated this in their decisions. Biotechnology inventions must satisfy the standard statutory requirements in the same way as any other invention. From the list of claimable inventions shown below, it is clear that biotechnology techniques have resulted in the production of inventions previously not obtainable by classical chemical methods.

Potential Biotechnology Inventions

Recombinant

- The protein per se
- Antibodies reacting specifically with the protein and anti-idiotype antibodies
- rDNA encoding the protein
- Expression systems
- Recombinant host cells containing the DNA
- Processes to make protein using recombinant host cells
- Processes for purifying the protein
- Processes to produce the antibody and anti-idiotype antibodies
- Methods of using the DNA sequence
- Pharmaceutical compositions of the protein
- Method of treatment

Monoclonal Antibodies

- Monoclonal antibody (Mab)
- Hybridoma producing Mab
- Process to prepare Mab
- Method to use the Mab
- Pharmaceutical composition of the Mab
- Novel antigen and related processes and methods

Requirements For Patentability

There are three basic requirements for patentability: novelty, nonobviousness or inventive step, and usefulness or industrial applicability. Each requirement may differ from country to country and is set forth by the statutes and regulations of each country.

Novelty

The first principle of patent law is that in order to obtain a patent, the invention must be new. The statutory requirements of novelty are set forth in Section 102 of the U.S. Patent Law and Article 54 of the European Patent Convention.

In the United States, Section 102 has several stated requirements. The first one is that the invention must not have been known or used by others in the United States or patented or described in a printed publication in the United States or any foreign country before the invention was made by the applicant. The second provision is that the invention must not have been patented or described in any printed publication anywhere in the world more than one year prior to the date of the application in the United States. This is the one-year grace period available in the United States but not in the rest of the world. These requirements are grouped under the term ''anticipation'' and mean that a single prior-art reference must show the invention being claimed in order to nullify novelty. If an essential part of the invention is not present in a single publication but is found in a second reference, anticipation does not exist (however, see the next section on obviousness.)

Article 54 of the EPC says an invention is ''new if it does not form part of the state of the art.'' It goes on to say that the state of the art comprises '' . . . everything made available to the public by means of a written or oral description, by use or in any other way before the date of filing . . . ''.

What constitutes prior art also varies from country to country. Novelty requirements of most countries can be classified as either absolute or relative. Absolute novelty means prior publications or public use or knowledge of the invention anywhere prior to filing the patent application. Relative novelty is divided in two classes: (1) prior publication anywhere or local public use, and (2) both prior publication or public use in the local country. In a country with local novelty it may be necessary to determine what was available in the country and when was it available in order to determine if the invention is novel. This may be difficult to determine.

In the United States, a ''printed publication'' is a publication which is available to the public. In a case dealing with a single thesis, the court found the thesis was a printed publication because the single copy was catalogued and available to the public in a library.

Nonobvious or Inventive Step

The requirement of nonobviousness, or inventive step as it is referred to in Europe, is the one which provides the most difficulty during the examination process in most cases. It is governed by Section 103 of the U.S. law and Article 56 of the European Convention. The general principle is that even though an invention is novel, the inventor is not entitled to a patent unless he or she has done something more than one would expect an ordinary person in the art or field to which the invention pertains to have been able to do. Two or more references can be used to make the case of what would have been obvious to the mythical person skilled in the art. In pharmaceutical art, chemical compounds are often known which are very close structurally and/or have similar utilities to the compounds claimed in the application. In these situations, the hurdle of proving nonobviousness is one of most concern during the examination process.

In the United States, the Supreme Court set forth a test for determining obviousness. It demands inquiry into the following facts:

1. The scope and content of the prior art,
2. The differences between the prior art and the patent claims in question,
3. The level of ordinary skill in the art, and
4. Whatever objective evidence may be present.

Objective evidence is viewed as a secondary consideration and may include such issues as commercial success, long-felt unsolved needs, failure of others, etc. The U.S. courts have further held that compounds and their properties are inseparable for purpose of patent law inquiry. Thus, if the compounds being claimed show superior and unexpected properties over similarly disclosed compounds, the invention will be found to be nonobvious.

Usefulness or Industrial Applicability

This requirement is covered by Section 101 of the U.S. Patent Law and Article 57 of the European Patent Convention.

In the United States, usefulness is a very broad concept and does not mean a commercial utility is in hand. In the pharmaceutical field, a showing of in vitro test results which have some nexus with treating a physiological condition is sufficient to meet this requirement. If, however, the invention is useful only as a scientific curiosity, this requirement is not met. Chemical intermediates may or may not have the required usefulness. If they are useful to prepare products which are themselves useful, they are patentable. However, intermediates are not patentable if they are useful only to prepare compounds with no utility.

In Europe, industrial applicability is required. The means, for example, that methods of medical treatment or diagnosis which are performed on a human or an animal are not capable of industrial application. Nevertheless, substances that are useful in these methods are patentable.

Obtaining A Patent

When an invention is made, a decision must be taken as to whether to obtain patent protection. The alternative to patent protection is maintaining the information as a trade secret.

After it has been decided to obtain patent protection, a patent application is prepared and filed. This first filing is referred to as a priority filing and the filing date as the priority date. This is the date against which the invention will be judged for purposes of determining whether a patent should be granted, as discussed above.

Filing Applications

The first patent application is usually filed in the home country of the inventors. Many countries have laws and/or regulations that require this or, if the inventor wants to file in another country first, certain requirements must be met. In the United States, there are regulations against exporting technology to other countries without government approval. An invention made in the United States must be filed first in the United States and not filed in any foreign country for six months after this filing without obtaining an export license from the U.S. Patent Office. If the applicant wishes to file first in another country, he or she must submit the application to the U.S. Patent Office and obtain this export license prior to filing in that country.

After the priority application is filed, the applicant must make what is often referred to as the foreign filing decision. This decision concerns in what additional countries the application should be filed during the 12-month convention period available under the Paris Convention. The cost of protecting the invention is directly proportional to the number of applications filed and the different language translations required by these filings. In these times of cost consciousness, the foreign filing decision is one which is not taken lightly.

Several options are available to the applicant at this time. The first is to obtain a patent only in the home country and not pursue patent protection elsewhere. The second possibility would be to proceed with foreign filing in one or more countries within the convention year. A final option would be to abandon the home country application and not pursue patent protection. An alternative strategy similar to this would be to abandon the first application and refile an application in the home country, thereby starting the 12-month convention period over again.

The choice among these options depends on many factors. If the invention is completely or almost completely understood and its commercial potential known, the decision as to which countries to file in can be made without much difficulty. Most pharmaceutical companies have listings of "filing groups" of countries, which are used depending on the projected commercial potential for the invention. These filing groups may contain a few major countries up to a large number of countries (30 to 50 countries or more). Each company develops its own set of filing groups based on numerous factors, including costs, strength of protection in each country, the company's markets, etc. Likewise, the selection of the filing group for each particular invention depends on factors such as type of invention, perceived commercial potential, projected market areas, and the like.

Alternatively, if the invention and its commercial potential is not fully understood, the applicant could abandon or abandon and refile. This process carries with it the danger that someone else may have filed a patent application between the applicant's priority date and the second priority date obtained through the refiling process. If this has occurred, the applicant has lost the rights to the invention in most countries of the world. This can be especially risky in highly competitive areas in which many people are conducting research.

An alternative strategy is to file the foreign applications under the provisions of the Patent Cooperation Treaty and through its provisions obtain an additional 18 months before significant costs of filing fees and translations would be incurred (see discussion under PCT.)

Even after the 12-month priority year has passed, the applicant may still file patent applications, provided that there has been no publication or public use of his invention. Applications filed in many countries, including the EPO and PCT, are published 18 months after the priority date. If the application has not been published and the applicant has not published in any scientific journal, he or she can still file within a country and obtain a patent. This is called a nonconvention filing because the applicant does not claim rights back to his first priority date. Therefore, if new information becomes available between the 12 and 18 month relating to the commercial potential of the invention, it should always be reviewed carefully and a decision made if nonconvention applications should be filed.

Examination of the Application

Once an application has been filed, each patent office examines it before granting a patent. The completeness of this examination differs from country to country. In some countries, it is a matter of merely checking if the application has all the proper formal papers required under the laws and regulations of that country. Other countries follow a rigorous examination as to the patentability of the invention, in addition to the formal matters of proper documents. The United States and European Patent Offices examine patent applications for all requirements of patentability. The U.S. PTO has set a goal of granting patents within approximately 18 months of filing, although biotechnology applications take much longer due to a large backlog. Currently, the European Patent Office starts the examination process approximately two to three years after the application is filed. Japan employs a deferred examination process. An application filed in the Japanese Patent Office lies dormant until the applicant requests the patent office to examine it. This request can be deferred up to seven years from the filing date. Once requested, the examination process in Japan normally takes two to three years to complete. On occasion this process can take significantly longer because Japan has a pregrant opposition system. This means that once the patent office makes a determination to grant an application, it is published and within 90 days of that publication date anyone may file an opposition to its grant. In this case, a lengthy proceeding can ensue, deferring the grant of the patent for many years.

Content of a Patent Application

Each country, through its laws and regulations, sets forth the requirements for a patent application. The United States uses Section 112 of the patent law for this purpose. It states that the application contains two parts: the specification and the claims. The requirements of the specification are set forth in the first paragraph of Section 112 as follows:

> The specification shall contain a written description of the invention and the manner and process of making and using it in such full, clear, concise and exact terms as to enable any person skilled in the art to which it pertains or with which it is most nearly connected to make and use the same and shall set forth the best mode contemplated by the inventor of carrying out his invention.

To summarize, there are three requirements: a written description, an enabling disclosure, and the best mode. A written description and an enabling disclosure are universal requirements. However, the best mode requirement is distinctive to the U.S. patent system and is one which causes much debate among patent practitioners. It is based on the theory that an applicant should not receive the privileges of patent protection if he or she has not disclosed the best methods of making and using the invention known to him at the time the patent application is filed. If the applicant fails to disclose the best mode, even unintentionally, the patent can be declared invalid.

Based on these disclosure requirements, the application normally contains the following:

1. An abstract,
2. A summary of the background useful in understanding the invention,
3. A summary of the invention, and
4. A detailed description of how to practice the invention including appropriate examples and any drawings.

The second paragraph of Section 112 requires that the applicant point out and distinctly claim the invention with a set of claims. Up to this point, a patent application has been a scientific paper which instructs other people in the same field how to make and use what the inventor has discovered. This is no different than a scientific journal article. The claims, however, set forth what the applicant considers to be the invention and for which patent protection is sought. During the examination process, the claims may be modified in order to overcome objections; therefore, as a result of the examination process, the allowed claims of a granted patent often define less subject matter than is disclosed in the specification. Since the claims define the subject matter protected by the patent, when asked a question regarding infringement, a patent attorney will turn immediately to the claims to begin his analysis as opposed to looking at the description within the specification.

Ownership

Patents are property whose ownership may be governed by law, contract, or statutory provision. In many employer–employee relationships a contract of employment has been signed by the employee. This contract states that the employer owns all inventions made by the employee. In some countries, most notably Germany, there are elaborate statutory provisions for compensation of inventors by the employer. In all countries, except the United States, the owner of the patent rights may file the patent application. The U.S. system has been based historically upon rewarding the inventor and therefore requires the inventor to apply for the patent. If the inventor is required by the contract of employment to assign inventions to the employer, the U.S. application is made in the inventor's name and an assignment noting transfer of rights to the employer is recorded in the patent office.

Inventorship

Throughout most of the world, inventorship of a patent may be relevant to the question of who owns the rights but not relevant to the validity of the patent. In fact, in some countries the inventor may never be mentioned or even appear on the patent. The one important exception is again the United States, where, as was noted above, the inventor or inventors must file the patent application. If the wrong inventor or inventors intentionally apply for the patent, this is grounds for declaring the patent invalid. Therefore, the proper inventors of the claimed invention are always determined according to the requirements of the U.S. law.

It must always be remembered that inventorship is different from authorship. Inventorship is based on legal requirements and must be followed strictly whereas authorship is more arbitrary. The determination of inventorship is based upon looking first at the invention and determining what person or persons made an "inventive" contribution to the conception and reduction to practice of this invention. Conception includes the mental steps taken at developing the invention. Reduction to practice is the physical process of taking the idea to the completed working invention. When two or more inventors, called joint inventors, are involved, each must contribute to the claimed invention but each does not have to have made a contribution to each claim.

Determination of inventorship is not always straight forward and simple in today's research environment. However, in order to make correct determinations, certain questions are asked. Did the alleged inventor do only routine work or experiments as directed by another or did he or she contribute something additional? Was the invention completed because of the specific activity of this person? Did this person proceed beyond specific directions? In today's modern pharmaceutical research atmosphere, where teams are involved in the discovery and development processes, the patent attorney may find the determination of the correct inventorship a very difficult aspect in preparation of a patent application. In a 1972 decision, where the issue of inventorship was in dispute, U.S. District Court Judge Newcomer made the following observation:

> The exact parameters of what constitutes joint inventorship are quite difficult to define. It is one of the muddiest concepts in the muddy metaphysics of patent law.

When Two or More Inventors Make the Same Invention

Some times two or more inventors make the same invention. Since only one patent will be issued, the question is who is granted the patent.

In all countries, except in the United States, the first to file a patent application is granted the patent for the invention. In the United States, the patent is granted to the first to make the invention. These two systems, "first to file" and "first to invent," are currently being debated as part of negotiations to harmonize patent systems throughout the world via a new WIPO-administered treaty.

In the United States, the first inventor is determined by a special administrative proceeding in the patent office called an interference. Evidence is presented by each applicant as to their earliest dates of conception and reduction to practice. Only activities in the United States can be used in these proofs. However, when the North American Free Trade Treaty becomes effective, activities in Mexico and Canada can also be used. The general rule is: the first to reduce the invention to practice is awarded the patent. The exception is when one applicant was first to conceive the invention but was last to reduce it to practice. This applicant will be granted the patent if he or she can prove diligence in activities to reduction to practice from the time just before the other party began activity until his or her completion of the invention.

In an interference, the proof requirements are very important. Activities or evidence given by the inventor or inventors must be collaborated in some manner. This is best done by evidence from noninventors although other forms of evidence have been successfully used in some cases. For this reason, research organizations institute policies and procedures governing notebook record keeping within their research laboratories. Frequently this policy consists of witnessing of research notebooks and written conception disclosures as a means of providing collaboration in an interference.

Interferences are very complex and expensive proceedings which can delay the grant of a patent for many years. Fortunately only less than 0.5% of all U.S. patent applications are involved in an interference. Nevertheless, the debate about changing the law from "first to invent" to "first to file" is a highly emotional issue because this law has been a part of the U.S. system for a long time. It may happen, however, as part of the global harmonization process.

Length of Patent Protection

The term of a grant of a patent is defined by the laws of each country, varying generally from 15 to 20 years. In some developing countries, patent terms are much shorter and are of little value to the pharmaceutical industry because the patent expires before the product can be marketed. Recently, most countries have adopted a standard patent life of 20 years from the date of filing. The notable exception is the United States where the term is 17 years from the date the patent is granted. Japanese patents have a 15-year term from the date of grant or 20 years from the date of filing, whichever is shorter.

Within the pharmaceutical industry the term of patent life is a very important factor. Since patents are filed very early in the life cycle of a new pharmaceutical product and much premarketing testing is needed before the health authorities permit public sale of a product, a large portion of patent life is lost. Often the term "effective patent life" is used for pharmaceutical products. Studies by the U.S. Pharmaceutical Manufacturers Association have shown that the effective patent life for pharmaceutical products averaged 15 years in the early 1960s and declined to eight years in the early 1980s. Studies in Japan and Great Britain gave similar results. In recent years, the laws of many important counties have been changed in order to provide for recapture of some of this lost patent life through patent-term extension provisions.

Patent-Term Extensions

Prior to 1980, patent extensions were obtainable upon petition at the end of the patent life in some countries, mainly those that were formerly part of the British Commonwealth. In order for a petition to be granted, the patent owner was required to show inability during the normal life of the patent to receive sufficient remuneration from the use of his patented invention. Under this system, patent extensions of four to ten years could be obtained based on the evidence presented.

In 1984, the United States passed the first patent term restoration statute as part of the Drug Price Competition and Patent Term Restoration Act of 1984 (often referred to as the Waxman-Hatch Act). This law is significant for the total pharmaceutical industry because it contains provisions important to both the research-based and generic sections of the industry. Under this act, generic companies were allowed to file abbreviated new drug applications (ANDA) and do the testing required in order to submit an ANDA before the patent expired without being liable for patent infringement. The second part provided for the innovator of a new pharmaceutical product to receive up to five years of patent extension based on the time required to receive marketing approval from the Food and Drug Administration. The extension can provide effective patent life for the product no longer than 14 years from the date of marketing approval.

The calculation of the allowed extension period (AEP) uses the following formula:

$$\text{AEP} = 1/2\,(\text{IND} - \text{X}) + (\text{NDA} - \text{X})$$

where IND is the testing period from the date of effective IND until NDA filing, NDA is the period from NDA filing to approval, and X is the period of time the applicant failed to act with due diligence.

Certain limitations apply to this calculation. First, periods before the patent is granted are not included in the calculation. Second, the AEP cannot exceed five years. Third, the patent term remaining on the date of NDA approval plus any AEP cannot exceed 14 years. For example, if the patent for which an extension is requested has ten years of its term remaining on the date of NDA approval and the calculated AEP is five years, the patent office will issue a patent term extension certificate for only four years. Finally, the law contained phase-in provisions for products approved after September 24, 1984, but which had an effective IND and a granted patent before this date. The extension for these products was limited to two years.

Other countries have followed the U.S. lead regarding patent-term extension. Japan enacted a provision effective January 1, 1986, where patents covering pharmaceutical products could be extended up to five years. The Japanese provisions differ from the U.S. law in several ways. First, more than one patent can be extended for each product. Furthermore, the Japanese law requires the patent to be granted two years prior to health authority approval of the product. Korea has enacted a patent-term extension law very similar to the Japanese system. Australia and Ireland have replaced their "lack of remuneration" system with a system based on regulatory delay.

Effective on January 1, 1993, the EC created a system of providing extended protection for pharmaceutical products called supplementary protection certificates (SPC). Such a certificate does not actually extend the patent per se but confers the same rights as the patent and is subject to the same limitations and obligations. The SPC provides protection only for the product covered by the granted marketing approval (MA) and any use of the product as a pharmaceutical product for humans or animals. If several patents protect the product, the owner must select the one patent which will be the basis for the SPC. The SPC goes into effect only after the normal patent term expires. The duration of the SPC is equal to the period of time from patent filing date until the first MA in a member country of the EC minus five years subject to the limitations that the SPC cannot be effective for more than five years or provide effective protection for more than 15 years from the date of the first MA.

The patent owner must request the SPC from the patent office of each country of the EC within six months of the first MA or six months of the patent grant date if it occurs after the first MA. The SPC will be granted if, at the time the application is filed, (1) the patent has not expired, (2) an MA has been granted, (3) the product has not previously been the subject of an SPC, and (4) the MA is the first authorization to market the product.

The regulations allowed Spain and Greece to delay accepting the SPC system for five years. In addition, transitional provisions were adopted which allowed each country to choose to make SPCs effective for products whose first MA was granted on January 1, 1982, June 1, 1985, or January 1, 1988.

Maintaining and Enforcing Patents

After a patent is granted, the owner must pay fees to keep it in force and may have to defend it from challenges to its validity and enforce it against infringers.

Maintenance Fees

A patent does not automatically stay in force in most countries of the world from the day it is granted until the end of its life. Most countries require payment of fees, referred to as renewal or maintenance fees, in order to keep the patent in force. In most countries these fees are paid on an annual basis. Until 1980, the United States was a notable exception. However, in 1980 the United States modified its patent laws to require a fee to be paid at three different time periods during the life of the patent. Specifically, renewal fees must be paid at 3.5, 7.5, and 11.5 years from the date the patent is granted. Although the amount of renewal fees varies from country to country, it is universal that the fees increase over the life of the patent. For example, the U.S. fees in 1993 are $930, $1870, and $2820 for the three periods, whereas Germany's fees begin at 100 DM and increase to 3000 DM for the 20th year. If the owner of the patent knows that it has no value to himself and others do not wish to license it, he or she generally stop paying the fees and allow the patent to lapse. Maintenance fees on a portfolio of patents can become very expensive, and therefore most companies have a program of regular review of their patent portfolio. Those patents which are no longer of value to them are lapsed.

Invalidation

Once a patent is granted, the patent owner is not guaranteed that it is valid. Challenges to the validity of the patent again vary from country to country, depending on the specific patent law.

In the United States, the patent law specifically provides that a granted patent carries with it a presumption of validity. Until 1980, the validity of a patent could be challenged only in a federal court as part of an infringement action or by suit for declaratory judgment of invalidity. This latter action could only be started by a party who was threatened by the patent owner, that is, the requisite legal dispute actually existed between the parties. In 1980, the patent law was amended to allow any person to file a request in the patent office for reexamination of a U.S. patent based on new prior art. The patent office studies the request and determines whether or not to grant reexamination. If reexamination is granted, the patentee has an opportunity to respond to the newly cited art and the party requesting examination then has an opportunity to comment on the patentee's response. This procedure is not used very often because the third party requestor has little opportunity to fully present his views as in a normal court trial. Specifically, if the patentee requests an interview with the examiner where clarification of positions often occur, the requestor may not be present.

Once a European patent is granted, there is a nine-month period during which opposition to its grant may be filed by interested parties. The opposition proceeding takes place within the European Patent Office and must be based on only the specific grounds set forth in the European Patent Convention. After the opposition period, the validity of a European patent, which, as noted above, is in fact a compilation of national patents, is determined in each country by the national courts according to the national laws. Although these laws have been harmonized along the same general requirements as in the EPC, application of these requirements can vary from country to country, and mixed results can be obtained.

Patent Infringement

A patent is infringed when someone makes, uses, or sells the claimed invention without the permission of the patent owner. When this occurs, the patent owner can bring a legal action against the infringing party.

In the United States this is a civil action brought in the federal courts. In which specific federal district court a patent owner can sue an infringer is governed by federal law. Patent litigation is very expensive and time-consuming. For this reason it is not entered into without careful consideration of the consequences and analysis of all options available. Various alternative dispute-resolution proceedings are being used more often in recent years.

Since patents are limited in their effect to the specific country granting them, a company with a pioneering drug may find itself suing patent infringers in a number of countries around the world. Usually these actions are in countries where the patent system is not as strong as in the United States and the major European countries. Direct costs of patent litigation are usually much lower than in the United States but time requirements can be just as extensive.

Patents to compounds or pharmaceutical compositions are infringed by their sale or use in the country of issuance. Patents to processes for preparation of a compound cause a different problem. There is no direct infringement if the compound is made by the process in a country without patent protection and then imported into the country where the process is patented. However, the laws of many countries specify that the sale or use of compounds made directly by a patented process is an infringement of the process patent. "Directly" means in most instances to be the final step to prepare the compound.

Such protection was not available in the United States until 1986 when the patent laws were amended. The amendment also had a provision whereby a party can ask the producer of a compound for a list of any U.S. process patents that are owned or licensed.

Government Intervention

After a patent is granted, governments can still intervene and affect the patent owner. This is especially true for owners of pharmaceutical patents in countries which do not have a strong patent system to protect pharmaceutical products. One form of intervention is to require "working" of the invention. In some countries, working can be demonstrated only by manufacture of the product in that country. Other countries allow a patent owner to satisfy the working requirement by importation of the product.

Countries that have working requirements usually also have a compulsory licensing provision which allows the government to grant a compulsory license to a third party if the patent owner fails to meet the working requirements. Until 1993, Canada had an especially harsh compulsory license provision limited to pharmaceuticals. Any party requesting a license would receive it. The licensee was required to pay the patent owner a royalty of 4% of its sales. If the product was protected by patents owned by two or more companies, this royalty was divided equally among them.

Other Forms of Protection

Although patents are the main source of defense to generic copying for the pharmaceutical industry, other forms of regulatory protection have been developed in recent years. Specifically, valuable periods of regulatory exclusivity have become available in the United States, Europe, and Japan. In addition, in the United States the Orphan Drug Act has provided a special kind of regulatory exclusivity.

Normal Regulatory Exclusivity

Generic manufacturers are able to reach the market quicker if they can refer to the originator's data when seeking regulatory approval. However, regulatory agencies find it is in the public interest to have a new drug distributed by the single originator for a period of time in order to monitor for any safety problems. To balance these two needs, a regulatory exclusivity system has emerged under which the health agency does not approve an abbreviated application for a limited period of time. These rights are acquired by operation of the law in each particular country rather than being applied for by the originating drug manufacturer. No certificate or other documentation are issued for these rights.

In 1980, Japan became the first country to have a regulatory exclusivity provision. The period is six years for new products, new combination products, or different routes of administration. For other modifications, such as a new indication or a new dosage regimen, the period of exclusivity is four years. If the second applicant does complete safety and efficacy studies, these periods of exclusivity do not apply.

In the United States, these regulatory exclusivity rights were part of the Waxman-Hatch Act. This law provides that no abbreviated new drug application (ANDA) can be submitted for a generic equivalent for a new compound entity (NCE) until five years after the approval date for the NCE. If the ANDA applicant certifies that the patent covering the NCE is invalid or not infringed, the period is four years. If an NCE is not involved or a pioneering supplemental NDA is approved, an ANDA can become effective only after a three-year period. Thus, for non-NCEs the regulatory period is reduced to three years. For an NCE, the five-year period is for submission of an ANDA and therefore the FDA processing time would extend this exclusivity period further.

Another interesting part of this law is that if a generic manufacturer challenges a patent and is successful, he or she is rewarded with a six-month period during which no other generic products will be approved.

In Europe, regulatory exclusivity is more complex. More specifically, the countries may choose between a ten-year or a six-year period. According to the European Community Directive 87/21, the national states can protect pharmaceutical products for six or ten years from first marketing approval in the European Community. An exception to this

TABLE 1 European Regulatory Exclusivity

10 years	6 years
UK	Denmark
France	Greece[a]
Germany	Ireland
Belgium	Luxembourg
Holland	Portugal[a]
Italy	Spain

[a]From 1.1.1992.

are biotechnology products where a ten-year period applies for all EC countries. The countries that have chosen ten or six years are shown in Table 1.

Orphan Drugs

Drugs that are used for treating rare diseases or conditions are referred to as orphan drugs. The U.S. Orphan Drug Act states that the FDA may not approve another application within seven years from approval of the first, unless the originator cannot assure availability to meet the needs of the patients. This law was amended in 1985 to apply to patented as well as nonpatented drugs. The requirements to be recognized as an orphan drug are (1) that the disease affects fewer than 200,000 persons in the United States, or (2) that recovery of the R&D costs from U.S. sales is unlikely. A request must be made to the FDA to obtain orphan drug status. The determination of eligibility is made as of the date of this request. This seven-year period of marketing exclusivity applies only to the individual uses of the compound or product and not to the compound itself.

Other countries in the world do not have exclusivity for orphan drugs at this time, although provisions exist in some countries for speedier approval. This is an area that is under study in Japan and new proposals may be forthcoming in the future.

Bibliography

Grubb, P. W., *Patents in Chemistry and Biotechnology*, Clarendon Press, Oxford, 1986.

Rosenstock, J., *The Law of Chemical and Pharmaceutical Invention, Patent and Nonpatent Protection*, Little, Brown and Company, Boston, 1993.

Wallerstein, M. B., Magee, M. E., and Schoen, R. A., eds., *Global Dimensions of Intellectual Property Rights in Science and Technology*, National Academy Press, Washington, 1993.

STUART R. SUTER

Pediatric Dosing and Dosage Forms

Introduction

The administration of medications to pediatric patients is in many ways difficult because health care providers and parents are faced with many challenges not experienced, or experienced to a lesser degree, when medications are prescribed and taken by adults. First, less information is available about the use of most drugs in pediatric patients. In 1975, Dr. John Wilson stated (as reported in Ref. 1) that only 22% of all prescription medications had labeling for use in pediatric patients. Over a decade later, in 1988, Rosa of the Food and Drug Administration (FDA) stated that approximately 50% of all prescription medications have some level of evaluation for use in infants. Of these, half were considered safe and efficacious for the pediatric population, with the remainder having a risk or caution statement in their labeling requirements [1]. Thus, information needed to make educated decisions on whether to administer a particular drug to a pediatric patient, especially if it is not FDA approved, is somewhat easier to find today than it was in the 1970s, but there are still many questions that need to be answered about drug administration to pediatric patients. For example, is the drug safe and effective for pediatric patients of various ages? What dose should be given and how frequently, what administration route followed, and what dosage form selected? How should the drug be monitored for effectiveness as well as for adverse effects. Information determined in adult medication studies may not be applicable to pediatric patients because of pharmacokinetic and pharmacodynamic differences as well as differences in disease states for which a particular drug might be used. Many questions about the use of particular drugs in various age groups of pediatric patients can only be answered through well designed, randomized controlled studies in pediatric patients who need certain medications for their health problems.

The FDA has proposed labeling for prescription products to include a pediatric-use section. It would include information on the use or limitations of the product for pediatric patients. The FDA may publish such labeling recommendations sometime in 1994.

This overview of pediatric dosing covers many issues that pediatric health care providers face daily, such as age-related drug pharmacokinetic and pharmacodynamic changes that occur secondarily to physiologic changes in the maturing neonate, infant, child, and adolescent that affect drug absorption from various routes of administration as well as drug distribution, metabolism, and elimination. To better monitor pharmacokinetic changes, therapeutic drug monitoring must be undertaken for drugs with narrow therapeutic indexes and for those for which pharmacodynamic data correlate with pharmacokinetic information. Also addressed will be drug administration by various routes including intravenous (iv), oral, intramuscular (im), subcutaneous (sc), percutaneous, rectal, otic, nasal, ophthalmic, and inhalation. Another issue discussed is product selection, for pediatric patients.

To better understand changes in drug disposition, the pediatric population needs to be categorized into various age groups (Table 1) because children vary markedly in their absorbtion, distribution, metabolism, and elimination of medications. This occurs because neonates, infants, children, adolescents, and adults have different body composi-

TABLE 1 Pediatric Age Groups Terminology

Terms	Definition
Gestational age	Time from the mother's last menstrual period to the time the baby is born; at birth, a Dubowitz score in weeks gestational age is assigned, based on the physical examination of the newborn
Postnatal age	Age since birth
Postconceptional age	Age since conception, i.e., gestational plus postnatal age
Neonate	First four weeks or first month of life
Premature neonates	Born at less than 37 weeks gestation
Fullterm neonates	Born between 37 and 42 weeks gestation
Postterm neonates	Born after 42 weeks gestation
Infant	One month to one year of age
Child	1 to 12 years of age
Adolescent	12 to 18 years of age

tions (i.e., as to their percentages of body water and fat) and have body organs in different stages of development.

Pediatric Pharmacokinetics and Pharmacodynamics

Effect of Developmental Physiologic Changes on the Pharmacokinetics and Pharmacodynamics of Drugs

Rational pediatric pharmacotherapy is primarily based upon the knowledge about a particular drug, including its pharmacokinetics and pharmacodynamics, that may be modified by physiologic maturation of the child from birth through adolescence. Physiologic changes that occur can affect drug absorption, distribution, metabolism, and elimination. The most dramatic physiologic changes occur during the neonatal period.

Oral Absorption

Drug absorption from the gastrointestinal (GI) tract is dependent on patient factors, physiochemical properties of the orally administered drug, and the drug formulation. Patient factors that affect GI absorption include gastric and duodenal pH, gastric emptying time, GI motility, enzyme activity, biliary function, absorptive surface area and the maturation of the mucosal membrane, bacterial colonization of the GI tract, and dietary intake [2–5]. Patient factors are influenced by rapid maturational changes that occur throughout early childhood, but which occur primarily during the first few months of life.

Most drugs are absorbed across the GI tract by passive diffusion, but a variety of drug physiochemical factors influence the extent of absorption. These factors include molecular weight, lipid solubility, dissolution rate, and pKa. In addition, drug absorption may be dependent on the drug form administered (e.g., a liquid, a tablet that may need to be crushed, or a sustained-release product), and the particular brand selected.

Gastric pH

When examining patient-specific factors, such as gastric pH, that affect oral absorption, it should be noted that infants born vaginally who are at least 32 weeks gestation, usually have at birth a gastric pH between 6 and 8 [2,5–7]. Gastric pH may be even higher in

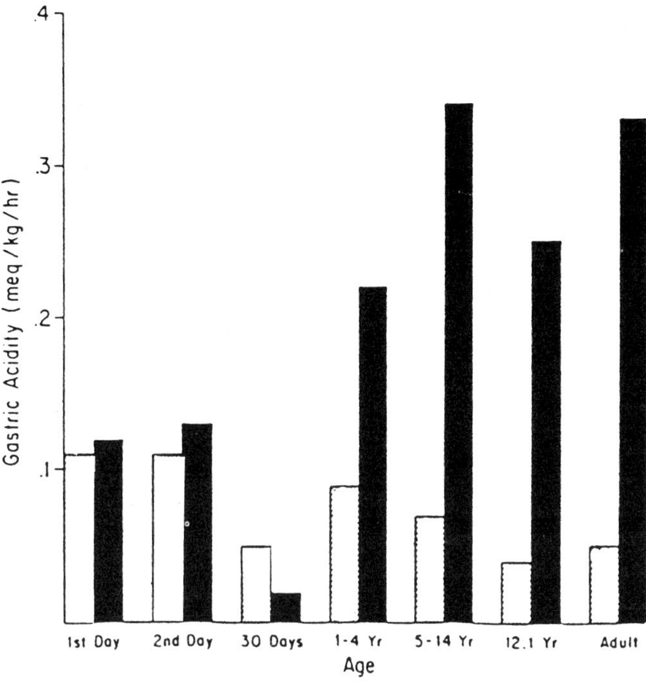

FIG. 1. Basal (□) and simulated (■) gastric acid secretion over the life cycle. (From Ref. 8.)

infants born by cesarean section [5]. Gastric pH then falls rapidly, and within a few hours after delivery the pH is below 3 [2,5–7]. The initial gastric pH is alkaline compared to that of adults and results from the presence of amniotic fluid in the infant's stomach [8,9]. Thereafter, gastric pH remains acidic until approximately day 10, when it again becomes alkaline because of decreased acid production. A nadir in acid production occurs between days 10 and 30 of life. Then gastric acid production begins to increase, but gastric pH and maximal gastric output may not mirror that of adults on a per kilogram (kg) basis until approximately three years of age [5,8]. Stewart and Hampton have described [8] basal and maximal gastric acid secretion in children from birth to age 14 years and have compared these values to those for adults (Fig. 1). It is thus important to know the gastric pH at a particular time in the neonatal period to determine differences in absorption based on acidity or alkalinity.

Gastric Emptying and Gastrointestinal Motility

Gastric emptying time in neonates, especially those less than 24 h of age, may be variable and prolonged when compared to that in adults [8]. It may not reach adult levels until six to eight months of age and may be associated with diet [10,11]. For example, gastric emptying appears to be shorter in infants who are fed breast milk rather than infant formula, but other studies have shown that gastric emptying in infants 5 to 27 days of age may be similar to that for adults, 25–87 min [12,13] and 22–53 min, respectively [14,15]. Varying viewpoints on this issue may be due to differences in study methodologies. Gastrointestinal transit time may be prolonged and peristaltic activity unpredictable in young infants [5,16]; both appear to depend on the feeding [16]. Lebenthal and colleagues noted that breast-fed infants, older than 45 days, had gastric transit times longer than 10 h, whereas formula-fed infants had gastric transit times less than 10 h [17]. It should also be noted that young infants have a propensity to reflux their gastric contents because of the immaturity of their esophagus as well as their GI motility. All of these factors affect the extent to which a drug may be absorbed.

Enzyme Activity in the Gastrointestinal Tract

Pancreatic enzyme activity is low at birth, but enzymes such as amylase, lipase, and trypsin develop to adult levels within the first year of life [3]. Premature infants appear to have lower amylase levels than full-term infants. Low amylase concentrations may be the reason why newborns have a decreased ability to hydrolyze drugs such as chloramphenicol palmitate [5]. Lipid-soluble drugs may not be well absorbed by neonates because of low lipase concentrations and bile acid pool [5]. Neonates appear to have higher concentrations of β-glucuronidase and UDP-glucuronyl transferase in their GI tracts.

Absorptive Surface Area

The surface area of the small intestine in young infants is proportionately greater than in adults; this may allow for increased drug absorption from the GI tract.

Other Factors

Little information is available about the effect of GI tract colonization on drug absorption. The GI flora changes with age. Initial colonization occurs by day 4 to 6 of life with adult bacterial colonization being observed by age five months to one year [16]. The rate and type of bacterial colonization is influenced by the infant's age and type of feeding (breast milk vs. infant formula and the specific type of formula fed). Infants and children may have diseases or health problems that can influence drug absorption. A problem that has a great effect on absorption is short-bowel syndrome which may reduce the absorptive surface. In addition, diseases that affect gastric emptying (pyloric stenosis, congestive heart failure), bile excretion (cholestatic liver disease), and intestinal transit time (thyroid disease, diarrhea) may influence drug absorption [16].

Intramuscular Absorption

When a pediatric patient is unable to take a medication orally or the drug is unavailable for oral use, there may be a need to administer it parenterally by the iv or im route. Of these, the latter is less desirable because of pain, irritation, and decreased drug delivery compared to iv administration. Drug absorption after im administration depends on various physiochemical and patient factors. Physiochemical factors that must be considered include lipid or water solubility, drug concentration, and surface area available for absorption. When addressing drug solubility, it should be noted that lipophilic drugs readily diffuse through capillary walls of endothelial cells whereas water-soluble drugs diffuse at fairly rapid rates from interstitial fluid to plasma via pores in capillary membranes [18]. A lipid-soluble drug may be more rapidly absorbed im, but a water-soluble drug may be more desirable because the drug must be stable in an aqueous solution until administered. After administration, the drug must be water soluble at physiologic pH until absorption occurs [18].

Drug absorption may also be dependent on concentration, but available data do not allow to determine whether an increased or decreased drug concentration results in better absorption. An increase in the osmolality of a pharmaceutical preparation secondary to the addition of another substance, such as an excipient, may decrease or slow im absorption [18]. Absorption occurs more rapidly when diffusion involves a large area of muscle or the drug spreads over a large muscle mass. The massaging of an injection site after im administration increases the rate of absorption [18].

A physiological determinant of im drug absorption is the adequacy of blood flow to muscle groups used for drug administration. Absorption rates vary at injection sites because blood flow varies among different muscle groups. For example, the absorption of a drug administered im in the deltoid muscle is faster than from the vastus lateralis which, in turn, is more rapid than from the gluteus [18,19]. This occurs because blood flow to the deltoid muscle is 7% higher than to vastus lateralis and 17% higher than to gluteal muscle groups [20]. Physiological conditions that reduce blood flow to a muscle group may adversely alter the rate and/or extent of a drug administered im. Decreased perfusion or hemostatic decompensation, frequently observed in ill neonates and young infants, may reduce im drug absorption. Drug absorption may also be adversely affected in neonates who receive a skeletal muscle-paralyzing agent such as pancuronium [18] because of decreased muscle contraction. In addition, a small muscle mass in neonates and young infants may reduce the ability of a drug to be adequately absorbed [2].

The injection technique may alter im absorption. This was noted when needles of different lengths were used. The use of a longer needle (38 vs. 31 mm, 1½ vs. 1¼ in.) for im administration in adult patients resulted in higher diazepam serum concentrations [20]. This occurred probably because the drug administered with the shorter needle was actually administered sc rather than im.

Some drugs are absorbed more slowly after im than after oral administration; examples include diazepam, digoxin, and phenytoin. This occurs probably because these drugs require a mixture of alcohol, propylene glycol, and water for solubility, and they are insoluble in the muscle after im administration [20].

Complications associated with im administration include nerve injury, muscle contracture, and abscess formation [21]. Less common problems include intramuscular hemorrhage, cellulitis, skin pigmentation, tissue necrosis, muscle atrophy, gangrene, and cyst or scar formation. In addition, injury may occur from broken needles and inadvertent injection into a joint or vein [21].

Subcutaneous Absorption

The sc route is used for the administration of drugs such as insulin that require slow absorption. Injection technique and patient factors, such as perfusion, fluid status, and physical build are important [20]. Exercise, elevation or warming of the injection site, or inadvertently administrating a drug im rather than sc, can increase absorption and be dangerous in some situations such as hypoglycemia occurring in the diabetic patient from excessive insulin absorption [20]. Adverse effects that can occur secondarily to sc administration include tissue ischemia, sterile and nonsterile abscesses, lipodystrophy, cysts, and granulomatous formation.

Intraosseous Drug Absorption

If an iv line cannot be placed, the intraosseous drug administration route can be used for pediatric patients during cardiopulmonary resuscitation (CPR) because drug delivery by this route is similar to that for iv administration [22]. If drug or fluid delivery by this route is sluggish, a saline flush can be used to clear the needle. Intraosseous administration has been used for the delivery of drugs such as epinephrine, atropine, sodium bicarbonate, dopamine, diazepam, isoproterenol, phenytoin, phenobarbital, dexamethasone, and various antibiotics [22].

Percutaneous Absorption

The percutaneous (topical) route for systemic drug delivery is used infrequently for pediatric patients. Medications are applied to the skin for their local effect. In the future, this route may be used more frequently for systemic effects as more transdermal systems are developed for drug delivery.

The percutaneous absorption of a drug occurs in the following manner. Initially the topically applied drug is absorbed into the stratum corneum and diffuses through that layer of the skin into the epidermis and then into the dermis where the drug molecules reach capillaries and enter the circulatory system. Diffusion through the stratum corneum is the rate-determining step unless skin perfusion is decreased. In the latter case, diffusion is controlled by the transfer of drug molecules into capillaries rather than by the diffusion process previously explained. Percutaneous absorption [23] is affected by:

- Patient age,
- Application site,
- State of hydration of the stratum corneum,
- Intactness of the stratum corneum,
- Solute, and
- Vehicle or solvent.

Drug diffusion may be explained by Eq. (1).

$$J = \frac{K_m \times D_m \times C_s}{l} \tag{1}$$

where J is flux, K_m is the partition coefficient, D_m is the diffusion constant under specific conditions such as temperature and hydration, C_s is the concentration gradient, and l is the length of thickness of stratum corneum [23].

Lipid-soluble drugs are better absorbed into the stratum corneum than are water-soluble drugs, but the latter do not easily traverse the stratum corneum itself. Thus, lipid-soluble drugs are more likely to be stored in the stratum corneum, whereas water-soluble drugs are more likely to diffuse across the stratum corneum to the epidermis and dermis [23].

Patient Age

Percutaneous drug absorption is not appreciably different in various age groups of patients, except for neonates less than 35 weeks gestation at birth. Drug absorption is increased in a premature neonate because the stratum corneum is not completely formed at birth. An example of increased drug absorption occurred in two premature neonates who were repeatedly washed with 3% hexachlorophene and developed encephalopathy secondary to drug absorption [23]. The absorption of the corticosteroid betamethasone valerate after topical application in children resulted in hypothalamus-pituitary-adrenal axis suppression. Children may have increased drug absorption from the percutaneous application of drugs not because of a higher absorption rate but because of a greater topical application or a larger dose per kilogram. Examples of deaths in children from percutaneous drug absorption include those caused by salicylic acid and phenol administration [23]. The percutaneous route has been used to deliver theophylline for the treatment of apnea in neonates less than 32 weeks gestation. A theophylline gel disk (not available in the United States) was the vehicle by which the drug was delivered [24].

Application Site

The ability of a drug to be absorbed percutaneously depends on the thickness of the stratum corneum. For example, absorption occurs more readily through abdominal skin than through skin on the plantar surface of the foot. Topical absorption may be enhanced from a particular site by the application of an occlusive dressing.

Hydration of the Stratum Corneum

Percutaneous absorption of a drug is enhanced by the hydration of the stratum corneum. Such hydration affects the absorption of hydrophilic drugs more than that of lipophilic drugs.

Status of the Stratum Corneum

Drugs penetrate damaged skin more readily than intact skin. Skin damaged because of dryness allows for increased drug penetration through areas where the skin is cracked or broken [23].

Solute

The penetration of the solute (or drug) depends on its polarity and on the polarity of the delivery vehicle.

Vehicle or Solvent

Drug-delivery vehicles typically used for topical application include lotions, ointments, creams, emulsions, and gels [23]. Substances may be added to the drug and vehicle such as an emulsifier to improve the texture of an emulsion, a stabilizer to preserve the stability of a drug, the vehicle, or both, a thickening agent to increase viscosity, or a humectant to draw moisture into the skin [23]. It is particularly important to consider the vehicle and other additives when selecting a topical drug preparation for a neonate, especially when premature, because of the greater possibility of absorption of not only the drug but also other product ingredients. Toxic reaction has occurred in neonates from ingredients considered "inactive."

Transdermal Drug-Delivery Systems

Drugs chosen for delivery via a transdermal drug-delivery system must adequately penetrate the skin in such a way that the system determines the delivery rate which should be fairly constant [23]. In addition, the drug must not irritate or sensitize the skin. It is hoped that in the future more drugs will be developed for transdermal delivery. This could be an alternative route for drug delivery to children who have difficulties with oral administration.

Endotracheal Absorption

The endotracheal (ET) route has been used to administer medications during CPR when other routes such as the iv route are unavailable [22]. It provides rapid access as well as rapid drug absorption and distribution [25]. Some studies have shown that the time to reach peak absorption is similar to that for the iv route, but the serum concentrations achieved were 10 to 33% of that achieved with iv administration, resulting in weaker response. A depot effect has been demonstrated for drugs such as epinephrine. Much work needs to be done to determine the optimal dose by this route, drug-delivery vehicle (e.g., saline), the most effective delivery technique (e.g., drug dilution with saline for administration vs. a saline bolus after administration), and the vehicle volume to be used [22].

Rectal Absorption

The rectal route is used for local and systemic therapy for the following reasons [26]:

- Nausea or vomiting,
- Rejection of oral medication because of its taste, texture, etc.,
- Upper GI disease that might affect absorption,
- Medication absorption affected by food or gastric emptying
- Medication is readily decomposed in gastric fluid but may be stable in rectal fluid, and
- First-pass effect of high-clearance drug may be partially avoided.

Absorption from the rectum depends on various physiological factors such as surface area, blood supply, pH, fluid volume, and possible metabolism by microorganisms in the rectum. The surface area of the rectum is smaller than that of the small intestine, primarily because the rectal epithelium is free of villi [26]. The rectum is perfused by the inferior and middle rectal arteries, whereas the superior, middle, and inferior rectal veins drain the rectum. The last two are connected directly to the systemic circulation; the superior rectal vein drains into the portal system. Therefore, drugs absorbed from the lower rectum are carried directly into the systemic circulation, whereas drugs absorbed from the upper rectum are subjected to a hepatic first-pass effect [26]. Therefore, a high-clearance drug should be more bioavailable after rectal than after oral administration. The volume of fluid in the rectum and the pH of that fluid may also affect drug absorption. Because the fluid volume is usually low compared to that in other areas of the GI tract, a drug may not be completely soluble. In addition, a variety of organisms colonize the rectum, and it is debatable whether these organisms are involved in drug metabolism [26]. Absorption is also influenced by the dosage form. For example, drugs are rapidly absorbed rectally from aqueous or alcoholic solutions, whereas absorption from a suppository depends on its base, the presence of a surfactant, particle size of the active ingredient(s), and drug concentration [26]. The following problems may be associated with the rectal route for drug administration [26].

- Decreased absorption secondary to defecation of the rectally administered pharmaceutical product,
- Less absorption rectally than orally because the absorbing surface area of the rectum is smaller,
- Dissolution problems for rectally administered medications because of a lower fluid volume in the rectum than in the stomach, duodenum, etc.,
- Microorganisms in rectum may cause degradation of some medications, and
- Patient or parent acceptability.

Distribution

A drug is distributed by moving from a patient's systemic circulation to various compartments, tissues, and cells. Distribution depends on patient factors, drug physiochemical properties, and the route of administration. Patient factors that influence drug distribution or the volume of drug distribution (V_d) include body composition, perfusion, protein- and tissue-binding characteristics, and permeability [2–5,8]. Many of these characteristics are age-dependent. Drug physiochemical properties that may influence distribution include molecular weight, pKa, and partition coefficient.

Differences in Body Composition

Age-related changes in body composition can alter the V_d of a drug. At birth, 85% of the weight of a premature infant may be water, compared to approximately 75% as total body water (TBW) in a full-term infant [16]. Neonates have the highest percentage of extracellular water (35–44% of TBW in full-term neonates vs. 20% in adults), and the highest ratio of extracellular to intracellular water (ICW); the ICW is more stable throughout life (i.e., 33% in neonates vs. 40% in adults) [16]. An infant's percentage of TBW approaches that of an adult male by one year of age (60% TBW); it reaches the same level about the time of puberty or 12 years of age [5]. Women have a lower percentage of TBW (50%) than men because of a higher concentration of body fat. Thus neonates, because of their high TBW, have a higher V_d for water-soluble drugs such as aminoglycosides than older children or adults. For example, the V_d for an aminoglycoside such as gentamicin approximates that of extracellular cellular fluid volume, 0.5–1.2 L/kg for a neonate, but only 0.2–0.3 L/kg for an older child or an adult [5].

Adipose tissue increases from as little as 0.5% in a premature infant to approximately 16% of body weight for a full-term infant [27,28]. Boys experience a spurt in body fat between the ages of 5 and 10 years, and then a gradual decrease in fat content until about 17 years of age; girls usually have a rapid increase in adipose tissue at puberty [8]. Thus one would expect neonates and young infants to have a decreased V_d for lipid-soluble drugs. This has been noted for diazepam in neonates who have exhibited an apparent V_d of 1.4–1.8 L/kg compared to 2.2–2.6 L/kg in adults [29].

Protein Binding

Neonates have lower concentrations of various plasma proteins (e.g., albumin concentrations are 80% of those in adults) for drug binding, but the albumin present may also have a lower affinity for binding drugs than noted for adults who are receiving the same medications. This lower affinity for binding drugs may result in a competition for various albumin-binding sites with substances such as bilirubin. Plasma protein binding noted in adults is usually achieved in children by age one year [16].

Acidic drugs have a high affinity for albumin binding, whereas basic drugs bind more readily to α-l-acid glycoprotein and lipoprotein. In neonates drugs such as penicillins, phenobarbital, phenytoin, and theophylline have lower protein-binding affinity than in adults. This may increase the concentration of free or pharmacological active drug in neonates, and may also change the apparent volume of distribution. Thus, neonates may require higher loading doses of these as well as other drugs to achieve therapeutic serum concentrations [30–33]. The increased free fraction may also lead to increased drug clearance from the blood.

In addition to binding to plasma proteins in the neonate, some drugs such as sulfonamides may displace plasma bilirubin from binding sites. This may increase an infant's risk for developing kernicterus. The significance of drugs displacing bilirubin is controversial because bilirubin may have a greater affinity for albumin than drugs have [4].

Free fatty acids (FFA) are present in high concentrations in the plasma of neonates, especially in those with gram-negative septicemia. The binding of drugs such as phenytoin to albumin is lower when FFA concentrations are elevated [16].

Tissue Binding

Binding of drugs to various body tissues appears to vary with age; for example, digoxin binding to erythrocytes is higher in neonates than in adults. This may be due to the increased number of binding sites on neonatal erythrocytes [34].

Drug Penetration into the Central Nervous System (CNS)

A drug is more likely to cross into the CNS of a neonate rather than that of an older child or an adult. This most likely occurs because its CNS is less mature and the blood-brain barrier is less formed. This is an important consideration when antimicrobial therapy is needed for the treatment of bacterial meningitis or an anticonvulsant for seizures [35,36].

Metabolism

Although drug metabolism can occur in various body organs including the lungs, GI tract, kidneys, and liver as well as in the blood, the liver is the primary organ for metabolism. Most drugs are metabolized from lipid-soluble parent compounds to more polar, less lipophilic metabolites that are more readily eliminated renally [8]. Occasionally, a drug is metabolized to an active drug from an inactive parent compound. Examples are the esterification of chloramphenicol succinate in the liver and other organs to free chloramphenicol or the cleavage in the GI tract of chloramphenicol palmitate to free chloramphenicol prior to absorption across the gut wall. In addition, some drugs are metabolized to more active compounds. This occurs when a neonate receives theophylline for apnea of prematurity. Theophylline is readily metabolized in neonates by N-methylation to caffeine, a compound equally, if not more effective, against apnea [4]. This type of metabolization occurs only to a small extent in older infants, children, and adults.

Hepatic Metabolism

Most drug metabolism occurs in the liver by phase 1 or phase 2 metabolic processes. Phase 1 reactions primarily biotransform an active drug to a more water-soluble compound that typically is inactive or has less activity than the parent compound. Oxidation, reduction, and hydrolysis are examples of phase 1 processes [5,8]. Oxidation is primarily catalyzed by a multiple monooxygenase system, the cytochrome P-450 system that has a multitude of isozymes. This system appears to be inhibited when the fetus is in utero, possibly by maternal progesterone or its metabolites [37,38] or by growth hormone [39].

Phase 2 reactions (glucuronidation, sulfation, acetylation, and glutathione conjugation) usually involve the conjugation of active drugs with endogenous molecules to form metabolites that are more water-soluble [18]; glucuronidation is the most thoroughly studied reaction. It is postulated that maternal glucocorticoids inhibit the development of glucuronyltransferase, the enzyme involved in glucuronidation in utero. After birth this metabolic system matures rapidly without the inhibition of maternal glucocorticoids [40,41]. Maturation of this pathway reaches adult levels by age two years [4]. Hyperbilirubinemia and toxicity secondary to chloramphenicol administration have occurred in neonates who were unable to adequately glucuronidate these compounds [8].

Sulfate conjugation appears to be fully developed immediately prior to or at the time of birth. Infants and young children readily sulfate acetaminophen; in adults the major metabolic route is glucuronidation [42]. Little is known about acetylation in neonates or infants. It is believed that neonates have an extremely low capacity for acetylation at birth, but this pathway is mature at approximately 20 days of age [4]. Figure 2 describes age-related hepatic maturation.

Neonates require close monitoring if their mothers received enzyme inducers such as phenytoin, phenobarbital, carbamazepine, or rifampin during pregnancy or if they need one of these drugs themselves [18]. Patients receiving medicines that inhibit drug metabolism must also be carefully monitored. Examples of drugs that inhibit the metabolism of other medications include cimetidine, erythromycin, and ketoconazole.

Renal Elimination

The kidneys are the major route for drug elimination, especially for water-soluble compounds or the metabolites of lipid-soluble drugs. Renal drug elimination is dependent

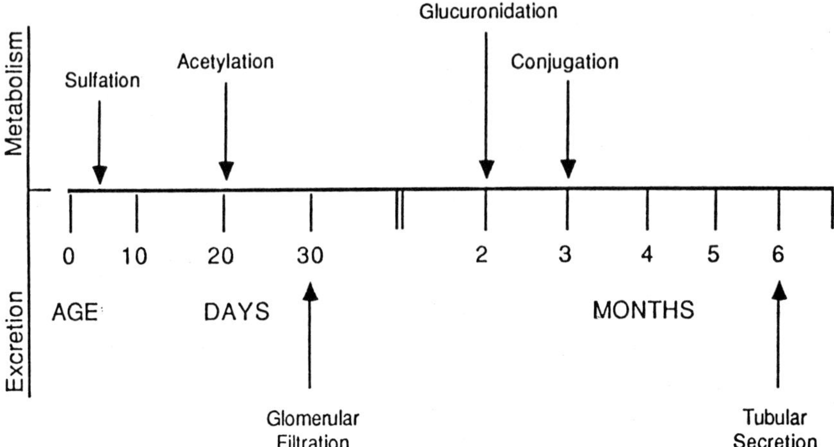

FIG. 2. Maturation of renal and hepatic function. (From Reed, M. D., and Besunder, J. B., Developmental pharmacology: Ontogenic basis of drug disposition, *Pediatr. Clin. North Am.*, 36:1053–1074 (1989).)

on renal blood flow, glomerular filtration, and tubular secretion and reabsorption. These functions appear to mature at different rates in the neonate and infant. Full-term infants achieve renal blood flow similar to that of adults by age 5 to 12 months; glomerular filtration approaches adult values by age three to five months [4,8]. Premature neonates exhibit lower rates for glomerular filtration at birth than do full-term neonates, and more time is required of them postnatally to develop filtration ability [43]. This is probably due to their lack of as many functional nephrons at birth. Tubular function is less mature in the neonate at birth than is glomerular filtration, and it matures at a slower rate. Tubular function begins to approach adult values by seven months of age. Renal function is equal to that of adults by one year of age. (See Fig. 2 for age-related maturation of renal and hepatic function.)

Aminoglycosides (gentamicin, tobramycin, amikacin) and digoxin are drugs whose elimination depends on renal maturation. The renal elimination of aminoglycosides in neonates and young infants parallels the maturation of glomerular function and correlates with creatinine clearance [44]. The renal elimination of digoxin also parallels kidney maturation. Dosage adjustment for this drug is necessary as renal function matures in neonates and young infants. In addition, older infants and children require higher mg/kg doses of digoxin than adults to achieve the same serum concentrations. This may be due to decreased digoxin absorption or increased renal elimination [5].

Therapeutic Drug Monitoring

Therapeutic drug monitoring should encompass the entire process including drug selection, product selection, route of administration, consideration of the patient's age, and appropriate dosing on a mg/kg or mg/m^2 basis, as well as monitoring serum concentrations when appropriate and observing the patient for optimal drug effect(s) and possible adverse effects.

Important Differences in Pediatric Serum Drug Concentrations

For many drugs, especially for those with narrow therapeutic indexes, serum concentration ranges have been determined that correlate to minimum and maximum therapeutic effects as well as to the development of toxicity. Therapeutic serum concentration ranges for various drugs have been developed for adults, and these data have been applied to pediatric patients including neonates. Such data may be appropriate to monitor drug therapy in children, but possibly not in children of all ages or possibly not in children at all. For example, Painter et al. [45] noted that neonates need higher serum phenobarbital concentrations than older children and adults to terminate seizures. Gilman et al. [46] observed that higher phenobarbital loading doses were needed to achieve serum concentrations in neonates that would reduce the occurrence seizures. Thus, there may be a need for different serum concentration ranges for various drugs needed by different age groups of patients for a similar pharmacodynamic or therapeutic outcome.

Free serum concentrations, rather than total concentrations, of some drugs such as phenytoin may need to be monitored in some patients, including neonates, who have low serum albumins. Gilman has advocated the possibility of using individualized dosing and serum concentration range for pediatric patients because children, especially neonates, have rapidly maturing functions of various organs and changes in albumin for drug binding [47].

Serum concentration monitoring of various drugs administered to pediatric patients may appropriately give information about the drug but not its metabolites. This may be a problem when children metabolize specific drugs differently than adults with resulting differences in metabolite concentrations or the presence of different metabolites. This has been noted when premature infants have been administered theophylline for central apnea. A major metabolite of theophylline in neonates is caffeine, although only small concentrations of this metabolite are noted in older children and adults [48–50]. Caffeine is effective in treating apnea, and thus may add to the effectiveness of theophylline. This may help explain why lower theophylline serum concentrations may be needed for apnea rather than asthma. In addition, the presence of the 4-en metabolite of valproic acid noted in the serum of infants and young children, but not adults, receiving this medication for seizures may be responsible for the hepatotoxicity of this drug in young pediatric patients [47,51].

Serum drug assays may be affected by interfering substances in the serum. For example, a digoxin-like immunoreactive substance has been found in the serum of neonates and infants that interferes with certain digoxin assays [52]. Similar interfering substances have been noted in the serum of pregnant women and in renal patients.

Serum Drug Concentrations

Because of the cost associated with therapeutic drug monitoring, serum drug concentrations must be drawn appropriately to provide useful information. Drugs typically followed pharmacokinetically are those with narrow therapeutic indexes for which there is an association between pharmacokinetic and pharmacodynamic data or toxicity. For many drugs, especially for those administered orally, the determination of trough concentrations (serum concentrations obtained prior to administration) may be most appropriate. This eliminates differences in absorption rates for orally administered drugs that could influence peak concentrations (e.g., orally administered phenobarbital, phenytoin, carbamazepine, or valproic acid). Trough concentrations may be important for drugs such as digoxin that take time to distribute to tissue receptors in such a way that serum concentrations reflect pharmacodynamic effects. Peak concentrations are best used for determining toxicity and therapeutic effects of drugs with short half-lives (aminoglycosides, theophylline).

Table 2 gives therapeutic serum concentrations and other pharmacokinetic information for some of the drugs administered to pediatric patients.

Technical Factors

Sample Size and Timing of Blood Drawing for Serum Concentration Determination

Because of the small blood volume and the small size of veins, it is technically difficult to draw blood from neonates, infants, and young children for therapeutic drug monitoring, and it is therefore important to determine the best drawing schedule. For example, when are peak and trough data needed compared to trough data only? For anticonvulsants administered orally or iv, trough concentrations are needed, whereas for aminoglycosides it may be important to obtain both peaks and troughs.

Chronopharmacokinetics should also be considered when determining serum concentrations for therapeutic drug monitoring. Chronopharmacokinetics is the difference in serum drug concentrations that may occur on a rhythmic or circadian basis. Phenytoin, theophylline, and carbamazepine have shown chronopharmacokinetic characteristics in children. This is an important factor to know about drugs used for pediatric patients because they typically have shorter half-lives in children and thus more fluctuation in peak and trough serum concentrations. Infants are less likely to exhibit chronopharmacokinetics because they sleep equally during the daytime and night and do not have established diurnal variation or a circadian rhythm. A list of drugs that possess chronopharmacokinetics is included in an article by Gilman [47].

Assay Accuracy

Assays should be used that are accurate, require small blood volumes, and are not affected by metabolites or interfering substances that might be found in a patient's serum. For the clinical laboratory, an assay that is easily and rapidly performed is also desired.

Dosing Regimens

Drugs for pediatric patients should be dosed on a mg/kg or a mg/m^2 basis, using information available for the patient's age group. In addition, the patient's renal and hepatic function must be considered. The route for administration must be determined based on the severity of the illness, the availability of the medication for a particular route of administration, and whether the patient is able to take a medication orally. For example, a patient who is comatose or is vomiting would be unable to take an oral medication.

TABLE 2 Pediatric Pharmacokinetic Data of Some Medications[a,b]

Drug	Therapeutic serum conc. (μg/mL)	Bioavailability (for oral drugs) (%)	Plasma Protein Binding (%)	V_d (L/kg)	$T_{1/2}$ (hours)
Carbamazepine	4–12	>70	40–90	1.5 (neonate) 0.8–1.9 (child)	8–25 (child), $T_{1/2}$ varies with multiple dosing
Clonazepam	20–80 ng/mL	>85	47–80	3.2 (child)	20–40 (child)
Ethosuximide	40–100	~100	0	0.6–0.7 (child)	24–36 (child)
Gentamicin	trough ≤2 peak 4–10	Not available	<30	0.4–0.6 (neonate) 0.3–0.35 (child)	3–11.5 (<1 wk) 3–6 (1 wk–6 mo) 1.2 (child)
Phenobarbital	15–40	80–100	40–60	0.6–1.2 (neonate) 0.7–1 (child)	45–173 (neonate) 37–72 (child)
Phenytoin	10–20	85–95	>90	1–1.2 (premature neonate) 0.8–0.9 (full-term neonate) 0.7–0.8 (child)	6–140 (<8 days)[d] 5–80 (9–21 days)[a] 2–20 (21–36 days)[d] 5–18 (child)[d]
Theophylline	5–15	up to 100%, depending on the formulation	32–40 (neonate) 55–60 (child	0.4–1 (premature neonate) 0.3–0.7 (child)	19.9–35 (neonate) 3.4 ± 1.1 (1–4 yrs)
Valproic acid	40–100 (150)[e]	100	>90[c]	0.2 (child)	23–35 (neonate) 4–14 (child)

[a]Adapted from Refs. 2 and 3 and Sagraves, R., Epilepsy and other convulsive disorders. In: *Pediatric Pharmacotherapy*, 2nd ed. (R. J. Kuhn, ed.), University of Kentucky, Lexington, 1993; Taketomo, C. K., Hodding, J. H., and Kraus, D. M., *Pediatric Dosage Handbook*, LEXI-COMP Inc., Hudson, OH, 1992; Kauffman, R. E., Drug therapeutics in the infant and child. In: *Pediatric Pharmacology: Therapeutic Principles in Practice* (S. J. Yaffe, and J. V. Aranda, eds.), W. B. Saunders Co., Philadelphia, 1992, pp. 212–219; Rane, A., Drug disposition and action in infants and children. In: *Pediatric Pharmacology: Therapeutic Principles in Practice* (S. J. Yaffe, and J. V. Aranda, eds.), W. B. Saunders Co., Philadelphia, 1992, pp. 10–19.

[b]Age or stage of life in parenthesis.

[c]May vary with serum concentration.

[d]Michaelis Menton Pharmacokinetics; $T_{1/2}$ varies with serum concentration.

[e]Upper end of the serum concentration range is not definitely established.

Clark's, Freid's, and Young's rules, found in some textbooks, have been used in the past to help determine doses for pediatric patients. They should, however, no longer be used because they do not take into consideration literature about pediatric dosing, body composition, and surface area, or pharmacokinetic considerations.

The bibliography contains a list of handbooks and other references that are useful sources of dosing information for neonatal and pediatric patients. *Drugdex* is also an excellent resource for such information as are drug information centers in pediatric hospitals or university settings.

Excipients and Additives in Medications

Pharmaceutical products may contain, in addition to the active or therapeutic agent(s), a variety of other ingredients, termed inactive or inert, which are categorized as excipients or additives (flavorings, sweeteners, preservatives, stabilizers, diluents, lubricants, etc.). The words inert or inactive may be misnomers for some excipients because some have been shown to cause adverse effects. Neonates and young children are at risk for such effects because they may not be able to metabolize or eliminate an ingredient in a pharmaceutical product in the same manner as an adult. In addition, patients of various ages have experienced allergic reactions to excipients such as tartrazine dyes.

Benzyl alcohol is a preservative contained in multidose vials of bacteriostatic sodium chloride and bacteriostatic water for injection and pharmaceuticals available in multidose vials for parenteral use. An association between benzyl alcohol in solutions used for flushing intravascular catheters and to reconstitute medications, and a "gasping syndrome" and deaths in neonates was first reported in the early 1980s [53,54]. In addition, neonates displayed clinical findings such as an elevated anion gap, metabolic acidosis, CNS depression, seizures, respiratory failure, renal and hepatic failure, cardiovascular collapse, and death. Those at highest risk were premature infants who weighed less than 1,250 g at birth [53–55]. In a study by Benda et al., premature neonates who survived benzyl alcohol administration were compared to neonates born after the use of benzyl alcohol-containing flush solutions was generally discontinued [56]. They noted that the survivors had a higher incidence of cerebral palsy (50%) compared to infants who did not receive benzyl alcohol flushes (2.4%) ($P < 0.001$). In addition, the incidence of cerebral palsy and developmental delay was 53.9 vs. 11.9% in the two populations ($P < 0.001$). The cause is probably neurotoxicity associated with benzyl alcohol use and the inability of neonates, especially those premature, to adequately metabolize benzyl alcohol [57]. The American Academy of Pediatrics [58], the Centers for Disease Control [59], and the FDA [60] recommend that the administration of products containing benzyl alcohol be avoided in infants. Preservative-free intravascular flush solutions are also recommended.

Initially, it was believed that benzyl alcohol was only toxic in neonates who received doses higher than 99 mg/kg [55], but it has been suggested that lower doses may also be toxic, resulting in kernicterus and intraventricular hemorrhage [61,62]. Therefore, pharmaceutical preparations and fluids containing benzyl alcohol should be avoided in premature neonates.

Benzoic acid and sodium benzoate are added in low concentrations to various pharmaceutical preparations as bacteriostatic and fungistatic agents. Hypersensitivity reactions to the benzoates have occurred when administered to allergic patients, such as those with asthma, those who do not tolerate aspirin, and those with a history of urticaria [57]. Hyperbilirubinemia and systemic effects attributable to benzyl alcohol may occur in premature neonates because benzyl alcohol is metabolized to benzoic acid [57].

Propylene glycol is found as a solvent in some iv multiple vitamin preparations (e.g., MVI-12) and a variety of pharmaceutical preparations for parenteral administration including phenytoin, digoxin, and diazepam. MacDonald et al. [63] noted that neonates who received MVI-12 (propylene glycol dose of approximately 3 g/day) vs. those who received MVI concentrate (propylene glycol dose of approximately 300 mg/day) exhibited a significant increase in seizures. In addition, infants in the first group suffered from hyperbilirubinemia and renal failure. (Although MVI concentrate is no longer on the market in the United States, it was used in the early 1980s).

Serum hyperosmolality has been reported in infants who received vitamin preparations [64] and in burn patients due to the topical absorption of propylene glycol-containing products [65,66]. In addition, burn patients have experienced metabolic acidosis with a high anion gap, decreased ionized calcium concentrations, acute renal failure, and death from topical propylene glycol absorption [57,67]. Problems associated with the oral ingestion of propylene glycol-containing products by children include CNS depression, seizures, and cardiac dysrhythmias [68]. Hypotension, cardiac dysrhythmias, respiratory depression, and seizures have occurred after the rapid administration of phenytoin which may be associated with propylene glycol [69].

In the early 1980s, reports appeared in the literature about deaths in neonates associated with the administration of IV E-Ferol, a product that contained vitamin E (dl-α-tocopherol) and the emulsifiers polysorbate 80 (9%) and polysorbate 20 (1%) [57]. Some infants who received this vitamin E product developed coagulopathy, renal failure, hepatic failure, and death. On autopsy, the infants who died from hepatic failure demonstrated cholestasis similar to that associated with parenteral nutrition. Toxic reactions may have occurred because of the high doses of vitamin E, the presence of polysorbate(s), a contaminant in the pharmaceutical preparation, or a combination of all three [57].

The American Academy of Pediatrics Committee on Drugs recommends that medications intended for pediatric use be ethanol free [70]. If, because of stability or solubility problems with the active ingredients(s), liquid medications need ethanol as an ingredient, they should not contain more than 5% v/v [70]. The Academy also recommends that ingestion of a single dose of an ethanol-containing product by a pediatric patient should not result in blood ethanol concentrations higher than 25 mg/100 mL, that the volume of a packaged liquid medication should be minimal so that its entire ingestion would not result in a lethal dose, and that safety closures should be on all medicinals containing more than 5% v/v ethanol. In addition, the Academy suggests that children under six years of age who need an ethanol-containing OTC preparation be under medical supervision and that doses of any ethanol-containing product be spaced at intervals to avoid ethanol accumulation [70].

The Academy of Pediatrics made their recommendations concerning ethanol exposure from medications based on potential acute and chronic ethanol-related problems. Acutely, the coadministration of ethanol may alter drug absorption or metabolism, and may result in drug interactions (e.g., increased sedation when taken with sedatives).

Disulfiram-like reactions have occurred after the ingestion of an alcohol-containing medication or when an ethanol-containing product is used in conjunction with medications such as metronidazole, sulfonamides, chloramphenicol, or cefamandole [70]. Central nervous system effects (muscle incoordination, a longer reaction time, behavioral changes) are the most commonly reported acute adverse reactions associated with ethanol ingestion. Such reactions have occurred with blood ethanol concentrations in the range of 1–100 mg/100 mL [70]. Lethal ethanol doses in children occur at approximately 3 g/kg although deaths due to ethanol-induced hypoglycemia have occurred at lower doses or because of interactions with other medications [70,71]. Chronic ethanol exposure may induce hepatic enzymes, and may thus alter the clearance of drugs such as phenytoin, phenobarbital, and warfarin [72]. Examples of other additives that have been problematic in pediatric patients include lactose [68], tartrazine dyes [57,68], and sulfites [68].

It is therefore important for health care professionals, and especially those who are responsible for selecting and administering medications to premature neonates, to examine pharmaceutical preparations for the presence of inactive ingredients as well as for the active drug. The provision of drugs should be based on choosing the safest preparations possible. Various brands of medications should be compared to ensure that products without hazardous excipients are selected. In the hospital setting, the Pharmacy and Therapeutics Committee and the pharmacy department play important roles in this process because they compare preparations for formulary selection. In the outpatient setting, physicians and pharmacists must responsibly select the most appropriate brand of a particular medication. Kumar et al. recommend that the labeling of pharmaceutical products should include the names and amounts of excipients as well as those of active ingredients to help health care professionals select the appropriate drug products for neonates [73].

Intravenous Administration

Without being properly instructed about methods used to administer iv medication to pediatric patients, health care personnel may give a medication incorrectly, resulting in an inappropriate or unexpected therapeutic response. Therefore, it is important that health care personnel (nurses, physicians, pharmacists) understand how medications are appropriately administered by this route to children.

The iv route is most frequently chosen for medication delivery when a patient's clinical condition requires that a medication be administered by the most expeditious and complete method possible. In addition, some drugs are only available for iv administration. Although this is the most reliable route for drug delivery to the systemic circulation, problems can occur that reduce and/or delay medication delivery because of the product selected, dosage volume needed, or frequency of administration, but problems can also be associated with the iv delivery system. The last occur most frequently when a small medication volume is administered at a slow rate as is often needed for a neonate or young infant. A brief discussion of problems associated with the delivery of iv medications to pediatric patients is given here. A thorough overview of iv drug administration to pediatric patients is given in Ref. 76 and in a recent review article [80].

A discussion of problems that can occur with iv drug administration to pediatric patients must include a review of the intrinsic factors, listed below, and of the disposable (e.g., tubing) and nondisposable equipment that can affect drug delivery [76].

- Location of the injection site in the iv tubing (i.e., sites on the iv tubing),
- Type of injection site (Y-site, T-type, T-connector, stopcock) used for drug administration,
- Iv tubing material,
- Intraluminal tubing diameter,
- Flow dynamics of the fluid in the intravenous system, and
- Filters.

Disposable IV Equipment, Effects on Drug Delivery

Infusion Rates and Location of Injection Sites

The first of many articles that have explored problems that can occur with iv drug delivery to pediatric patients was published in 1979 by Gould and Roberts [74]. They demonstrated in their study of an in vitro system for drug administration (Fig. 3) that infusion rates as well as the location of the injection sites in the infusion system influence the infusion profile of iv-administered medications. Figure 4 shows the effects of different iv-fluid rates on the length of time to infuse 95% of a gentamicin dose administered at various injection sites in the infusion system [74]. Gould and Roberts reported that at a low infusion rate of 3 mL/h, a drug takes longer to be infused and that the infusion time depends on the site of administration (i.e., the further the drug injection site from a

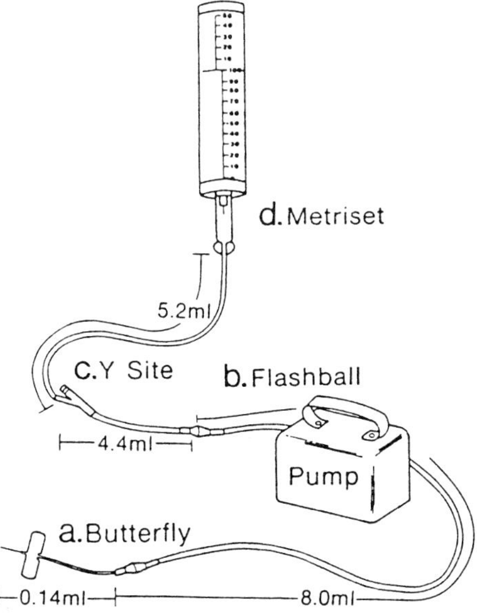

FIG. 3. Intravenous administration system used by Gould and Roberts. (From Ref. 74.)

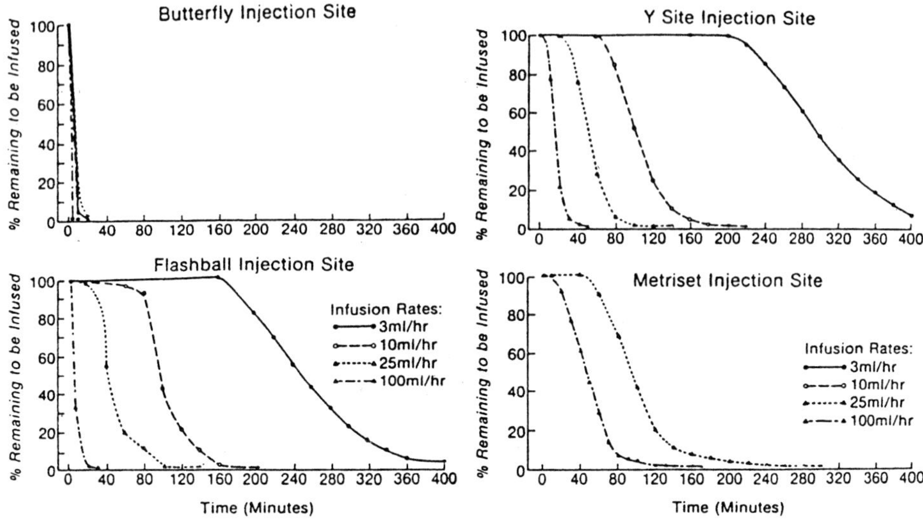

FIG. 4. Influence of iv flow rate on the infusion profile of gentamicin. (From Ref. 74.)

patient, the longer it takes to administer 95% of the medication, see Figs. 4–6). Thus, it took Gould and Roberts approximately 400 min to infuse gentamicin at a rate of 3 mL/h via the Y-site in their administration system. However, the same drug administered at the butterfly injection site at the same flow rate, reduced the length of time to administer 95% of the drug to less than 20 min. Figure 5 shows further differences in infusion

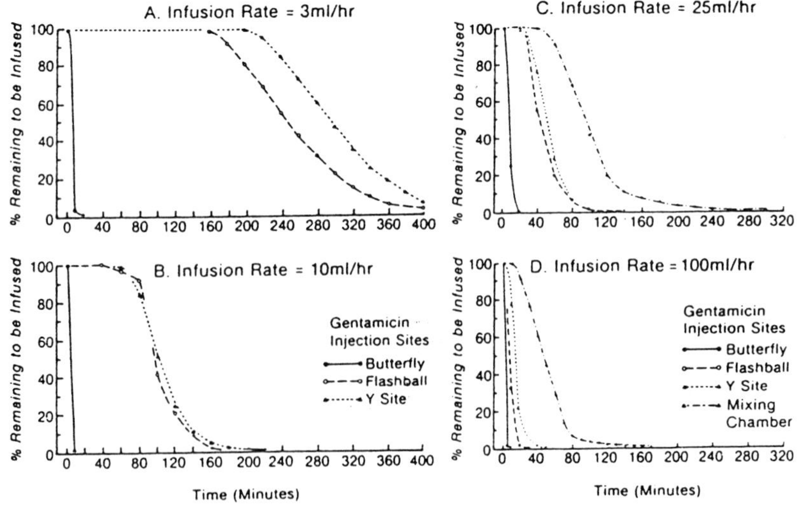

FIG. 5. Influence of location and injection sites on the infusion profile of gentamicin. (From. Ref. 76.)

A.

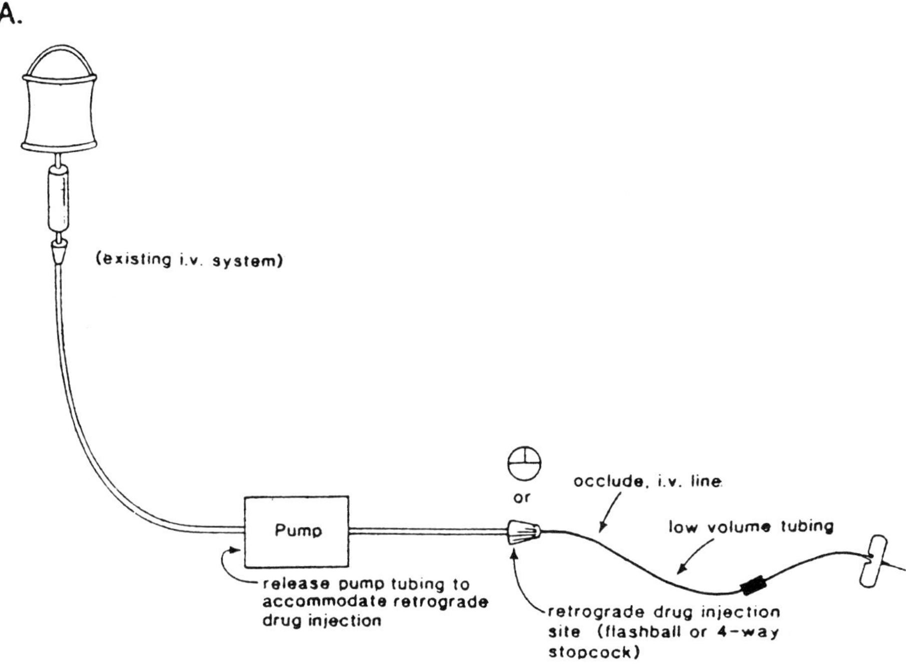

B.

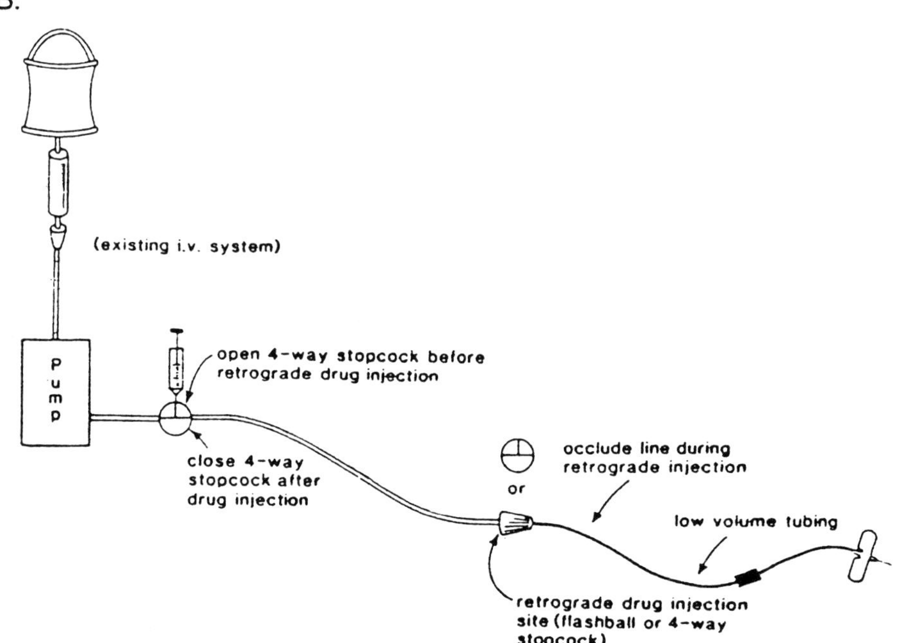

FIG. 6. Examples of retrograde system setups. (From Leff, R. D., and Roberts, R. J., Methods for intravenous drug administration in the pediatric patient, *J. Pediatr.*, 98:631–635 (1981).)

profiles for gentamicin administered at various injection sites located at various distances from a patient. Gould and Roberts also stated that the time needed for drug administration in their iv system was longer than expected [74].

Nahata et al. [75] demonstrated that the injection site chosen for drug administration could affect serum drug concentrations in pediatric patients. Peak serum chloramphenicol succinate and free chloramphenicol concentrations were significantly higher when the drug was administered at a flashball site than in a Buretol (mixing chamber) at a significant distance from the patient. In addition, peak serum concentrations occurred earlier at the flashball site. However, no statistical differences were observed between trough concentrations or areas under the curve when the two injection sites were compared.

Type of Injection Site

Leff and Roberts [76] demonstrated that the amount of drug received by a pediatric patient and the drug-delivery rate are influenced by the type of injection site (Y-site, T-type, T-connector, stopcock) and the volume (dead space) contained in that particular site. For the delivery of small dosage volumes (less than 1 mL) the iv tubing should have "micro" injection sites (Y-sites, T-connectors, etc.) that hold a minimum volume of fluid to prevent a drug from being sequestered in the injection site. In addition, the amount of iv fluid needed to adequately flush microinjection sites to clear the drug would be less than needed to flush injection sites found on macrobore tubing used to administer drugs to adults.

Manufacturers' Materials and Intraluminal Tubing Diameter

The material used by the manufacturer of iv tubing, and the intraluminal diameter of the tubing affects drug delivery. Drugs such as diazepam, insulin, and nitroglycerin can adsorb to polyvinyl chloride plastic iv tubing and filters; insulin can also adsorb to polyethylene and glass [76]. Kubajak et al. [77] demonstrated that the diameter and length of iv tubing affects the rate of drug administration as does the flow rate of the iv fluid in the system.

Fluid Flow Dynamics

Another characteristic of iv tubing that affects drug delivery is the fluid flow dynamics. It appears that flow in iv tubing is best characterized by laminar flow, and that the radius of the tubing has the greatest influence on the drug flow rate and thus on the drug-delivery time. Poiseuille's law describes flow in iv tubing as in Eq. (2).

$$q_v = \frac{Pr^4}{4nL} \tag{2}$$

where q_v is the volumetric flow rate, P is the pressure change in the tubing, r is the radius of the tubing, n is the viscosity of the fluid, and L is the length of the tubing.

Thus, for iv drug delivery to pediatric patients, microbore tubing with an intraluminal diameter of <0.06 in. (1.5 mm) should be used rather than macrobore tubing. The use of microbore tubing allows lengthening the tubing without significantly increasing delivery time.

Filters

A filter, especially one with a large reservoir volume, may prolong and/or reduce drug delivery. This occurs if the drug and its diluent are of different densities and the drug separates in a layer in the filter [78]. Therefore, a filter with a small reservoir volume should be chosen.

Drug and Fluid Considerations for Intravenous Drug Administration

Characteristics of the drug and the fluid such as drug volume, osmolality, pH, and density may affect iv drug delivery. The frequency and duration of drug administration is also important as is the need for the infusion system to handle multiple drugs. This may lead to drug incompatibilities, and problems in medication scheduling.

Osmolality and pH

Osmolality and pH must be considered when preparing a drug solution for iv administration to pediatric patients. Problems such as tissue irritation, pain on injection, phlebitis, electrolyte shifts, and even intraventricular hemorrhages in neonates have been associated with the administration of drug solutions with high osmolalities [79]. The drug solutions should have osmolalities similar to serum osmolality. To control osmolality, a drug can be diluted with a vehicle selected for iv infusion via a syringe infusion system [79] or the iv flow rate can be adjusted to achieve a particular drug–vehicle osmolality [76]. Although pH may also be a causative factor for the development of phlebitis and pain at the injection site, it is difficult to adjust the pH because changing it may affect the solubility and stability of the drug.

Density

If the density of a drug is significantly different from that of the diluent, the drug may layer out on a filter or in the iv tubing. The latter occurs more frequently with macrobore tubing, a low flow rate, or if the tubing is in a particular position. A density problem can be avoided by using microbore tubing which promotes mixing; this is especially important when iv flow rates are low, as are needed for neonates or young infants.

Frequency and Duration of Drug Administration; Multiple Drugs

To ensure that frequent doses are administered at appropriate intervals or that multiple drugs are administered to avoid drug incompatibilities, a syringe infusion pump can be used to administer drug volumes over a specific length of time. This also avoids a situation where part of a dose is left in the tubing when the iv set is changed, as has been reported for manual administration techniques. More than one syringe pump can be used to simultaneously administer compatible drugs in a parallel system into a micro-Y-site or stopcock.

Types of Intravenous Administration

Drugs may require iv administration as continuous infusions or at intermittent intervals (q4h, q6h, q12h, etc.). Manual methods require the administration of the drug into the iv system at an injection site (Y-site, T-connector, stopcock, etc.), added to the iv solution in a mixing chamber, or added to an iv bag to be administered by gravity. A mechanical device such as a syringe pump, controller, or infusion pump may be used for drug administration. All the mechanical devices may have utility for continuous drug infusions, but a syringe pump is best for administering a drug at intermittent intervals.

Manual Administration

Manual administration is not as accurate as using a syringe pump for drug administration. It can be used for small volumes of medication (<3 mL), a low flow rate (< 20 mL/hr), or if the antegrade (forward toward the patient) injection of a drug bolus is safe [76]. If a medication is to be administered antegrade, it should be administered slowly into a microinjection site (stopcock, micro-Y-site, etc.) toward the patient; microbore tubing should be placed between the injection site and the patient to reduce the time to get the drug to the patient. Leff and Roberts [76] recommend that the volume of the drug to be injected by the antegrade technique should be smaller than the tubing fluid volume between the injection site and the patient. If the medication volume is too large to be safely given by antegrade administration, but the fluid flow rate is low (<20 mL/hr), the drug may be administered by a retrograde technique (Fig. 6). Advantages of retrograde administration include no need for additional fluid to administer the medication and no need to change the flow rate [80]. Disadvantages include that the drug volume should not exceed half the volume in the retrograde tubing and that the delivery of the medication to the patient may be slower than anticipated [80].

Mechanical System for Drug Administration

If a mechanical system is chosen for drug administration, the appropriate infusion device must be selected, based on operating mechanism, flow accuracy, flow continuity, and the ability to detect occlusions. Other important factors include an alarm system, ease of operation, ability to be cleaned easily, and safety from children inadvertently trying to change pump settings. A syringe pump is best for administering small dosage volumes and when intermittent intervals are needed for medications. It is the mechanical device most often chosen for medication administration because it can be used for intermittent administration of small and large doses, or for the continuous infusion of medications at low rates. The drug can be administered separately of the primary iv fluid flow rate with the drug and the fluid mixing for only a short distance thereafter in microbore tubing (Fig. 7) before reaching the patient or the drug can be delivered via microbore tubing between the syringe pump and a micro-T-connector, where for a short distance the drug is mixed with the iv fluid from the primary iv (Fig. 8). In addition to being able to more accurately deliver drugs than by manual methods, syringe pump systems have the advantages of enabling nurses to separate the administration of incompatible drugs, reduce the difficulties associated with the administration of multiple doses of a particular medication, and shorten nursing time.

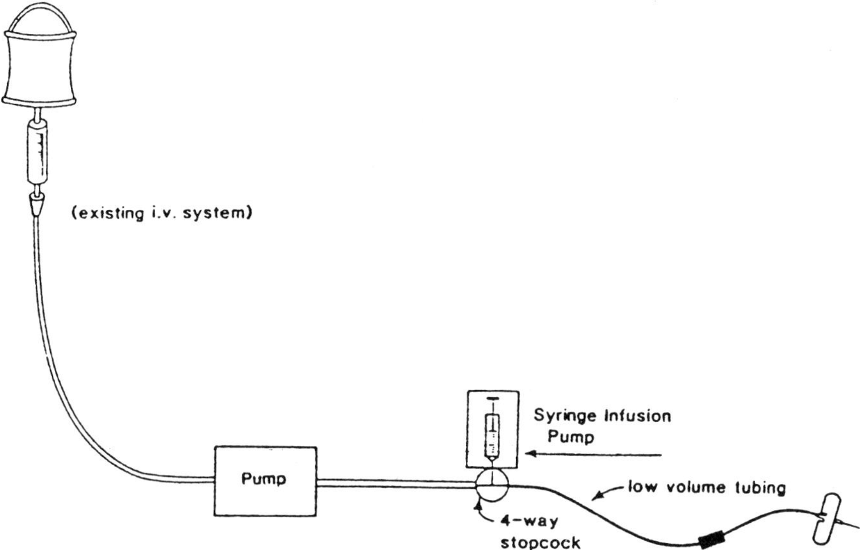

FIG. 7. Syringe pump setup with drug administered separately of the primary iv fluid flow rate. Mixing of the drug and iv fluid occurs at a stopcock and for a short distance in microbore tubing. (From Leff, R. D., and Roberts, R. J., Methods for intravenous drug administration in the pediatric patient, *J. Pediatr.*, 98:631–635 (1981).)

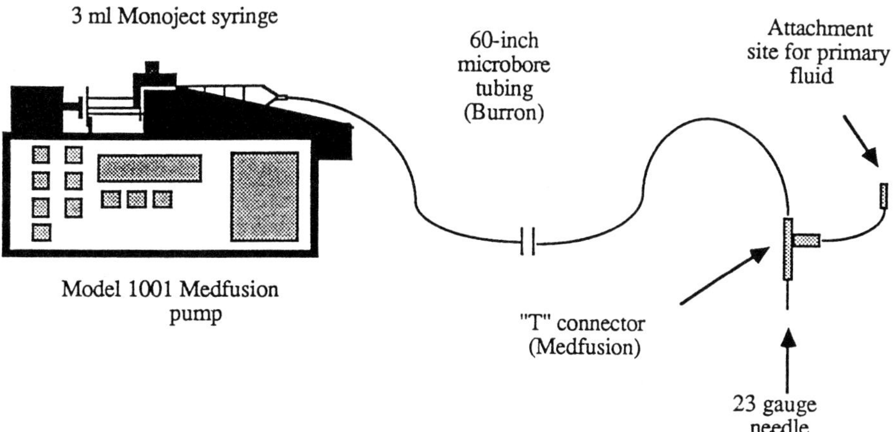

FIG. 8. Drug delivered via microbore tubing between the syringe pump and a micro-T-connector where for a short distance the drug is mixed with iv fluid from the primary iv. (From Roberts, G., Smith, C. L., Sagraves, R., Kamper, C., and Hampton, E. M., *An in vitro evaluation of gentamicin delivery to neonates*, ASHP Midyear Clinical Meeting Abstracts, New Orleans, 1991 (December); P-61R Abstract, in preparation for publication.)

At Children's Hospital of Oklahoma, a syringe pump setup is used as depicted in Fig. 8. Medication syringes are prepared in the pharmacy (drugs prepared in appropriate diluents at set concentrations to achieve desired osmolalities) for iv administration, and preparation does not need to be undertaken in a patient-care area. For more information on iv drug administration to pediatric patients, the reader is referred to Leff, R. D., and Roberts, R. J., *Practical Aspects of Intravenous Drug Administration*, American Society of Hospital Pharmacists (ASHP), Bethesda, MD, 1992. This publication also covers information on programmable infusion, patient-controlled infusion, closed-loop infusion devices, and pulsatile infusion.

Administration of Oral Medications

The oral route is typically the preferred route for medication administration to pediatric patients. Other routes may be used, if for example, the patient cannot take a medication orally because of vomiting or being unable to swallow, or the medication is unavailable for oral use. In addition, for specific problems it may be better to deliver the medication directly to the area being treated, for example, inhalation, ophthalmic administration, or otic administration.

Dosage Forms

Oral Liquids

Liquid medications are the most commonly administered oral medications to pediatric patients because of the ease of swallowing by infants and young children who cannot swallow solid dosage forms. However, the availability of some medications as liquid formulations may be limited. If not available in liquid form, a solid dosage form may need to be modified by the pharmacist, another health care provider, or by the parent at home. If a solid dosage form is modified, for example, a suspension is prepared, will the drug be stable and for how long, and will it be absorbed differently than the original dosage form? These are just a few questions that must be answered about the extemporaneous preparation of a drug product for a pediatric patient.

Alcohol-free products should be chosen for pediatric patients whenever possible. Furthermore, the inactive ingredients or excipients contained in a particular oral preparation should be identified. This is especially important if the patient had an adverse reaction to a particular excipient or there is another reason to avoid a particular additive in a medication. In 1985, the Committee on Drugs of the American Academy of Pediatrics recommended that pharmaceutical products contain a qualitative listing of inactive ingredients in order that products containing these ingredients could be avoided in patients who had problems with specific adjuvants [68]. A recent article by Kumar et al. [73] contains lists of inactive ingredients (sweeteners, flavorings, dyes, and preservatives) found in many liquid medications such as analgesics, antipyretics, antihistamine decongestants, cough and cold remedies, antidiarrheal agents, and theophylline preparations. The authors of this article and Golightly et al. have reviewed adverse effects associated with many inactive ingredients [57,73].

TABLE 3 Osmolalities of Liquid Pharmaceuticals for Oral Administration[a]

Liquid Preparation	Osmolality (Mean ± SEM)
Propylene glycol	8326 ± 1467
Saccharin-containing drugs	
Albuterol	65
Haloperidol	47
Suspensions	2500 ± 246
Sugar-containing[b] drugs	5574 ± 594

[a]Adapted from Ref. 83.
[b]Sucrose, mannitol, glucose, and others.

Liquid medications, taken orally, may cause diarrhea and other GI symptoms, or they may aggravate a GI distress that a patient is already experiencing. These GI effects can be associated with the high osmolality of some oral liquids. The addition of theophylline to enteral feedings increases the osmolality of the feeding [81] and has resulted in diarrhea [82]. Bloss and Sybert [83] determined the osmolalities of various oral liquids and noted that osmolalities are especially high in preparations containing propylene glycol or sugars (e.g., sucrose, mannitol, glucose), or were listed as suspensions (see Table 3). It is important to compare various brands of liquid medications because they may contain different excipients and may have different osmolalities.

Sustained-Release Preparations

Most medications have shorter half-lives in children than in adults, and therefore children may need sustained-release products to maintain serum concentrations in the therapeutic range. For example, a sustained-release theophylline product may be needed for a child with asthma. It may need to be administered every 8 h compared to every 12 h for a healthy, nonsmoking adult to maintain therapeutic serum concentrations. When choosing a sustained-release theophylline preparation for a child, it must be remembered that because of differences in release properties, theophylline sustained-release products are not interchangeable. A product selected for the pediatric asthma patient should be reliably absorbed with minimal serum concentration fluctuation (Slo-bid Gyrocaps) and not a preparation that has exhibited a two-fold difference in bioavailability when administered with or without food (e.g., Theo-Dur Sprinkle) [84–86].

For asthmatic children unable to swallow solid dosage forms, Slo-bid Gyrocaps are useful. They are available in variety of strengths for accurate mg/kg dosing and their contents can be sprinkled on a small amount of food (e.g., apple sauce) for administration. Sustained-release products should never be chewed, crushed, or made into a liquid preparation such as a suspension. Any of these practices would change the release characteristics and could result in a rapid release of the active ingredients, possibly resulting in toxicity. Reference 87 is an excellent resource on what solid dosage forms should not be crushed for oral administration.

Extemporaneous Liquid Preparations

Because many medications are not available as liquid preparations, there are times when powder papers or suspensions must be prepared. In addition, capsules must sometimes be opened and the contents taken orally. An excellent source of information about the preparation of liquid dosage forms for pediatric patients can be found in Nahata, M. C., and Hipple, T. F., *Pediatric Drug Formulations*, 2nd ed., Harvey Whitney Books, Cincinnati, 1992, pp. 1–79. Of the products included in this book, Nahata estimates that approximately 70% have little stability data. This is a major problem that can only be reconciled with the availability of more commercial liquid products for pediatric use or with an increase in stability information provided via research.

Product Selection

Products for oral administration should be in the dosage form most readily taken by the child. If the child is old enough to participate in the decision-making process, he or she may state a preference for a liquid, chewable tablet, tablet, or capsule, if the needed drug is available in a variety of dosage forms and appropriate dosage. If a liquid medication is needed, a product should be chosen based on texture, taste, and ease of administration. Other factors that must be considered is the absence of alcohol and dyes, and an osmolality that should be close to physiologic (280-290 mOsm/kg). Are there excipients or adjuvants in the product, and if so, what are they and what is their concentration? Is there bioavailability information or pharmacokinetic information for the oral medication in pediatric patients, and if so, in what age groups? Is there information about the extemporaneous product that is to be prepared?

Ms. Wheeler Chater, a pharmacist in North Carolina whose pharmacy is in a pediatric clinic, recommends that pediatric patients be involved in medication counseling in order to improve their understanding of why the medication is needed. In the counseling process, the word medication should be used and not the word drug because of the connotation associated with the latter in today's society [88,89]. Wheeler recommends that, when possible, a product be selected that requires the fewest number of doses administered per day, for example, every 12 h dosing rather than every 8 h, so that the medication does not have to be taken to school or day care for administration. If a medication must be given outside of the home, she recommends that two small labeled bottles be dispensed or one large bottle with a small empty bottle labeled to be used for medication administration at day care or school.

Health care providers including nurses, pharmacists, and physicians should demonstrate to parents and older children how medications should be administered and offer appropriate dosing devices (oral syringe, dropper, cylindrical medication spoon, or a small-volume doser with attachable nipple) to enable parents to accurately measure liquid products. A household teaspoon or tablespoon should not be used for medication administration because they are inaccurate.

Administration Techniques

The following information is given here to help health care providers counsel parents and older children on how medications should be administered by various routes.

Oral Liquids

An oral liquid medication needed for an infant or young child should be shaken well, if required, and accurately measured using an oral syringe, dropper, cylindrical medication spoon, or a small-volume doser with attachable nipple. If a dropper or an oral syringe is used, the liquid should be administered toward the inner cheek. Administration at the front of the mouth may allow the child to spit out the medication, whereas administration toward the back of the mouth may result in gagging or choking. Therefore, the oral syringe should be of an appropriate size to allow for administration into the inner cheek [88,89].

Oral Solid Dosage Forms (Tablets, Capsules)

A medication available only as a solid dosage form may be prepared as an extemporaneous liquid (e.g., suspension) or it may be modified for oral use, for example, by crushing. As mentioned previously, a sustained-release product should not be crushed or chewed. For a solid, nonsustained-release medication, the product can be crushed and mixed with a small amount of food just prior to administration. Examples of foods that may be used for mixing include applesauce, yogurt, or instant pudding, but the medication should not be added to an entire dish of food or to infant formula because the infant or child may not ingest the entire portion and thus not receive the total amount of medication.

Other Routes

Before and after administering a medication, the health care provider must wash his or her hands thoroughly.

Intramuscular Administration

Absorption of im administered medications depends on the injection site because the perfusion of individual muscle groups differs. For example, drug absorption from the deltoid muscle is faster than that from the vastus lateralis which is more rapid than that from the gluteus [18,19]. In addition, lower perfusion or hemostatic decompensation, frequently observed in ill neonates and young infants, may reduce im drug absorption. It may also be decreased in neonates who receive a skeletal muscle-paralyzing agent such as pancuronium because of reduced muscle contraction. In addition, the small muscle mass of neonates and young infants provides a small absorptive area [2].

The injection technique and the length of the needle used may affect drug absorption and thus serum concentrations. For example, using a longer needle (3.8 vs. 3.1 cm or 1½ vs. 1¼ in.) for im administration resulted in higher diazepam serum concentrations in adult patients [20]. Therefore, it is important to select the appropriate site for drug administration as well as the appropriate length and needle bore. Sites that can be used for im drug administration include the anterior thigh and vastus lateralis, the gluteal area, ventrogluteal, and the deltoid.

The midanterior thigh (rectus femoris) and the middle third of the vastus lateralis are used for im administration to young infants as well as to older children [21]. These sites are better developed and larger than other muscle groups that are used for drug administration to older children or adults. The technique is shown in Fig. 9 [21]. With the patient lying supine, the "needle should be inserted in the upper lateral quadrant of the

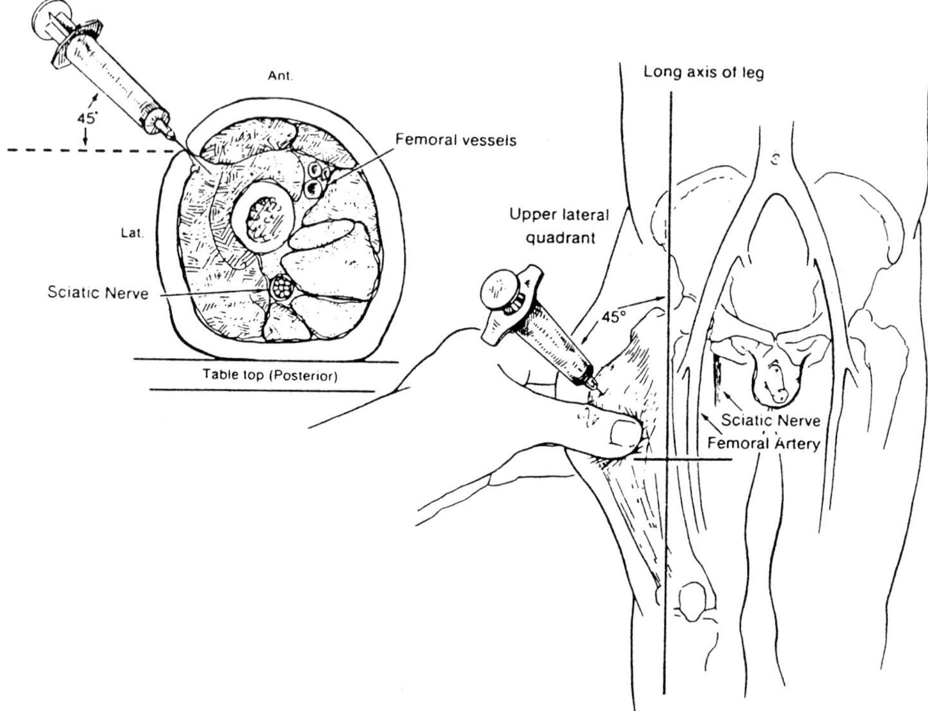

FIG. 9. A technique for anterior lateral-thigh intramuscular injection. (From Ref. 21.)

thigh, directed inferiorly at an angle of 45° with the long axis of the leg and posteriorly at a 45° angle'' [21] to the surface on which the patient is lying. The person administering the injection should compress the tissues of the injection site to help stabilize the extremity. A 1-in. (2.5-cm) needle has been recommended for all pediatric age groups for im administration by Bergeson et al. [21], whereas Newton et al. [20] recommend a 23–26 gauge 1½ in. (3.8-cm) needle. The volume of drug that can be administered in this manner is 0.1–1 mL in infants and 0.1–5 mL in older children and adults [20].

The gluteal musculature develops as the infant or child increases its mobility; it becomes a more suitable injection site in children who are walking [20,21]. Damage to the sciatic nerve is the major problem associated with this injection site, and it occurs more commonly in infants because of their lack of gluteal muscle mass [90]. Injury to the gluteal nerve, resulting in muscle atrophy, has occurred even when the injection technique was appropriately performed [21]. Other nerves including the pudendal, posterior femoral cutaneous, and the inferior cluneal nerves have been damaged because of poor injection technique [21]. Additional adverse effects associated with this drug administration route are discussed by Bergeson et al. [21].

A technique for gluteal administration is shown in Fig. 10, although other techniques are also used [21]. All techniques involve the determination of the upper outer quadrant (see Fig. 10 for anatomical landmarks). After the location of the upper outer quadrant is determined, the needle should be inserted at a 90° angle to the surface on which the

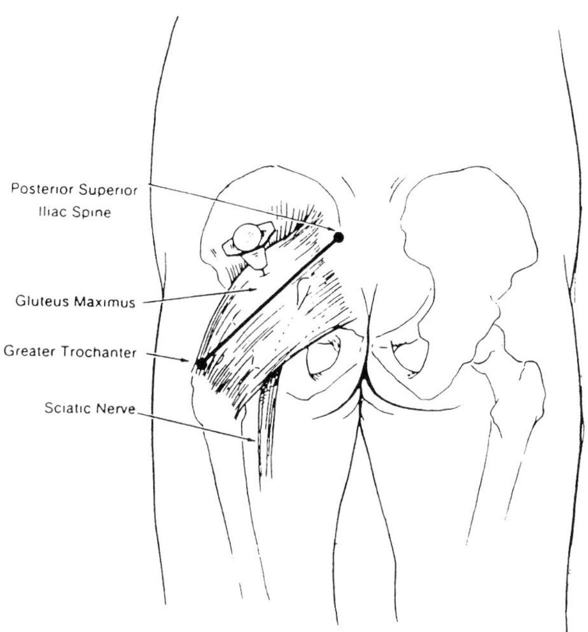

FIG. 10. A technique for gluteal-area intramuscular injection. (From Ref. 21.)

patient is lying, not to the patient's skin [21]. This site can be used for older children. A 1-in. (2.5-cm) needle has been recommended [21]. The volume of drug that can be administered in this manner is 0.1–5 mL for older children and adults [20].

The ventrogluteal (gluteus medius and minimus) site may be less hazardous for im administration than the dorsogluteal (gluteus maximus) site [21]. The technique is shown in Fig. 11 [21]. The person administering a drug im ventrogluteally, should first note the anatomical landmarks (the anterior superior iliac spine, tubercle of the iliac crest, and the upper border of the greater trochanter). The needle is inserted into a triangular area bounded by these landmarks while the patient is in the supine position. The location for this injection can be determined ''by placing the palm over the greater trochanter, the index finger over the anterior superior iliac spine, and spreading the index and middle fingers as far as possible'' [21].

The deltoid muscle can be used for im injections in older children, but is not an option for young infants and children because of their limited muscle mass. Although there are few complications associated with this administration route, nerve injury can occur [21]. The technique is shown in Fig. 12 [21]. The area for deltoid administration should be fully visible, so that the anatomical landmarks can be visualized. The needle for deltoid injection should enter the muscle halfway between the acromium process and the deltoid tuberosity to avoid hitting the underlying nerves [21]. The volume of drug that can be administered by this route to older children and adults is 0.1–2 mL [20]. The recommended needle length for older children is 1 in. (2.5 cm).

Newton et al. review the methods for minimizing pain associated with im injection [20].

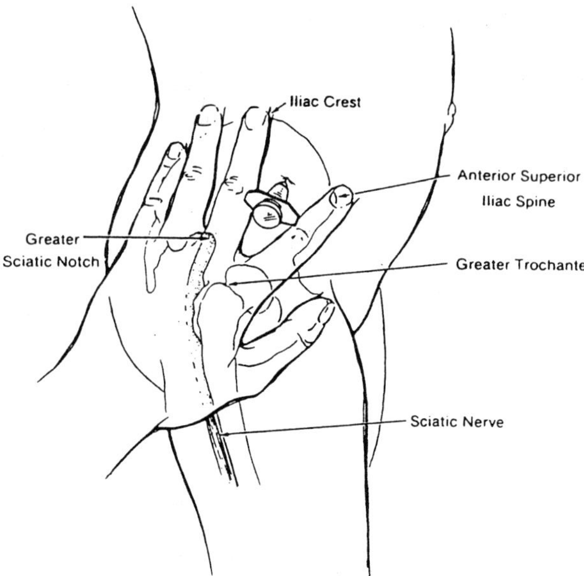

FIG. 11. von Hochstetter technique for ventrogluteal intramuscular injection. (From Ref. 21.)

Subcutaneous Administration

The sc route is used for the administration of drugs such as insulin that require slow absorption. It is not commonly employed for pediatric patients but is used for specific drugs. Typically a ½- or 1-in. (1.25- or 2.5-cm) needle is used with the volume of drug that can be administered by this route ranging from 0.1 to 1 mL (the volume of drug administered by this route may depend on patient size).

Percutaneous Administration

The skin should be thoroughly cleaned prior to applying a topical ointment, cream, etc. A thin layer of ointment or cream should be applied to the prescribed area to reduce the possibility of a toxic reaction. The area of the skin where the medication is applied should not be covered or occluded unless instructed to do so by the physician because this procedure may increase drug absorption. Specific information should be given on how to cover the area.

Rectal Suppositories

Before administration of a rectal suppository, the child's rectal area should be thoroughly cleaned. The infant or child should be placed on its side or stomach. The wrapper should be removed from the suppository and its pointed end should be inserted into the rectum above the anal sphincter. (If only half a suppository is prescribed, the suppository should be cut lengthwise.) A finger cot or finger wrapped in plastic can be used for administering the suppository. Because an infant or small child cannot adequately retain the sup-

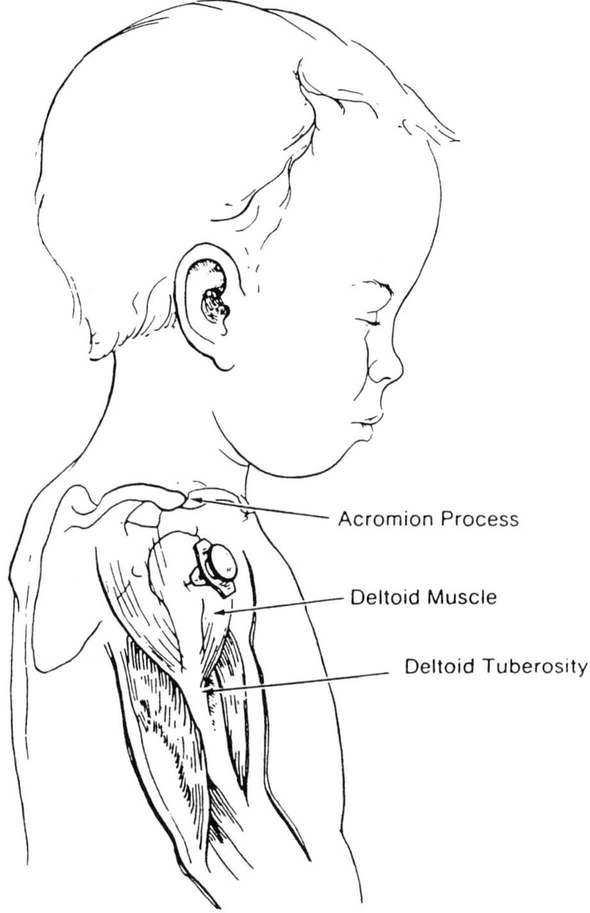

FIG. 12. A technique for deltoid intramuscular injection. (From Ref. 21.)

pository in the rectum, the buttocks should be held together firmly for a few minutes after rectal administration to hold the suppository in place [91].

Otic Preparations

Otic preparations should be at room temperature prior to administration. If the otic product is a suspension, it should be gently shaken for approximately 10 s before administration. The child should be lying on its side, and the earlobe should be gently pulled down and back to straighten the outer ear canal (for adults the earlobe is pulled up and back). Then the prescribed number of drops should be instilled in the ear without placing the dropper in the ear canal. The patient should be kept in a position with the ear tilted for approximately 2 min to help keep the ear drops in the ear [92]. This procedure may be repeated for the treatment of the other ear if needed. In some cases, the physician or pharmacist may recommend insertion of a cotton plug into the ear to retain the drug [91]. The tip of the dropper should be wiped clean after use.

Nasal Preparations

For adults, the first step in administering nose drops or a nasal spray is blowing the nose to clear the nasal passages of mucus and other secretions, but infants and young children are unable to do this. Therefore, the nasal passages may need to be cleared with a bulb syringe prior to medication administration. A child should lie down on its back, or a young infant or child should be placed in a lying position, and the head should be tilted slightly backward. An appropriate amount of medication should then be placed in each nostril. Thereafter, the infant or child should remain quiet for a few minutes to allow the medication to be absorbed. The dropper should be rinsed with hot water before return to the medication container.

Ophthalmic Preparations

An ophthalmic medication should be at room temperature prior to administration. If the eye drops are in a suspension, the container should be gently shaken before administration. A child old enough to follow directions should tilt its head slightly backward and to the side so that the eye drops will not drain into the tear ducts near the nose. The eyelids should be separated and the patient should be asked to look up. The appropriate amount of medication is instilled into the lower eyelid using the medication dropper, which should not touch the eyelids. The patient should look downward for a few seconds after drug administration. The eye(s) should then be closed for several minutes in order to spread the medication across the eyeball and be absorbed if the effect is to be systemic [93]. In addition, it has been recommended to gently put pressure on the inside corner of the eye for at least one minute to retard drainage of the medication [91]. If a squeeze bottle is used, the appropriate amount of medication should be gently squeezed into the eye(s). For each of these methods, the dropper or the tip of the squeeze bottle should be kept away from the eye or skin to avoid contamination of the administration device [93]. The dropper should not be rinsed after use because this could contaminate the dropper and the medication. The package insert should be reviewed for specific product information.

An alternative method, proposed by Smith [94], recommends that eyedrops be applied to the inner canthus of the eye while the patient keeps the eyes closed until told to open them after medication administration. Approximately 66% of the medication administered in this fashion is absorbed. In addition, this method may increase compliance and make children more cooperative [94].

For the administration of an ophthalmic ointment to a child who can cooperate the child should tilt its head backward and look up. After the hands have been washed, the person administering the medication should gently pull down the child's lower eyelid(s) for drug administration. A thin layer of ointment should then be placed in the lower eyelid(s). Afterward, the eyelid(s) should be closed for 1 to 2 min to allow for the spreading of the medication and absorption. During this process, the tip of the ophthalmic applicator should not touch the eye. After administration is completed, the tip of the applicator tube should be cleaned and tightly capped [93]. The package insert should be reviewed for specific product information.

Inhalers

For the use of inhaled medications (e.g., $\beta 2$ agonists, corticosteroids, or cromolyn for asthma), it is crucial for the child and parents to fully understand the mechanism of the metered-dose inhaler (MDI). A spacer may need to be used with the medication canister. The spacer, attached to the inhaler, provides a reservoir for the spray that is released from the inhaler, depositing the drug in the lungs rather than in the mouth. The following steps should be observed in the use of an MDI (adapted from Ref. 84).

- Read the instructions for the MDI that is to be used and modify the following instructions for that particular product; a child may need to use the MDI with a spacer
- Shake the MDI canister
- Remove the cap from the canister and hold the inhaler upright
- Tilt the head backward and place the mouthpiece between the lips
- Exhale
- Actuate the MDI with a slow, deep breath
- Hold a full inspiration for 10 s
- Exhale
- Repeat the process, if needed, after at least 1 min
- If the MDI is used for corticosteroid administration, the mouth should be rinsed with water after inhaling

Bibliography

Benitz, W. E., and Tatro, D. S., *The Pediatric Drug Handbook*, 2nd ed., Year Book Medical Publisher, Inc., Chicago, 1988.

Covington, T. R., and Lawson, L. C., eds., *Handbook of Nonprescription Drugs*, 10th ed., American Pharmaceutical Association, Washington (1993).

Leff, R. D., and Roberts, R. J., *Practical Aspects of Intravenous Drug Administration*, American Society of Hospital Pharmacists, Bethesda, 1992.

Levin, D. L., and Farrington, E., *Essentials of Pediatric Intensive Care: A Pocket Companion*, Quality Medical Publishing, Inc., St. Louis, 1990.

Nahata, M. C., and Hipple, T. F., *Pediatric Drug Formulations*, 2nd ed., Harvey Whitney Books, Cincinnati, 1992.

Nelson, J. D., *Pocketbook of Pediatric Antimicrobial Therapy*, 10th ed., Williams & Wilkins, Baltimore, 1993.

PDR for Nonprescription Drugs, Medical Economics, Montvale, NJ (yearly).

Phelps, S., and Cochran, E., eds., *Guidelines for Administration of Intravenous Medications to Pediatric Patients*, 4th ed., American Society of Hospital Pharmacists, Bethesda, 1993.

Physicians' Desk Reference, Medical Economics, Montvale, NJ (yearly).

Taketomo, C. K., Hodding, J. H., and Kraus, D. M., eds., *Pediatric Dosage Handbook*, 2nd ed., Lexi-Comp, Inc., Hudson, OH, 1993.

The Harriet Lane Handbook, 13th ed., Johns Hopkins Hospital, Mosby Year Book, St. Louis, 1993.

Young, T., and Magnum, O. B., eds., *Neofax '93: A Manual of Drugs Used in Neonatal Care*, 6th ed., Wake AHEC, Raleigh, NC, 1993.

Package inserts are also excellent sources of information.

References

1. Yaffe, S. J., and Aranda, J. V., Introduction and historical perspectives. In: *Pediatric Pharmacology: Therapeutic Principles in Practice* (S. J. Yaffe, and J. V. Aranda, eds.), W. B. Saunders, Philadelphia, 1992, pp. 3–9.

2. Besunder, J. B., Reed, M. D., and Blumer, J. L., Principles of drug biodisposition in the neonate: A critical evaluation of the pharmacokinetic-pharmacodynamic interface (Part I), *Clin. Pharmacokinet.*, 14:189–216 (1988).
3. Kearns, G. L., and Reed, M. D., Clinical pharmacokinetics in infants and children: A reappraisal, *Clin. Pharmacokinet.* 17 (Suppl. 1):29–67 (1989).
4. Reed, M. D., and Besunder, J. B., Developmental pharmacology: Ontogenic basis of drug disposition, *Pediatr. Clin. North. Am.*, 36:1053–1074 (1989).
5. Milsap, R. L., Hill, M. R., and Szefler, S. J., Special pharmacokinetic considerations in children. In: *Applied pharmacokinetics: Principles of therapeutic drug monitoring*, 3rd ed. (W. E. Evans, J. J. Schentag, and W. J. Jusko, eds.), Applied Therapeutics, Vancouver, WA, 1992, pp. 10.1–10.32.
6. Grand, R. J., Watkins, J. B., and Torti, F. M., Development of the human gastrointestinal tract: A review, *Gastroenterol.*, 70:790–810 (1976).
7. Agunod, M., Yomaguchi, N., Lopez, R., Lubby, A. L., and Glass, G. B. J., Correlative study of hydrochloric acid, pepsin and intrinsic factor secretion in newborns and infants, *Am. J. Dig. Dis.*, 14:400–414 (1969).
8. Stewart, C. F., and Hampton, E. M., Effect of maturation on drug disposition in pediatric patients, *Clin. Pharm.*, 6:548–564 (1987).
9. Christie, D. L., Development of Gastric Function During the First Month of Life. In: *Infancy* (E. Lebenthal, ed.), Raven Press, New York, 1981, pp. 109–120.
10. Cavell, B., Gastric emptying in preterm infants, *Acta Paediatr. Scand.*, 68:725–730 (1979).
11. Cavell, B., Gastric emptying in infants fed human milk or infant formula, *Acta Paediatr. Scand.*, 70:639–641 (1981).
12. Blumenthal, I., Edel, A., and Pides, R. S., Effect of posture on the pattern of stomach emptying in the newborn, *Pediatrics*, 62:532–632 (1979).
13. Blumenthal, I., The significance of gastric emptying time studies, *Pediatrics*, 66:480–481 (1980).
14. Hunt, J. N., Gastric emptying and secretion in man, *Physiol. Rev.*, 39:491–533 (1959).
15. Benmair, Y., Dreyfuss, F., Fischel, B., Frei, E. H., and Gilat, T., Study of gastric emptying using a ferro-magnetic tracer, *Gastroenterol.*, 73:1041–1045 (1977).
16. Blumer, J. L., and Reed, M. D., Principles of neonatal pharmacology. In: *Pediatric Pharmacology: Therapeutic Principles in Practice* (S. J., Yaffe, and J. V. Aranda, eds.), W. B. Saunders Co., Philadelphia, 1992; pp. 164–177.
17. Lebenthal, E., Lee, P. C., and Heitlinger, L. A., Impact of the development of the GI tract on infant feeding, *J. Pediatr.*, 101:1–9 (1983).
18. Greenblatt, D. J., and Koch-Weser, J., Intramuscular injection of drugs, *N. Engl. J.* Med., 295:542–546 (1976).
19. Evans, E. F., Proctor, J. D., Frantkin, M. J., Velandia, J., and Wasserman, A. J., Blood low in muscle groups and drug absorption, *Clin. Pharmacol. Ther.*, 17:44–47 (1975).
20. Newton, M., Newton, D., and Fudin, J., Reviewing the big three injection routes, *Nursing 92*, 1992 (Febr.):34–42.
21. Bergeson, P. S., Singer, S. A., and Kaplan, A. M., Intramuscular injections in children, *Pediatrics*, 70:944–948 (1982).
22. Sagraves, R., and Kamper, C., Controversies in cardiopulmonary resuscitation: Pediatric considerations, *DICP, Ann. Pharmacother.*, 25:760–772 (1991).
23. Ghadially, R., and Shear, N. H., Topical Therapy and Percutaneous Absorption. In: *Pediatric Pharmacology: Therapeutic Principles in Practice* (S. J. Yaffe, and J. V. Aranda, eds.), W. B. Saunders Co., Philadelphia, 1992, pp. 72–77.
24. Evans, N. S., Rutter, N., and Hadgraft, J., Percutaneous administration of theophylline in preterm infant, *J. Pediatr.*, 107:307–311 (1985).
25. Ward, J. T., Jr., Endotracheal drug therapy, *Am. J. Emerg. Med.*, 1:71–82 (1983).

26. de Boer, A. G., Moolenaar, F., de Leede, L. G. J., and Breimer, D. D., Rectal drug administration: Clinical pharmacokinetic considerations, *Clin. Pharmacokinet.*, 7:285–311 (1982).
27. Iob, V., and Swanson, W. W., Mineral growth of the human fetus, *Am. J. Dis. Child.*, 47:302–306 (1934).
28. Widdowson, E. M., and Spray, C. M., Chemical development in utero, *Arch. Dis. Child.*, 26:205–214 (1951).
29. Morselli, P. L., Clinical pharmacokinetics in neonates, *Clin. Pharmacokinet.*, 1:81–98 (1976).
30. Pitlick, W., Painter, M., and Pippenger, C., Phenobarbital pharmacokinetics in neonates, *Clin. Pharmacol. Ther.*, 23:346–350 (1978).
31. Painter, M. J., Pippenger, C., MacDonald, H., and Pitlick, W., Phenobarbital and diphenylhydantoin levels in neonates with seizures, *J. Pediatr.*, 92:315–319 (1978).
32. Giacoia, G., Jusko, W. J., Menke, J., and Koup, J. R., Theophylline pharmacokinetics in premature infants with apnea, *J. Pediatr.*, 89:829–832 (1976).
33. Kraus, D. M., Fischer, J. H., Reitz, S. J., Keeskes, S. A., Yeh, T. F., McCulloch, K. M., Tung, E. C., and Cwik, M. J., Alterations in theophylline metabolism during the first year of life, *Clin. Pharmacol. Ther.*, 54:11–19 (1993).
34. Kearin, M., Kelly, J. G., and O'Malley, K., Digoxin "receptors" in neonates: An explanation of less sensitivity to digoxin in adults, *Clin. Pharmacol. Ther.*, 28:346–349 (1980).
35. Assael, B. M., Pharmacokinetics and drug distribution during postnatal development, *Pharmacol. Ther.*, 18:159–197 (1982).
36. Cornford, E. M., Pardridge, W. M., Braun, L. D., and Oldendorf, W. H., Increased blood-brain barrier transport of protein-bound anticonvulsant drugs in the newborn, *J. Cereb. Blood Flow Metab.*, 3:280–286 (1983).
37. Kardish, R., and Feuer, G., Relationship between maternal progesterone and the delayed drug metabolism in the neonate, *Biol. Neonate*, 20:58–67 (1972).
38. Feuer, G., Action of pregnancy and various progesterones on hepatic microsomal activities, *Drug Metab. Rev.*, 9:147–169 (1979).
39. Wilson, J. T., Developmental pharmacology: A review of the application to clinical and basic science, *Annu. Rev. Pharmacol.*, 12:423–450 (1972).
40. Wishart, G. J., and Dutton, G. J., Precocious development of UDP-glucuronyltransferase activity in cultured fetal rat liver brought about by glucocorticoids and requiring amino acid incorporation into protein, *Biochem. Biophys. Res. Commun.*, 73:960–964 (1976).
41. Wishart, G. J., and Dutton, G. J., Regulation of onset of development of UDP-glucuronosyltransferase activity towards O-aminophenol by glucocorticoids in late-foetal rat liver in utero, *Biochem. J.*, 168:507–511 (1977).
42. Levy, G., Khanna, N. N., Soda, D. M., Tsuzuki, O., and Stern, L., Pharmacokinetics of acetaminophen in the human neonate: Formation of acetaminophen glucuronide and sulfate in relation to plasma bilirubin concentration and d-glucaric acid excretion, *Pediatrics*, 55:818–825 (1975).
43. Siegel, S. R., and Oh, W., Renal function as a marker of human fetal maturation, *Acta Paediatr. Scand.*, 65:481–485 (1976).
44. Siber, G. R., Smith, A. L., and Levin, M. J., Predictability of peak serum gentamicin concentration with dosage based on body surface area, *J. Pediatr.*, 94:135–138 (1978).
45. Painter, M. J., Pippenger, C. E., Wasterlein, C., Barmada, M., Pitlick, W., Carter, G., and Aberin, S., Phenobarbital and phenytoin in neonatal seizures: Metabolism and tissue distribution, *Neurology*, 31:1107–1112 (1981).
46. Gilman, J. T., Gal, P., Duchowny, M. S., Weaver, R. L., and Ransom, J. L., Rapid sequential phenobarbital treatment of neonatal seizures, *Pediatrics*, 83:674–678 (1989).
47. Gilman, J. T., Therapeutic drug monitoring in neonate and paediatric age group. Problems and clinical pharmacokinetic implications, *Clin. Pharmacokinet.*, 19:1–10 (1990).

48. Bory, C., Baltassat, P., Porthault, M., Bethenod, M., Frederich, A., and Aranda, J. V., Metabolism of theophylline to caffeine in premature newborn infants, *J. Pediatr.*, 94:988–993 (1979).
49. Tserng, K. Y., Takieddine, F. N., and King, K. C., Developmental aspects of theophylline metabolism in premature infants, *Clin. Pharmacol. Ther.*, 33:522–528 (1983).
50. Lonnerholm, G., Lindstrom, B., Paalzow, L., and Sedin, G., Plasma theophylline and caffeine and plasma clearance of theophylline during theophylline treatment in the first year of life, *Eur. J. Clin. Pharmacol.*, 24:371–374 (1983).
51. Dreifuss, F. E., Santilli, N., Langer, D. H., Sweeney, K. P., Moline, K. A., and Menander, K. B., Valproic acid hepatic fatalities: A retrospective review, *Neurology*, 37:379–385 (1987).
52. Phelps, S. J., Kamper, C. A., Bottorff, M. B., and Alpert, B. S., Effect of age and serum creatinine on endogenous digoxin-like substances in infants and children, *J. Pediatr.*, 110:136–139 (1987).
53. Gershanik, J. J., Boecler, B., George, W., Sola, A., Leitner, M., and Kapadia, C., The gasping syndrome: Benzyl alcohol (BA) poisoning? *Clin. Res.*, 29:895A (Abstract) (1981).
54. Brown, W. J., Buist, N. R. M., Gipson, H. T. C., Huston, R. K., and Kennaway, N. G., Fatal benzyl alcohol poisoning in neonatal intensive care unit, *Lancet*, 1:1250 (Letter) (1982).
55. Gershanik, J. J., Boecler, B., Ensley, H., McCloskey, S., and George, W., The gasping syndrome and benzyl alcohol poisoning, *N. Engl. J. Med.*, 307:1384–1388 (1982).
56. Benda, G. I., Hiller, J. L., and Reynolds, J. W., Benzyl alcohol toxicity: Impact on neurologic handicaps among surviving very low birth weight infants, *Pediatrics*, 77:507–512 (1986).
57. Golightly, L. K., Smolinske, S. S., Bennett, M. L., Sutherland, E. W., III, and Rumack, B. H., Pharmaceutical excipients. Adverse effects associated with inactive ingredients in drug products (Part I), *Med. Toxicol.*, 3:128–165 (1988).
58. American Academy of Pediatrics, Committee on Fetus and Newborn and Committee on Drugs, Benzyl alcohol: Toxic agents in neonatal units, *Pediatrics*, 72:356–358 (1983).
59. Centers for Disease Control, Neonatal death associated with use of benzyl alcohol—United States, *MMWR*, 31:290–291 (1982).
60. Anon., Benzyl alcohol may be toxic to newborns, *FDA Drug Bull.*, 12:10–11 (1982).
61. Hiller, J. L., Benda, G. I., Rahatzad, M., Alen, J. R., Culver, D. H., Carlson, C. V., and Reynolds, J. W., Benzyl alcohol toxicity: Impact on mortality and intraventricular hemorrhage among very low birth weight infants, *Pediatrics*, 77:500–506 (1986).
62. Jadine, D. S., and Rogers, K., Relationship of benzyl alcohol to kernicterus, intraventricular hemorrhage, and mortality in preterm infants, *Pediatrics*, 83:153–160 (1989).
63. MacDonald, M. G., Getson, P. R., Glasgow, A. M., Miller, M. K., Boeckx, R. L., and Johnson, E. L., Propylene glycol: Increased incidence of seizures in low birth weight infants, *Pediatrics*, 79:622–625 (1987).
64. Glascow, A. M., Boeckx, R. L., Miller, M. K., MacDonald, M. G., and August, G. P., Hyperosmolality in small infants due to propylene glycol, *Pediatrics*, 72:353–355 (1983).
65. Berkeris, L., Baker, C., Fenton, J., et al., Propylene glycol as a cause of an elevated serum osmolality, *Am. J. Clin. Pathol.*, 72:633–636 (1979).
66. Fligner, C. L., Jack, R., Twigg, G. A., and Raisys, V. A., Hyperosmolality induced by propylene glycol, *JAMA*, 253:1606–1609 (1985).
67. Kulick, M. I., Lewis, N. S., Bansal, V., and Warpeha, R., Hyperosmolality in the burn patient: Analysis of an osmolal discrepancy, *J. Trauma*, 20:223–228 (1980)
68. American Academy of Pediatrics Committee on Drugs, "Inactive" ingredients in pharmaceutical products, *Pediatrics*, 76:635–643 (1985).
69. Louis, S., Jutt, H., and McDowell, F., The cardiocirculatory changes caused by intravenous dilantin and its solvent, *Am. Heart J.*, 74:523–529 (1967).

70. American Academy of Pediatrics Committee on Drugs, Ethanol in liquid preparations intended for children, *Pediatrics*, 73:405–407 (1984).
71. Rumack, B. H., and Spoerke, D. G., *Poisindex Information System*, Denver, CO, Micromedex, Inc.
72. Hoyumpa, A. M., and Schenker, S., Major drug interactions. Effect of liver disease, alcohol, and malnutrition, *Annu. Rev. Med.*, 33:113–149 (1982).
73. Kumar, A., Rawlings, R. D., and Beaman, D. C., The mystery ingredients: Sweeteners, flavorings, dyes, and preservatives in analgesic/antipyretic, antihistamine/decongestant, cough and cold, antidiarrheal, and liquid theophylline preparations, *Pediatrics*, 91:927–933 (1993).
74. Gould, T., and Roberts, R. J., Therapeutic problems arising from the use of the intravenous route for drug administration, *J. Pediatr.*, 95:465–471 (1979).
75. Nahata, M. C., Powell, D. A., Glazer, J. P., and Hilty, M. D., Effect of intravenous flow rate and injection site on in vitro delivery of chloramphenicol succinate and in vivo kinetics, *J. Pediatr.*, 99:463–466 (1981).
76. Leff, R. D., and Roberts, R. J., *Practical Aspects of Intravenous Drug Administration*, American Society of Hospital Pharmacists, Bethesda, MD, 1992.
77. Kubajak, C. A. M., Leff, R. D., and Roberts, R. J., Influence of physical characteristics of intravenous systems on drug delivery, *Dev. Pharmacol. Ther.*, 11:189–195 (1988).
78. Rajchgot, P., Radde, I. C., and MacLeod, S. M., Influence of specific gravity on intravenous drug delivery, *J. Pediatr.*, 99:658–661 (1981).
79. Santeiro, M. L., Sagraves, R., and Allen, L. V., Osmolality of small-volume iv admixtures for pediatric patients, *Am. J. Hosp. Pharm.*, 47:1359–1364 (1990).
80. Nahata, M. C., Intravenous infusion conditions: Implications for pharmacokinetic monitoring, *Clin. Pharmacokinet.*, 24:221–229 (1993).
81. Holtz, L., Milton, J., and Sturek, J. K., Compatibility of medications with enteral feedings, *JPEN*, 11:183–186 (1987).
82. Edes, T. E., Walk, B. E., and Austin, J. L., Diarrhea in tube-fed patients: Feeding formula not necessarily the cause, *Am. J. Med.*, 88:91–93 (1990).
83. Bloss, C. S., and Sybert, K., Osmolality of commercially available oral liquid drug preparations, ASHP Annual Meeting, 48 (June):P-35 (Abstract) (1991).
84. Maish, W., and Sagraves, R., Childhood asthma, *US Pharmacist*, 1993 (January):36–58,105.
85. Hendeles, L., Weinberger, M., and Szefler S., Safety and efficacy of theophylline in children with asthma, *J. Pediatr.*, 120:177–183 (1992).
86. Hendeles, L., and Weinberger, M., Selection of a slow-release theophylline product, *J. Allergy Clin. Immunol.*, 78:743–751 (1986).
87. Mitchell, J. F., and Pawlicki, K. S., Oral dosage forms that should not be crushed, 1992 revision, *Hosp. Pharm.*, 27:690–692, 695–699 (1992).
88. Martin, S., Catering to pediatric patients, *Am. Pharm.*, NS32:47–50 (1992).
89. Chater, R. W., Pediatric dosing: Tips for tots, *Am. Pharm.*, NS33:55–56 (1993).
90. Gilles, F. H., and Matson, D. D., Sciatic nerve injury following misplaced gluteal injection, *J. Pediatr.*, 76:247–254 (1970).
91. Administration Guides, *Drugstore News*, 13 (Dec.):7–14 (1993).
92. Otic Preparations Monograph. In: *Facts and Comparisons* (B. R. Olin, ed.), J. B. Lippincott Co., St. Louis, 1992 (Nov.), p. 517.
93. Topical Ophthalmic Monograph. In: *Facts and Comparisons* (B. R. Olin, ed.), J. B. Lippincott Co., St. Louis 1993 (May), pp. 477b–477c.
94. Smith, S. E., Eyedrop instillation for reluctant children, *Br. J. Ophthalmol.*, 75:480–481 (1991).

ROSALIE SAGRAVES

Pelletization Techniques

Introduction

Historically, the word pellet has been used by a number of industries to describe a variety of agglomerates produced from diverse raw materials, utilizing different pieces of manufacturing equipment. These agglomerates include fertilizers, animal feeds, iron ores, and pharmaceutical dosage forms, and hence do not only differ in composition but also encompass different sizes and shapes. As a result, pellets mean different things for different industries. In the pharmaceutical industry, pellets can be defined as small, free-flowing, spherical particulates manufactured by the agglomeration of fine powders or granules of drug substances and excipients using appropriate processing equipment. Although pellets have been used in the pharmaceutical industry for more than four decades, it is only since the late 1970s, with the advent of controlled-release technology, that the full impact of the inherent advantages of pellets over single-unit dosage forms have been realized. Not only has research focused on refining and optimizing existing pelletization techniques, but also on the development of novel approaches and procedures of manufacturing pellets employing innovative formulations and processing equipment. As a result, a number of pelletized products are being designed to maximize the in vivo performance of medications already in the market and to meet all regulatory requirements, including cGMPs (current Good Manufacturing Practices).

Pellets provide the development scientist with a high degree of flexibility during the design and development of oral dosage forms. They can be divided into desired dose strengths without formulation or process changes, and can also be blended to deliver incompatible bioactive agents simultaneously or particles with different release profiles at the same site or at different sites within the gastrointestinal tract. In addition, pellets have numerous therapeutic advantages over traditional single units, such as tablets and powder-filled capsules. Taken orally, pellets generally disperse freely in the gastrointestinal tract, and consequently maximize the drug absorption, minimize local irritation of the mucosa by certain irritant drugs because of the small quantity of drug available in a single pellet, and reduce inter- and intrapatient variability [1]. As the advantages of pellets over single units became clear, the pharmaceutical industry as a whole started to devote resources to conduct research in pellet technology and, whenever possible, acquire advanced equipment suitable for the manufacture of pellets.

Although a variety of techniques are available, the most commonly used pelletization processes are solution layering, suspension layering, powder layering, and extrusion–spheronization; they are discussed at length in this article. Other technologies that are used occasionally, such as balling, spray congealing and drying as well as emerging technologies such as cryopelletization and melt spheronization, are described briefly.

Layering

Layering processes are probably the most well-controlled and straightforward pelletization techniques that have been used over the years. They are classified into three categories: solution layering, suspension layering, and powder layering.

Solution and suspension layering involve the deposition of successive layers of solutions and suspensions of drug substances, respectively, on starter seeds which may be inert materials or crystals or granules of the same drug. In principle, the factors that control coating processes apply directly to solution or suspension layering, and, as a result, require basically the same processing equipment. Over the years, conventional coating pans, fluid-bed centrifugal granulators, and Wurster coaters have been used to manufacture pellets by solution and suspension layering. Depending upon the equipment design and the accompanying processing parameters, the processing time needed to manufacture a batch of pellets varies from minutes to hours and even days. In addition, the efficiency of the process and the quality of the pellets produced is in part related to the type of equipment employed. Although the equipment and process that provide the desired pellets can easily be identified and utilized, it is usually the availability of the equipment that dictates the decision-making process.

During solution or suspension layering, all the components of the formulation are dissolved or suspended in the application medium and hence determine the solids content and the viscosity of the liquid sprayed. As the solution or suspension is sprayed onto the product bed, the droplets impinge on the starter seeds or cores and spread evenly on the surface, provided that the drying conditions and fluid dynamics are favorable. This is followed by a drying phase which allows dissolved materials to crystallize and form solid bridges between the core and initial layer of the drug substance as well as among the successive layers of drug substance. The process continues until the desired layers of drug and hence the target potency of the pellets are achieved. The rate of particle growth is rather slow due to the incremental addition of the dissolved or suspended drug. In this process, though the particle population remains the same, the size of the pellets increases as a function of time and, as a result, the total mass of the system increases.

Powder layering involves the deposition of successive layers of dry powder of drug and/or excipients on preformed nuclei or cores with the help of a binding liquid. Because powder layering involves the simultaneous application of the binding liquid and dry powder, not all the pelletization equipment that is routinely used to prepare pellets by solution or suspension layering can be employed, although the reverse is true. The main equipment-related requirement in a powder layering process is that the product container should have solid walls with no perforations in order to avoid powder loss underneath the product chamber before the powder is picked up by the wet mass of pellets that are being layered upon.

During powder layering, a binding solution and a finely milled powder are added, simultaneously, to a bed of starter seeds at a controlled rate. In the initial stages, the drug particles are bound to the starter seeds and subsequently to the forming pellets with the help of liquid bridges originated from the sprayed binding liquid. These liquid bridges are eventually replaced by solid bridges derived either from a binder in the application medium or from any material, including the drug substance, that is soluble in the binding liquid. Successive layering of the drug and binder solution continues until the desired pellet size is reached. Throughout the process, it is extremely important to deliver the powder accurately at a predetermined rate and in a manner that maintains an equilibrium between the binder liquid application rate and the powder delivery rate. If the powder delivery rate is not maintained at predetermined levels, overwetting or dust generation, as the case may be, occurs, and neither the quality nor the yield of the product can be maximized.

Equipment

The most common pieces of layering equipment employed by the pharmaceutical industry are the standard or conventional coating pans, the Wurster coaters, and the centrifugal fluid-bed granulators.

Coating Pans

Coating pans can be classified broadly as conventional and modified coating pans. Conventional pans have been used by pharmaceutical firms for a long time, mainly for sugar coating. During the 1950s, however, the industry, in an attempt to prolong the release of drugs from solid oral dosage forms, explored various technologies for the manufacture of multiparticulate drug-delivery systems. The turning point came when candy seeds, which had been employed for topping decorations in foodstuffs like pastries, were used as starter seeds to develop sustained-release pellets in conventional coating pans [2]. The process was similar to that used to manufacture the candy seeds themselves, and involved the successive layering of powder and binder solution on sugar crystals tumbling in a coating pan [3]. Subsequently, the standard pan was used not only to manufacture nonpareils which serve as starter seeds for layering processes, but also to develop sustained-release products of a number of prescription drugs.

The conventional pan is generally the equipment of choice simply because it has been used for years for sugar coating by the industry and hence is accessible. This obviates the need to purchase new pieces of equipment with a huge capital investment. Where it is not accessible, the conventional pan is inexpensive compared to other advanced pelletization equipment. Conventional pans have many advantages but also drawbacks. Labor costs are high, processing times are long, and yields are low. Above all, the conventional pan coating process still remains more of an art rather than a well-controlled process that can be easily validated.

Although conventional coating pans generally consist of circular metal pans that are mounted at an angle relative to the horizontal, they are marketed in a variety of shapes, including spherical, pear, hexagonal, and elliptical, and in a variety of sizes, ranging in diameter from 15 to 230 cm [4]. The internal walls of the pans are smooth, and the pellets tend to slide rather than roll over during the layering process. As a result, the pans are sometimes modified to include baffles of different shapes and sizes to enhance the mixing action. The spray gun is positioned at an angle to allow perpendicular spraying onto the cascading bed. The distance between the spray gun and the bed can be adjusted to satisfy the evaporative requirements of the sprayed liquid. Conventional coating pans are equipped with an inlet drying-air duct which is positioned immediately above the tumbling pellets at or near the lower quadrant of the pan, and with an exhaust air duct which is positioned above the bed in the top third or quarter of the pan. In spite of this arrangement, one of the main limitations of conventional pans has been the poor drying efficiency. A schematic diagram of a typical conventional pan with the inlet and exhaust air ducts is shown in Fig. 1 [5].

Over the years, attempts have been made to improve the drying capabilities of conventional pans; a good example is the Glatt Immersion Sword designed by Glatt Air Techniques (Fig. 2). The system consists of a perforated metal sword that is inserted into the bed to allow the introduction of drying air directly into the cascading bed. The moisture

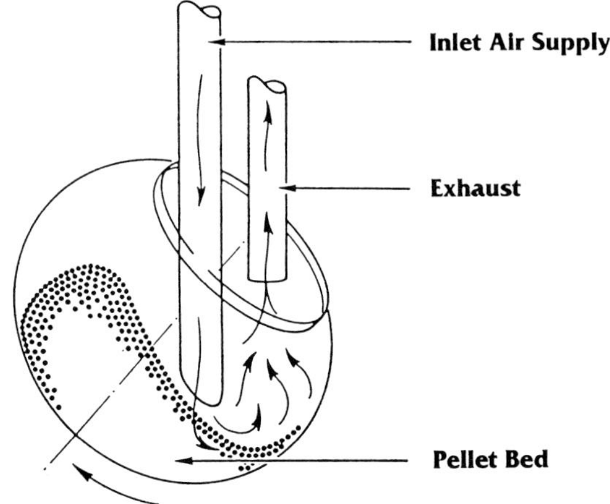

FIG. 1. Schematic diagram of a conventional pan. (From Ref. 5.)

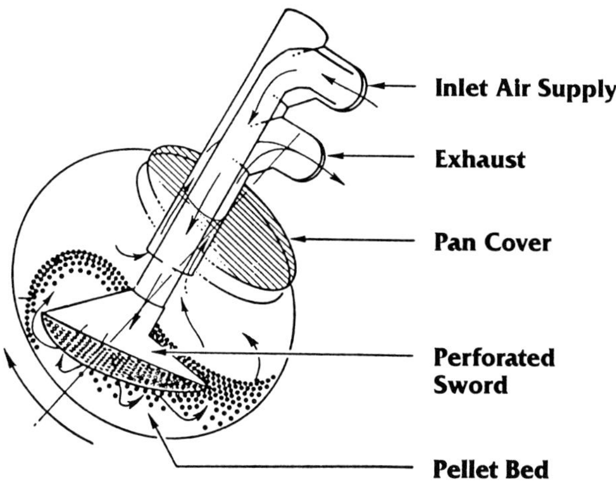

FIG. 2. Schematic diagram of a Glatt Immersion Sword. (From Ref. 5.)

or solvent-laden air exits through an exhaust duct located above the product bed. Since such a setup forces the drying air to flow through the bed, it maximizes exposure of the pellets to the heated air, thereby significantly reducing the drying time. Another approach that significantly improved drying efficiency was developed by Strunck GmbH; it is known as a Strunck Immersion Tube (Fig. 3). It utilizes an assembly of inlet air duct and a spray-gun system enclosed within a tube and immersed in the cascading bed of pellets. The liquid is atomized into the pocket of air created by the drying air. The air then passes through the bed of pellets and is exhausted from the top of the bed as is the case with the conventional pan. The immersion sword and immersion tube were designed to improve the drying efficiency of the air-handling system while leaving the pan body intact.

The next family of coating pans introduced into the market were redesigned to modify the body of the pan itself. Most of these pans consist of perforated drums enclosed within a housing and rotate around a horizontal axis. The drying air is introduced from the top

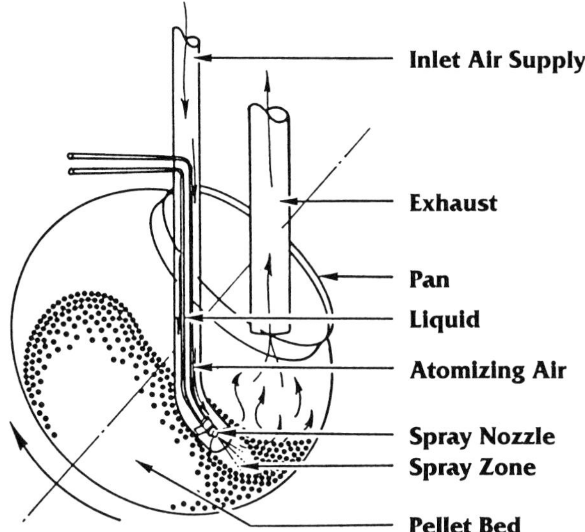

FIG. 3. Schematic diagram of a Strunck Immersion Tube. (From Ref. 5.)

or bottom of the perforated pan, flows through the product bed, and exits through the exhaust air duct. Because of the high volume of air that traverses the bed, the drying efficiency of these pans is much better than that of conventional pans, and therefore they have replaced the latter as the mainstay of tablet coating in the pharmaceutical industry. Although these pans could be modified to allow manufacture of pellets, for instance, by placing a finer screen on the pan to prevent loss of pellets to the exhaust, to-date they have had limited use. As a result, from the coating pan category, conventional pans are still the pelletization equipment of choice.

Wurster Coaters

Although the Wurster coating process was invented about 30 years ago, it has been applied only recently to manufacture and coat pellets of different sizes after elaborate design modifications and refinement. The high drying efficiency inherent in a fluid-bed equipment coupled with innovative and efficient design features allow the machines to hold a center stage in pharmaceutical processing technology. Not only have manufacture and coating of pellets of varying drug loadings become routine and efficient, but the scale-up, which is key to the viability of any processing technique, proved to be predictable and economically feasible.

The main feature that distinguishes Wurster coaters from other fluid-bed equipment is the inclusion of a cylindrical partition within the product chamber. At the base of the product chamber is a perforated plate that has large holes underneath the partition (Fig. 4). The diameter of the partition is half the diameter of the cylindrical wall of the product chamber. Immediately above the product chamber is the expansion chamber, which is an inverted cone structure that has its smallest diameter at the point of contact with the product chamber. The spray gun is located at the center of the air distributer or orifice plate (Fig. 5) just below the partition. Depending upon the process requirements,

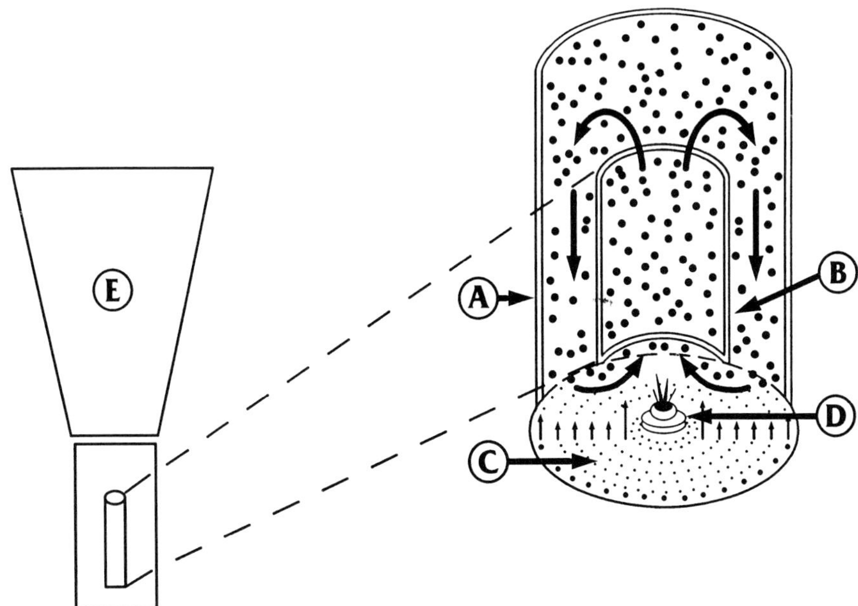

FIG. 4. Schematic representation of the Wurster product chamber and process. A = product chamber, B = partition, C = orifice plate, D = nozzle, and E = expansion chamber. (Adapted from Ref. 6.)

the partition can be raised or lowered to provide the desired particle motion. As the size of the Wurster equipment is increased to accommodate bigger batches, it is the number of partitions within the product chamber rather than the inner diameter of the partition that is increased. For instance, the 18-in. Wurster (45.7 cm) has one 9-in. diameter (22.8-cm) partition, whereas the 32-in. Wurster (81.3 cm) and the 46 in. Wurster (116.8 cm) have three and seven partitions, respectively, of the same diameter. Smaller Wurster coaters for research and development have smaller-diameter partitions. The partitions are designed to keep their functional characteristics equivalent, that is, the particle motion in the up bed within the partition and the down bed outside the partition is the same. Wurster coaters that are used to manufacture pellets have longer expansion chambers than those used to coat tablets. Technically, the Wurster process is a variation of a spouted fluid-bed process. A detailed description of Wurster equipment and accessories is given in Ref. 6.

Centrifugal Granulators

Although tangential spray equipment was originally developed to perform granulation processes, its applications was later expanded to cover other unit operations including the manufacture and coating of pellets. Over the years, these pieces of equipment have been perfected to such an extent that they have become not only standard manufacturing units for various operations but have also proved to be most versatile and efficient. They are routinely used to manufacture pellets by solution, suspension, and powder layering as well as to produce high potency pellets in a few minutes or hours in contrast to the long processing times required in a coating pan process, particularly during powder layering.

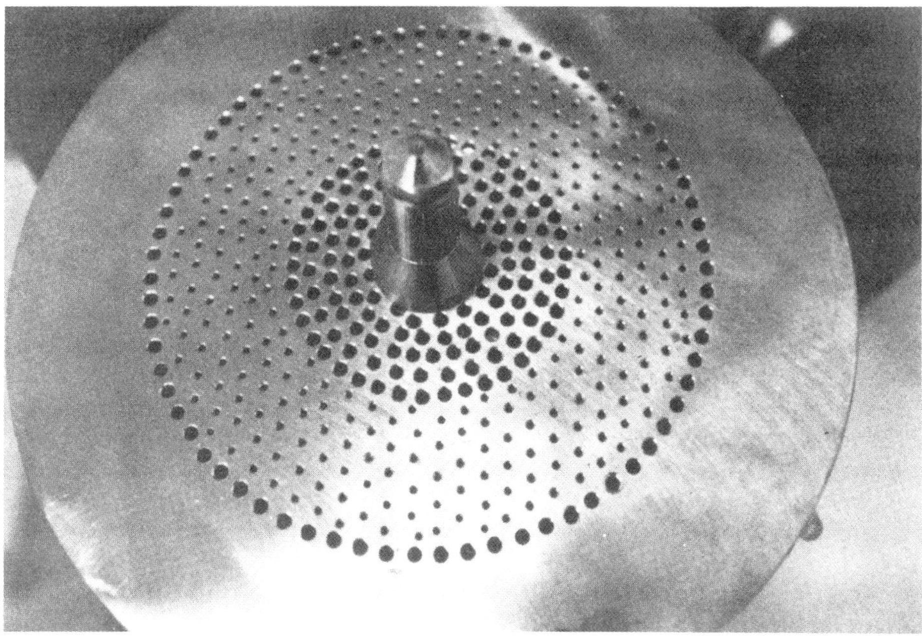

FIG. 5. Air distributer or orifice plate of a Wurster coater. (From Ref. 6.)

Centrifugal fluid-bed granulators can be classified as single- and double-chamber rotary granulators. Most of these granulators utilize a single-walled product chamber with a rotating disk at the base (Fig. 6). The rotational speed of the disk is variable, whereas the height is variable or fixed. The slit width is adjustable by raising or lowering the disk. The nozzle is located at the bottom of the vertical wall of the product container immediately above and tangential to the disk to allow the liquid to be sprayed concurrent with the tumbling bed.

Another version of centrifugal fluid-bed granulators consists of a product container that has an inner and outer processing chambers, known as the forming and drying zones, respectively (Fig. 7) [7]. The two chambers are separated by an inner wall which could be configured in a closed position where the product remains within the inner chamber, or in the open position where the inner wall is lifted pneumatically or mechanically to create an opening that allows the product to pass from the inner chamber to the outer chamber. The base of the outer portion of the product chamber is perforated to permit the flow of a high volume of fluidization air.

Auxiliary Equipment

Other than the air-handling system, which is not discussed here, the most important pieces of auxiliary equipment are the powder-delivery devices and the spray systems.

Powder Feeders. During the manufacture of pellets by powder layering, two types of feeders are routinely used, volumetric and loss-in-weight feeders. In volumetric feeders, the rate at which the powder is delivered is controlled by means of an auger and is a

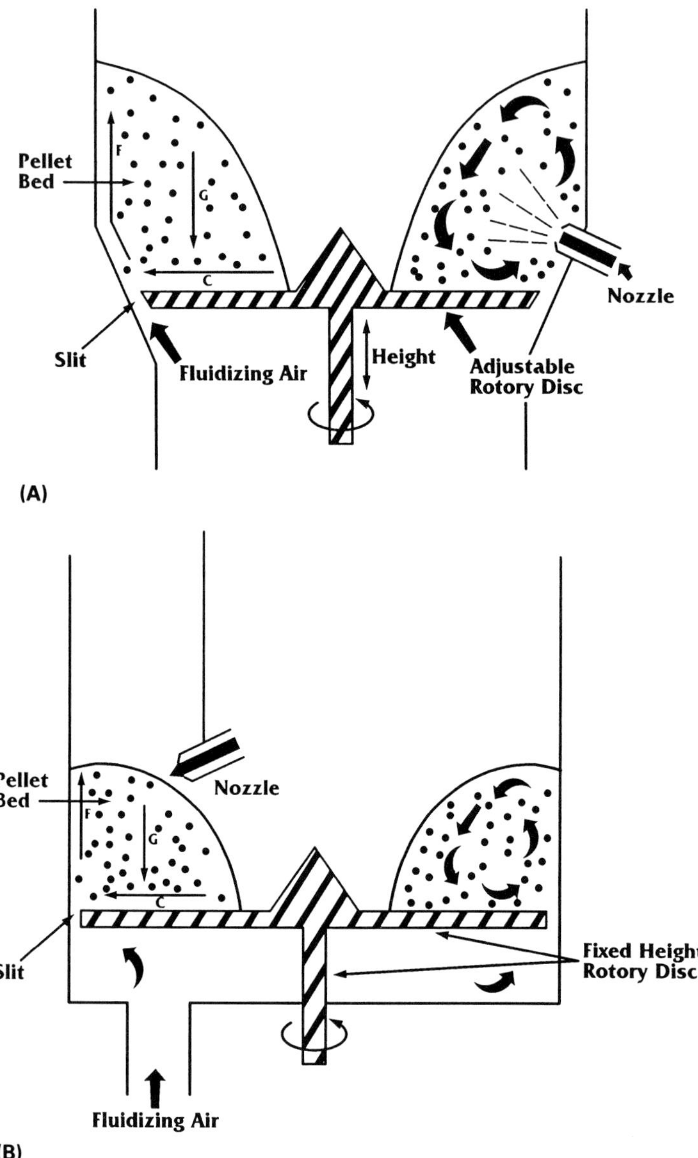

FIG. 6. Schematic representation of centrifugal fluid-bed equipment and process with a single-walled product chamber. A: Glatt GPCG and GRG Granulators. B: Freund CF-Granulators. (Adapted from Ref. 9.)

function of the rotational speed and the diameter of the screw. Accurate feed rate is achieved only when the auger remains filled at all times. Since volumetric measurements are influenced by differences in physical properties such as powder particle size distribution and bulk densities, it is critical to evaluate the flow characteristics of powders before the layering process is initiated. Extrapolation of feed rate parameters in the absence of critical evaluation could potentially lead to processing failures. The more accurate feeders are the loss-in-weight feeders. They are equipped with a counterbalanced

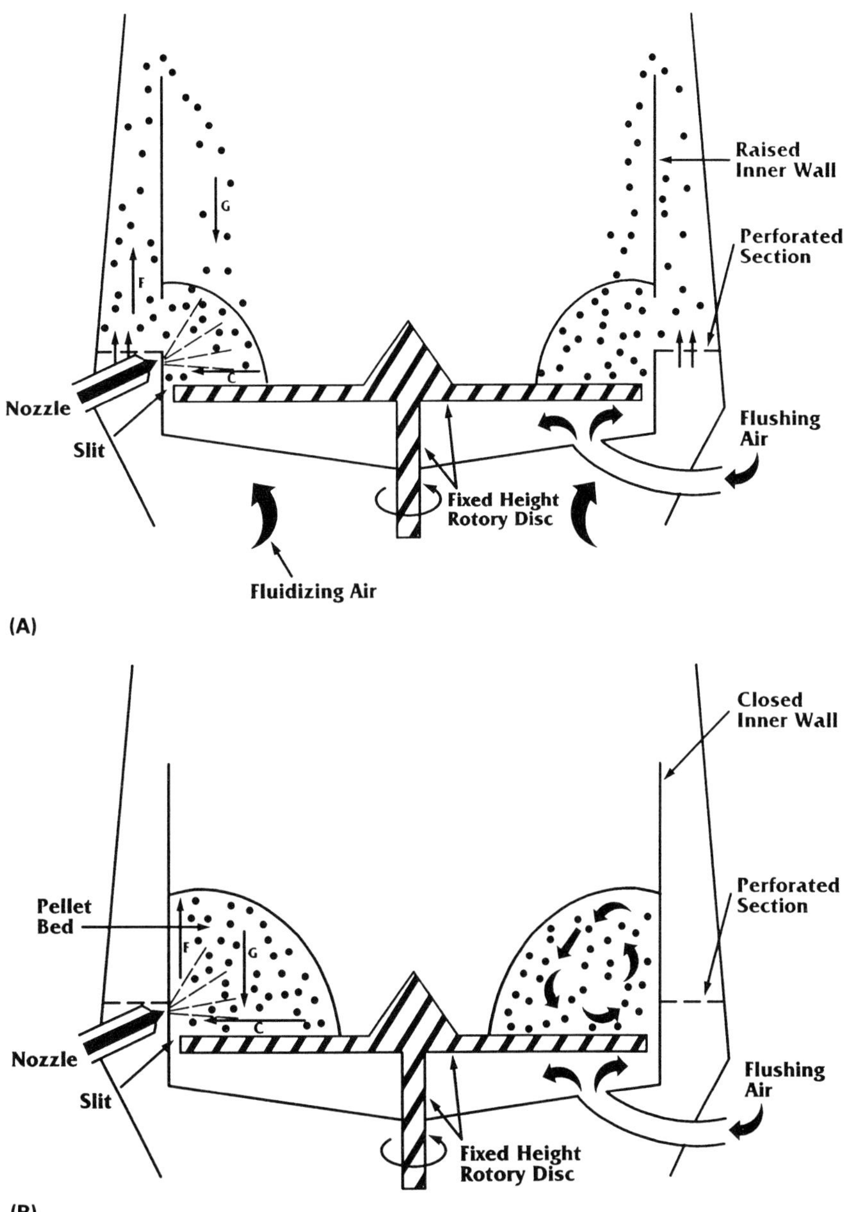

FIG. 7. Schematic representation of centrifugal fluid-bed equipment and process with a double-walled product chamber (Niro-Aeromatic). A: Open position. B: Closed position. (Adapted from Ref. 7.)

scale under the base which measures weight loss during powder delivery. The target feed rate is adjusted by means of a microprocessor.

Spray Systems. Pelletization technologies use two liquid spray systems: the hydraulic (airless) systems and the pneumatic (air-atomized) systems. The former, mainly used in a production setting, utilize pressure to atomize liquid droplets through a nozzle orifice. The droplet size is therefore determined by the applied pressure and the nozzle orifice diameter. The flow rate is uniform and the droplets are less susceptible to spray drying. Pneumatic spray systems utilize an air stream at high pressure to atomize the droplets, and may contribute to premature drying. Pneumatic spray systems are preferred in the laboratory because of their high accuracy at low flow rates.

Process

Though the formulation requirements for the manufacture of pellets by solution, suspension, and powder layering are somewhat different, the basic operational principles of the three processes are similar, and are discussed together while, at the same time, emphasizing the critical processing aspects of each. For the sake of clarity, the processes are discussed on the basis of the type of pelletization equipment employed.

Coating Pans

As indicated earlier, the main disadvantage of coating pans as pelletization equipment and, for that matter, tablet-coating equipment, is the poor drying condition that limits the efficiency of the overall process. Every processing variable has to be optimized to accommodate this limitation. Thus, if a given layering process is to succeed, the other variables, particularly the extent of mixing must be maximized. The extent of mixing is a function of the pan shape, the tilt angle with respect to the horizontal, the baffle arrangement, and the rotational speed of the pan itself. These parameters must be optimized to provide uniform drying and sufficient particle movement to eliminate the potential formation of dead spots during the operation which can adversely affect the end product. For instance, during pelletization, elliptical pans tend to have fewer stagnant spots than cylindrical pans, and are preferentially used to reduce the formation of dead spots [4]. Formation of dead spots can also be minimized by reducing the tilt angle. If the rotational speed of the pan is too slow, segregation may occur due to percolation and induce the preferential layering of drug solution or suspension onto larger particles. In addition, the time the particles spend in contact with one another could be long enough to allow bonding bridges to form among the particles. Therefore, not only will tacky surfaces stick to one another, but even particles that are held together through liquid bridges can eventually lead to agglomeration.

Another critical process parameter is the application rate of the solution or suspension. Because of the low drying capacity of conventional coating pans, the liquid application rate is kept low in order to establish an equilibrium between heat and mass transfer on the surface of the pellets. This equilibrium should be maintained even when the pellet size, and hence the surface area, increases as a function of time. As a result, layering processing times in coating pans are invariably long and tedious. In an attempt to improve the drying efficiency, reduce the processing time, and prevent agglomeration, the rotational speed of the pan could be increased. However, if the pan speed is too high, attrition could be a problem, and pellet growth could be severely compromised. A balance must, therefore, be established between conditions that favor pellet growth and those that reduce agglomeration. During any layering process, it is likely that some of the fines that form due to potential interparticle and wall-to-particle friction may appear in the final product and lower the yield. The problem can be overcome if the application medium is sprayed on the cascading pellets at the end of the layering process, thereby increasing the moisture level at the pellet surface, which in turn facilitates the layering of the fines on the pellets. Since the liquid being sprayed, if delivered at the same rate, does no longer contain dissolved or suspended solids, it may easily wet the product bed and should be adjusted accordingly. Therefore, all the parameters cited earlier must be carefully selected to obtain mixing conditions, spray rates, and drying conditions that provide the desired end product. In an ideal process the processing variables would be optimized in such a way that the particle population at the end of the process is the same as that of the starter seeds or cores, the only difference being an increase in the size of the pellets and the total mass in the coating pan.

Wurster Coaters

As mentioned earlier, the main features that distinguish the Wurster equipment from other fluid-bed equipment are the cylindrical partition located in the product chamber and the configuration of the air distributor plate, also known as the orifice plate (Figs. 4 and 5). The latter is configured to allow most of the fluidization or drying air to pass at high velocity around the nozzle and through the partition, carrying with it the particles being layered upon. Once the particles leave the partition, they enter the expansion chamber where the velocity of the air is reduced below the entrainment velocity and the particles fall back to the area surrounding the partition, referred to as the down bed. The down bed is kept aerated by the small fraction of air that passes through the small holes on this section of the orifice plate. The particles in the down bed are transported horizontally through the gap between the air distributor plate and the partition by the suction generated by the high air velocity that prevails around the nozzle and immediately below the partition. The amount of air that passes through the down bed outside the partition is just enough to bring about modest particle movement, and cycling into the partition, and hence the spray zone, can proceed unimpeded. Because the spray direction is concurrent with particle movement and particle motion is well organized under optimum conditions, uniform layering of drug is consistently achieved. Since the partition height, i.e., the gap between the partition and the orifice plate, controls the rate at which the particles enter the spray zone, it is an important variable that needs to be optimized for a specific batch size. For instance, at a given load size and fluidization air volume, the partition height can be reduced or increased to provide, a well-controlled particle motion that produces the desired pellet characteristics or a bubbling down bed that leads to disorganized particle movement and hence an inefficient process, respectively.

The worst disadvantage of the Wurster process is the inaccessibility of the nozzles. If at any time during the layering process, the nozzles clog, the operation has to be interrupted and the spray guns must be removed for cleaning. Screening of the solution or suspension or employing a spray gun with a bigger nozzle, if the processing conditions permit, may help alleviate the problem. Although the position of the nozzle is fixed, the spray zone can be expanded or reduced, using the air cap.

During scale-up, the number of partitions in the product container is increased with an increase in batch size; the diameter of the partitions, however, is kept the same. The intent is to maintain the particle movement and processing dynamics that were established during the development phase for a Wurster equipment containing a single partition. Increase of the fluidization air volume to compensate for the increase in the number of spray zones should be adjusted to create a well-organized particle movement in all partitions. If the fluidization air volume is too high, it will create a bubbling bed and adversely affect the layering process. The fluidization air volume also dictates the scale-up factor of the overall process since the liquid application rate is determined by the volume of drying air passing through the product bed rather than the batch size.

Centrifugal Granulators

Though there are variations in the design of centrifugal or rotary granulators, the basic operational principle that determines the degree of mixing and hence the efficiency of the process is the same, and involves centrifugal force, fluidization air velocity, and gravitational force (Figs. 6 and 7). During a layering process, these three forces act in concert to generate a spiral, rope-like motion of the particles in the product bed. The rotating disk, which may have fixed or variable speeds, creates a centrifugal force that pushes the particles toward the vertical wall of the product chamber or stator. The fluidization air, which is directed toward the slit between the perimeter of the disk and the stator, generates a force strong enough that it carries the particles vertically along the wall of the product container into the expansion chamber. The particles lose their momentum and cascade down toward the center of the rotating disk due to gravitational force. The cycle repeats itself, bringing about an intense mixing that makes this type of granulators unique. The degree of mixing depends upon the fluidization air volume and velocity, the slit width, the bed size, and the disk speed. These variables coupled with the liquid and powder application rates, atomization air pressure, fluidization air temperature, and degree of moisture saturation determine desired yield and quality of the pellets.

During solution, suspension, or powder layering, the quantity of starter seeds or cores charged initially into the machine should be at least enough to cover the nozzles. Otherwise, the sprayed liquid droplets coat the wall of the product container and get entrained in the fluidization air where potentially spray drying occurs. If the droplets survive, they can get entrapped in the filters, thereby complicating the equipment cleanup. In either case, the yield and, probably, the quality of the pellets will dramatically be reduced. As the size of the pellets being formed increases, the mass in the bed increases, and the fluidization air volume is continuously increased to provide optimum expansion and mixing of the product bed. This process continues until either the desired drug loading is obtained or the fluidization air volume is not high enough to bring about the required spiral, rope-like motion of the bed. If such particle movement cannot be achieved, the bed load is excessive and the process should be stopped. During layering in a centrifugal fluid-bed equipment, the product bed expands both vertically and horizontally, and, consequently, a several-fold increase in batch weight can be realized in a single step.

As mentioned earlier, the key process variable that determines the success of any pelletization process in centrifugal fluid-bed granulators is the degree of mixing which is partly dictated by the radial velocity of the disk. At low radial velocities, the extent of mixing becomes inadequate, as indicated by the loss in the spiral, rope-like motion of the particles. Thus, the rate at which the particles traverse the spray zone is prolonged and could potentially lead to excessive agglomeration. Caking is another serious problem encountered during powder layering. At high radial velocities, the particle-to-particle and particle-to-wall frictional forces become intense with a very rapid pellet turnover. Generally, this condition leads to an uncontrollable, wobbly bed resulting in severe particle attrition. That is, the forces that contribute to particle growth through layering are overcome by the breaking forces, and the pelletization process cannot proceed as intended. In this process, not only a large amount of fines is generated, but some of the attrited particles may agglomerate to form nuclei that are subsequently layered upon. Since the drug content of the pellets that contain inert starter seeds and those that utilize the newly formed nuclei is different, the process may create content uniformity problems. The optimum radial velocities of the disk are generally 3 to 8 m/s, irrespective of the granulator size [8]. At the initial stages of the pelletization process, the radial velocity may be kept low and increased as the batch size increases. After the layering process is completed, the radial disk velocity is usually reduced to avoid particle attrition during the drying step.

Another parameter that plays a key role during layering is the disk clearance or slit width. In some centrifugal granulators, the slit width is fixed, and the fluidization air velocity can be varied only with a change in the fluidization air volume. In others, the slit width is variable and is adjusted to meet the processing requirements. As the disk clearance is increased, the air velocity decreases and pellet turnover is reduced. Conversely, as disk clearance decreases, the air velocity increases, resulting in a rapid pellet turnover. Therefore, for maximum process efficiency, the disk clearance is chosen not only to avoid loss of pellets through the gap between the disk and the vertical wall into the plenum and to minimize the loss of powder into the exhaust system, but also to generate an air velocity that provides the desired degree of pellet turnover.

During solution or suspension layering, much like in a coating process, the sprayed droplets must have the necessary rheological properties to spread evenly over the surfaces they impinge upon. This must be followed immediately by a very rapid evaporation of the application medium to avoid overwetting and agglomeration, though the evaporation rate should not be too high to impair binder effectiveness. During powder layering, the condition is somewhat complicated. The rheological properties of the binding liquid, the liquid application rate and drying air temperature should be optimized to produce the desired product temperature. In addition, the powder should be delivered at a rate that maintains a balance between the surface wetness of the cores and powder adhesion. If the product bed temperature is high, powder is lost to the exhaust system, and if it is too low, it leads to agglomeration and possibly the formation of new nuclei that are subsequently layered upon. Therefore, the product temperature should be optimized to keep the particle population the same throughout the layering and subsequent drying steps.

Aside from the rotory disk, the other unique feature of the centrifugal equipment is the spray method. During layering, the liquid is sprayed tangentially to and concurrent with particle movement. This feature accounts mostly for the high yield that is typically obtained from a process involving this type of equipment. The distance the droplets travel before they impinge on the particles is short, and consequently the droplets are picked up by the particles almost completely, with little, if any, loss to the wall of the product chamber or due to spray drying, assuming that the other process variables are optimized.

The powder delivery rate is a critical parameter that must be carefully evaluated. It must be precisely controlled in a manner that maintains an optimum level of solvent or moisture on the surface of the particles. Since the surface moisture or amount of solvent dictates the binding between the forming pellets and the powder being layered upon, the powder delivery rate and the liquid application rate should be adjusted to establish an equilibrium that provides a critical moisture level. It is important that the powder delivery rate is not affected, whether air flow is mediated by suction (negative pressure) as in the Glatt centrifugal granulators or by positive air flow as with the Freund CF-granulators. The barrel and screw design requirements are more stringent for a powder feeder that is employed with an equipment that operates by suction. The clearance between the barrel wall and the screw apex has to be tight, and the flight of the screws should be such that, following an initial burst of powder into the bed, the delivery rate should be well controlled and adjustable during the process as needed.

With a double-walled centrifugal granulator, the process is carried out with the inner wall in the open or closed position [7]. During solution or suspension layering, the inner wall is raised to allow faster drying of the layered pellets. With powder layering, the inner wall is closed so that simultaneous application of liquid and powder could proceed until the pellets have reached the desired size. The inner wall is then raised and the spheres enter the drying zone. The pellets are lifted by the fluidization air up and over the inner wall back into the forming zone. The cycle is repeated until the desired residual moisture level in the pellets is achieved.

Scaling-up of a layering process from the laboratory to production equipment is straightforward. As is true with all fluid-bed equipment, the most critical parameter that need to be met, in addition to the spiral, rope-like motion of the particles, are the density of the particles and the droplet size within the spray zone. Since more than one spray gun is used in production equipment, the spray gun must be positioned around the perimeter of the base of the product chamber in such a way that optimum drying of the layered drug is attained prior to the pellets entering the next spray zone. Generally, the rate-limiting step in the process is saturation of the fluidization air by the application media. Sometimes, depending upon the equipment employed, the spiral, rope-like motion of the particles could be lost during scale-up, and baffles must be inserted to enhance particle motion [9].

Formulation

Although optimization of process variables is critical for the successful development of a pelletized product, it can only be manufactured routinely on a large scale if the formulation is not sensitive to slight variations in processing parameters. It is, therefore, imperative during the development phase that the formulation characteristics are carefully identified and optimized, both qualitatively and quantitatively. These include drug solubility, type and concentration of the binder, and the viscosity of the solution or suspension. The working viscosity range usually dictates the solid content of the formulation that can successfully be sprayed onto the starter seeds and the forming pellets.

Solution layering is usually employed when the potency of the desired pellets is low, since production of high potency pellets using solution layering from a low solids content formulation is not economically feasible. The most important factor that needs to be considered during suspension layering is the particle size of the drug. Micronized drug particles tend to provide pellets that are smooth in appearance, a property that is extremely desirable during subsequent film coating, particularly for controlled-release applications. If the particle size of the drug in the suspension is large, the amount of binder required to immobilize the particles onto the cores will be high, and consequently pellets of low potency are produced. The morphology of the finished pellets tends to be rough and may adversely affect the coating process and the coated product. Moreover, since the particles detach easily from the core they are being layered upon due to frictional forces, the yield is usually low.

Although it is possible to produce pellets from a formulation that does not contain binders, especially during solution layering, almost invariably the layers of drug applied tend to delaminate or break off from the cores in the later stages of the layering process or the subsequent drying step. Therefore, binders are consistently utilized during solution and suspension layering to impart strength to the pellets. They are usually low molecular weight polymers that are compatible with the drug substance. They should not increase the viscosities of the formulations appreciably, and should not, unless intended to do so, modify the release characteristics of the pellets.

The viscosity requirements of the binders in powder layering are not as stringent as with solution and suspension layering since the drug is applied separately in powder form, and hence only the binder is dissolved in the application medium, where, under standard binder concentrations, the viscosity is relatively low. In fact, the viscosity of the binder solution is not a serious problem as long as the solution can be pumped and atomized easily. Nevertheless, binders must have a high binding capacity to easily pick up the powdered particles and immobilize them onto the cores. Micronizing or finely milling the drug prior to layering improves the efficiency of the layering process significantly and provides morphologically smooth pellets that are suitable for film coating.

During powder layering, it is absolutely essential that the powder delivery rate be as precise as the liquid application rate to avoid overwetting or underwetting. This implies that the powder has to have excellent flow characteristics, which, however, is not usually the case, especially when the particle size is reduced to maximize the efficiency of the layering process and to satisfy the morphological requirements of the finished pellets. It is likely, therefore, that during processing, powders may adhere to the sides of the hopper or the feed screw, and may even form rat holes within the hopper. To improve the flow properties of the drug substance, glidants are incorporated into the powder prior to processing. Chemically, glidants could be hydrophobic or hydrophilic and are chosen based on the type of formulation utilized.

Extrusion–Spheronization

Extrusion–spheronization as a pelletization technique was developed in the early 1960s, and since then has been extensively researched and discussed. Interest in the technology is still strong as witnessed by the extent of coverage of the topic in scientific meetings and symposium proceedings as well as in the scientific literature. The technology is unique in that it is not only suitable for the manufacture of pellets with a high drug loading, but it can also be used to produce extended-release pellets in the same step in certain situations, and hence obviate the need for subsequent film coating.

Equipment

Many types of equipment are utilized in the extrusion–spheronization process such as blenders, granulators, and sieve sizers. The most unique and critical processing equipment that, in effect, dictates the outcome of the overall process are the extruders and the spheronizers [10].

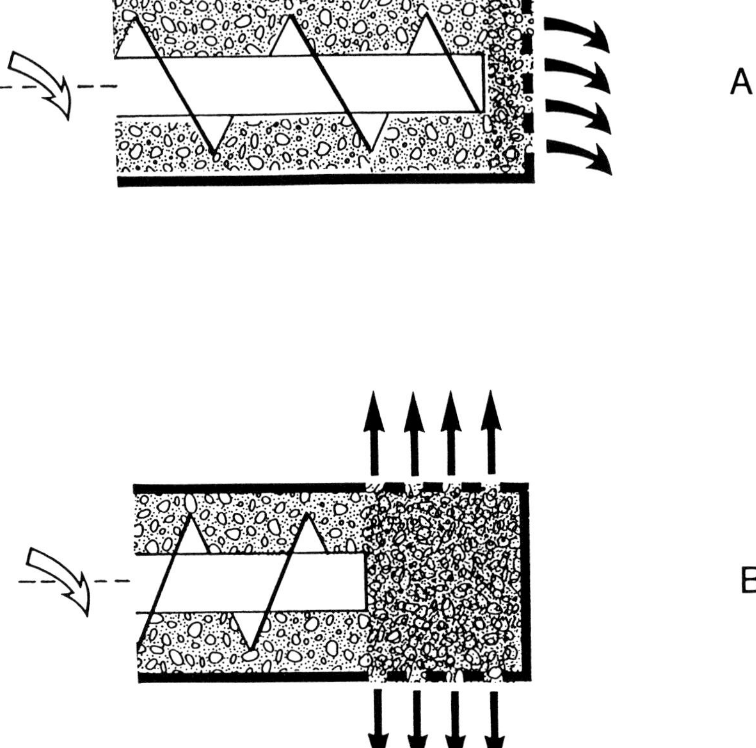

FIG. 8. Schematic representation of screw-fed extruders. A: Axial extruder. B: Radial extruder.

Extruders

A variety of extruders are currently on the market, differing in design features and operational principles. These can be classified as screw-fed extruders, gravity-fed extruders, and ram extruders.

Screw-fed extruders have screws that rotate along the horizontal axis and hence transport the material horizontally; they may be axial or radial screw extruders (Fig. 8). Axial extruders which have a die plate that is positioned axially, basically consist of a feeding zone, a compression zone, and an extrusion zone. The temperature of the product during extrusion is controlled by a jacket barrel. In radial extruders, the transport zone is short, and the material is extruded radially through screens that are mounted around the horizontal axis of the screws.

Gravity-fed extruders include the rotary cylinder and rotary gear extruders, which differ mainly in the design of the two counterrotating cylinders (Fig. 9). In the rotary-cylinder extruder, one of the two counterrotating cylinders is hollow and perforated, whereas the other cylinder is solid and acts as a pressure roller. In the so-called rotary-gear extruder, there are two hollow counterrotating gear cylinders with counterbored holes.

In ram extruders, probably the oldest type of extruders, a piston displaces and forces the material through a die at the end (Fig. 10). Ram extruders are preferentially used in

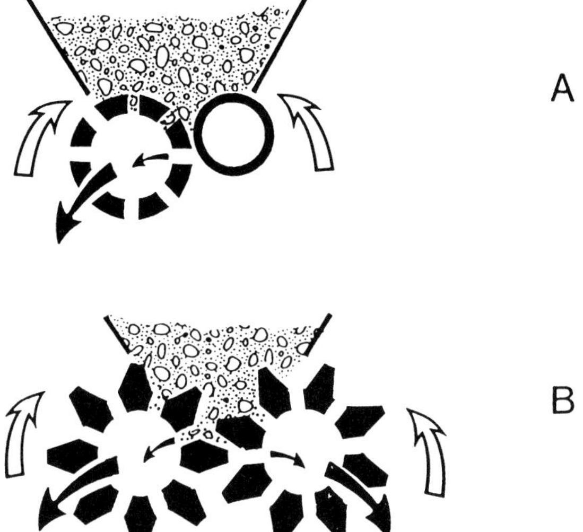

FIG. 9. Schematic representation of gravity-fed extruders. A: Rotary-cylinder extruder. B: Rotary-gear extruder.

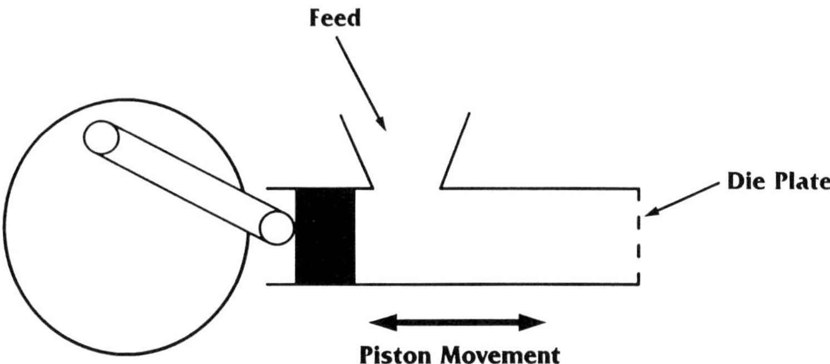

FIG. 10. Schematic representation of a ram extruder. (From Ref. 10.)

the development phase, because they can also be used to measure the rheological properties of formulations [11–13].

Since extruders were initially developed to serve industries other than the pharmaceutical industry, only few of them meet cGMP requirements; these are usually custom-made. To meet all aspects of GMP, all the parts of the extruder that come in contact with the product must be of high quality stainless steel and the construction must be such that the machine can be easily cleaned. In addition, it should be possible to document all critical process parameters, such as pressure at the die plate, product temperature, inlet and outlet temperature of the coolant, power consumption or torque of the driving unit, and rotational speed of the screw. Recently, a qualification procedure for an extruder that is suitable for the manufacture of clinical samples has been proposed [14,15].

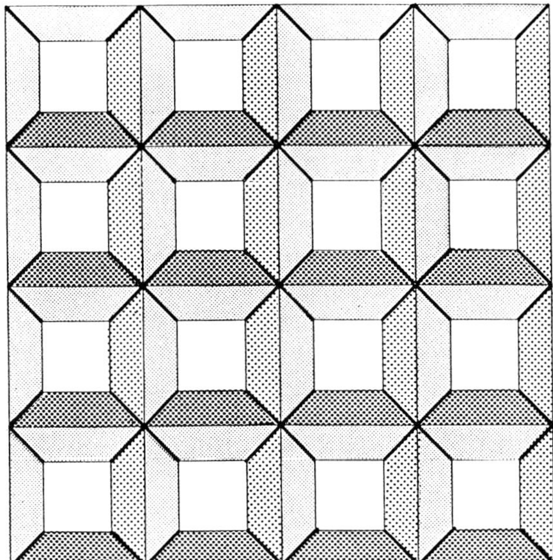

FIG. 11. Schematic representation of a spheronizer friction plate with a cross-hatch pattern.

Spheronizers

The spheronization technology was introduced by Nakahara in 1964 [16]. Since then, the technology has been modified and improved so much that currently well-designed spheronizers of different sizes are commercially available. A spheronizer, known as Marumerizer, consists of a static cylinder or stator and a rotating friction plate at the base. The stator can be jacketed for temperature control. The friction plate, a rotating disk with a characteristically grooved surface, is the most important component of the equipment. A standard friction plate with a cross-hatch pattern, where the grooves intersect at a 90° angle, is shown in Fig. 11. The width of the grooves should be selected according to the pellet diameter, and is, in general, 1.5 to twice the target pellet diameter. The diameter of the friction plate is about 20 cm in laboratory-scale equipment and up to about 1 m in production-scale units. The rotational speed of the friction plate is variable, ranging from 100 to 2000 rpm, depending on the diameter of the unit. In air-assisted spheronizers, a conditioned air-stream is introduced into the product from underneath the rotating disk and passes through the gap or slit between the cylindrical wall and the rotating friction plate; these are also available commercially.

Process

The extrusion–spheronization process is a multistep procedure, involving dry mixing, wet granulation, extrusion, spheronization, drying and (if necessary) screening (Fig. 12). The first step is dry mixing of the drug and excipients in suitable mixers followed by wet granulation, which converts the powder into a plastic mass that can be easily extruded. The extruded strands are transferred into a spheronizer where, when upon contact with the rotating friction plate, they are instantaneously broken into short cylindrical rods and are pushed toward and up the stationary wall of the processing chamber by centrifugal

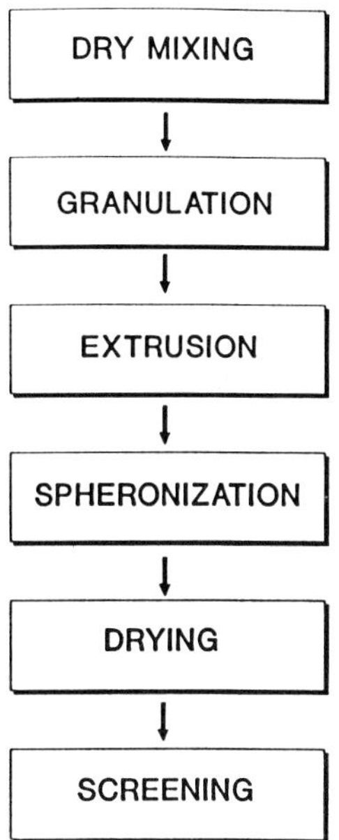

FIG. 12. Flow chart of a typical extrusion–spheronization process.

force. Finally, due to gravity, the particles fall back to the friction plate and the cycle is repeated until the desired sphericity is achieved.

Single-screw extruders tend to produce extrudates with slightly higher densities. Twin-screw extruders have better material transport characteristics and higher capacity or throughput. Radial-type extruders increase throughput even further. They produce extrudates that are less dense than those obtained from an axial type extruders. The product temperature increases very little during the extrusion step, probably because of a shorter compression zone and shorter depth of die openings. This is very important because absence of heat build up during processing prevents evaporation of the granulation fluid, which invariably appears to have a detrimental effect on the quality of the spheronized product. In addition, it allows the processing of thermolabile drug substances.

Inherently, the extrusion step is a continuous process with a very high throughput. However, the subsequent steps (spheronization, drying, and sizing) are batch processes and thus are rate-limiting. As a result, the extrusion–spheronization process is a multistep batch process rather than a continuous process. If necessary, however, it can be used as a semi-continuous process by arranging two spheronizers and an extruder in such a way that the extrudates are alternately fed into the spheronizers. Thus, one of the spheronizers is operational while the other is being charged.

In a batch process, a defined quantity of extrudate is fed into the spheronizer from the top and the spheronized particles are discharged by centrifugal force via a discharge chute positioned in the vertical wall of the cylinder. The process is repeated until the batch is completed. The extrudate is spheromized by interparticle collisions and particle-to-wall frictional forces. The various stages of the spheronization process are depicted in Fig. 13. The spheronizing time is usually 2–15 min, depending on the formulation characteristics. Processing time is reproducible when the composition of the extrudate, including the water content, is kept constant. Since relatively high amounts of water or

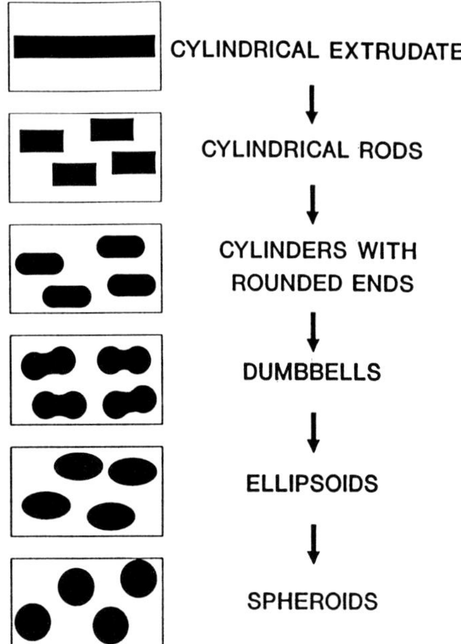

FIG. 13. Shape transitions during a spheronization process.

solvent are incorporated in the formulation, the final pellets contain significant quantities of residual moisture or solvent. They are dried either on trays or in a fluid-bed dryer prior to further processing. A sizing step might be necessary to separate the various fractions if the particle size distribution is wider than intended. In a batch process, the pellets are generally spherical in shape with a narrow particle size distribution. The most critical process parameters in the spheronization step that influence the yield and quality are the design and rotational speed of the friction plate and the residence time of the pellets.

Formulation

In the extrusion–spheronization process the excipients incorporated in the formulation for a specific function, such as fillers, lubricants, and pH modifiers, play a critical role to produce pellets with the desired attributes. The granulated mass should be plastic and sufficiently cohesive and self-lubricating during the extrusion step.

The extruded material should have characteristics, such as moisture content that are desirable for the spheronization step. The degree of liquid saturation of the granulation is one of the most critical factors in the formulation, and must be just high enough to bring about the optimum surface plasticity required for spheronization. Very dry granulated material may generate extrudates that produce large quantities of fines during the spheronization step. Very wet granulated material results in extrudates that may adhere to each other and form bundles of strands that cannot be processed further. Even if the extrudates remain separate following the extrusion step, they tend to form agglomerates readily during spheronization. Therefore, the extrudates must have sufficient mechanical strength to form strands during the extrusion, but must also be easily broken into uniform rods during spheronization to provide pellets with a narrow particle size distribution.

Generally, the liquid content of the wet powder mixture is about 20 to 30% (w/w). Solvents, such as ethanol or mixtures of water and ethanol, may be used as granulating liquids when pure water is not suitable, for instance, for stability or solubility reasons. However, the more volatile the granulation liquid is, the more difficult it is to control the spheronization process.

Excipients play a critical role during extrusion–spheronization [17]. They impart strength and integrity to pellets following drying and govern final pellet formation. Microcrystalline cellulose is one of the most important and widely investigated excipients in extrusion–spheronization. It is used as a filler and a spheronization aid, regulating the water content and distribution in the granulation. In effect, it modifies the rheological properties of the formulation and imparts plasticity to the pellets. Lactose is another excipient that has been studied extensively and used occasionally to evaluate the mechanism and process of pelletization by extrusion–spheronization.

In contrast to layering processes, which are mainly utilized to produce pellets that are coated with a functional membrane to control the rate of drug release, extrusion–spheronization can be used to manufacture pellets with sustained-release characteristics without a membrane. For instance, matrix-type pellets can be produced with the help of mixtures of microcrystalline cellulose and sodium carboxymethylcellulose [18,19]. Organic acids can be incorporated into the pellet matrix to stabilize sensitive drug substances or modify the release characteristics, especially if the solubility of the drug substance being formulated is pH dependent [20]. Although water or other granulation media act as lubricating agents during the extrusion process, lubricants are sometimes incorporated to improve processing [21].

It is no surprise that the drug substance itself plays an important role in the pelletization process, particularly at high drug loading. Physical properties such as particle size and polymorphism, and chemical properties such as pKa and solubility determine the amount of active ingredient which can be incorporated in the formulation and influence the quality of the final pellet with respect to shape and surface smoothness. These properties must be carefully characterized during the development program.

Extrusion–spheronization is a very complex manufacturing process that depends on a number of formulation and processing factors (Table 1). As a result, various workers have attempted to determine the significance of these factors based on multifactorial statistical designs [14,15,22–25].

Cryopelletization

In cryopelletization droplets of a liquid formulation are converted into solid spherical particles or pellets by employing liquid nitrogen as the fixing medium. The technology, which was initially developed for the nutrition industry to lyophilize viscous bacterial suspensions, can be used to produce drug-loaded pellets by allowing droplets of a solution or suspension to come in contact with liquid nitrogen at $-160°C$. The procedure permits instantaneous and even freezing of the material being processed due to the rapid heat transfer that occurs between the droplets and the liquid nitrogen. The pellets are dried in conventional freeze-dryers. The small size of the droplets, and hence the large surface area, facilitate the drying process. The amount of liquid nitrogen required for manufac-

TABLE 1 Critical Factors in Extrusion–Spheronization

	Characteristic	Significance[a]	References
Drug substance	particle size	+++	
	particle size distribution	++	
	particle shape	+++	
	solubility	++	26
Formulation	water content	+++	23–25, 27, 28
	water temperature	+	25
	excipients type	+++	13, 18, 19, 24, 26
	excipients concentration	++	24, 26
	excipients particle size	++	12, 13, 28
Extrusion	extruder type	++	13
	extruder speed	++	14, 15, 22, 23, 25
	extrusion screen size	+++	22, 24
	thickness of the die plate	+	14, 15, 30
Spheronization	spheronizer speed (rpm)	+++	23–25, 27, 29
	spheronizer load	+	23, 24
	spheronization time	+++	23–25
	friction plate design	+	

[a]Relative significance: +, low; ++, medium; +++, high.

turing a given quantity depends on the solids content and temperature of the solution or suspension being processed. It is usually, between 3 and 5 kg per kg of finished pellets.

The equipment consists of a container equipped with perforated plates at the bottom. Immediately below the plates at a predetermined distance is a reservoir of liquid nitrogen in which a conveyor belt with transport baffles is immersed. The conveyor belt has a variable speed and can be adjusted to provide the residence time required for freezing the pellets. The frozen pellets are transported out of the nitrogen bath into a storage container at −60°C prior to drying. Equipment of different sizes, ranging from laboratory scale to production size, is available commercially. A detailed description is given in Refs. 31 and 32.

The most critical step in cryopelletization is droplet formation, which is influenced not only by formulation-related variables such as viscosity, surface tension, and solids content, but also by equipment design and the corresponding processing variables. The diameter and design of the shearing edge of the holes on the container plates are critical. For instance, the diameter of the holes determines the flow rate, which in turn is governed by the viscosity of the formulation. The diameter of the holes also influences the size and shape of the pellets. The smaller the nozzle diameter, the smaller the pellets produced.

The shape of the droplets depends on the distance the droplets travel before contacting the liquid nitrogen. This distance has to be long enough to allow the drops to become spherical, but not too long to lead to deformation when the droplets contact the liquid nitrogen. When all processing parameters are carefully characterized and optimized, smooth, spherical pellets can be routinely manufactured. In cases where the desired pellet diameter is less than 2 mm, the liquid nitrogen should be stirred to prevent agglomeration.

Solutions or suspensions that are suitable for cryopelletization must have a high solids content and viscosity values that should not exceed a critical limit which depends on the formulation. Another important property is the surface tension of the liquid formulation which partly determines the pellet size. Addition of a surfactant to the formulation reduces the surface tension and results in smaller particle size. Pellet size also depends on the surface activity of the drug substance.

Immediate-release formulations typically consist of the drug substance, fillers like mannitol and lactose, and binders like gelatin, gelatin hydrolysates, and polyvinylpyrrolidone. Cross-linked biopolymers based on collagen derivatives are used for sustained-release pellets. A detailed discussion on the formulation and processing variables is given in Refs. 32 and 33.

Balling

Balling, or spherical agglomeration, is a pelletization process in which powders, upon addition of an appropriate quantity of liquid, are converted to spherical particles by a continuous rolling or tumbling action. The liquid may be added prior to or during the agitation stage. Over the years balling has been carried out in horizontal drum pelletizers, inclined dish pelletizers, and tumbling blenders; a more recent technology uses rotary fluid-bed granulators. Although balling has been routinely practiced in the iron ore and fertilizer industries, its application in the pharmaceutical industry is marginal at best. Nevertheless, the process is one of the most thoroughly investigated pelletization processes, and, as a result, a number of mechanisms describing the various phases of pellet formation and growth during balling have been proposed [34].

As powders come in contact with a liquid phase, they form agglomerates or nuclei which initially are bound together by liquid bridges that are subsequently replaced by solid bridges derived from the hardening binder or any other dissolved material within the liquid phase. The nuclei formed collide with other adjacent nuclei and coalesce to form larger nuclei or pellets. The coalescence process continues until a condition arises where the bonding forces are overcome by the breaking forces. At this point, coalescence is replaced by a layering process where small particles adhere to much larger particles and increase the size of the latter until pelletization is completed. Simultaneously, particles undergo nucleation and coalescence to form differently sized nuclei admixed with the larger pellets. As a result, balling tends to produce pellets with a wide particle size distribution.

The rate and extent of agglomerate formation depend, in part, upon formulation variables, such as particle size of the powder, the degree of liquid saturation, and the viscosity of the liquid phase. The moisture content is particularly critical, since it determines whether nucleation occurs to initiate pelletization, or whether the nuclei formed have the necessary plasticity to bring about coalescence following collisions between two nuclei. Furthermore, layering of fine particles on the larger nuclei or pellets occurs only if the surface moisture is above the critical level. The rate and extent of agglomerate formation also depend upon processing variables which are specific to a given equipment. In the case of pelletizers, drum speed, residence time, load size, and angle of inclination relative to the horizontal are critical process variables that need to be optimized. Variables critical to a balling process using centrifugal fluid-bed granulators are disk speed, load size, residence time, fluidization air volume and temperature, and disk clearance. A detailed discussion on the formulation and processing aspects as well as the mechanism of pellet formation and growth during balling is given in Ref. 35.

Melt Spheronization

In melt spheronization drug substances and excipients are converted into a molten or semi-molten state and subsequently shaped using appropriate equipment to provide solid spheres or pellets. Melt spheronization can be carried out in a single piece of equipment, such as a jacketed, high-shear mixer where certain components of a formulation are melted to generate spherical particles. The process is similar to wet granulation, except that the binder is in the molten state and hence does not require water or other solvents to liquify it. Due to the randomness of the interparticle collisions that occurs during the process, the particle size distribution of the pellets tends to be wide as is commonly observed with balling. In fact, the process is considered a variation of the balling process.

Melt spheronization can also be carried out with several pieces of equipment, such as blenders, extruders, cutters (known as pelletizers in the plastic industry), and spheronizers. The drug substance is first blended with the appropriate pharmaceutical excipients, such as polymers and waxes, and extruded at a predetermined temperature. The extrusion temperature must be high enough to, at least, melt one or more of the formulation components. The extrudate is cut into uniform cylindrical segments with a so-called pelletizer. The segments are spheronized in a jacketed spheronizer to generate uniformly sized pellets. The spheronization temperature should be high enough that it partially softens the extrudate to facilitate its deformation and eventual spheronization. Depending upon the formulation components, pellets that exhibit immediate or sustained-release characteristics can be manufactured in a single step. However, the process is still at the development stage and additional work is needed before the process becomes a viable pelletization technique.

Spray Drying and Spray Congealing

Spray drying and spray congealing, known as globulation processes, involve atomization of hot melts, solutions, or suspensions to generate spherical particles or pellets. The droplet size in both processes is kept small to maximize the rate of evaporation or congealing, and consequently the particle size of the pellets produced is usually very small. During spray drying, drug entities in solution or suspension are sprayed, with or without excipients, into a hot air stream to generate dry and highly spherical particles. As the atomized droplets come in contact with hot air, evaporation of the application medium is initiated. This drying process continues through a series of stages where the viscosity of the droplets constantly increases until finally almost all of the application medium is driven off and solid particles are formed. Generally, spray-dried pellets tend to be porous. For a thorough discussion on spray drying technology, see Ref. 36.

During spray congealing, a drug substance is allowed to melt, disperse, or dissolve in hot melts of waxes, fatty acids, etc., and sprayed into an air chamber where the temperature is below the melting temperatures of the formulation components, to provide under appropriate processing conditions spherical congealed pellets. A critical requirement in a spray congealing process is that the formulation components have well-defined, sharp melting points or narrow melting zones. Since the process does not involve evaporation of solvents, the pellets produced are dense and nonporous. A detailed description of the formulation and processing requirements of spray congealing as a pelletization technique is given in Ref. 37.

References

1. Bechgaard, H., and Nielson, G. H., Controlled release multiple units and single unit doses, *Drug Dev. Ind. Pharm.*, 4:53–67 (1978).
2. Special Delivery: Advances in drug therapy, *The Research News*, University of Michigan, 1986, p. 1.
3. Cimicata, L. E., How to manufacture and polish smallest pan goods—nonpareil seeds, *Confectioners J.*, 41–43 (1951).
4. Chambliss, W. C., Conventional and Specialized Coating Pans. In: *Pharmaceutical Pelletization Technology* (I. Ghebre-Sellassie, ed.), Marcel Dekker, Inc., New York, 1989, pp. 16–17.
5. Seitz, J. A., Mehta, S. P., and Yeager, J. L., Tablet Coating. In: *Theory and Practice of Industrial Pharmacy*, 3rd ed. (L. Lachman, H. A. Liberman, and J. L. Kanig, eds.), Lea & Febiger, Philadelphia, 1976, p. 350.
6. Olsen, K. W., Fluid Bed Equipment. In: *Pharmaceutical Pelletization Technology* (I. Ghebre-Sellassie, ed.), Marcel Dekker, Inc., New York, 1989, pp. 39–69.
7. Niro-Aeromatic Product Manual, 1992, Niro-Aeromatic, Inc., Columbia, MD.
8. Jones, D. M., Solution and Suspension Layering. In: *Pharmaceutical Pelletization Technology* (I. Ghebre-Sellassie, ed.), Marcel Dekker, Inc., New York, 1989, pp. 158–159.
9. Jan, S., and Goodhart, F. W., Dry Powder Layering. In: *Pharmaceutical Pelletization Technology* (I. Ghebre-Sellassie, ed.), Marcel Dekker, Inc., New York, 1989, pp. 182–183.
10. Hicks, D. C., and Freese, H. L., Extrusion Spheronization Equipment. In: *Pharmaceutical Pelletization Technology* (I. Ghebre-Sellassie, ed.), Marcel Dekker, Inc., New York, 1989, pp. 71–100.
11. Harrison, P. J., Newton, J. M., and Rowe, R. C., The characterization of wet powder masses suitable for extrusion/spheronization, *J. Pharm. Pharmacol.*, 37:686–691 (1985).
12. Fielden, K. E., Newton, J. M., and Rowe, R. C., The effect of lactose particle size on the extrusion properties of microcrystalline cellulose-lactose mixtures, *J. Pharm. Pharmacol.*, 41:217–221 (1989).
13. Fielden, K. E., Newton, J. M., and Rowe, R. C., A comparison of the extrusion and spheronization behavior of wet powder masses processed by a ram extruder and a cylinder extruder, *Int. J. Pharm.*, 81:225–233 (1992).
14. Dietrich, R., and Brausse, R., Erste Erfahrungen und Validierungsversuche an einem neu entwickelten GMP-gerechten und instrumentierten Pharma-extruder, *Pharm. Ind.*, 50(10): 1179–1186 (1988).
15. Dietrich, R., Food technology transfers to pellet production, *Manuf. Chem.*, 8:29–33 (1989).
16. Nakahara, N., Method and apparatus for making spherical granules, U. S. Pat. 3,277,520 (1964).
17. Harris, M. R., and Ghebre-Sellassie, I., Formulation Variables. In: *Pharmaceutical Pelletization Technology* (I. Ghebre-Sellassie, ed.), Marcel Dekker, Inc., New York, 1989, pp. 217–239.
18. O'Conner, R. E., and Schwartz, J. B., Spheronization II: Drug release from drug diluent mixtures, *Drug Dev. Ind. Pharm.*, 11(9,10): 1837–1857 (1985).

19. Ghali, E. S., Klinger, G. H., and Schwartz, J. B., Modified drug release from beads prepared with combinations of two grades of microcrystalline cellulose, *Drug Dev. Ind. Pharm.*, 15(9): 1455–1473 (1989).
20. Bianchini, R., Bruni, R., Gazzaniga, A., and Vecchio, C., Influence of extrusion/spheronization processing on the physical properties of d-indobufen pellets containing pH adjusters, *Drug Dev. Ind. Pharm.*, 18(14): 1485–1503 (1992).
21. Mesiha, M. S., and Valles, J., A screening study of lubricants in wet powder masses suitable for extrusion-spheronization, *Drug Dev. Ind. Pharm.*, 19(8): 943–959 (1993).
23. Hasznos, L., Langer, I., and Gyarmathy, M., Some factors influencing pellet characteristics made by an extrusion/spheronization process. Part I: Effects on size characteristics and moisture content decrease of pellets, *Drug Dev. Ind. Pharm.*, 18(4): 409–439 (1992).
24. Hileman, G. A., Goskonda, S. R., Spalitto, A. J., and Upadrashta, S. M., A factorial approach to high dose product development by an extrusion/spheronization process, *Drug Dev. Ind. Pharm.*, 19(4): 483–491 (1993).
25. Ku, C. C., Joshi, Y. M., Bergum, J. S., and Jain, N. B., Bead manufacture by extrusion/spheronization. A statistical design for process optimization, *Drug Dev. Ind. Pharm.*, 19(13): 1505–1519 (1993).
26. Baert, L., Fanara, D., Remon, J. P., and Massart, D., Correlation of extrusion forces, raw materials and sphere characteristics, *J. Pharm. Pharmacol.*, 44:676–678 (1992).
27. Battaille, B., Rahman, L., and Jacob, M., Etude des parametres de formulation sur les characteristiques physico-techniques de granules de theophylline obtenus par extrusion–spheronisation, *Pharma. Acta Helv.*, 66(8): 223–236 (1991).
28. Newton, J. M., Chow, A. K., and Jeewa, K. B., The effect of excipient source on spherical granules made by extrusion/spheronization, *Pharm. Tech.*, 3:166–174 (1993).
29. Bataille, B., Ligarski, K., Jacob, M., Thomas, C., and Duru, C., Study of the influence of spheronization and drying conditions on the physico-mechanical properties of neutral spheroids containing Avicel PH 101 and lactose, *Drug Dev. Ind. Pharm.*, 19(6): 653–671 (1993).
30. Helen, L., Yliruusi, J., and Muttonen, E., Process variables of the radial screen extruder, Part II: Size and size distribution of pellets, *Pharm. Tech. Int.*, 1:44–53 (1993).
31. Europ. Pat. EP 0 081 913 (1985).
32. German Pat. DE 37 11 169 (1988).
33. Knoch, A., Cryopelletization. In: *Multiparticulate Oral Drug Delivery* (I. Ghebre-Sellassie, ed.), Marcel Dekker, Inc., New York, 1994, pp. 35–50.
34. I. Ghebre-Sellassie, Mechanism of Pellet Formation and Growth. In: *Pharmaceutical Pelletization Technology* (I. Ghebre-Sellassie, ed.), Marcel Dekker, Inc., New York, 1989, pp. 123–143.
35. Wan, L. S. C., Manufacture of Core Pellets by Balling. In: *Multiparticulate Oral Drug Delivery* (I. Ghebre-Sellassie, ed.), Marcel Dekker, Inc., New York, 1994, pp. 1–15.
36. Masters, K., *Spray Drying Handbook*, 4th ed., John Wiley & Sons, New York, 1985.
37. Atilla Hincal, A., and Suheyla Kas, H., Preparation of Micropellets by Spray Congealing. In: *Multiparticulate Oral Drug Delivery* (I. Ghebre-Sellassie, ed.), Marcel Dekker, Inc., New York, 1994, pp. 17–34.

ISAAC GHEBRE-SELLASSIE
AXEL KNOCH

Peptide and Protein Drug Delivery

Introduction

In order to survive, the human body needs to nourish itself with the basic nutrients, that is, carbohydrates, fats, proteins, vitamins, minerals, and water. The proteins in food are digested in the stomach to smaller fragments or into its building blocks, the amino acids, which are absorbed. The body can also synthesize amino acids, except for the eight essential amino acids, which must be obtained from food. From the 20 naturally occurring amino acids, the body can construct proteins by joining these amino acids by amide linkages, also known as peptide bonds. Proteins thus consist of amino acids strung together like the beads of a necklace. These chains of amino acids, if short, are called peptides; longer chains are called proteins. The distinction between peptides and proteins is somewhat arbitrary, with a molecular weight of about 5,000 Daltons (5kDa, about 50 amino acid residues) generally being the criterion. Taking a typical small protein to be one with 60 amino acids, the number of proteins that can be made from the 20 naturally occurring amino acids is $20^{60} = 10^{78}$. This is an enormous number, perhaps higher than the total number of atoms in the universe. The human body makes only a tiny fraction of this number, even though this fraction happens to be about 100,000 different proteins in the human body. Although many of these proteins are structural units in muscle, skin, bone, etc., others serve as mediators that enable the whole organism to adjust to the demands of a changing environment. These include hormones, neurotransmitters, and others.

In the past, the traditional drug discovery process relied on an extensive screening of organic compounds to discover their therapeutic potential, mostly on a trial basis. However, the drugs of the future are expected to be designed based on our understanding of cellular phenomena at the molecular level, and will be tied in with basic biochemistry. For some time now, scientists have realized that physiological peptides and proteins play a key role in the well-being of the human body and that various disease states may be associated with a change in the balance; for example, insulin-dependent diabetes may be caused by the inability of the body to produce adequate insulin. A more recent development, which has enabled scientists to use these physiological peptides and proteins in therapeutic applications, has been the advances in recombinant-DNA technology and the arrival of the biotechnology industry.

Biotechnology-derived drugs are produced by recombinant-DNA technology, known as genetic engineering or gene cloning, whereby human genes responsible for the production of a protein, are transferred to a organism such as *E. Coli* bacterium. *Escherichia Coli* is then cultured by fermentation for the large-scale production of therapeutic proteins on a commercially viable scale. The biotechnology industry originated in the 1970s and has undergone tremendous growth since then. Today, the number of companies involved in biotechnology research is at least 1100, with a total revenue of $5.8 billion for 1991.

Through the advances in recombinant-DNA technology, many new and biologically active proteins and peptides are now commercially available for their potential use as drugs in the therapeutic management of a variety of pathological conditions and diseases that are poorly controlled now. The success story of this modern era began with the approval of the first drug of biotechnology, human insulin (marketed as Humulin by Eli

Lilly), by the FDA in 1982. Since then, the growth of the biotechnology industry has been exponential. Today, there are about 24 biotechnology products on the market with more than 132 products in the pipeline, either in human clinical tests or at the FDA for review and approval. These biotechnology drugs are effective against a variety of ailments, including diabetes, hypertension, autoimmune diseases, memory impairment, mental disorders, and certain cardiovascular and metabolic diseases. Biotechnology is now providing an impetus to search for cures for cancer and AIDS, which are providing a major challenge to our society today.

Although several such products are being rapidly made available, their therapeutic utility is limited by the lack of convenient methods for their effective delivery. Peptide–protein drugs are not active by oral administration because they are rapidly degraded by the proteolytic enzymes and the acid conditions of the gastrointestinal tract. In addition, their macromolecular dimensions and hydrophilic nature prevent effective absorption through the mucosa of the gastrointestinal tract or the mucosa at the alternative routes. Currently, these drugs are formulated as parenterals. However, repeated injections are often required because of their extremely short biological half-lives. A great and urgent need thus exists to develop viable delivery systems for these biotechnologically derived peptide–protein drugs. This article presents a discussion on various barriers to the delivery of such drugs, current status of drug administration by various routes, and some strategies to overcome the barriers to their absorption.

Formulation and Delivery of Peptides and Proteins

The challenges (or opportunities) facing the formulator of peptides and proteins are to:

1. Maximize physical and chemical stability,
2. Prolong half-life,
3. Decrease antigenicity,
4. Increase rate of absorption, and
5. Minimize metabolism.

Proteins are amphiphilic molecules which respond to their environment by changing conformation in order to have the most energetically favorable interactions with their environment. Unfortunately, this new conformation may not have the desired therapeutic efficacy. Much of the most recent literature reports on formulation techniques which minimize conformational changes during processing and shelf-life. Lyoprotectants, such as sucrose, dextran, glycols, glycerols, and cyclodextrins have been found to minimize physical instability in solution and freeze-dried formulations of luteinizing hormone releasing hormone (LHRH) analogues [1], monoclonal antibodies [2], tumor necrosis factor [3], and β-galactosidase [4]. Pikal [5,6] has discussed the mechanism and requirements for a good lyoprotectant. Optimizing pH, type and concentration of buffer, processing conditions, water content, and of course storage temperature also affects physical stability.

Manning [7] lists the most common routes for chemical instability as deamidation, racemization, hydrolysis, oxidation, beta elimination, and disulfide exchange. Asparaginyl residues are subject to deamidation, which can be followed by isomerization and racemization. The rate and pathway of this reactions is pH dependent [8–11]. Methionine oxidation and asparagine deamidation and aggregation are responsible for the decomposition of freeze-dried human growth hormone. Optimization of pH and of sodium phosphate concentration and addition of amorphous glycine minimize this decomposition [12]. The mechanism of decomposition of interleukin-1β in aqueous solution is temperature dependent. Autooxidation of the two cysteine residues predominates above 39°C, whereas deamidation predominates below 30°C [13]. Metal ions can contribute to protein stability. Loss of intrinsic zinc atoms from certain metalloproteases reduces biological activity, whereas metal ions such as manganese, copper, and iron catalyze oxidation of protein thiol groups [14,7].

The circulating half-life of peptides and proteins is typically very short. Protecting proteins with polymers, such as polyethylene glycol and dextran, increases half-life and reduces antigenicity [15–17]. Other examples are given below in the section on invasive routes of delivery.

Increasing absorption rate and minimizing metabolism at the site of delivery are the major stumbling blocks to noninvasive delivery routes. In a systematic analysis of the problem, Harris and Robinson [18] estimated the permeability coefficients and elimination rates for a number of peptide drugs. They demonstrated that for larger proteins with low permeability and very short half-life, maintaining the protein at the delivery site with a bioadhesive does not improve bioavailability. A permeation enhancer and/or an enzyme inhibitor is necessary to achieve therapeutic blood levels.

The choice of delivery site can be crucial to success. Rojanasakul et al. [19] characterized the permeability and permselectivity of the shunt pathway of the nasal, tracheal, bronchial, buccal, rectal, vaginal, corneal, epidermal, duodenal, jejunal, ileal, and colonic epithelia. Potassium chloride diffusion potential measurements were used to quantitate membrane permselectivity or charge discrimination. Membrane permeability was determined by measuring both the flux of a hydrophilic fluorescent probe and the electrical conductance. All epithelia were found to be selective to positively charged solutes to approximately the same degree. Wide variability was found with respect to membrane permeability. The rank order from highest to lowest was: intestinal $=$ nasal $\geq$ bronchial $\geq$ tracheal $>$ vaginal $\geq$ rectal $>$ corneal $>$ buccal $>$ skin [19].

The following describes some recent advances in how pharmaceutical scientists have turned the challenge of peptide and protein delivery into an opportunity.

Invasive Delivery Routes, Parenteral Administration

Most therapeutic peptides and proteins are currently available as parenteral preparations. Due to stability reasons, many of these are on the market as freeze-dried or lyophilized powders which are reconstituted before administration as intravenous (iv), subcutaneous (sc), and intramuscular (im) injections. Generally speaking, protein drugs are likely to be marketed as a freeze-dried powder (due to stability reasons) along with a suitable bulking agent, whereas peptide drugs are available in ready-to-use injectable solutions [20]. Typical preservatives used in solutions include phenol, benzyl alcohol, and chlorobutanol. Aggregation needs to be avoided during formulation. Much of the expertise for formulating proteins is still evolving and relevant papers have appeared in the recent literature.

If the peptide–protein drug undergoes substantial degradation at the im or sc site, iv administration remains the only viable route. However, in some studies, investigators have tried to stabilize the drug at the sc or im site with the help of a protease inhibitor. Takeyama et al. [21], for example, found that application of an ointment containing protease inhibitors prior to subcutaneous injection of insulin increased the plasma immunoreactive insulin levels and the hypoglycemic effects of insulin in healthy volunteers. Since peptide–protein drugs have extremely short half-lives (on the order of a few minutes), repeated injections are often required. Much effort has thus been directed toward the development of controlled-release parenteral dosage forms, which is discussed below.

Parenteral Delivery

Currently, peptide–protein drugs administered parenterally are given as conventional multiple daily injections. Due to the short half-life of these drugs, a better control on drug therapy may be achieved by a continuous infusion. However, many of these drugs, such as luteinizing hormone releasing hormone (LHRH), vasopressin, etc., are secreted in the body in a pulsatile manner. This may have important implications for their delivery. For example, pulsatile administration of LHRH causes a sustained secretion of gonadotropins, but continuous delivery may inhibit gonadotropin release, a fact now utilized to employ LHRH as a potential contraceptive. Pulsatile delivery may be open loop or closed loop [22]. A closed-loop delivery system involves a biofeedback mechanism to control delivery, and self-regulating systems are under development for insulin delivery which will control the insulin release in response to changing blood glucose levels. Since these have not yet been commercialized, the marketed systems for pulsatile delivery are open-loop systems, such as those consisting of an infusion pump and a program for insulin delivery. Portable pumps for continuous subcutaneous delivery of insulin have been in use for several years. A pump differs from other diffusion-based drug-delivery systems in that the primary driving force for delivery is pressure difference rather than a concentration gradient. The Alza Osmotic minipump (Alzet) is an implantable pump which uses osmotic action to create a pressure difference. It has been used in research studies for the delivery of several peptide–protein drugs [22].

Biodegradable Polymers

At present the most promising polymers for controlled-release parenterals are the biodegradable hydrophobic polymers, including poly(D,L-lactide-*co*-glycolide) (PLGA), poly(ortho esters) and polyanhydrides [23]. The PLGA polymers are hydrolyzed in the body to lactic and glycolic acids, which are easily metabolized by the body. Thus, PLGA polymers are biocompatible, and they have been extensively investigated. These polymers undergo bulk erosion, whereas the poly(ortho ester)s and polyanhydrides undergo surface erosion. Innovative strategies can be used to control drug release from these polymers. In PLGA polymers, the biodegradation rate is dependent on the mole ratio of lactide to glycolide. The erosion rates of polyanhydride can be controlled, taking advantage of the fact that the hydrolysis rates of aliphatic and aromatic polyanhydrides are different.

Polymeric Microspheres

Microspheres are spherical particles of less than 125 μm diameter which can be easily suspended in a vehicle for parenteral administration through a conventional syringe and needle. The drug is dispersed in the polymeric particle, which is often composed of one of the biodegradable polymers discussed earlier. The most common microencapsulation process is either solvent evaporation or phase separation. In a recent study by Tabata et al. [24], several proteins of different molecular sizes were slowly released from polyanhydride microspheres at a near constant rate. It was also found that encapsulation of enzymes inside these microspheres can protect them from activity loss.

The PLGA microspheres have also been extensively investigated [25–27] and are perhaps the most promising from a regulatory point of view. Release of a peptide from PLGA microspheres often follows a triphasic release profile [23]. The initial release represents diffusion of the peptide from the surface layer. This is followed by a latent period during which the polymer is being hydrolyzed. Eventually, porosity is generated and the peptide drug is slowly released again. Outside of the United States, a peptide microsphere formulation (Decapeptyl) was marketed in 1986 by Ipsen Biotech of France. It contains microspheres of the LHRH agonist, [D-Trp^6]-LHRH and 50:50 poly(D,L-lactide-*co*-glycolide) as the polymeric excipient [28]. With a single injection, this product delivers 3.75 mg of the peptide over a one-month period for the treatment of prostate cancer. A similar product is under development in the United States for Nafarelin, an LHRH agonist. Nafarelin is useful in indications responsive to the suppression of circulating levels of sex hormones, such as endometriosis and uterine fibroids in women and prostatic cancer in men. The PLGA–nafarelin controlled-release system was evaluated in humans by im injection [29]. As seen in Fig. 1, the release for a 2% loading was predominantly in the tertiary erosion-controlled phase. At 4 and 7% loadings, the release increased in the primary phase as its mechanism shifted from an erosional to a diffusional phase.

Subdermal Polymeric Implants

A subdermal polymeric implant can provide controlled release of the peptide–protein drug for a prolonged period [30]. The biocompatibility of subdermal polymeric implants is an important concern since these implants may reside in the body for an extended period of time. Ethylene–vinyl acetate copolymer (EVAc), a nondegradable hydrophobic polymer, has been investigated for the preparation of a polymer matrix to control polypeptide delivery. EVAc is biocompatible and has already been used in some nonparenteral controlled-release drug-delivery systems approved by the FDA for human applications, for example, the Ocusert system for ocular drug delivery. However, this system is nondegradable, and if used as an implant, has to be surgically removed once delivery is complete. The implantable osmotic minipump, mentioned before, provides another delivery approach which is not dependent on polymers. Biodegradable polymers are also being investigated for implants, which have the advantage that they need not be surgically removed after drug delivery.

Liposomes for Sustained and Targeted Delivery

Liposomes, upon iv injection, are taken up by the reticuloendothelial system (RES) because of their particulate nature, and this can be exploited to target drugs to the RES. On the other hand, an sc or im injection of liposomes can provide a sustained release of the drug as the liposomes forms a depot at the injection site [31]. The release rate depends upon the type of liposome and the lipid composition. Peptide–protein drugs have hydrophobic regions, and if these regions insert into the bilayer membranes, the sustained re-

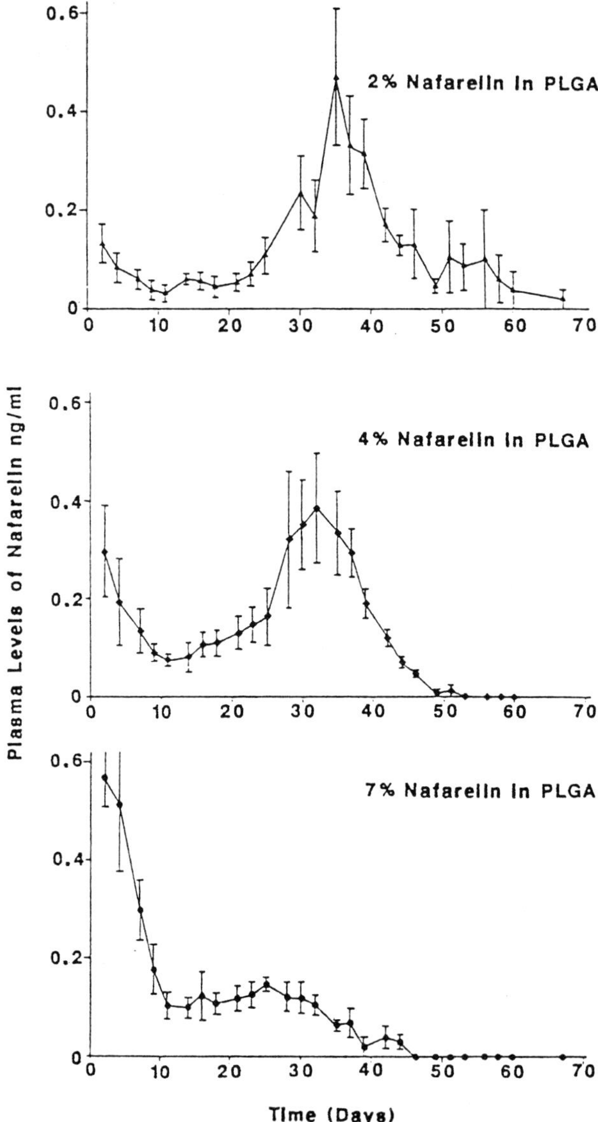

FIG. 1. Mean plasma levels of nafarelin in male subjects receiving 4 mg nafarelin controlled-release injectable. (From Ref. 29 with permission.)

lease can continue even after the liposome vesicles have released their aqueous contents. It is also possible to attach antibodies covalently to liposomes, which increases their cell specificity and provides another pathway for drug targeting. Yet another method is to use liposomes containing ultrafine magnetite, which can be targeted to tumors or other sites by an external magnetic field. Although liposomes, for the most part, are biocompatible, stability and manufacturing issues need to be resolved before commercialization of this technology.

Noninvasive Delivery Routes

Chronic parenteral administration, requiring repeated injections may give rise to problems of patient compliance. Noninvasive delivery routes, if feasible, can overcome these drawbacks because no injection is required and steady input from the mucosae or skin can provide a controlled drug release, thereby overcoming the drawback of short biological half-lives. A comparison of insulin absorption from various nonconventional mucosal sites has been reported [32]. The efficacy of different routes of administration in the presence of sodium glycocholate, an absorption-promoting adjuvant, had the rank order of nasal > rectal > buccal > sublingual, with nasal and rectal insulin being roughly half as efficacious as an intramuscular injection.

Ocular Delivery

The ocular route may potentially be used for the systemic delivery of proteins and peptides. The early finding that insulin, when topically administered to the eye, produces a sustained lowering of blood glucose, supports the potential usefulness of the ocular route for systemic delivery of peptide–protein drugs. Although earlier investigators incorrectly assumed that insulin was absorbed through the conjunctiva at the cul de sac, it is now known that absorption occurs primarily through the nasolacrimal system, as the drug is swept away from the conjunctival sac by incoming tears and comes in contact with the nasal mucosa, where it is systemically absorbed. Although longer-lasting formulations might be prepared for ocular inserts, ointments, gels, etc., this may be difficult for intranasal preparations. Besides insulin, thyrotropin releasing hormone (TRH), LHRH, enkephalins, calcitonin, and glucagon have been administered via the ocular route [33].

The ocular availability of topically applied proteins and peptides is expected to be even lower than that of conventional small drug molecules because of their unfavorable molecular size, hydrophilicity, and susceptibility to degradation by peptidases in various tissues of the eye. However, the systemic absorption is relatively fast and the absorbed polypeptides bypass the portal circulation to the liver, thus avoiding the first-pass metabolism by the liver. Although the acceptability of the ocular route for systemic delivery is in question [34], the topical use of growth factors to heal eye injury is very likely, as the eye heals very slowly because of a lack of blood supply [35].

Nasal Delivery

Peptide drugs have been commercially available in nasal dosage forms for routine clinical use for quite some time. These include lypressin (Diapid), desmopressin (Concentraid), oxytocin (Syntocinon), and the LHRH agonist Nafarelin (Synarel). Several other peptides as well as protein drugs, including insulin, calcitonin, growth hormone, etc., are currently under investigation for intranasal delivery.

The intranasal delivery of a given peptide or protein depends on the size of the molecule. Peptides with a molecular weight of less than 1000 are easily absorbed. Larger peptides or proteins are less easily absorbed unless they are mixed or concomitantly administered with nasal absorption promoters such as surfactants and bile salt derivatives [36]. The permeation enhancer, sodium tauro-24,25-dihydrofusidate (STDHF) was found to greatly enhance the delivery of human growth hormone after intranasal administration in the rat, rabbit, and sheep [37]. Cyclodextrins have also been investigated as enhancers of nasal delivery of protein drugs such as insulin [38]. The safety of enhancers must be evaluated because some can cause morphological damage, as evidenced by their effect on the ciliary beat frequency of nasal epithelial tissue [39].

Although the nasal route is an efficient means of achieving systemic effects, it presents a number of barriers to systemic drug absorption:

- The mucous layer consisting of mucins and enzymes,
- The mucociliary transport system,
- The epithelial cell layer consisting of ciliary cells, and
- The capillary endothelial cells.

Even so, the intranasal route is one of the most promising noninvasive routes of peptide–protein delivery.

Buccal Delivery

The buccal route [30] offers promise for the absorption of small peptides, though it is likely to be ineffective in delivering protein drugs. Mucosal adhesive dosage forms, which also incorporate a penetration enhancer, have been investigated for the delivery of insulin with partial success [40]. Some of the advantages of this route include a large surface area of the oral mucosa for the placement of delivery systems, including adhesive tablets, gels, and patches. It also provides easy accessibility although the site should be chosen carefully, considering permeability differences. Furthermore, some sites must be avoided because of the functions of the mouth, that is, mastication, swallowing, and salivary secretion.

Transdermal and Topical Administration

Transdermal Delivery

Administration of drugs through the skin, called transdermal delivery, is currently providing a route for the delivery of several drugs. Transdermal products on market include drugs such as scopolamine, nitroglycerin, clonidine, estradiol, and, most recently, nicotine. Transdermal delivery offers many advantages:

- Bypass hepatic ''first-pass'' effect, enhancing therapeutic efficacy,
- Constant absorption and metabolism (in contrast to oral administration),
- Use of drugs with short biological half-lives,
- Rapid termination of the medication as and when needed, and
- A simplified therapeutic regimen with improved patient compliance.

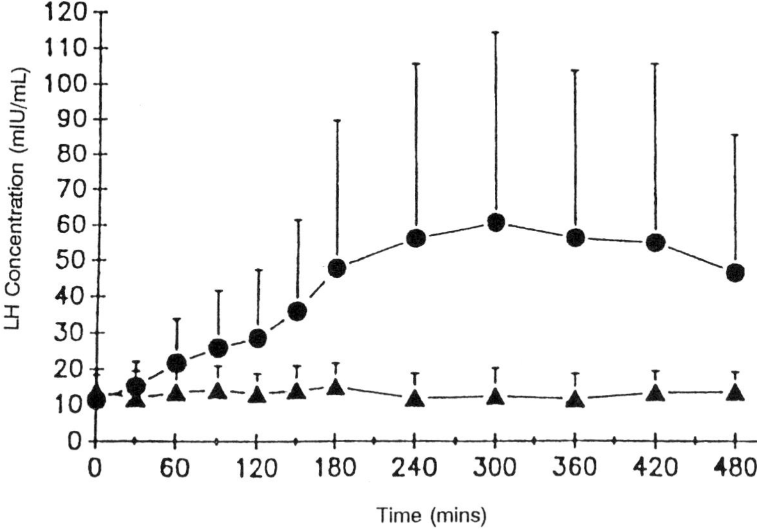

FIG. 2. Mean serum LH concentrations in volunteers receiving active (●) or passive (▲) patches containing leuprolide, an LHRH analogue. (Modified from Ref. 45 with permission.)

Although the transdermal route may be feasible for delivery of peptide–protein drugs, these molecules are too big and too hydrophilic to pass through the skin by themselves. Their delivery, therefore, has to be assisted in some way. Permeation across the stratum corneum can be improved by absorption enhancers such as dimethyl sulfoxide, azone, and surfactants [41]. A physical force can also be used; phonophoresis, for example, involves the transport of drug molecules, contained in a contact agent, through the skin under the influence of ultrasound [42].

An alternative method, called iontophoresis, employs a minute amount (< 1 milliampere) of physiologically safe electric current [43,44]. Conceptually, the applied electrical potential may alter the molecular arrangement of the skin, especially of the stratum corneum, resulting in changes in the skin's permeability. Recently, successful transdermal administration of therapeutic doses of a leuprolide, a 9-amino acid LHRH analog, to normal human subjects was reported [45]. As seen in Fig. 2, the delivery of the leuprolide resulted in a significant elevation of serum LH concentrations with active patches compared to those of passive controls, the active patches being the ones to which the current was applied. Research is also underway to explore the feasibility of iontophoretic delivery of insulin to diabetics. Factors affecting the rate of transdermal iontophoretic delivery of peptide–protein drugs include the physico-chemical properties of the formulation, such as pH, ionic strength, and electrolyte concentration, and the electronic variables of the iontophoretic technique, such as intensity of the applied voltage, wave form, frequency, and treatment time. The ultimate goal is to develop disposable, battery-operated skin patches that will be operated and controlled by microchips to deliver the drugs at the desired rate. The technique of transdermal iontophoresis is expected to result in a marketed product in the very near future. According to Dr. Burton H. Sage [46] of Becton Dickinson & Company, "it seems only a matter of time now before the appearance of prefilled iontophoretic skin patches for home use."

Topical Skin Delivery

Peptide–protein drugs could also provide local effects on the skin, an example being the potential use of growth factors to accelerate wound healing. Since more than 90% of wounds result from surgical procedures, enhanced wound healing could shorten hospital stays with substantial cost savings and improved quality of life [47]. Clinical trials are underway with epidermal (EGF) and other growth factors, with an estimated annual market of $1 billion by the end of the century. Since proteolytic activity at the wound site may degrade the growth factors, stabilization with a protease inhibitor may enhance the efficacy of growth factors to heal wounds [48].

Oral Delivery

The oral route, traditionally believed to be the least likely site for peptide and protein delivery, is still actively researched because of the popularity and convenience of this route. The following approaches have received the most attention:

1. The peptide carrier system for small peptides;
2. Delivery of nanoparticles to the Peyers patches; and
3. Polymers or prodrugs that protect the protein until degraded in the colon by indigenous bacteria.

Di- and tripeptides, including some small peptide-like drugs (β-lactam antibiotics and angiotensin-converting enzyme (ACE) inhibitors) are transported via a carrier-mediated process [49]. The number of peptide transport enzymes is unknown; to date only one has been isolated. The peptide-carrier system has broad specificity; Bai et al. [50] studied a series of dipeptide analogues without the *N*-terminal α-animo group and determined that it is not required for transport to occur via this mechanism. Information on the carrier system was used by Sinko et al. [51] to model the intestinal absorption and metabolism of peptides and analogues. Using numerical routines for carrier-mediated absorption and enzymatic reaction, the model was applied to tripeptide analogues and insulin. The simulations suggest that insulin is permeability limited, and therefore the co-administration of enzyme inhibitors may not increase the extent of oral absorption beyond 2%.

A number of investigators have shown that proteins protected in nanocapsules or liposomes can pass through the Peyers patches into the underlying lymphoid tissue [52–57]. This site of delivery is especially useful to target sites in the lymph system. Eldridge et al. have utilized this approach for the delivery of a vaccine [53,54].

A number of polymers resistant to enzymes in the gut and intestine, have been utilized to deliver proteins to the colon, where they are degraded by the colonic bacteria. Rubenstein et al. [58] used calcium pectinate as carrier. It is degraded by pectinolytic enzymes of the bacterial flora of the colon. Hydrogels prepared from *N*, *N*-dimethylacrylamide, *N*-*t*-butylacrylamide, or acrylic acid, cross-linked with azoaromatic compounds [59], functioned by swelling at increasing pH in the intestine in such a way that once in the colon, the cross-links are accessible to azoreductase systems in the colon. Van den Mooter et al. [60] prepared azo polymers of 2-hydroxyethyl methacrylate and methyl methacrylate in the presence of bis(methacryloylamino)azobenzene. The rate of decomposition in the presence of colonic flora was dependent on polymer composition.

Although proteolytic enzymes are less concentrated in the colon than in other parts of the gastrointestinal tract, the permeability of proteins across the colonic membrane is still low, and coadministration of permeation enhancers may be required. Then the question as to whether the enhancers will also allow undesired substances (e.g., colonic bacteria or toxins) to permeate remains.

Pulmonary Delivery

Delivery of proteins to the lungs offers some advantages over other routes. The walls of the alveoli in the deep lung are extremely thin (0.1–1 μm) compared to the capillary walls (7 μm) or red blood cells (8 μm). They are an order of magnitude thinner than typical mucosal or epithelial membranes, which are several millimeters thick. In addition, the surface area of the lung is extremely large, approximately 75 m^2 for a 70 kg male [61].

Although the lungs are rich in enzymes, they also contain several proteinase inhibitors. There is some evidence that exogenous proteins may be protected from proteolytic degradation by these inhibitors [62–64].

The mechanics of delivery to the lungs are perhaps more complex than for other routes. The fraction of drug that reaches the lungs depends on a number of factors, including amount and rate of air inhaled, respiratory pause, and particle size and characteristics. Particle size and characteristics can be combined into a measure known as the "mass median aerodynamic diameter" (MMAD). It must be approximately 5 μm or less in order for drug particles to reach the lung [61]. In spite of these complex mechanics, pulmonary delivery of a number of drugs, such as bronchodilators and steroids have enjoyed great success.

Fortunately, the advantages of this route of delivery have been recognized, and the number of researchers in the field has increased steadily. Genetech has recently completed clinical trials on a nebulized form of the enzyme DNase. This protein helps to break down the thick mucous clogging the lungs of cystic fibrosis patients [65].

Delivery of insulin to the lung has been encouraging. Liu et al. [66] observed a hypoglycemic effect by intratracheal instillation of insulin to rats. Insulin encapsulated in liposomes (dipalmitoylphosphatidyl choline:cholesterol, 7:2) enhanced the hypoglycemic effect, although a physical mixture of insulin with liposomes resulted in a similar effect.

Colthorpe et al. [67] delivered an aqueous solution of insulin to rabbits by iv, intratracheal instillation, and aerosol administration via a nebulizer. The particle size was characterized by a multi-stage liquid impinger and laser light scattering. Gamma scintigraphy was used to visualize the extent and site of deposition and to calculate the exact dose of insulin delivered. The aerosol delivered much more to the peripheral lung than intratracheal instillation (Fig. 3). Bioavailability values relative to iv administration were 5.6 ± 3.3% and 57.2 ± 28.5% for intratracheal and aerosol delivery, respectively.

Encouraging results in the pulmonary delivery of insulin to rabbits were also reported by Sakr [68]. In this case, nebulized insulin was compared to subcutaneous injection (Fig. 4). A dose response in the plasma glucose levels was observed with the nebulized insulin. Faster absorption and more rapid onset of action was evident with pulmonary vs. subcutaneously delivered insulin, and the bioavailability was 50%.

To avoid stability problems associated with holding proteins in solution for their entire shelf-life, researchers at Inhale Therapeutic Systems developed a method for aerosolizing peptides and proteins from a powder formulation. Approximately 55–60% of

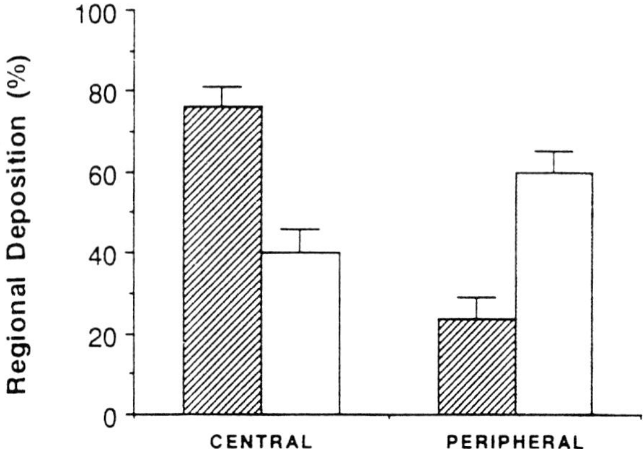

FIG. 3. Distribution of activity in the central and peripheral zones across a horizontal profile of the right side of the lung following intracheal (hatched bars) and aerosol (open bars) administration, as determined by gamma scintigraphy. (From Ref. 67 with permission).

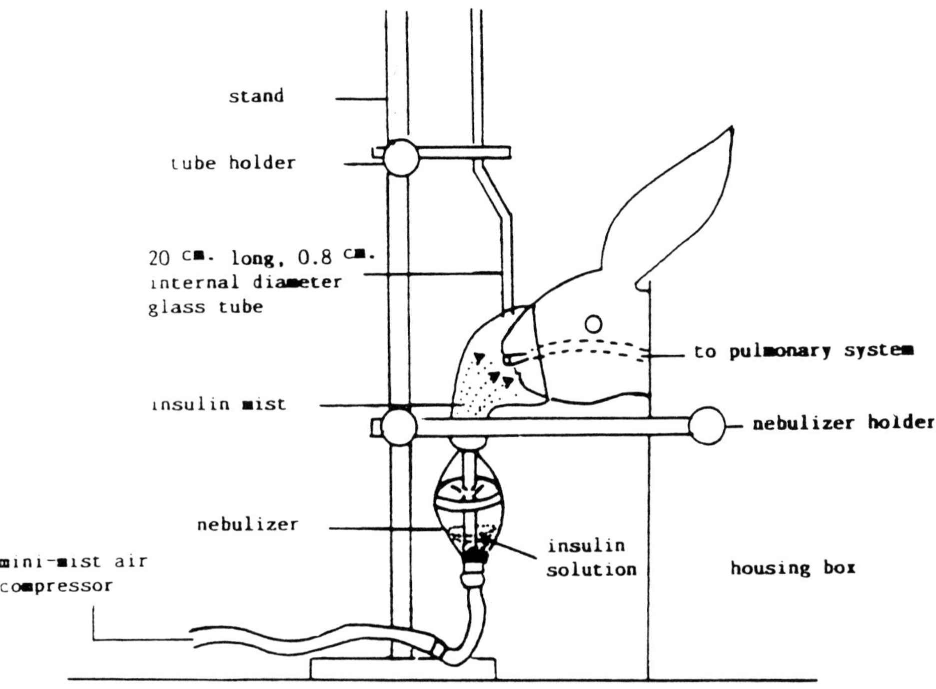

FIG. 4. Nebulizer fittings for the delivery of insulin mist to rabbit pulmonary system. (From Ref. 68 with permission.)

aerosolized α-interferon and granulocyte colony-stimulating factor were absorbed into the bloodstream through the lung epithelium in animal studies [65].

Schreier et al. [69], reviewed the use of liposomes for pulmonary delivery. The retention of encapsulated drug during nebulization is dependent on the formulation and the liposome size. Formulations containing cholesterol retained their contents better than those without, and large, unextruded multilamellar vesicles lost much more of their contents than vesicles with diameters of less than 0.2 μm. Pulmonary delivery of liposomes to animals and humans did not result in any untoward effects, although systematic toxicological studies were not reported. Pulmonary delivery of liposomally encapsulated small molecules, such as cytosine arabinoside and metaproterenol, reduced the side effects of the drug and the release rates which could be controlled by varying the liposomal formulation. The author has shown that alveolar macrophages do take up liposomes in vitro, and other investigators have demonstrated uptake in vivo using fluorescence-labeled liposomes. Delivery of liposomes to pulmonary epithelial cells has been demonstrated in vitro by the author by designing an artificial respiratory syncytial viral envelope which entered essentially 100% of an HEp-2 cell culture within 1 h [69]. See also the article Liposomes as Pharmaceutical Dosage Form by Barenholz and Crommelin, Vol. 9, pp. 1–39, of this encyclopedia.

Outlook

Gene Therapy

Until very recently, gene therapy was considered an experimental and perhaps esoteric field. The success of gene therapy in treating children with adenosine deaminase (ADA) deficiency paved the way for its application to other disorders. Over 40 proposals for gene therapy have been approved to date by the FDA and NIH, and nearly a dozen companies have entered the field. As of March 1993, a total of five proposals for the application of gene therapy to cystic fibrosis have been approved by the NIH gene therapy review board. In these trials, genes will be delivered in vivo directly to human lungs or nasal cavities. Early methods utilized ex vivo techniques, which involved the delivery of genes to cells in a culture dish and then implanting the cells back into the patient [70].

Although treatment of genetic diseases is the obvious market for gene therapy, the applications have extended to other diseases. Cancer therapy may be aided by several approaches:

1. Modification of cancer cells in such a way that the immune system can recognize and destroy them more readily,
2. Modification of lymphocytes to improve their ability to attack cancers, and
3. Insertion of a herpes virus gene into tumor cells, followed by an antiviral drug, which kills all cells expressing the gene [70].

Delivering the gene into the cell in an efficient manner is no easy task, and many of the protein drug-delivery techniques reviewed have been tried, some successfully, for the transfection procedure. The early trials utilized modified retroviruses to infect cells and deliver the desired DNA. In the cystic fibrosis trials, a modified adenovirus (one of the viruses responsible for colds) was used because of the ease with which this virus infects the upper respiratory tract [70].

Other techniques include driving DNA-coated gold beads into the skin via an electric current, and attaching DNA to a carrier protein which is recognized by receptors on liver cells, thus targeting the DNA specifically to the liver [70]. The ubiquitous liposome also offers a method of transfecting cells. Legendre and Szoka [71] compared pH-sensitive with cationic liposomes for the delivery of plasmid expression vectors in different mammalian cell lines. They found that the cationic liposomes were superior because they achieved higher cell-associated levels of plasmid DNA of high molecular weight. Furthermore, several pathways of DNA delivery are possible, including endocytosis and membrane fusion.

Abbreviated Proteins

The difficulty in manufacturing and delivering proteins, as well as the unexpected side effects that have turned up, in spite of their being ''natural'' drugs, has caused a rebirth in traditional synthesis of small drugs which are similar in structure to the active sites of therapeutic proteins. A better understanding of the structure of proteins and their receptors, gained through biotechnology, may have brought us to a full circle. An indicator of this interest is the growth of the synthetic chemistry department at Genetech, a pioneer of gene-cloning technology. Currently the researchers of this company are attempting to develop a small molecule to simulate the desirable properties of human growth hormone (hGH), without the unwanted side effects of diabetes and lactation. One of the difficulties in this approach is that hGH binds to two receptors, and finding a single small molecule that could reach both is a challenge [72].

Prodrugs of peptides may offer another solution to delivery. The peptides are smaller overall, and therefore can permeate more readily. Several investigators have developed bioreversible derivatives of the functional groups occurring in peptides and amino acids. These include imidazolidinones for the α-aminoamide group in peptides [73]; 5-oxazolidinones for the α-amidocarboxy moiety [74]; *N*-acylation and *N*-aminomethylation of the pyroglutamyl moiety to protect against pyroglutamyl aminopeptidase [75]; and *N*-α-hydroxyalkylation of the peptide bond as a way to protect the peptide bond against cleavage by enzymes such as carboxypeptidase A [76]. Subsequently, Bundgaard and co-workers showed that esterification of the hydroxyl group to give *N*-α-acyloxyalkyl derivatives released the parent peptide in a two-step reaction. This derivatization allows modification of the peptide stability profile as well as its lipophilicity [77].

Esterification of the tyrosine phenolic group in α-*N*-acylated tyrosine amide model compounds improved their stability in the presence of α-chymotrypsin. A similar approach was taken with the antidiuretic hormone desmopressin. Various aliphatic carboxylic acid esters of the tyrosine phenolic group were synthesized. All were converted to the parent compound in human plasma and rabbit liver homogenates. However, only the sterically hindered pivalate ester was more stable to α-chymotrypsin hydrolysis [78].

A better understanding of receptor structure has also led to the development of small molecules which block those receptors and thus prevent disease. Examples of this approach are the studies by Sterling Winthrop researchers of the small synthetic drugs disoxaril and WIN 54954 that bind to the ''pockets'' in the rhinovirus which causes the common cold and prevents its attachment to cellular receptor, the adhesion molecule

ICAM. In a similar approach, a number of researchers are attempting to block receptor binding of the AIDS virus to CD4 receptor molecules on T cells. Soluble CD4 receptors have not performed well in the clinic. However, another path, such as that used by workers at Procept, Inc. of Cambridge, MA, would be to synthesize drugs to which the CD4 receptor could attach [72].

Summary

Progress has been made in overcoming or circumventing the problems associated with peptide and protein delivery. It appears that therapeutic effect of a given peptide–protein drug can be obtained by:

1. Enhancing delivery through one or a combination of the various approaches discussed above,
2. Gene therapy to allow the body to produce its own protein, and
3. Substitution of a small molecule, often modeled at the active site of the therapeutic protein, which interacts with the appropriate receptors and results in the same therapeutic effect.

It will be interesting to observe in the next decade which path proves commercially most viable. In all of them, pharmaceutical scientists will play a key role.

References

1. Powell, M. F., Sanders, L. M., Rogerson, A., and Si, V., *J. Pharm. Res.*, 8:1258–1263 (1991).
2. Ressing, M. E., Jiskoot, W., Talsma, H., van Ingen, C. W., Bwuvery, C., and Crommelin, D. J. A., *J. Pharm. Res.*, 9:226–270 (1992).
3. Hora, M. S., Rana, R. K., and Smith, F. W., *J. Pharm. Res.*, 9:33–36 (1992).
4. Izutsu, K. I., Yoshioka, S., and Terao, T., *Int. J. Pharm.*, 90:187–194 (1993).
5. Pikal, M. J., *BioPharm.*, 3:18–27 (1990a).
6. Pikal, M. J., *BioPharm.*, 3:26–30 (1990b).
7. Manning, M. C., Patel, K., and Borchardt, R. T., *Pharm. Res.*, 6:903–918 (1989).
8. Bhatt, N. P, Patel, K., and Borchardt, R. T., *Pharm. Res.*, 7:593–599 (1990a).
9. Patel, K., and Borchardt, R. T., *Pharm. Res.*, 7:703–711 (1990).
10. Patel, K., and Borchardt, R. T., *Pharm. Res.*, 7:787–793 (1990.
11. Oliyai, C., and Borchardt, R. T., *Pharm.* Res., 10:95–102 (1993).
12. Pikal, M. J., Dellerman, K. M., Roy, M. L., and Riggin, R. M., *Pharm. Res.*, 8:427–436 (1991).
13. Gu, L. C., Erdos, E. A., Chiang, H. S., Calderwood, T., Tsai, K., Visor, G. C., Duffy, J., Hsu, W. C., and Foster, L. C., *Pharm. Res.*, 8:485–490 (1991).
14. Creighton, T. E., *Proteins*, W. H. Freeman and Co., New York, 1984, pp. 376–380.
15. Yoshinobu, T., Fujita, T., Hashida, M., Maeda, H., and Sezaki, H., *J. Pharm. Sci.*, 78:219–222 (1989).

16. Tsuji, J. I., Hirose, K., Kasahara, E., Naitoh, M., and Yamamoto, I., *Immunopharmac.*, 7:725–730 (1985).
17. Hershfield, M. S., Buckley, R. H., Greenberg, M. L., Melton, A. L., Schiff, R., Hatem, C., Kurtzberg, J., Markert, M., Kobayashi, R., Kobayashi, A., and Abuchowski, A., *N. Eng. J. Med.*, 316:589–596, 623–624 (1987).
18. Harris, D., and Robinson, J. R., *Biomaterials*, 11:652–655 (1990).
19. Rojanasakul, Y., Wang, L. Y., Bhat, M., Glover, D. D., Malanga, C. J., and Ma, J. K. H., *Pharm. Res.*, 9:1029–1034 (1992).
20. Wang., Y. J., Parenteral Products of Peptides and Proteins. In: *Pharmaceutical Dosage Forms: Parenteral Medications* (K. E. Avis, H. A. Lieberman, and L. Lachman, eds.), Marcel Dekker, Inc., New York, 1992, pp. 283–319.
21. Takeyama, M., Ishida, T., Kokubu, N., Komada, F., Iwakawa, S., Okumura, K., and Hori, R., *Pharm. Res.*, 8:60–64 (1991).
22. Banerjee, P. S., Hosny, E. A., and Robinson, J. R., Parenteral Delivery of Peptide and Protein Drugs. In: *Peptide and Protein Drug Delivery* (V. H. L. Lee, ed.), Marcel Dekker, Inc., New York, 1991, pp. 487–543.
23. Heller, J., *Adv. Drug Deliv. Rev.*, 10:163–204 (1993).
24. Tabata, Y., Gutta, S., and Langer, R., *Pharm. Res.*, 10:487–496 (1993).
25. Sanders, L. M., Kent, J. S., McRae, G. I., Vickery, B. H., Tice, T. R., and Lewis, D. H., *J. Pharm.* Sci., 73:1294–1297 (1984).
26. Sah, H. K., and Chien, Y. W., *Drug Develop. Ind. Pharm.*, 19:1243–1263 (1993).
27. Cohen, S., Yoshioka, T., Lucarelli, M., Hwang, L. H., and Langer, R., *Pharm. Res.*, 8:713–720 (1991).
28. Tice, T. R., and Tabibi, S. E., Parenteral Drug Delivery: Injectables. In: *Treatise on Controlled Drug Delivery* (A. Kydonieus., ed.), Marcel Dekker, New York, 1992, pp. 315–339.
29. Sanders, L. M., McRae, G., Vitale, K., Burns, R., Hoffman, P., and Shek, E., *J.. Pharm. Sci.*, 78:888–890 (1989).
30. Banga, A. K., and Chien, Y. W., *Int. J. Pharm.*, 48:15–50 (1988).
31. Weiner, A. L., *Adv. Drug Del. Rev.*, 3:307–341 (1989).
32. Aungst, B. J., Rogers, N. J., and Shefter, E., *J. Pharmacol. Exp. Therap.*, 224:23–27 (1988).
33. Chiou, G. C. Y., *Annu. Rev. Pharmacol. Toxicol.*, 31:457–467 (1991).
34. Lee, V. H. L., *Pharm. Technol.*, April:26–38 (1987).
35. Ratafia, M., *Pharm. Executive*, Sept:74–80 (1988).
36. McMartin, C., Hutchinson, L. E. F., Hyde, R., and Peters, G. E., *J. Pharm. Sci.*, 76:535–540 (1987).
37. Baldwin, P. A., Klingbeil, C. K., Grimm, C. J., and Longenecker, J. P., *Pharm. Res.*, 7:547–552 (1990).
38. Schipper, N. G. M., Romeijn, S. G., Verhoef, J. C., and Merkus, F. W. H. M., *Pharm. Res.*, 10:682–686 (1993).
39. Merkus, F. W. H. M., Schipper, N. G. M., Hermens, W. A. J. J., Romeijn, S. G., and Verhoef, J. C., *J. Control. Rel.*, 24:201–208 (1993).
40. Nagai, T., and Machida, Y., *Pharm. Int.*, 6:196–200 (1985).
41. Ghosh, T. K., and Banga, A. K., *Pharm. Technol.*, 17(4):62–90 (1993).
42. Tyle, P., and Agrawala, P., *Pharm. Res.*, 6:355–361 (1989).
43. Wearley, L. L., Tojo, K., and Chien, Y. W., *J. Pharm. Sci.*, 79:992–998 (1990).
44. Banga, A. K., and Chien, Y. W., *Pharm. Res.*, 10:697–702 (1993).
45. Meyer, B. R., Kreis, W., and Eschbach, J., *Clin. Pharmacol. Ther.*, 44:607–612 (1988).
46. Sage, B. H., Iontophoresis. In: *Encyclopedia of Pharmaceutical Technology*, Vol. 8 (J. Swarbrick and J. C. Boylan, eds.), Marcel Dekker, Inc., New York, 1993, pp. 217–247.
47. Lenz, G. R., and Mansson, P. E., *Pharm. Technol.*, 15 (Jan):34–40 (1991).

48. Okumura, K., Kiyohara, Y., Komada, F., Iwakawa, S., Hirai, M., and Fuwa, T., *Pharm. Res.*, 7:1289–1293 (1990).
49. Bai, J. P. F., and Amidon, G. L., *Pharm. Res.*, 9:960–978 (1992).
50. Bai, P. F., Subramanian, P., Mosberg, H. I., and Amidon, G. L., *Pharm. Res.*, 8:593–599 (1991).
51. Sinko, P. J., Leesman, G. D., and Amidon, G. L., *Pharm. Res.*, 10:271–275 (1993).
52. Damge, C., Michel, C., Aprahamian, M., Couvreur, P., and Devissauguet, J. P., *J. Control. Rel.*, 13:233–236 (1990).
53. Eldridge, J. H., Gilley, R. M., Staas, J. K., Moldoveanu, Z., Muelbroek, J. A., and Tice T. R., *Curr. Top. Microbiol. Immunol.*, 146:59–66 (1989).
54. Eldridge, J. H., Hammond, C. J., Muelbroek, J. A., Staas, J. K., Gilley, R. M. and Tice, T. R., *J. Control. Rel.*, 11:205–214 (1990).
55. Jani, P., Halbert, G. W., Langridge, J., and Florence, A. T., *J. Pharm. Pharmacol.*, 41:809–812 (1989).
56. Jani, P., Halbert, G. W., Langridge, J., and Florence, A. T., *J. Pharm. Pharmacol.*, 42:821–826 (1990).
57. Tomizawa, H., Aramaki, Y., Fujii, Y., Hara, T., Suzuki, N., Yachi, K., Kikuchi, H., and Tsuchiqa, S., *Pharm. Res.*, 10:549–552 (1993).
58. Rubinstein, A., Radae, R., Ezra, M., Pathak, S., and Rokem, J. S., *Pharm. Res.*, 10:258–263 (1993).
59. Brondsted, H., and Kopecik, J., *Pharm. Res.*, 9:1540–1545 (1992).
60. Van den Mooter, G., Samyn, C., and Kinget, R., *Int. J. Pharm.*, 87:37–46 (1992).
61. Wearley, L. L., Recent progress in protein and peptide delivery by noninvasive routes, *Crit. Rev. Ther. Drug Carrier Syst.*, 8:331–394 (1991).
62. Debs, R. J., Fuchs, H. J., Philip, R., Brunette, D., Duzgunes, N., Shellito, J. E., Liggitt, D., and Patton, J. R., *Cancer Res.*, 50:375 (1990).
63. Schankar, L. S., Mitchel, E. W., and Brown, R. A., *Drug Metab. Dispos.*, 14:79 (1986).
64. Boudier, Pelletier, A., Gast, A., Tournier, J. M., Pauli, G., and Bieth, J. G., *Hoppe Seyler's Biol. Chem.*, 368:981 (1987).
65. Wallace, B. M., and Lasker, J. S., *Science*, 260:912–913 (1993).
66. Liu, F. Y., Shao, Z., Kildsig, D. O., and Mitra, A. K., *Pharm. Res.*, 10:228–232 (1993).
67. Colthorpe, P., Farr, S. J., Taylor, G., Smith, I. J., and Wyatt, D., *Pharm. Res.*, 9:764–768 (1992).
68. Sakr, F., *Int. J. Pharm.*, 86:1–7 (1992).
69. Schreier, H., Gonzalez-Rothi, R. J., and Stecenko, A. A., *J. Control. Rel.*, 24:209–223 (1993).
70. Culotta, E., *Science*, 260:914–915 (1993).
71. Legendre, J. Y., and Szoka, F. C., *Pharm. Res.*, 9:1235–1242 (1992).
72. Moffat, A. S., *Science*, 260:910–912 (1993).
73. Klixbull, U., and Bundgaard, H., *Int. J. Pharm.*, 20:273–284 (1984).
74. Buur, A., and Bundgaard, H., Prodrugs of peptides, *Int. J. Pharm.*, 46:159–167 (1988).
75. Bundgaard, H., and Moss, J., *J. Pharm. Sci.*, 78:122–126 (1989).
76. Bundgaard, H., and Rasmussen, G. J., *Pharm. Res.*, 8:313–322 (1991).
77. Bundgaard, H., and Rasmussen, G. J., *Pharm. Res.*, 8:1238–1242 (1991).
78. Kahns, A. H., Buur, A., and Bundgaard, H., *Pharm. Res.*, 10:68–74 (1993).

LORRAINE L. WEARLEY
AJAY K. BANGA

Percutaneous Absorption

Introduction

Like all epithelial systems of the body, the skin serves as a barrier to keep water and other vital substances in and foreign material out. However, skin is the only epithelial system that must function in a hostile, nonaqueous environment [1]. Whereas the epithelial linings of the gastrointestinal or genitourinary tracts, for example, are bathed by interstitial fluid on the inside and another aqueous phase (gastric juices or urine) on the outside, skin is without aqueous contact on the outside under most environmental conditions. To survive and protect its own integrity from the ravages of desiccation and to fulfill its functional obligations to the body, skin has developed a specialized structure of unique physical-chemical composition, the stratum corneum.

The stratum corneum, which is the outermost layer of skin, is a multilayered structure consisting of flat anucleate cells totally devoid of normal intracellular structures. It is metabolically inactive in the usual sense, though some very critical enzymatic activities persist. That the "barrier" properties of skin do indeed reside in the stratum corneum was not clearly demonstrated until the work of Winsor and Burch [2]. Through a series of simple in vitro experiments in which water loss through cadaver skin was measured gravimetrically, they showed that following separation of skin into its two constituent layers (epidermis and dermis), the barrier to water loss resided in the outermost layer (epidermis). Water movement across the isolated dermal layer was roughly equivalent to the rate of loss from bulk water. Subsequently, they demonstrated that destruction of the outermost portion of the epidermis, the stratum corneum, resulted in loss of barrier properties to water movement.

Since those elegantly simple initial studies, a more definitive experiment has been performed. Water permeation through isolated stratum corneum has been measured, and it was found that all the resistance of water movement through full-thickness skin is accounted for by the resistance residing in the stratum corneum [3]. It is, therefore, the rate-limiting barrier of skin.

Subsequent work during the last few decades has served to better define the nature of the stratum corneum barrier and has shown that it is also the rate-limiting barrier to the diffusion of most molecular species. An observation frequently made by many investigators over the years has been the tendency for lipid-soluble molecules to permeate the skin better than water-soluble molecules. This is now known to be related to the presence of lipid bilayers in the intercellular space of the stratum corneum and represents a structural feature not seen in other epithelial systems [4]. Concurrently, the concept of the barrier has changed dramatically. Whereas skin was commonly thought of as being a barrier of low permeability to most substances, it is now recognized as a barrier of variable permeability. In some instances, it has been the portal of entry for toxic substances, resulting in serious adverse systemic reactions and death. It is now used as a route for delivery of therapeutic agents to the systemic circulation.

Anatomy and Biochemistry of Skin

Skin Structure

Skin is one of the largest organs of the body, 15,000–20,000 cm^2 in area in most adults, varying in thickness from approximately 1.5 to 4 mm, and weighing approximately 2 kg [5]. It consists of two parts: the cellular outermost layer, the epidermis, and the inner, relatively acellular, connective tissue layer, the dermis (Fig. 1). Lying between these two layers is a submicroscopic structure, the basal lamina or basement membrane zone, which serves as the anchoring structure by which the epidermis and dermis are held together. The blood supply to the skin resides exclusively in the dermis, and the nutritional needs of the epidermis are met entirely by diffusion.

The epidermis is composed of two parts (Fig. 2): the living cells of the Malpighian layer, which in turn can be divided into several strata, and the dead cells of the stratum corneum, commonly referred to as the horny layer because it also forms specialized structures such as hair, nails, and the horns of animals. The prime function of the viable cells of the epidermis is to move progressively through a process of differentiation, eventually to die (terminal differentiation), and through this mechanism generate the barrier layer. As cells undergo differentiation and move from inner to outer epidermis, many identifiable biochemical and structural changes take place:

- Loss of mitotic activity,
- Synthesis of new organelles (lamellar and keratohyalin granules) and subsequent loss of all cell organelles,
- Total remodeling of cell architecture as cells increase in width, flatten, and lose most of their water content,
- Modification of cell membrane and cell surface antigens and receptors, and
- Synthesis of new lipids, as well as structural and enzymatic proteins.

Epidermis

The epidermis is a continually renewing, stratified squamous epithelium covering the entire outer surface of the body. Over most of the body it ranges in thickness from 0.06 to 0.1 mm, though it is much thicker over the palms and soles because of the increased thickness of the horny layer. The principal cell (80%) of the epidermis is the keratinocyte, so named because of the family of fibrous proteins (keratins) contained within. Other cells include the melanocyte, the source of melanin pigment which gives the skin its color and affords protection from the damaging effects of ultraviolet radiation; the Langerhans cell, which is part of the immune surveillance system and serves in host defense; and the Merkel cell, which is thought to function as a mechanoreceptor for the sensation of touch.

Keratinocytes are characterized by the presence of submicroscopic (7–10 nm) filaments (keratins) and desmosomes, specialized structures occurring at irregular intervals on the cell membrane that serve as points of attachment for adjacent cells, analogous to spot welds.

The mitotically active keratinocytes reside in the basal layer or stratum germinativum (Fig. 3). As daughter cells move outward through the other strata of the epidermis, they begin to flatten and assume a polyhedral shape. When viewed by light microscopy, the

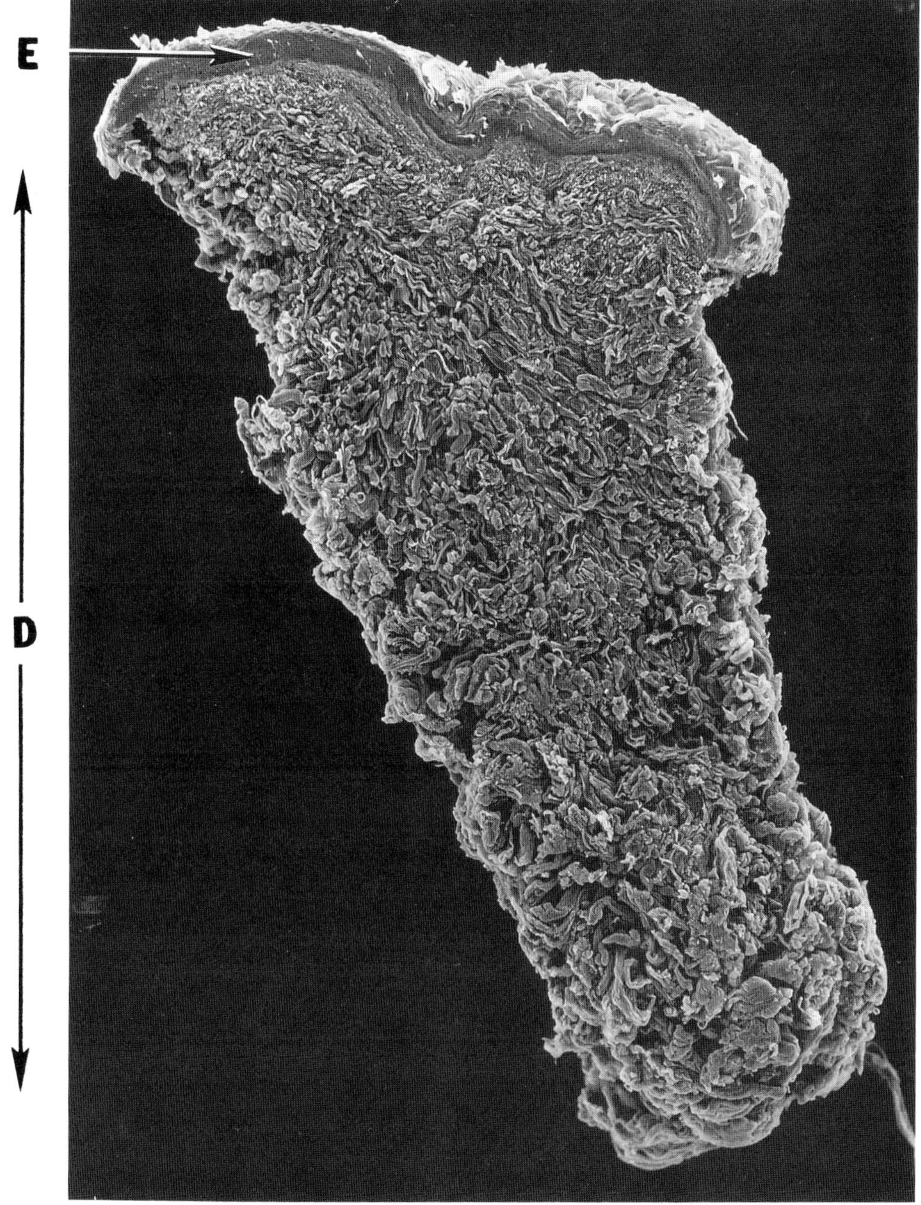

FIG. 1. Low magnification (× 80) scanning electron micrograph of skin from upper back, showing relative thinness of epidermis (E) and fibrous nature of dermis (D). (Reprinted with permission from Ref. 1.)

cells appear to have spines (stratum spinosum) due to the dehydration and shrinkage caused by routine histological preparation. They pull away from each other, except where firmly attached by desmosomes. In the spinous layer, keratin filaments become more prominent and a shift toward the synthesis of higher molecular weight keratins begins. Also in this layer a new organelle appears, the lamellar granule (membrane-coating gran-

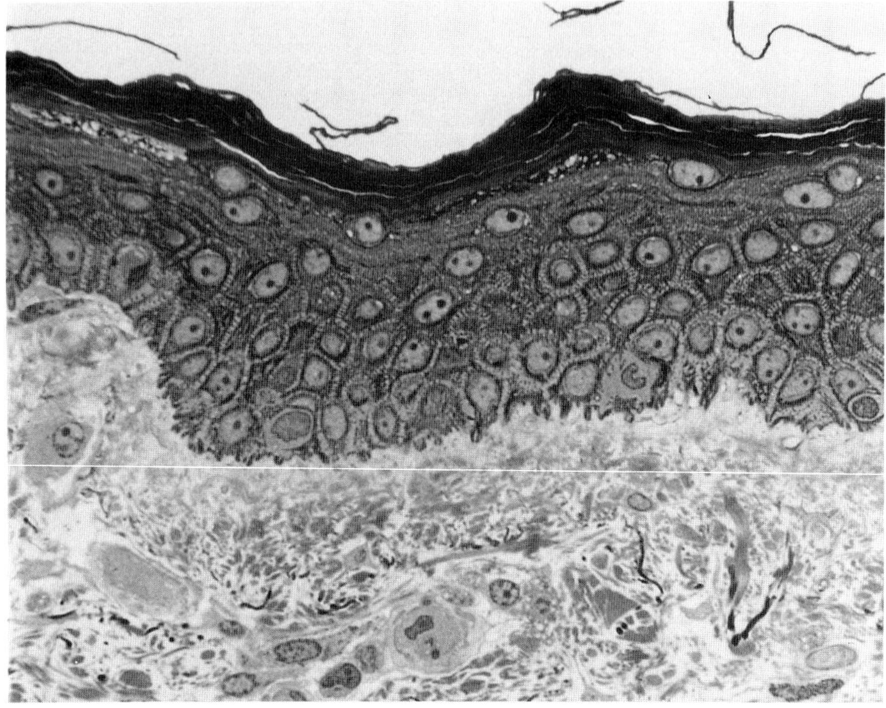

FIG. 2. Photomicrograph (× 250) illustrating cellular nature of epidermis and a portion of the relatively acellular upper dermis. The dark amorphous layer at the top is the stratum corneum. (Reprinted with permission from Ref. 1.)

ule, Odland body). These organelles (0.1–0.3 μm diameter) contain large amounts of lipid and are distinguished by the presence of alternating lamellae (Fig. 4a and b). It is the extrusion of these lipids into the intercellular space of the next strata, the granular layer, that initiates formation of the barrier.

Major changes in cellular architecture occur in the granular layer, named for the basophilic granules (keratohyalin granules) that are so prominently seen under both light and electron microscopy. The cells of this layer continue to flatten and become much wider than the underlying cells, and new proteins appear. The principal new protein is a high molecular weight, histidine-rich precursor, profilaggrin, which is contained in the keratohyalin granule. It will be converted to filaggrin and serve as the matrix in which the keratin filaments are enmeshed in the stratum corneum. Another protein, cystine-rich involucrin, first appears. It will become a major component of the thickened cell envelope of stratum corneum cells.

Lamellar granules become more numerous in the granular layer, where they migrate to the cell membrane and release their contents into the intercellular space. This is the first step in the formation of a barrier which is unique to skin. Studies have shown that large molecular weight substances such as lanthanum and horseradish peroxide, which diffuse freely from the dermis through the intercellular space of the basal and spinous layers, do not penetrate the granular layer [6,7].

The transition from granular layer to horny layer must occur abruptly, as intermediate cell types are seldom seen. The nucleus and all cell organelles (microsomes, mitochon-

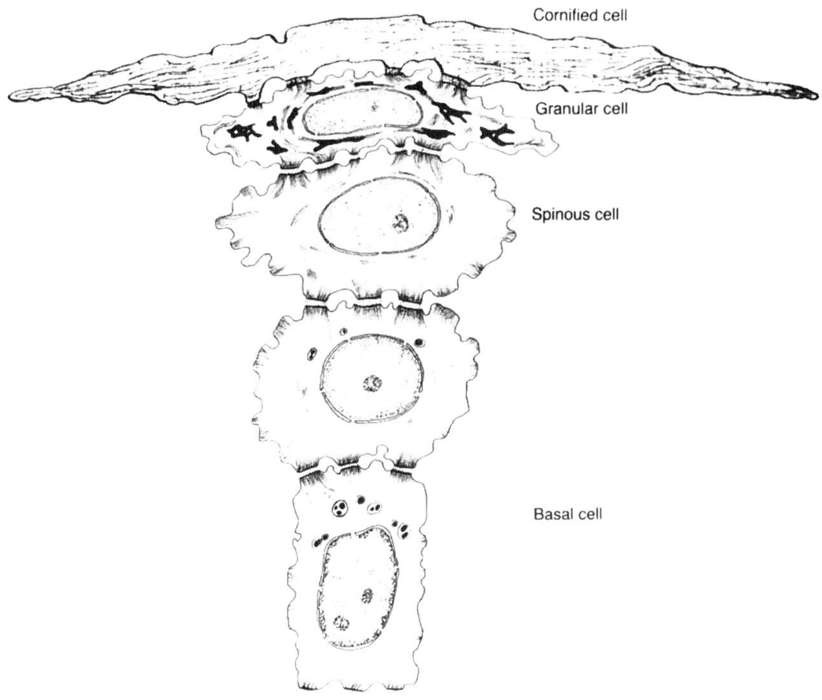

FIG. 3. Schematic of epidermal differentiation, showing transformation of mitotically active, vertically oriented basal cell to "dead," horizontally oriented corneocyte. (Reprinted with permission from S. L. Moschella, and H. J. Hurley, eds., *Dermatology*, 3rd ed., W. B. Saunders Co., Philadelphia, 1993.

dria, etc.) are broken down, a thick band of protein is deposited on the inner surface of the cell membrane to form the cell envelope, and the entire cell is filled with keratin filaments and associated matrix proteins.

The stratum corneum is the end product of epidermal differentiation and consists of 15 to 25 cell layers over most of the body surface (Fig. 5), though it is much thicker over the palms and soles [8]. Each cell (corneocyte) is approximately 0.5 μm in thickness and 30–40 μm in width, the largest cell in the epidermis. It contains no organelles but is filled with protein, 80% of which is high molecular keratin (>60,000 Daltons). The intercellular space is filled with lipids organized as bilayers. These lipids are of unusual composition and constitute approximately 14% by weight of the stratum corneum. In addition, the stratum corneum has a very low water content, though it can take up to five times its weight in water when placed in an aqueous environment [9].

Formation of the stratum corneum is also accompanied by the deposition of a thick band of protein on the inner surface of the plasma membrane which becomes cross-linked through the formation of both disulfide bonds and transglutaminase-dependent isopeptide linkages between the side chains of glutamine and lysine residues [10,11]. As this band forms, an unusual ω-hydroxyceramide becomes covalently attached to the external surface, and the phospholipids, which normally make up a large component of cell membranes, are degraded, leaving the barrier layer with little or no phospholipid content [12]. Thus, corneocytes are left with a compound cell envelope, consisting of a highly insol-

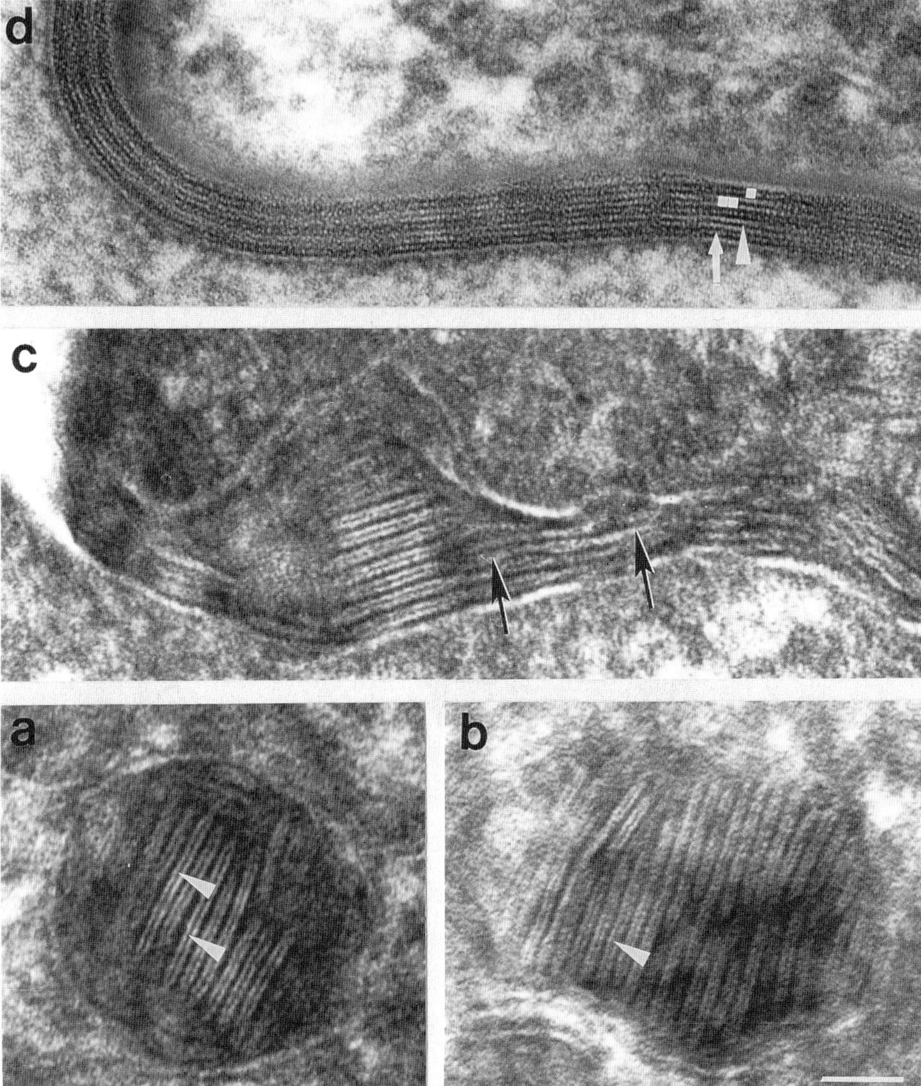

FIG. 4. Electron micrograph of lamellar granules from neonatal mouse skin, showing their changing structure. In a and b they appear intracellularly as "stacked disks" in the granular layer. In c, following extrusion to the intercellular space, fusion of disks (between arrows) begins to occur. In d, in the outer stratum corneum, only broad lamellar sheets are seen and the appearance of the dense and lucent bands is changed. Bar = 50 nm. (From Madison, K. C., et al., *J. Invest. Dermatol.*, 88:714–718 (1987).

uble, cross-linked protein inner surface and a hydroxyceramide monolayer outer surface. The lipid coating may serve as an anchor for the intercellular lipid bilayers and serve to influence their organization as well [13,14].

The corneocytes are joined together by modified desmosomes and overlap with each other at their edges to form a mechanically strong layer. All the mechanical strength of the epidermis derives from the stratum corneum which can be prepared in pure form as an intact "membrane" suitable for permeability studies [15].

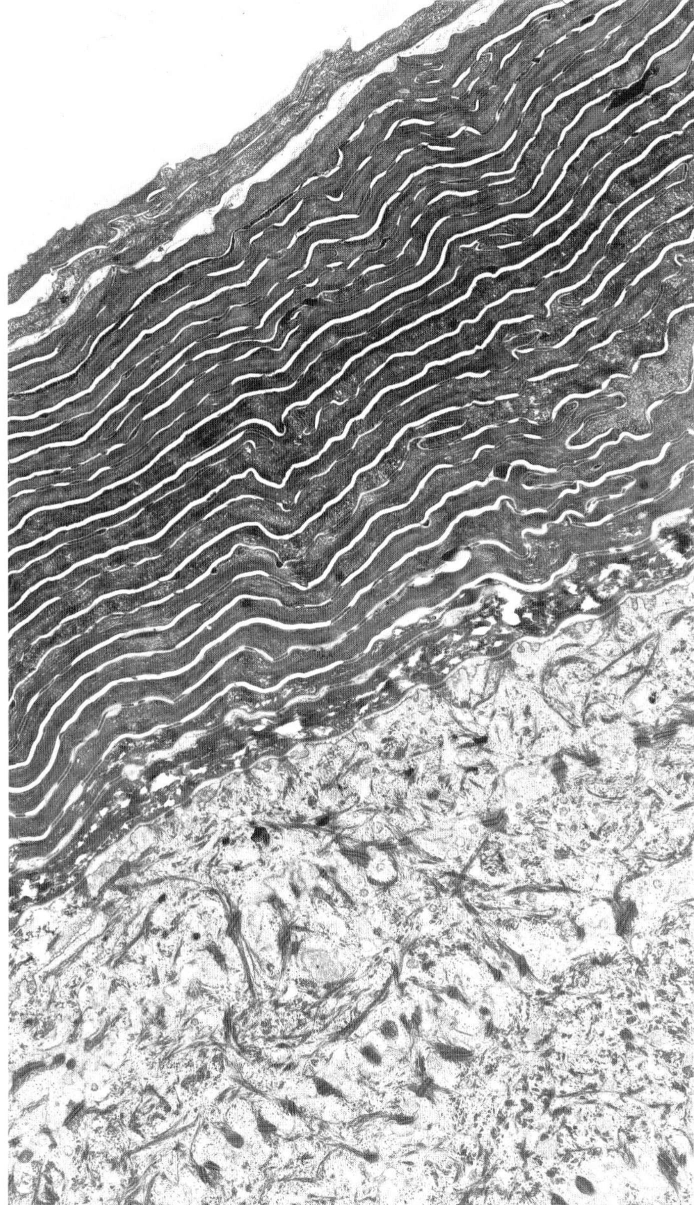

FIG. 5. Electron micrograph (× 96,000) through full thickness of stratum corneum and upper layers of the living epidermis. The multilayered nature of the barrier and the relative thinness of individual cells are apparent. The absence of structure in the intercellular space is due to lipid solvents used to prepare the specimen. (Reprinted with permission from Ref. 1.)

A particularly intriguing feature of stratum corneum architecture is its orderly arrangement into columns or stacks [16], a feature not seen in routine histologic preparations of the skin in which defatting solvents have been used. However, when frozen sections of unfixed skin are swollen (hydrated) with dilute acid or alkali, the cells of the horny layer are neatly aligned (Fig. 6). This is most evident in regions where the epi-

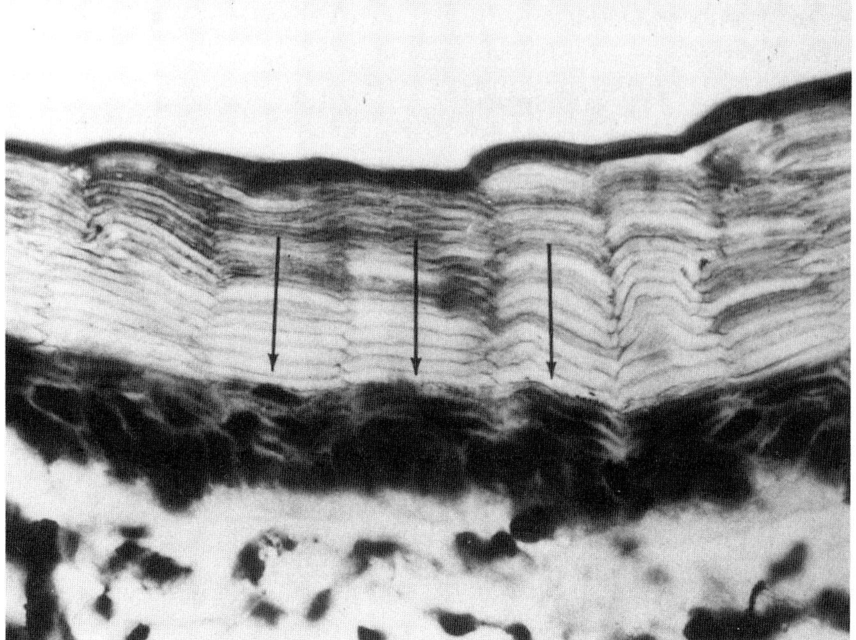

FIG. 6. Light micrograph of alkali-swollen mouse ear skin, showing corneocytes arranged in vertical columns. (Reprinted with permission from Ref. 1.)

dermis is thin (and in animal skin) and the turnover rate is low. It is not seen in areas such as the palms and soles, where the stratum corneum is unusually thick and the turnover rate high. This orderly arrangement of corneocytes may have some relationship to barrier function, as the diffusion coefficient of water in palmar and plantar skin is much higher than elsewhere [17].

The turnover time of the stratum corneum, the time for a newly formed cell to move from inside to outside and be sloughed, has been found to be approximately 14 days, using two separate techniques. Impregnation of the stratum corneum with the fluorescent dye tetrachlorsalicylanilide, which stains the entire thickness of the stratum corneum, revealed that the surface of the skin lost its fluorescence in approximately 10 to 15 days in regions such as the abdomen, back, and forearm [18]. A separate approach, in which the cells of the viable epidermis were labeled with ^{14}C-glycine, revealed that the first labeled cells (those coming from the granular layer) reached the skin surface in 13 to 14 days [19]. It should be noted, however, that there is a significant regional variation in stratum corneum renewal.

Dermis

The dermis is largely an integrated fibroelastic, acellular structure consisting of interwoven fibrous, filamentous, and amorphous connective tissue. It is the largest component of skin and it is from this layer that the skin derives its mechanical strength. The dermis is divided into two parts: the upper, papillary dermis, and the lower, reticular dermis. The papillary dermis is the thinner of the two and is distinguished from the reticular dermis by fiber bundles of much smaller diameter. Its interface with the epidermis is irregular and thrown into folds. The most elevated portions of the papillary dermis are referred to as dermal papillae; each contains a capillary loop arising from the underlying arteriole plexus. As skin ages, there is loss of dermal papillae and a reduction in the number of capillary loops.

Collagen is the principal fibrous protein of the dermis, accounting for more than 70% of its dry weight. Bundles of collagen fibers are woven into a network within the dermis, which accounts for the great tensile strength of skin. Interwoven among the collagen fabric is a network of elastic fibers which give skin its resilience, that is, the ability to restore normal structure following deformation by external forces. Elastin constitutes only 1–2% of the dry weight of the dermis. Other nonfibrous components of the dermis are the glycosaminoglycans (the amorphous ground substance) and the finely filamentous glycoproteins; both contribute to the water-binding properties of dermis.

From the standpoint of percutaneous absorption, perhaps the most important element of the dermis is its vasculature which serves as the sink for absorption. The blood supply to the skin comes from cutaneous branches of musculoskeletal arteries, which ascend from the underlying musculature, penetrate the subcutaneous fat, and enter the dermis. In the deeper regions of the dermis, branches spread horizontally to form a deep vascular plexus running parallel to the surface of the skin. In addition, the parent vessel ascends to the papillary dermis and divides into smaller arterioles which form a superficial plexus. Arising from the superficial plexus are smaller arterioles that give rise to capillary loops running at right angles to the surface of the skin and traversing the dermal papillae to within a few micrometers of the basement membrane (Fig. 7).

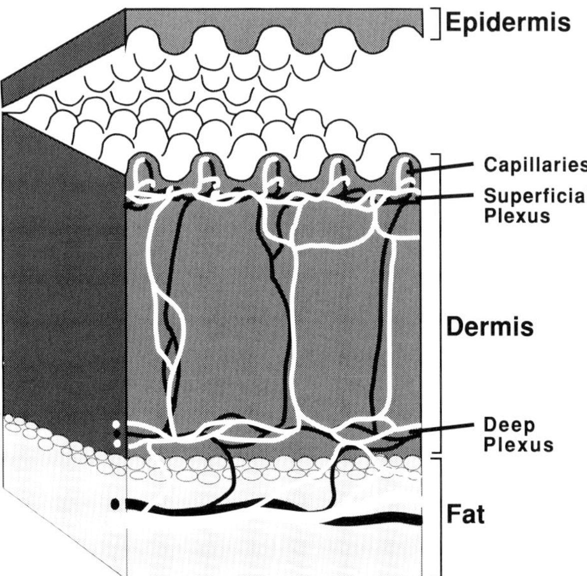

FIG. 7. Schematic illustration of cutaneous vasculature, showing both a superficial and deep plexus. Capillary loops arise from the superficial plexus and serve as the nutritional source for the living epidermis and the sink for percutaneous absorption. (Reprinted with permission from Ref. 1.)

The Role of Lipids in Barrier Function

An important element underlying the impermeability of skin is the hydrophobic nature of the stratum corneum. Recent data derived from morphologic, histochemical, and biochemical studies provide strong evidence that the stratum corneum can be viewed as a "heterogeneous two-compartment system of protein-enriched cells embedded in lipid-laden intercellular domains" [4]. The term "bricks and mortar" is now widely used to describe this organizational model and the lipids (mortar) are thought to be the principal element underlying barrier function, particularly to water and other hydrophilic materials.

Major changes in the lipid composition of the epidermis occur as cells differentiate and move from the basal layer to the horny layer (Fig. 8). There is a shift from polar lipids to neutral lipids and almost complete loss of phospholipids. With respect to barrier function, the most important changes occur in the granular layer just beneath the horny layer, and lead to the deposition of lipids in the intercellular space. These lipids, derived from lamellar granules, which have fused with the cell membrane to discharge the contents, first appear as broad disks (Fig. 4c and d). As this material moves up into the stratum corneum, modifications occur resulting in the formation of broad multilaminate

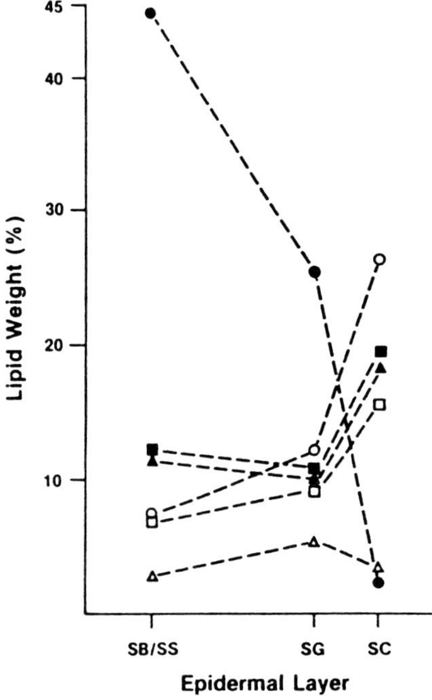

FIG. 8. The composition of lipid species within the human epidermis change as cells differentiate and move from the stratum basale/stratum spinosum (SB/SS), to the stratum granulosum (SG), and the stratum corneum (SC). ■ = Phospholipids; △ = cholesterol sulfate; □ = free fatty acids; ○ = sphingolipids; ▲ = free sterols; □ = nonpolar: SE = sterol esters, WE = wax esters, Sq = squalene, HC = hydrocarbons. (Reprinted with permission from Ref. 20.)

sheets, not unlike those normally seen in cell membranes. Synchronous with this change in morphology are major biochemical changes in lipid composition, which can best be characterized as movement from a ''polar'' to a nonpolar lipid profile. Nature's intent seems clear: The prime function of the horny layer is to serve as a barrier to water loss and this is accomplished through the generation of a domain of very high hydrophobicity. The resulting biochemical and morphological structures created are unique to skin.

Changes in the lipid content of human skin with differentiation are known from the work of Lampe et al. [20]. A complete analysis of the lipids obtained from abdominal skin was made at three levels within the epidermis. Total lipids were extracted from each layer, fractionated, and quantified by thin-layer chromatography (Table 1). It was found that generation of a fully formed stratum corneum is accompanied by an enrichment of neutral lipids and sphingolipids (ceramides) and virtual elimination of the most polar lipids, the phospholipids. Whereas the neutral lipids and ceramides make up less than 60% of the combined basal and spinous layers, they account for more than 95% of the horny layer. Virtually identical results have been obtained with the epidermis of pig skin using a similar experimental design [21]. Thus, it can be assumed that the same phenomena are operative in the skin of most mammals.

Regional variation in stratum corneum lipid content was evaluated at four sites (face, abdomen, leg, plantar) known to have different permeability properties [22]. Total lipid content varied among the four sites, with face skin having the greatest and plantar skin the lowest lipid content (Table 2). Neutral lipids comprised the largest percentage of stratum corneum lipids at all four sites, varying from 60 to 78%, and sphingolipids the next largest percentage, 18 to 35%. In trying to correlate these observations with known regional differences in percutaneous absorption of water [23], an inverse relationship between neutral lipid content and permeability is noted. Neutral lipids are highest in the

TABLE 1 Variations in Lipid Composition During Human Epidermal Differentiation and Cornification[a,b]

Fraction	Strata basale/spinosum (n = 5)	Stratum grandulosum (n = 7)	Stratum corneum Whole (n = 4)	Stratum corneum Outer (n = 8)
Polar lipids	44.5 ± 3.4	25.3 ± 2.6	4.9 ± 1.6	2.3 ± 0.5
Cholesterol sulfate	2.4 ± 0.5	5.5 ± 1.3	1.5 ± 0.2	3.4 ± 0.5
Neutral lipids	51.0 ± 4.5	56.5 ± 2.8	77.7 ± 5.6	68.4 ± 2.1
Free sterols	11.2 ± 1.7	11.5 ± 1.1	14.0 ± 1.1	18.8 ± 2.1
Free fatty acids	7.0 ± 2.1	9.2 ± 1.5	19.3 ± 3.7	15.6 ± 3.0
Triglycerides	12.4 ± 2.9	24.7 ± 4.0	25.2 ± 4.6	11.2 ± 1.5
Sterol/wax esters[c]	5.3 ± 1.3	4.7 ± 0.7	5.4 ± 0.9	12.4 ± 1.9
Squalene	4.9 ± 1.1	4.6 ± 1.0	4.8 ± 2.0	5.6 ± 2.1
n-Alkanes	3.9 ± 0.3	3.8 ± 0.8	6.1 ± 2.6	5.4 ± 0.8
Sphingolipids	7.3 ± 1.0	11.7 ± 2.7	18.1 ± 2.8	26.6 ± 2.3
Glucosylceramides I	2.0 ± 0.3	4.0 ± 0.3	trace	trace
Glucosylceramides II	1.5 ± 0.3	1.8 ± 0.2	trace	trace
Ceramides I	1.7 ± 0.1	5.1 ± 0.4	13.8 ± 0.4	19.4 ± 0.5
Ceramides II	2.1 ± 0.3	3.7 ± 0.1	4.3 ± 0.4	7.2 ± 0.5
Total	99.1	101.1	99.3	100.7

[a]From Ref. 20 with permission.
[b]Weight percent ± SEM.
[c]Sterol/wax esters present in approximately equal quantities, as determined by acid hydrolysis.

TABLE 2 Regional Variations in Lipid Weight Percent and Distribution of Major Lipid Species[a]

	Abdomen (n = 4)	Leg (n = 4)	Face (n = 3)	Plantar (n = 3)
Lipid weight % present	6.5 ± 0.5	4.3 ± 0.8	7.2 ± 0.4	2.0 ± 0.6
Major lipid species				
Polar lipids	4.9 ± 1.6	5.2 ± 1.1	3.3 ± 0.3	3.2 ± 0.89
Cholesterol sulfate[b]	1.5 ± 0.2	6.0 ± 0.9	2.7 ± 0.3	3.4 ± 1.2
Neutral lipids	77.7 ± 5.6	65.7 ± 1.8	66.4 ± 1.4	60.4 ± 0.9
Sphingolipids[c]	18.2 ± 2.8	25.9 ± 1.3	26.5 ± 0.9	34.8 ± 2.1

[a]Reprinted with permission from Ref. 22

[b]Significant differences: abdomen vs. leg, $P < 0.01$; leg vs. face, $P < 0.02$; abdomen vs. face, $P < 0.02$; face vs. plantar, $P < 0.01$; abdomen vs. plantar, $P < 0.01$; plantar vs. leg, $P < 0.02$. Cholesterol sulfate: leg > plantar > face > abdomen.

[c]Significant differences: abdomen vs. leg, $P < 0.05$; abdomen vs. face, $P < 0.05$. Sphingolipids: plantar > face > leg > abdomen.

abdomen, where water permeability is lowest, and lowest in plantar skin, where water permeability is highest. Also noted is the fact that sphingolipids show a direct correlation to water permeability, having just the opposite distribution as the neutral lipids at the same two sites. (It should be remembered that plantar, as well as palmar, skin has a paradoxical permeability profile. Though more permeable to water than other body sites, it is less permeable to most drugs because of its thicker stratum corneum.)

A comparison of oral epithelium with skin also points up the important relationship between lipids and barrier properties. Oral epithelium is similar to skin in that it differentiates to form a stratum corneum containing intercellular lipid lamellae, yet is an order of magnitude more permeable to water than skin [24]. In the pig, oral epithelium was found to have approximately 15% less total lipid content per cm^2 surface area than skin, not enough difference to account for the tenfold permeability difference. More importantly, it contained a lower percentage of ceramides (21 vs. 39%), particularly the linoleate-rich acylceramide unique to keratinizing epithelia and thought to be critical to barrier function. Linoleic acid deficiency has long been known to be associated with the formation of an abnormal barrier with increased water permeability [25]. Oral epithelium was also found to contain one-tenth the level of covalently bound cell-envelope hydroxyceramide as skin, and still retained significant levels of phospholipids, 13% vs. none in skin. Thus, qualitative changes in lipid composition can clearly affect barrier function.

Kinetics of Absorption

In the process commonly referred to as percutaneous absorption, a drug moves sequentially from the surface of the skin through the stratum corneum, viable epidermis, dermis, and finally into the blood stream. Access to the systemic circulation can presumably take place at different levels of the dermis because of its unusual distribution of blood vessels, including the capillary loops in the high portion and superficial and deep plexuses in the mid and deeper portions. Indeed, there is some evidence that drugs can permeate directly into the deeper tissues, such as muscle or joints [26].

Although percutaneous absorption is a multistep process, resistance to penetration through this composite barrier is not equally distributed among all layers. Numerous studies have shown that, for most substances, movement through the stratum corneum is the rate-limiting step [3]. Therefore, the kinetics of drug absorption through the skin can often be understood solely on the basis of an understanding of the kinetics of movement through the stratum corneum.

Finite Dose

Clear differentiation must be made between topical drugs (where the therapeutic effects are intended for the skin immediately under the area of application) and transdermal drugs (where the therapeutic effects are intended for distant organs). Excluding transdermal drugs from further consideration, it is safe to say that most topical drug formulations (and cosmetics) are applied to the skin in very small doses. For creams and ointments the dose is 2–3 mg/cm^2 of formulation containing only microgram amounts of drug, that is, a finite dose [27]. Generally, within minutes of application, excipients volatilize or disappear into the fine wrinkles and crevices of the skin and no evidence of application is visible. Drug is now present in some poorly defined microscopic layer on the surface of the barrier, the stratum corneum. The appropriate solution [28] to the diffusion equation for a finite dose is given in Eqs. (1) to (3).

$$J = 2hpDC_0 \sum_{n=1}^{\infty} \frac{\alpha_n e^{-D\alpha_n^2 t}}{\sin \alpha_n l[l(\alpha_n^2 + h^2) + h]} \tag{1}$$

$$h = \frac{p}{v} \tag{2}$$

$$\alpha_n = \text{roots of } [\alpha l \tan \alpha l] = hl \tag{3}$$

where J = rate of absorption,
D = diffusion coefficient,
C_0 = concentration at $t = 0$,
p = partition coefficient,
v = thickness of applied formulation, and
l = stratum corneum thickness

The rate of absorption (flux) of drug from the film into the living epidermis and subsequently into the systemic circulation follows the pattern depicted in Fig. 9. The process can be divided into three phases, indicated in Fig. 9B by a, b, and c.

1. Lag Phase. Initially, there is a period of time in which no absorption is detected. Drug is moving from surface film into and through the stratum corneum, but none has penetrated the entire thickness of the barrier to allow detection in the systemic circulation (in vivo) or into the dermis or dermal bathing solution (in vitro). In fact, during this period significant movement of drug across the interface is rapidly occurring, as is shown in Fig. 10a with a hypothetical drug of $D = 1 \times 10^{-10}$ cm^2/s and $p = 5$. Within the first 8 min drug content in the surface film has fallen 50%, yet virtually none has reached the deeper layers of skin and the flux is still zero. After 24 min the drug content in the surface film has fallen 75%, yet the flux is just barely measurable.

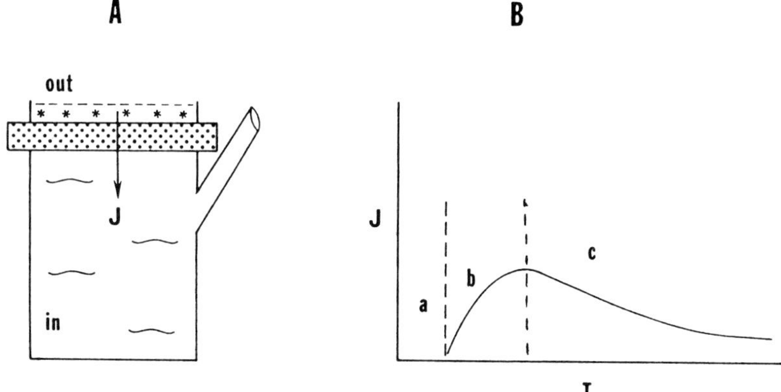

FIG. 9. A. Schematic showing application of a thin film or "finite dose" to skin mounted in vitro in a one-chambered diffusion cell, and B. theoretical flux (J) of drug from thin film into receptor fluid, bathing underside of skin.

The flux profile within the stratum corneum, arbitrarily dividing the barrier into quarters, is shown in Fig. 10b. Peak drug concentration occurs somewhat later and is much lower in the inner than in the outer barrier. Drug concentration in the inner quarter of the barrier is the driving force for the flux into the deeper tissues and, thus its time course will closely match the flux time course.

2. Rising Phase. With increasing time, the initial front of drug penetrates the entire thickness of the barrier and shortly thereafter enters the living epidermis, dermis, and capillaries, thus making the process measurable by standard in vitro or in vivo methods. As the concentration of drug in the barrier layer continues to increase due to continual supply from the surface film, the rate of efflux from this layer into the deeper layers and systemic circulation also increases. This accounts for the rising portion of the absorption curve.

3. Falling Phase. Obviously the movement of drug from surface film to stratum corneum cannot continue indefinitely if the dose is finite. The supply eventually becomes depleted, a process that begins the instant a drug is applied to the skin. Thus, under finite dose conditions, a drug is at its maximum concentration in the surface film at the moment of application and is always decreasing thereafter (Fig. 10a). The falling portion of the curve reflects a decreasing drug concentration in the stratum corneum which, in turn, reflects a decreasing drug concentration on the surface of the skin. Though drug concentration in the surface film is always decreasing subsequent to dosing, the concentration in the stratum corneum initially increases for a period of time (Fig. 10b) supporting the rising phase of the absorption profile, then falls as the rate of influx cannot keep pace with the rate of efflux.

The time course of absorption following application of a finite dose is most strongly affected by the diffusion coefficient and the thickness of the stratum corneum. (Fig. 10c) As D increases, or l decreases, the peak rate of absorption occurs earlier and is higher. A change in barrier thickness has a disproportionately greater effect on the flux profile than D, since l appears in the finite-dose equation as l^2. Thus, a threefold decrease in l has approximately the same effect as a ninefold change in D. This is one reason why animals, which generally have a thinner horny layer than humans, are poor models with respect to percutaneous absorption.

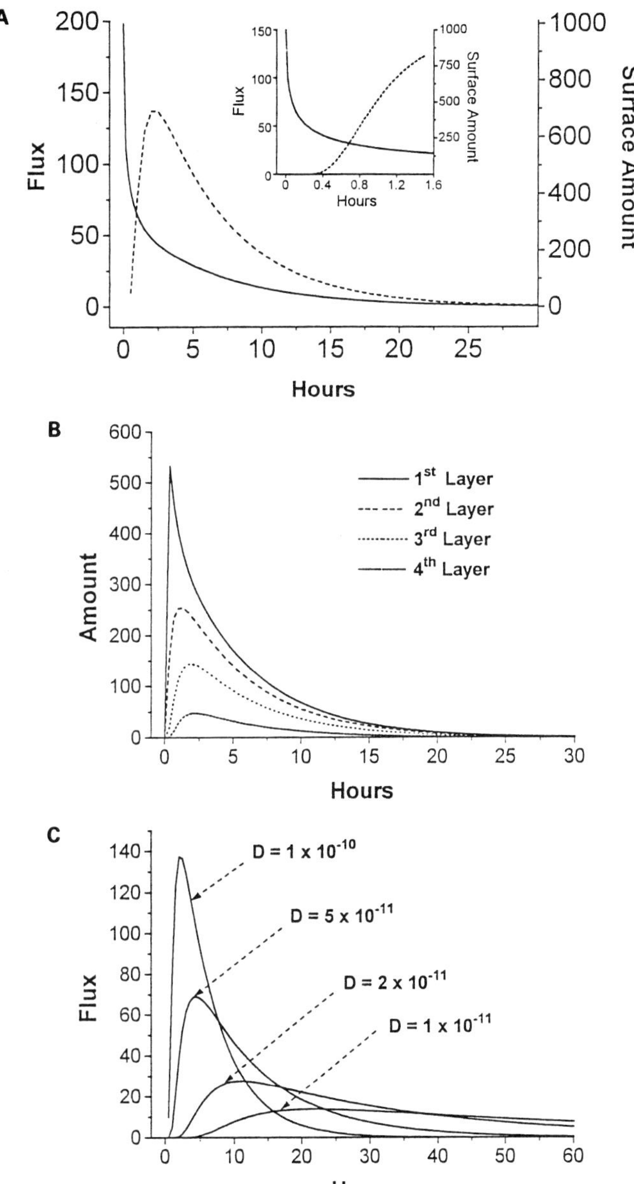

FIG. 10. A. Rate of drug loss from a thin film (solid line) and flux into receptor phase (dashed line) where $D = 1 \times 10^{-10}$ cm^2/s, $p = 5$, $v = 0.001$ cm, $l = 0.002$ cm and the dose is 1000 units; the inset expands the first 1.6 h to show the delay in drug appearance in the receptor. B. Drug distribution in stratum corneum a function of time; the barrier is arbitrarily divided into four quarters and all parameters are same as above. C. Effect of diffusion coefficient D on the flux profile; all other values are the same as above.

Infinite Dose

What has been described thus far characterizes percutaneous absorption as a nonsteady-state phenomenon; the flux rises to a peak and then declines. A constant rate of absorption is never attained. Although this is the situation which most closely mimics the clinical use of topical medications, application of an infinite dose to attain a steady-state rate of absorption is frequently used in the laboratory setting as an investigative tool because of certain advantages it offers, particularly that of simplicity. Indeed, historically, use of an infinite dose has been the dominant approach to the study of membrane permeability and this is true for the field of percutaneous absorption as well. The early studies of skin permeability, underlying most of the current dogma, were all done under steady-state conditions [3].

The major factor that determines the development of steady-state or nonsteady-state kinetics is the amount of drug applied to the skin. In theory, when the amount is small (finite dose), it will be depleted, and the kinetics shown in Fig. 9 hold. However, if the amount applied is so large as to be inexhaustible (infinite dose), a steady-state rate of absorption results (Fig. 11). Thus, the difference between steady-state and nonsteady-state kinetics is more a function of the amount of drug applied than of the drug itself. Drugs of very low permeability are an exception. Even application of a finite dose may lead to a constant absorption rate.

The relationship between the two conditions, finite or infinite dose, is shown in Fig. 12. As the dose of a hypothetical drug is increased by raising its concentration in the

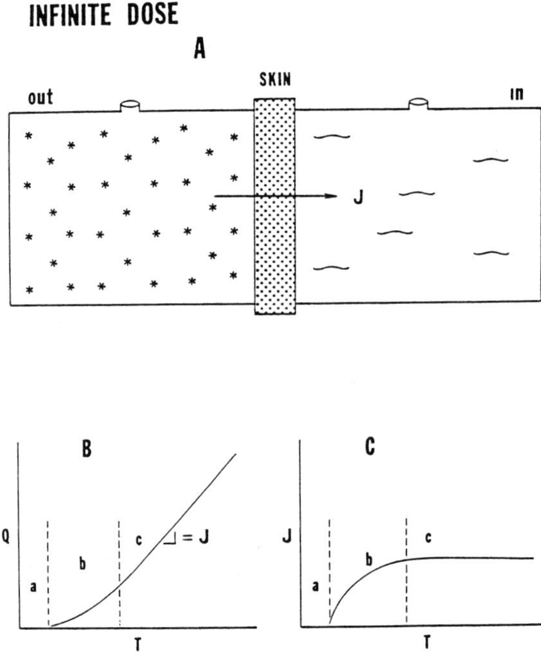

FIG. 11. A. Schematic showing application of "infinite dose" to skin mounted in vitro in side-by-side diffusion cells. Experiment can be run and/or data plotted to determine: B. cumulative amount of drug Q in receptor as function of time, or C. rate of absorption J into receptor as function of time.

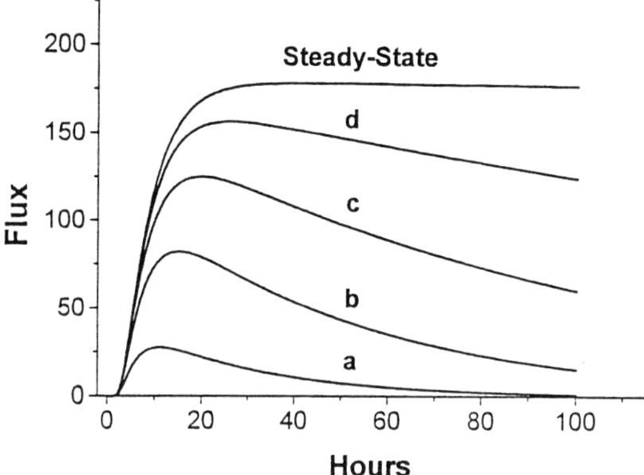

FIG. 12. Theoretical relationship between rate of absorption (flux) and amount of drug applied, i.e., finite vs. infinite dose. As the layer thickness increases, the flux increases (a to d), until the layer becomes large enough (infinite dose) to sustain a steady-state rate of absorption.

formulation or the amount of formulation applied, the rate of absorption also increases. Eventually the amount applied is sufficiently large to sustain a constant rate of absorption over the period of study. Equations (4) to (7), describing the rate of absorption at steady-state, are well known and widely used.

$$\text{Steady-state slope} = \text{Flux } (J) \tag{4}$$

$$J = K_p C \tag{5}$$

$$K_p = \frac{DP}{l} \tag{6}$$

$$T_{lag} = \frac{l^2}{6D} \tag{7}$$

where K_p = the permeability coefficient,
C = the applied concentration,
D = the diffusion coefficient,
P = the partition coefficient,
l = the thickness of the stratum corneum, and
T_{lag} = is the x-axis intercept of the slope

In theory, for simple membranes, it is possible to calculate all the parameters controlling absorption from the type of experiment depicted in Fig. 11 B, where drug is allowed to accumulate in the receptor solution of an in vitro chamber. From J, the steady-state rate of absorption, the permeability coefficient (K_p) can be calculated from Eq. (5). The diffusion coefficient is calculated from the lag time, Eq. (7) and, assuming the thickness of the barrier is known, the partition coefficient can be calculated from Eq. (6).

For a more complete discussion of the kinetics of absorption through skin and other equations which can be used to describe this process, the reader is referred to an earlier article by Flynn [29].

In Vitro Methods of Absorption

Since the rate-limiting barrier to the movement of substances into and through the skin is a layer of mechanically tough, but mitotically ''dead'' cells whose functions no longer require intracellular organelles such as microsomes and mitochondria, it has become common practice to employ in vitro techniques for the study of percutaneous absorption. The barrier properties remain intact for many days under in vitro conditions and the fact that skin can be stored frozen for long periods of time gives this method great flexibility. Another advantage is that of simplicity, in comparison to in vivo experiments. Sampling and analysis of the relatively small, ''clean'' volume of receptor fluid bathing the undersurface of the skin is much easier to deal with from many considerations than the chemically complex blood–urine–fecal specimens provided in vivo. In addition, cost and regulatory considerations greatly favor in vitro experimentation. In the drug development process, the initial screening of many different topical formulations for maximum bioavailability can largely be done in vitro, thus avoiding the need for human volunteers [30,31].

Methodological Considerations

Skin Preparation

Skin sections for in vitro investigation can be prepared in different thicknesses:

1. Full thickness (epidermis and complete dermis), 1–4 mm for human skin
2. Split thickness, in which a portion of the dermis is removed (0.25–0.5 mm)
3. Isolated epidermis (~0.1 mm)
4. Isolated stratum corneum (~0.02 mm)

From a theoretical standpoint, split-thickness or isolated epidermal preparations should be ideal since the distance from skin surface to receptor solution most closely approximates the distance from skin surface to blood stream in vivo. From a practical standpoint, the question is only important when dealing with drugs of low water solubility. Since the dermis offers little resistance to the movement of water-soluble materials, its presence or absence has only a small effect on the rate of absorption of these compounds. Indeed, the original studies, demonstrating agreement between in vitro and in vivo data, used full-thickness skin preparations (and water-soluble compounds) throughout [32].

The situation is quite different with compounds of low water solubility. The dermis, which consist of approximately 70% water, can become the rate-limiting step to absorption of these compounds. Thus, the inclusion of an additional 1–2 mm of dermis, which the compound does not have to permeate in vivo, can introduce a significant error into in vitro data.

Because of the above considerations, the recommendation of the FDA/AAPS Workshop on the Principles and Practices of In Vitro Percutaneous Penetration Studies is that thinly dermatomed (< 0.5 mm) or isolated epidermal preparations be used for in vitro studies [33]. For water-soluble compounds, full-thickness preparations should also prove acceptable. Studies requiring isolated stratum corneum are rare and usually limited to the identification of the contribution of each skin layer to the overall diffusional resistance of a drug, or the contribution of each skin layer to the overall metabolism of a drug in the skin.

Full-thickness skin is the easiest to prepare since it requires only the removal of adherent subcutaneous fat, generally absent in animal skin; this can be done by blunt dissection with a No. 11 scalpel blade. With human skin, the fat layer can be many times the thickness of the skin itself and care must be taken not to contaminate the skin surface with a film of oil from this underlying layer. Placing the skin face down on a moistened paper towel while shaving the fat with a motion parallel to the skin surface is generally adequate to prevent surface contamination. When necessary, at the end of the procedure, the surface can be washed with warm water to remove blood and fat, and blotted several times with absorbent paper towels or tissues. The surface should never be washed with soap and water as the surfactants may affect barrier properties.

Split-thickness skin is prepared with the help of a dermatome (e.g., the Padgett Electrodermatome, Padgett Instruments, Kansas City) [34]. This technique can be used with hairless or haired skin, as well as fresh skin without impairment of viability. The skin to be dermatomed should be pinned, epidermis down, on the surface of a styrofoam block. Styrofoam is ideal because it can be cut to any size and easily accepts pins. The width of the styrofoam block should be smaller than that of the dermatome blade, and the skin should overlap the block in such a way that when stretched taut and pinned (on the side rather than the top) the pins do not obstruct the movement of dermatome. Prior to cutting, it is helpful to stretch the skin lengthwise to prevent wrinkling or bunching up in front of the advancing blade. The depth of the cut is controlled by a lever on the dermatome, and current recommendations are that skin less than 0.5 mm be used for in vitro studies. Actual thickness can be checked with a micrometer (Mitutoyo micrometer, L. A. Benson, Inc., Baltimore).

Pure epidermal membranes can be prepared by heat separation [15]. Full-thickness skin is placed in water at 60°C and held there for 1–2 min or, between aluminum blocks which had been preheated to 60°C. The skin is placed epidermal side up on a block, where it can be stretched and pinned, and the epidermis is peeled off the dermis with forceps. It helps to scratch the skin surface initially with one edge of the forceps or with a scalpel blade, to lift an edge of epidermis to grasp. The length of time the skin is heated greatly affects the ease of separation, that is, 2 min give better results than 1 min, although this varies considerably from donor to donor.

Intact sheets of epidermis cannot be prepared from haired animal skins. Since the hair follicles are embedded deeply in the dermis, holes are created as the epidermis is pulled over hairs which remain attached at their roots. Likewise, this procedure may not be suitable for metabolic studies as the viability of the skin may be affected.

Intact stratum corneum can be prepared by two methods [15]. In a two-step procedure isolated epidermis is prepared by heat separation, as above, and treated with a proteolytic enzyme such as trypsin to disrupt the integrity of the living cells and facilitate their removal from the underside of the stratum corneum with a moistened cotton-tipped applicator. Alternatively, isolated stratum corneum can be prepared directly from human subjects using the blistering agent cantharidin. It causes the skin to split at the mid-epidermis, leaving a blister top which is almost pure stratum corneum. The remnants of the living epidermis, still adherent to the underside of the barrier layer, can be easily rubbed off with a moistened cotton-tipped applicator without prior enzymatic treatment.

Skin Storage and Validation

If specimens of valuable human skin obtained at autopsy or from surgical procedures cannot immediately be used, storage at −20°C or lower in impermeable plastic material generally preserves barrier function for many months. Storage at refrigerator temperature for up to 48 h also appears to be without deleterious effect on barrier integrity. When stored frozen, some workers have found no appreciable change in barrier properties for up to one year [32,35]. This subject is not without controversy, however, and some method to validate barrier integrity should always be used no matter what the method of storage or length of time.

Tritiated water (^3H_2O) has been recommended as a means by which to check the integrity as well as the normalcy of any skin preparation. Several methods are available, and it is apparent that the variability inherent in absorption studies can be greatly reduced by first screening each skin section with ^3H_2O [36,37]. This allows skin sections to be discarded which, though perfectly normal in appearance, clearly have microscopic holes. This also limits what is acceptable for any given experimental objective, and serves as a means by which data can be compared.

Since freezing and thawing leads to the disruption of the metabolically active cells in the skin, viability is not preserved by ordinary freezing. Therefore, this type of preparation should not be used for metabolic studies. Likewise, animal skin seems much more susceptible to damage following freezing and reduction in barrier function has been reported [35]. Thus, again, validation of skin integrity is imperative.

Cell Design

Many different types of diffusion cells are available to suit all possible needs. They fall into two categories: one-chambered, vertical cells, depicted schematically in Fig. 9, and two-chambered, horizontal (side-by-side) cells, depicted schematically in Fig. 11. The latter are used for traditional steady-state, infinite-dose experiments and were favored by early investigators in the field who came from a physical-chemical background. Today, this cell is commonly used in studies of absorption mechanism and transdermal drug delivery.

The one-chambered cell is of more recent origin. It was developed specifically for the study of drug permeation under clinical conditions. Topical medications, both drugs and cosmetics, are applied in the same small amounts (finite dose) generally used by patients and consumers. The outer surface of the skin is not enclosed but is exposed to normal ambient conditions just as it is in vivo. The prime purpose of this type of cell, as originally designed, was to duplicate the physical conditions found in vivo and maintain the two most important physical factors controlling absorption under physiological conditions [32]. Thus, both the temperature and relative humidity gradients that normally exist across the skin are maintained by this design.

This type of chamber can also be used for studies of transdermal delivery, since any type of formulation can be applied to the outer surface, even a patch. It also accepts application of an infinite dose since the outer half-cell (chimney) can be sufficiently tall to hold large volumes of material. (The term one-chambered cell is slightly misleading since what is actually meant is that the top chamber has been left open to the atmosphere.) In fact, the top half-cell can be modified to allow for the trapping of volatile materials in the formulation. In the design of mosquito repellents, for example, pharmacologic activity is dependent upon the volatility of the drug substance. In this unique situation, the rate and extent of volatilization of the active moiety becomes the true measure of "bioavailability," not the rate and extent of absorption [38].

A useful variant of the one-chambered design is the flow-through cell which allows for automated sample collection [39]. In this design, receptor fluid is continually pumped from a reservoir into the receptor chamber beneath the skin, the volume of this chamber being quite small to allow for an adequate turnover rate, and then into a collection device such as a commercial fraction collector. Since the old receptor fluid is continually being diluted by fresh receptor fluid, the kinetics of the absorption are different from those obtained in a "static" (noncirculating cell) and dependent upon the pumping rate. However, it is possible to mathematically adjust for this artifact and calculate the true rate of absorption [40].

A good review of the many types of cells available for skin absorption studies is given in Ref. 41.

In Vitro–In Vivo Comparison

Though the ultimate goal of most studies of percutaneous absorption relates to humans, such in vivo studies are not always possible or desirable. In numerous situations human experimentation would be too costly and time-consuming or unwise for ethical reasons. Certainly some compounds are too toxic for application to humans. For these reasons as well as for simplicity, in vitro methods are preferred. A critical question, then, is how relevant are in vitro data. Are they a true and accurate reflection, both qualitatively and quantitatively, of percutaneous absorption as it occurs in humans?

Although comparative studies of in vitro and in vivo absorption through human skin are limited, the existing data strongly support the relevance of in vitro data. In a study of the permeation of 12 organic compounds from an acetone vehicle [32,42], excellent agreement between the two methods was found both with respect to total absorption (Table 3) and the rate of absorption. This is most easily seen with compounds that are rapidly excreted from the body, for example, benzoic acid and hippuric acid, where the similarity between the in vivo rate of excretion profile and the in vitro rate of absorption profile is striking (Fig. 13).

TABLE 3 In Vitro and In Vivo Human Absorption Data[a]

	Percent of Dose Absorbed	
Compound	In Vivo	In Vitro
Hippuric acid	1.0	1.3
Chloramphenicol	2.0	2.9
Nicotinic acid	2.1	2.3
Thiourea	3.7	4.6
Phenol	4.4	10.9
Urea	6.0	11.1
Nicotinamide	11.1	28.8
Acetylsalicylic acid	21.8	40.5
Caffeine	22.1	24.1
Salicylic acid	22.8	12.0
Benzoic acid	42.6	44.9
Dinitrochlorobenzene	53.1	27.5

[a]Data from Refs. 32 and 42.

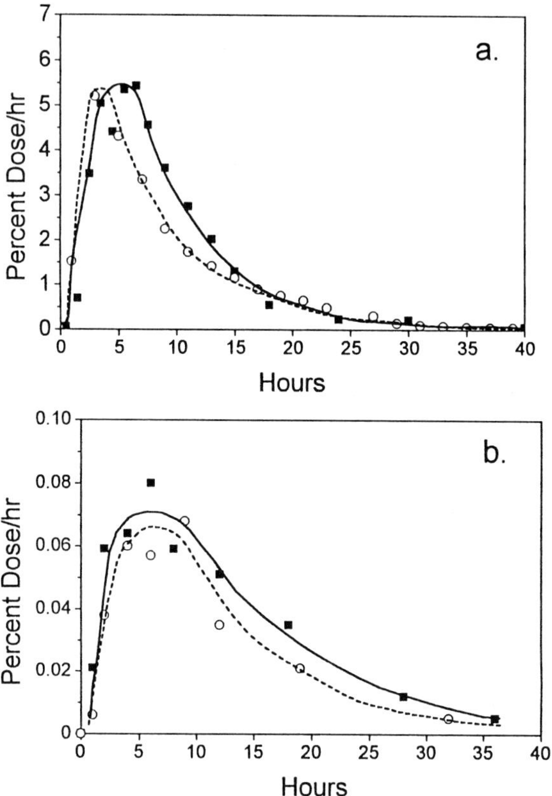

FIG. 13. Correlation between in vitro rate of absorption through cadaver skin (open circles) and in vivo rate of excretion (solid squares) in human subjects for: a. benzoic acid applied in petrolatum, and b. hippuric acid applied in acetone. Both rates expressed as percent dose/h.

In a similar comparative study in which the absorption of caffeine and testosterone from three different vehicles was measured [43], good agreement between the in vitro and in vivo data was found (Table 4). In these and the two studies mentioned before [32,42], great care was taken to ensure that the experimental conditions were as identical as possible. The major parameters that must be considered are temperature, relative humidity, region of application, length of application (time of wash-off), formulation dose, and drug dose. Studies with animal skin have also tended to show good agreement between in vitro and in vivo data [44].

Animal Models

The problem of identifying an animal model whose skin has barrier properties similar to those of humans has been addressed by many investigators for more than 30 years. A conclusion reached by most is that human skin is unique and that there is no universally acceptable animal model. Indeed, the recommendation of the FDA/AAPS Workshop on the Principles and Practices of In Vitro Percutaneous Penetration Studies is that human

TABLE 4 In Vitro and In Vivo Human Absorption Data from Different Vehicles[a]

Compound and Vehicle	Percent of Dose Absorbed	
	In Vivo	In Vitro
Caffeine		
Petrolatum	40.6	40.6
Ethylene glycol gel	55.6	32.3
Water gel	4.0	5.1
Testosterone		
Petrolatum	49.5	39.4
Ethylene glycol gel	36.3	23.7
Water gel	49.2	41.4

[a]Data from Ref. 43.

skin is to be preferred for in vitro studies but, realizing its limited availability, does not discourage the use of animal skin in product development work [33].

Recent work suggests that the barrier properties of pig skin most closely resemble those of human skin. Reifenrath [45] studied the percutaneous absorption of nine compounds in female weanling Yorkshire pigs in vivo and compared the results to published human data (Table 5). Agreement was reasonably good and much better than generally seen with other animal skin. Other in vitro comparisons between pig and human skin gave similar results [46,47].

Many other animal models have been investigated. The conflicting nature of the data obtained is somewhat puzzling. For some compounds good agreement between animal model and human skin can be obtained, yet for other compounds the same animal model fails to duplicate the human data. Clearly, the animal models are unreliable. As a generalization, it is safe to say that rabbit and rodent skins tend to have barrier properties most dissimilar to those of human skin [44]. Rabbit skin, in particular, often gives results an order of magnitude greater than that of human skin. Hairless mouse skin, another popular model for which extensive data can be found in the literature, has likewise been shown to be a poor model [48]. More recent animal models, such as the hairless guinea pig, may prove useful but current data are insufficient to draw a conclusion.

TABLE 5 In Vivo, Absorption Data Pig and Human[a]

Compound	Percent of Dose Absorbed	
	Pig	Human
Fluocinolone acetonide	5.9	1.3
Malathion	4.5	8.2
Lindane	8.4	9.3
Parathion	19.2	9.7
Progesterone	9.4	10.8
Testosterone	5.9	13.2
Diethyltoluamide	9.4	16.7
Benzoic Acid	29.3	42.6
Caffeine	23.3	47.6

[a]Data from Ref. 45.

In Vivo Methods of Absorption

Most studies of percutaneous absorption use animal or in vitro models. However, as extrapolation of results to humans and clinical situations is often the goal, some questions are best addressed by human in vivo experimentation. Though the latitude of human experimental design is often restricted, these limitations are seldom crucial and are more than balanced by data which are eminently relevant and not subject to extrapolation error. In fact, when combined with suitably designed in vitro or animal experiments, data from limited but well targeted human in vivo studies may not only confirm the other studies but also lead to a more comprehensive understanding of the drug or issue in question.

Historical Perspective

The systematic investigation of the permeability of human skin did not begin until the 1950s and was largely the result of radioactive tracers becoming available for medical use. The first human study of percutaneous absorption which successfully demonstrated that the skin was permeable to topically applied drugs was conducted by Malkinson and Ferguson [49]. Using ^{14}C-hydrocortisone incorporated at 2.5% in an ointment base, they showed that topical application of a finite dose to the forearms of two subjects results in the appearance of radioactivity in the urine over the entire collection period of six days. Total urinary excretion of hydrocortisone was estimated to be less than 1% of the applied dose, and the peak rate of urinary excretion of radioactivity occurred during the second day. Other studies from the same laboratory demonstrated limited percutaneous absorption of other steroid compounds such as cortisone acetate, triamcinolone acetonide, and testosterone [50,51].

These workers also tried to quantify percutaneous absorption by simply measuring loss of radioactivity from the surface of the skin, the "disappearance" technique. By holding a thin end-window, gas-flow beta detector over the skin surface to monitor the count rate, absorption could be continuously monitored. However, sensitivity was not sufficient to detect the small changes normally seen with slowly absorbed compounds such as corticosteroids, for example, from 100 to 99% of initial count rate. Across skin whose barrier had been removed by tape stripping, however, absorption was easily measured by the disappearance technique.

A number of conclusions could be drawn from the early human in vivo studies. It was evident that the use of radioisotopes made the detection of low levels of absorption possible. However, the technique employed is of critical importance. Compounds having a slow rate of absorption (corticosteroids such as hydrocortisone and triamcinolone acetonide) cannot be measured with the disappearance technique which lacks the necessary sensitivity. Presumably, for compounds displaying a very rapid rate of absorption, or in situations where absorption through damaged skin is being studied, this technique might prove adequate. It has the advantage of great simplicity, since it does not require the quantitative collection of urine or feces, nor is there need for the processing and analysis of numerous specimens.

However, a major disadvantage is that it equates disappearance with absorption. There are numerous situations where this assumption is invalid. Obviously, compounds that exhibit any degree of volatility could never be accurately measured with this technique. Likewise, loss of topically applied materials to the environment can occur through the normal physiological process of exfoliation, whereby the outer cells of the stratum corneum are shed as new cells form at the inner surface. Thus, even if the site of application is protected to prevent wash-off or rub-off, the continuous microscopic shedding of corneocytes results in loss of surface material which could erroneously be perceived as "absorption." This becomes an even greater problem in diseases with increased epidermal turnover such as psoriasis. Overall, the disappearance technique is potentially subject to many errors and, therefore, its general utility greatly limited. In special situations, however, it can be a useful technique.

The successful application of urinary excretion by Malkinson as a means by which to quantify topical drug absorption in living humans set the stage for subsequent investigators and, to this day, remains the standard method for the assessment of percutaneous absorption.

Urinary Excretion Method

Studies of percutaneous absorption in humans are still relatively limited, but the most detailed, systematic investigations have been those of Feldmann and Maibach [52–55]. Like in the earlier investigations, many of the compounds studied were corticosteroids, and the basic protocol involved application to the skin of compounds labeled with a radioisotope and the measurement of urinary excretion of radioactivity. Many modifications of the basic technique have subsequently been made by others to better suit the compound, formulation, or conditions of application (or exposure in the case of toxicants), but the basic elements of the protocol have remained the same and are presented in detail below.

In the Feldmann and Maibach protocol, the compound of interest was dissolved in acetone and applied to a defined area on the volar forearm at a dose of 4 $\mu g/cm^2$. This dose was chosen because it approximates the very small doses of corticosteroids received by patients in a clinical setting. The size of the application site varied from compound to compound and was determined by the interplay of three factors:

1. the specific activity of the compound under study (μCi/mg),
2. the radioactive dose (total amount of μCi to be applied), and
3. the drug dose (4 $\mu g/cm^2$).

Compounds having a low specific activity required larger areas of application in order to achieve the desired radioactive dose, yet not exceed the target drug dose. On the other hand, compounds of very high specific activity required dilution with cold drug if the 4 $\mu g/cm^2$ dose was to be maintained without exceeding the desired or safe radioactive dose.

Following application of the compound under study in an acetone vehicle, the acetone was gently blown dry and did not remain on the skin for more than 15 s. This brief exposure to a lipid solvent such as acetone was not regarded to be damaging to the lipid barrier of the skin. The application site was then left unprotected, and the subjects were instructed not to bathe for 24 h. All urinary output was collected over the next 5 to 10 days and analyzed for radioactive content. In order to correct for radioactivity excreted via other routes, an intravenous (iv) dose of the same compound was given. Determination of the fraction of an iv dose excreted in the urine allows for the calculation of total absorption following a topical dose, according to the following equation.

$$\text{Total absorption} = \frac{\text{total urinary excretion (topical dose)}}{\text{fractional urinary excretion (iv dose)}}$$

Thus, this technique is based on the assumption that the relationship between the routes of excretion following an intravenous dose is the same as when the drug enters the systemic circulation through the skin. If 75% of drug molecules entering the systemic circulation via an intravenous dose are excreted in the urine, then 75% of drug molecules entering the systemic circulation percutaneously are assumed to be excreted in the urine.

Although the literature contains no critical evaluation of this assumption, one situation of potential concern can be envisioned. When the compound of interest is directly injected into the circulation, it is the unmetabolized parent compound which is injected. When the same compound is applied to the skin, it cannot be assumed that it is only the unmetabolized species that enter the bloodstream. The skin is known to have significant metabolic activity and there are a number of studies which have demonstrated simultaneous metabolism and absorption of topically applied drugs [56,57]. Thus, one critical assumption underlying the use of the urinary excretion method needs further study. An alternative, of course, would be the measurement of both urinary and fecal excretion of radioactivity and this will be discussed subsequently.

Proper use of the urinary excretion method, or modifications thereof, requires that consideration be given to a number of specific details. Among these are site of application, the size of the dose, application time, collection time, and fecal collection. Since all of these factors can significantly affect the results, lack of adequate consideration can lead to results which are either erroneous or not directly applicable to the clinical or use situation.

Site of Application

Since it is well established that there are regional differences in percutaneous absorption, the site chosen for the application of the test medication should reflect its intended site of use [53,58]. This is particularly true for products intended for the face or scalp where absorption is generally much higher than elsewhere on the body, often five- to tenfold higher. Intertriginous areas (axillae, groin) also deserve special consideration since the increased hydration of the skin at those sites results in significantly increased absorption. A specialized area of skin that has invariably been found to be of unusually high permeability is the scrotum [59]. It appears to be the most permeable of all integumentary sites. Generally, differences in absorption observed over the rest of the body (trunk and extremities) are not as great as those of the previously mentioned sites, with the exception of the palms and soles which tend to show somewhat lower rates of absorption.

The forearm is the most popular site of application because it is the most convenient site for both subject and investigator. It is also convenient for the design and construction of relatively simple devices to protect the applied material from rub-off. This is an important consideration from the standpoint of both experimental design and control and, if radioisotopes are being used, from the standpoint of radiation containment and safety. Inexpensive devices can be made from materials obtained at a hardware store. For example, a forearm device can be constructed from heavy aluminum screen (0.63 × 1.27 cm grid), a dense soft rubber floor mat (2.5 cm thick), and Velcro closure strips. The

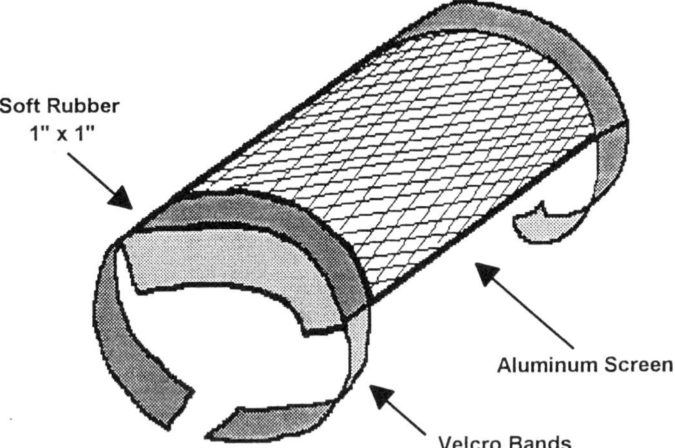

FIG. 14. A simple device, easily constructed, to protect a topical application to the forearm.

materials are cut to the desired dimension and assembled with cyanoacrylate adhesive (Fig. 14).

The forearm as the site of application, aside from the relevance issue, has the disadvantage of a relatively small available surface area. When a larger area is required, for example, because of radiation dosimetry considerations or the need to apply large amounts of drug for the determination of blood levels, the trunk is the next logical choice.

Repeated Applications

Since most topical preparations involve multiple applications to the same site, it may be of importance to determine if repeated applications result in changes in the absorption profile. This is especially critical when there is reason to believe that chronic use may lead to barrier alteration or damage.

Several human studies have been conducted with labeled drugs in which percutaneous absorption has been measured first through previously untreated skin and, approximately one week later, through skin that has received daily treatments with an unlabeled version of the same formulation [60,61]. No evidence of a significant change in absorption was noted after one week of continuous treatment (Table 6). Since the limited number of compounds examined to date does not allow extrapolation with confidence to other compounds, this procedure should be routine for most topical medications.

TABLE 6 Effect of Repeated Applications on Percutaneous Absorption[a]

	Percent of Dose Absorbed			
Doses[b]	Minoxidil	Hydrocortisone	Testosterone	Estradiol
1	3.9 ± 2.9	2.6 ± 0.7	22.1 ± 6.9	9.9 ± 2.3
2	2.4 ± 1.0	3.4 ± 1.4	20.2 ± 6.8	10.8 ± 4.7

[a]Data from Refs. 60 and 61.
[b]Administered one week apart.

Drug and Formulation Dose

Since percutaneous absorption is known to obey Fick's law, careful consideration must be given to the drug concentration in the dosing formulation. For the data to be meaningful, drug concentration should approximate the use condition. In the case of commercial or development formulations, the concentration is usually fixed and not subject to experimental variation. However, what may be overlooked is the equally important issue of formulation dose. Though the concentration of the test drug is fixed (e.g., 1%), total drug dose to the skin ($\mu g/cm^2$) is a function of the amount of formulation applied (Fig. 12). Relevant data can only be obtained when the formulation dose approximates use conditions. For creams and ointments, it has been observed that patients and consumers generally apply 2-3 mg of product per cm^2 of skin [27].

However, the tendency in protocol design is often to apply much larger amounts of formulation since ease and accuracy are better in the application of larger doses, and the analytical task is made easier. The fallacy in this approach is, however, that both the rate of absorption and total absorption are a function of the size of the applied dose under finite dose conditions. Thus, inappropriately large formulation doses can lead to a significant overestimation of total systemic absorption, as well as of maximum flux rate and peak blood level.

Application Time

It is advisable to apply the test formulation for a specific period of time and then remove it. The length of time may be dictated by radiation dosimetry considerations but, even if not, it is generally relevant to experimental objectives. Most topically applied compounds are poorly absorbed through the skin. The source of the flux, even after many hours, continues to be drug remaining on the surface of the skin and not that below the surface (Fig. 15). Thus, physical removal of the surface source (e.g., by washing) results in a rapid decline of the flux.

When trying to duplicate clinical or use conditions, the length of time the product would normally remain on the skin should be considered. For many products, removal may be linked to the daily bathing routine, and 24 h is a reasonable application time. For others, such as facial products applied at night (e.g., retinoic acid), removal at 8–12 h seems more appropriate, since this would approximate the timing of a morning face wash. Drugs to which the skin is exposed via shampoo or a bath would obviously have even shorter contact times.

Collection Time

Urinary collections should be continued until background levels of radioactivity are reached. Although this is commonly within 5 to 6 days, longer times may be necessary for some compounds (those with long turnover times). Failure to appreciate this factor can result in significant experimental error; two examples from the literature illustrate this point.

Total absorption of nicotinic acid and thiourea following application from an acetone vehicle were originally determined to be 0.3 and 0.9% of the applied dose, respectively [55]. These data were based on a five-day collection period. Subsequent experiments found that measurable levels of radioactivity could be found in the urine for at least 21

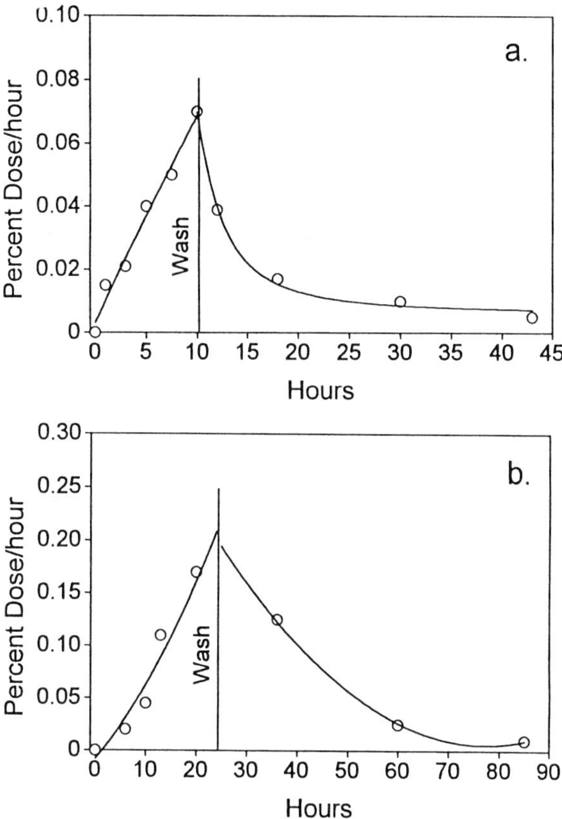

FIG. 15. The effect of a skin surface wash with soap and water on the rate of urinary excretion of topically applied drugs: a. wash of face 10 h following a single application of 0.05% retinoic acid cream [69], and b. wash of trunk 24 h following two applications (q 12 h) of sulconazole nitrate cream [68].

days, and the total absorption was, in fact, fourfold higher for thiourea and tenfold higher for nicotinic acid [42]. (A portion of the error in the original estimate of nicotinic acid absorption was also due to an erroneous intravenous correction factor.)

Compounds for which the rate of excretion continues at low levels for long periods of time must be dosed with sufficiently high levels of radioactivity to make long collection times feasible; this may require a large area of application. This type of situation can be often anticipated from animal studies or if the drug has been administered intravenously in humans prior to topical administration. Increasing the application area allows an increased total radioactive dose while at the same time maintaining any desired drug dose ($\mu g/cm^2$) or formulation dose (mg/cm^2).

Another important issue related to collection time is the collection frequency, particularly during the early phase of the experiment. Accurate determination of the absorption kinetics of rapidly absorbed compounds is possible only if urine specimens are collected frequently at early times (Fig. 13); 1-h collection intervals are recommended for at least the first 4 to 6 h. This can be accomplished by having the subjects drink 150-300 mL (5–10 fl. oz) of water prior to drug application and every 2 h thereafter. By pushing fluids it is generally possible for volunteers to void by the clock at hourly intervals.

Fecal Collection

Simultaneous collection of feces should be incorporated into the protocol when this represents a significant route of excretion for the compound under study. This will be known from animal studies or a prior human intravenous study. Although fecal collection is also important from the standpoint of mass balance, in practice fecal data are often of little consequence to the overall pharmacokinetic profile of a drug following topical application. For drugs that are poorly absorbed through the skin and minimally excreted in the feces, given the infrequency of stool samples and the greater error associated with fecal (as opposed to urine) analysis, collection of these data may be unnecessary.

Fecal collection is absolutely essential in cases where this route represents the main path of excretion and only limited amounts of drug are excreted in the urine. When the yield via the urinary route is very low, the iv correction factor can become quite large and subject to high variability. This has the potential to introduce significant error into the calculation of total absorption, if urinary excretion data are the only basis of calculation. DDT is a compound that illustrates the problem. In the monkey, Bartek and LaBudde [62] found that only 0.4% of an iv dose was excreted in the urine, giving a correction factor for topical application of 250 (100/0.4). Use of this factor to estimate total absorption of DDT in the rhesus monkey following topical application led to the absurd value of 375% of the applied dose. Thus, the larger the iv correction factor, the greater the error introduced into the calculation of total absorption when using only urinary excretion data.

Blood Collection

Although the determination of blood levels is an essential component of studies involving other routes of administration, its utility in topical drug studies is problematic because of the combination of low total absorption and low absorption rates. Blood levels are usually extremely low following topical application, in fact, often below detectable limits. For this very reason the use of radio-labeled drugs and urinary measurement of radioactivity has become the method of choice.

Highly sensitive assay methods are generally needed for the identification of plasma levels of topically applied materials. A case in point is that of topically applied retinoids. Isotretinoin 0.05% gel (13-cis retinoic acid, Isotrex) was applied twice daily for four weeks at an excessive dose to 1900 cm^2 of skin in order to determine steady-state blood level [63]. However, at no time during the study were detectable levels found in any of the volunteers using a high-pressure liquid chromatographic (HPLC) assay sensitive to 20 ng/mL. The same was found to be true for the all-trans isomer of retinoic acid (tretinoin, Retin-A) in a similar, but not identical, subchronic dosing study [64]. Subsequently, it was found with radioactive all-trans retinoic acid that the maximum blood level (assuming all radioactivity in the parent drug) was less than 0.1 ng/mL [65]. These results are in contrast with those of oral studies of isotretinoin (Accutane) absorption in which steady-state blood levels of 160 ng/mL and a peak level over 400 ng/mL were measured (*Physicians Desk Reference*, Medical Economics, Oradell, NJ, 1993).

As more sensitive analytical methods are developed, measurement of blood levels of topically applied drugs may become possible. For example, the technique of radioimmunoassay (RIA) was sensitive enough for the detection of plasma levels of the corticosteroid betamethasone 17-benzoate (0.3–5 ng/mL), following its application under occlusion (plastic wrap) for seven days to patients with eczema and psoriasis [66].

Mass Balance Method

A recently introduced modification of the urinary excretion method is the mass balance technique, which has the advantage that it accounts for all the topically applied material [67]. This method is based on the same principles as the original Feldmann and Maibach protocol. Radioactive compounds at a dose of 4 $\mu g/cm^2$ are applied to the forearm of human volunteers. Percutaneous absorption is assessed from the excretion of radioactivity in urine corrected for excretion via other routes. The application site is covered with a semirigid polypropylene chamber (Hilltop Research, Inc., Cincinnati, OH) which is taped to the skin. Absorption can be measured under occluded or nonoccluded conditions by employing the chamber in either closed or vented status, respectively. To vent the chamber, holes are drilled in such a way that approximately 50% of the surface area is open to the atmosphere. To prevent drug loss from the surface through exfoliation, the holes are covered with a 0.2-μm pore size Gore-Tex membrane (W. L. Gore and Associates, Inc., Elkton, MD). This material does not retard transepidermal water loss and therefore does not increase hydration of the stratum corneum, which would increase the absorption rate.

The chamber is removed and analyzed for trapped radioactivity 24 h after application, and the site is washed by a standard washing procedure. All wash material is analyzed for radioactive content. The application site is covered with a new chamber which remains in place for six days. At the end of this period, the chamber is removed and analyzed for radioactive content and washed again. Following the wash, the application site itself is stripped ten times with adhesive tape (Scotch Brand Tape, 3M, St. Paul) and the tape is analyzed for radioactive content.

This new method allows accounting for the single biggest source of loss following topical application, that which is lost from the surface of the skin due to exfoliation, rub-off, and wash-off. In addition, tape stripping the stratum corneum at the end of the experiment recovers any test compound remaining (possibly bound) within the barrier. In principle, it should be possible to account for all of the applied radioactivity material and thus avoid one of the questions that always accompanies the estimation of topical percutaneous absorption: Where is all of the unrecovered material?

The validity of this new method, designed to obtain a true mass balance, can be seen from the results in Table 7 on four steroid compounds [67]. For comparison, data obtained in human subjects on three other drugs using the standard urinary excretion method are shown [60,68,69]. Total recovery of the four steroid compounds using the mass balance technique with vented (nonoccluded) chambers ranged from 89 to 100% of

TABLE 7 Total Recovery with Mass Balance and Standard Urinary Excretion Methods[a]

Method and Compound	Total Absorption (%)	Total Recovery (%)
Urinary Excretion		
Minoxidil	3.9	47
Sulconazole	6.7	43
Retinoic acid	1.1	51
Mass Balance		
Hydrocortisone	4.4	89
Estradiol	3.4	100
Progesterone	13	96
Testosterone	18	96

[a]Data from Refs. 60 and 67–69.

TABLE 8 Disposition of Topically Applied Steroids[a]

Compound	Chamber (%)	Wash (%)	Strip (%)	Absorbed (%)	Total (%)
Hydrocortisone	30	54	2.5	4.4	89
Estradiol	39	58	0.1	3.4	100
Progesterone	55	27	n.d.	13	96
Testosterone	47	30	n.d.	18	96

[a]Data from Ref. 67.

the dose, with three of the four compounds showing recovery of 96% or more. In contrast, total recovery of three commonly used topical drugs using the standard urinary excretion method was only 51% or less. That material lost from the surface of the skin does indeed represent a significant portion of the total applied dose is shown in Table 8. Of the four steroid compounds shown in Table 7, the amount that was trapped in the chamber accounts for 30–55% of the recoverable radioactivity.

Stratum Corneum Stripping Method

Techniques other than those related to urinary excretion can be used to measure percutaneous absorption in vivo. The disappearance technique with all its limitations, mentioned earlier, is one example. Another technique, introduced by Rougier's laboratory, utilizes a unique approach [70], where the total absorption is quantified by measuring the stratum corneum uptake. Total absorption can be accurately estimated by stripping and analyzing the stratum corneum for drug content 30 min following application of the test drug. They have furthermore shown that the accuracy of the technique is independent of factors known to influence percutaneous absorption. Such complications as variation in dose, vehicle, application time, or anatomical site do not invalidate the method. It has also been shown to be valid in animals as well as humans.

The basis for the technique is quite simple and follows logically from the known properties of the stratum corneum barrier. The stratum corneum is unique among biological barriers in that its dimensions are of the order of micrometers not nanometers. The fact that it is a thick barrier with low internal diffusivity results in permeating species being contained within the interstices for a substantial period of time. Thus, the application of a test compound to the skin is followed by a period of time during which the fraction that has partitioned into the stratum corneum is totally contained within. If the stratum corneum is quantitatively removed before significant diffusional loss to the lower layers occurs, total absorption can be measured. However, this method does not yield data pertinent to the absorption rate, such as the time to maximum rate or steady-state, or the magnitude of either of those parameters.

An example of the relationship between stratum corneum content and total absorption is shown in Fig. 16. An almost perfect correlation is observed between absorption of the four compounds (benzoic acid, benzoic acid sodium salt, caffeine, and acetylsalicylic acid) at various sites in human subjects, measured by the traditional urinary excretion method, and their stratum corneum content 30 min after application.

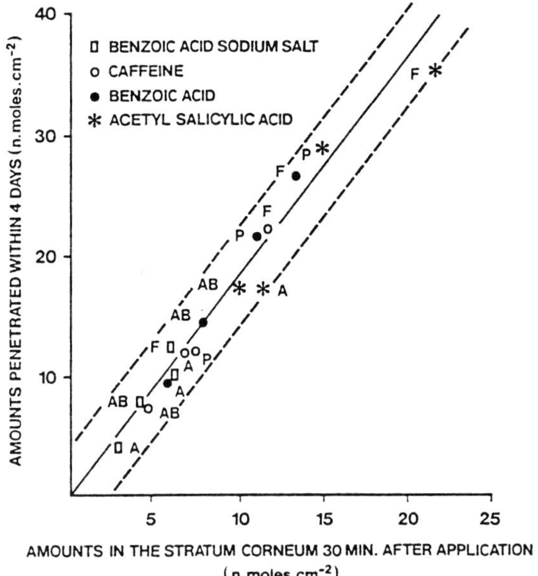

FIG. 16. Correlation of total absorption, based on urinary excretion at 4 days, and stratum corneum content at 30 min. A good linear relationship exists which is independent of the compound studied or anatomical site. Key: □ = benzoic acid sodium salt; ○ = caffeine; ● = benzoic acid; * = acetyl salicylic acid; $y = 1.83 \times - 0.52$; $r = 0.97$, $p<0.001$; A = arm (upper, outer); AB = abdomen; P = postauricular; F = forehead. (Reprinted from Ref. 70 with permission).

References

1. Franz, T. J., Tojo, K., Shah, K. R., and Kydonieus, A., Transdermal Delivery. In: *Treatise on Controlled Drug Delivery* (A. Kydonieus, ed.), Marcel Dekker, Inc., New York, 1991, pp. 341–421.
2. Winsor, T., and Burch, G. E., *Arch. Int. Med.*, 74:428–436 (1944).
3. Scheuplein, R. J., and Blank, I. H., *Physiol. Rev.*, 51:702–747 (1971).
4. Elias, P. M., *J. Invest. Dermatol.*, 80:44s–49s (1983).
5. Rushmer, R. F., Buettner, K. J., Short, J. M., and Odland, G. F., *Science*, 154:343–348 (1966).
6. Squier, C. A., *J. Ultrastruc. Res.*, 43:160–177 (1973).
7. Elias, P. M., McNutt, N. S., and Friend, D. S., *Anat. Rec.*, 189:577–594 (1977).
8. Holbrook, K. A., and Odland, G. F., *J. Invest. Dermatol.*, 62:415–422 (1974).
9. Scheuplein, R. J., and Morgan, L., *Nature*, 214:456–458 (1969).
10. Rice, R. H., and Green, H., *Cell*, 11:417–422 (1977).
11. Banks-Schlegel, S., and Green, H., *J. Cell Biol.*, 90:732–737 (1981).
12. Swartzendruber, D. C., Wertz, P. W., Madison, K. C., and Downing, D. T., *J. Invest. Dermatol.*, 88:709–713 (1987).
13. Wertz, P. W., Madison, K. C., and Downing, D. T., *J. Invest. Dermatol.*, 92:109–111 (1989).
14. Swartzendruber, D. C., Wertz, P. W., Kitko, D. J., Madison, K. C., and Downing, D. T., *J. Invest. Dermatol.*, 92:251–257 (1989).
15. Kligman, A. M., and Christophers, E., *Arch. Dermatol.*, 88:702–705 (1963).
16. Menton, D. N., *Am. J. Anat.*, 145:1–21 (1976).

17. Blank, I. H., *J. Invest. Dermatol.*, 21:259–271 (1953).
18. Baker, H., and Kligman, A. M., *Arch. Dermatol.*, 95:408–411 (1967).
19. Rothberg, S., Crounse, R. G., and Lee, J. L., *J. Invest. Dermatol.*, 37:497–504 (1961).
20. Lampe, M. A., Williams, M. L., and Elias, P. M., *J. Lipid Res.*, 24:131–140 (1983).
21. Gray, G. M., and Yardley, H. J., *J. Lipid Res.*, 16:441–447 (1975).
22. Lampe, M. A., Burlingame, A. L., Whitney, et al., *J. Lipid Res.*, 24:120–130 (1983).
23. Scheuplein, R. J., and Bronaugh, R. L., Percutaneous Absorption. In: *Biochemistry and Physiology of Skin*, 1st ed. (L. A. Goldsmith, ed.), Oxford University Press, New York, 1983, p. 1280.
24. Wertz, P. W., Kremer, M., and Squier, C. A., *J. Invest. Dermatol.*, 98:375–378 (1992).
25. Hansen, H. S., and Jensen, B., *Biochim. Biophys. Acta*, 878:357–363 (1985).
26. Guy, R. H., and Maibach, H. I., *J. Pharm. Sci.*, 72:1375–1380 (1983).
27. Schlagel, C. A., and Sanborn, E. C., *J. Invest. Dermatol.*, 42:253–256 (1964).
28. Carslaw, H. S., and Jaeger, J. C., *Conduction of Heat in Solids*, 2nd ed., Oxford University Press, London, 1959, p. 128.
29. Flynn, G. L., Dermal Diffusion and Delivery Principles. In: *Encyclopedia of Pharmaceutical Technology*, Vol 3 (J. Swarbrick, and J. C. Boylan, eds.), Marcel Dekker, Inc., New York, 1990, pp. 457–503.
30. Ostrenga, J., Steinmetz, C., and Poulsen, B. J., *J. Pharm. Sci.*, 60:1175–1179 (1971).
31. Mallory, S. B., Lehman, P. A., Vanderpool, D. R., and Franz, T. J., *Ped. Dermatol.*, 10:370–375 (1993).
32. Franz, T. J., *J. Invest. Dermatol.*, 64:190–195 (1975).
33. Skelly, J. P., Shah, V. P., Maibach, H. I., et al., *Pharm. Res.*, 4:265–267 (1987).
34. Bronaugh, R. L., and Collier, S. W., Preparation of Human and Animal Skin. In: *In Vitro Percutaneous Absorption: Principles, Fundamentals, and Applications* (R. L. Bronaugh, and H. I. Maibach, eds.), CRC Press, Boca Raton, FL, 1991, pp. 1–6.
35. Reifenrath, W. G., and Kemppainen, B. W., Skin Storage Conditions. In: *In Vitro Percutaneous Absorption: Principles, Fundamentals, and Applications* (R. L. Bronaugh, and H. I. Maibach, eds.), CRC Press, Boca Raton, FL, 1991, pp. 115–127.
36. Bronaugh, R. L., Stewart, R. F., and Simon, G., *J. Pharm. Sci.*, 75:1094–1097 (1986).
37. Franz, T. J., and Lehman, P. A., *J. Invest. Dermatol.*, 94:525 (1990).
38. Reifenrath, W. G., and Robinson, P. B., *J. Pharm. Sci.*, 71:1014–1018 (1982).
39. Bronaugh, R. L., and Stewart, R. F., *J. Pharm. Sci.*, 74:64–67 (1985).
40. Sclafani, J., Nightingale, J., Liu, P., and Kurihara-Bergstrom, T., *Pharm. Res.*, 10:1521–1526 (1993).
41. Frantz, S. W., Instrumentation and Methodology for In Vitro Skin Diffusion Cells. In: *Methods for Skin Absorption* (Kemppainen, B. W., and Reifenrath, W. G., eds.), CRC Press, Boca Raton, FL, 1990, pp. 36–59.
42. Franz, T. J., The Finite Dose Technique as a Valid In Vitro Model for the Study of Percutaneous Absorption in Man. In: *Current Problems in Dermatology*, Vol. 7 (Simon, G., Paster, Z., Klingberg, M., and Kaye, M., eds.), S. Karger, Basel, 1978, pp. 58–68.
43. Bronaugh, R. L., and Franz, T. J., *Br. J. Dermatol.*, 115:1–11 (1986).
44. Bronaugh, R. L., and Collier, S. W., In Vitro Methods for Measuring Skin Permeation. In: *Skin Permeation: Fundamentals and Application* (J. L., Zatz, ed.), Allured Publishing Corp. Wheaton, IL., 1993, pp. 93–111.
45. Reifenrath W. G., Chellquist, E. M., Shipwash, E. A., Jederberg, W. W., and Krueger, G. G., *Br. J. Dermatol.* (Supp. 3) 27:123–135 (1984).
46. Bronaugh, R. L., Stewart, R. F., and Congdon, E. R., *Tox. Appl. Pharmacol.*, 62:481–488 (1982).
47. Hawkins, G. S., and Reifenrath, W. G., *Fund. Appl. Toxicol.*, 4:S133–144 (1984).
48. Rigg, P. C., and Barry, B. W., *J. Invest. Dermatol.*, 94:235–240 (1990).
49. Malkinson, F. D., and Ferguson, E. H., *J. Invest. Dermatol.*, 25:281–283 (1955).

50. Malkinson, F. D., *J. Invest. Dermatol.*, 31:19–26 (1958).
51. Malkinson, F. D., and Kirschenbaum, M. B., *Arch. Dermatol.*, 88:427–436 (1963).
52. Feldmann, R. J., and Maibach, H. I., *Arch. Dermatol.*, 91:661–666 (1965).
53. Feldmann, R. J., and Maibach, H. I., *J. Invest. Dermatol.*, 48:181–183 (1967).
54. Feldmann, R. J., and Maibach, H. I., *J. Invest. Dermatol.*, 52:89–94 (1969).
55. Feldmann, R. J., and Maibach, H. I., *J. Invest. Dermatol.*, 54:399–404 (1970).
56. Kao, J., Patterson, F. K., and Hall, J., *Toxicol. Appl. Pharmacol.*, 81:502–516 (1985).
57. Bronaugh, R. L., Stewart, R. F., and Storm, J. E., *Toxicol. Appl. Pharmacol.*, 99:534–543 (1989).
58. Maibach, H. I., Feldmann, R. J., Milby, T. H., and Serat, W. F., *Arch. Environ. Health*, 23:208–211 (1971).
59. Rosenberg, E. W., Blank, H., and Resnik, S., *J. Am. Med. Assoc.*, 179:809–811 (1962).
60. Franz, T. J., *Arch. Dermatol.*, 121:203–206 (1985).
61. Bucks, D. A. W., Maibach, H. I., and Guy, R. H., *J. Pharm. Sci.*, 74:1337–1339 (1985).
62. Bartek, M. J., and LaBudde, J. A., Percutaneous Absorption In Vivo. In: *Animal Models in Dermatology* (H. I. Maibach, ed.), Churchill-Livingstone, New York, 1975, pp. 102–120.
63. Jensen, B. K., McGann, B. A., Kachevsky, V., and Franz, T. J., *J. Am. Acad. Dermatol.*, 24:425–428 (1991).
64. Chiang, T., *J. Chromatogr.*, 182:335–340 (1980).
65. Franz, T. J., Lehman, P. A., and Franz, S. F. *J. Invest. Dermatol.*, 100:490 (1993).
66. Mizuchi, A., Miyachi, Y., Tamaki, K., and Kukita, A., *J. Invest. Dermatol.*, 67:279–282 (1976).
67. Bucks, D. A. W., McMaster, J. R., Maibach, H. I., and Guy, R. H., *J. Invest. Dermatol.*, 91:29–33 (1988).
68. Franz, T. J., and Lehman, P. A., *J. Pharm. Sci.*, 77:489–491 (1988).
69. Franz, T. J., and Lehman, P. A., *J. Cut. Ocul. Toxicol.*, 8:517–524 (1989).
70. Rougier, A., and Lotte, C., Correlation between Horny Layer Concentration and Percutaneous Absorption. In: *Pharmacology and the Skin: Skin Pharmacokinetics*, Vol. 1 (B. Shroot, and H. Schaefer, eds.), S. Karger, Basel, 1987, pp. 82–102.

THOMAS J. FRANZ
PAUL A. LEHMAN

Permeation Enhancement through Skin

Introduction

Transdermal drug delivery (percutaneous absorption) can provide potential advantages for some drugs, including avoidance of first-pass gut and hepatic metabolism, fewer side effects, and relative ease of drug input termination in problematic cases [1,2]. A typical example is estradiol, which has been developed in several types of transdermal delivery patches to treat menopausal symptoms and for the prevention of postmenopausal osteoporosis. The increasing popularity of such products as Estraderm TTS is partially due to the slight effects on hepatic proteins upon percutaneous hormone administration and the more normal estrone to estradiol serum concentration, as confirmed in the clinic [3–7]. Other drugs selected for transdermal delivery include scopolamine (hyoscine) [7,8], clonidine [9–12], propranolol [13,14], fentanyl [15–17], nicotine [18,19], and testosterone [20,22]. However, transdermal delivery of most drugs is often not feasible because of the barrier nature of human skin. Various methods for increasing the percutaneous absorption of drugs have been developed, including ionotophoresis [23,24], occlusion [25], vehicle manipulation [26,27], and ultrasound [28]. Yet another approach is to employ penetration enhancers (accelerants or absorption enhancers). These are agents that partition into, and interact with, skin constituents to induce a temporary, reversible increase in skin permeability. Researchers thus aim to broaden the range of therapeutic agents that may be delivered by the transdermal route for both local and systemic action by the coadministration of penetration enhancers.

Percutaneous Absorption

Before discussing the various types and mechanisms of action of penetration enhancers, it is suitable to survey the essential structures of human skin and drug diffusion as these apply to percutaneous absorption. This section also briefly reviews most of the experimental techniques used when studying transdermal permeation.

Anatomy and Function of Human Skin

Human skin provides an excellent barrier between the external environment and the body. It is a self-repairing composite membrane which protects against physical, chemical, microbial, and radiological attack and performs a homeostatic role by controlling moisture and heat loss from the body. It also serves as a food reserve and a sensory organ transmitting external environmental information. Human skin may be subdivided into three mutually dependent layers (Fig. 1):

- The subcutaneous fatty layer (hypodermis),
- The overlying dermis, and
- The epidermis, the outermost stratum of the skin.

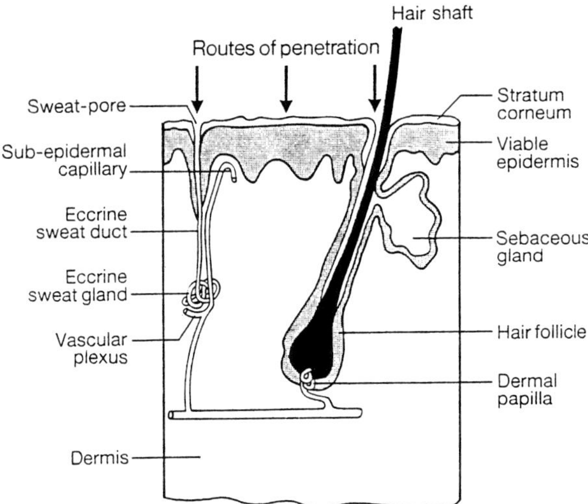

FIG. 1. Simplified structure of human skin, with potential routes for drug permeation indicated.

The fatty subcutaneous tissue merges with the overlying dermis. The hypodermis supplies a layer of adipose tissue over most of the body that provides thermal insulation, mechanic protection, and a reserve of readily available high energy molecules. It carries the principal blood vessels and nerves to the skin and may contain sensory pressure organs.

The dermis (or corium) is 3 to 5 mm thick and is composed of a matrix of connective tissue in which predominant bundles of collagen fibrils interlace with elastic tissue (approximately 4%) and sparse reticular fibers (approximately 0.4%). This composite is embedded in an amorphous mucopolysaccharide ground substance comprising approximately 20% of the dermal mass [29]. The dermis encloses cutaneous appendages (eccrine sweat glands, apocrine glands, and pilosebacious units) and is penetrated by blood vessels, lymphatics, and nerves. The cutaneous blood supply has an essential function in the regulation of body temperature. It delivers oxygen and nutrients to the skin while removing toxins and waste products; the vasculature is vital in repairing damaged skin. Capillaries reach to within 0.2 mm of the skin surface and provide sink conditions for most molecules penetrating the skin barrier (other than extremely lipophilic molecules). The blood supply thus keeps the dermal concentration of a penetrant usually very low, and the resulting concentration difference across the epidermis provides the essential driving force for transdermal permeation.

The superficial, multilayered epidermis varies in thickness from 0.06 mm on the eyelids to 0.8 mm on the palms. The epidermal cells divide in the basal layer and migrate toward the exterior, undergoing keratinization to form the outermost layer, the stratum corneum [30–32].

The stratum corneum (or horny layer) typically comprises 10 to 15 cell layers and is approximately 10 μm thick when dry (but swells to several times this thickness when fully hydrated). This membrane, consisting of dead, anucleate, keratinized cells embedded in a lipid matrix, is essential for controlling the percutaneous absorption of most drugs and other chemicals. The barrier nature of the horny layer depends critically on its constituents: 75–80% proteins, 5–15% lipids, and 5–10% unidentified material on a dry

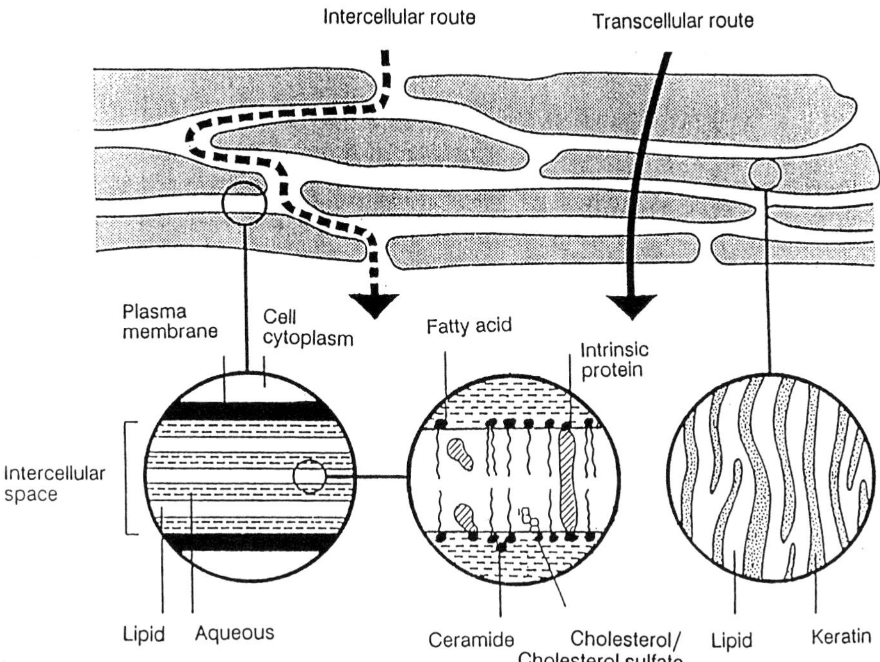

FIG. 2. The "brick-and-mortar" model of the stratum corneum.

weight basis [29]. The protein fraction predominantly comprises α-keratin (approximately 70%) with some β-keratin (10%) and the cell envelope (5%). The lipid constituents vary with body site; the abdomen comprises neutral lipids (75%), sphingolipids (18%), polar lipids (5%), and cholesterol sulfate (2%) [33]. Phospholipids are largely absent, a unique feature for a mammalian membrane. The lipid composition of the intercellular domain of the stratum corneum has been well researched [34–38].

The architecture of the horny layer may be modeled as a brick-and-mortar structure [35,38–41]. In this model, the keratinized corneocytes function as protein "bricks" embedded in a lipid "mortar" (Fig. 2). The lipids construct multiple bilayers [42,43], despite the minimal charged phospholipid content, and it has been proposed that there is sufficient amphiphilic material in the lipid fraction, such as polar free fatty acids and cholesterol sulfate, to maintain a bilayer form [35,44].

The precise molecular arrangement of intercellular lipid bilayers in the horny layer is still being investigated. Lipids covalently bound to the surface of corneocytes may play a part in determining the barrier function of the membrane [45–48]. Additionally protein molecules may be intrinsically or extrinsically incorporated into the lipid bilayers [49–51].

Permeation Pathways through Human Skin

A molecule may use two diffusional routes to penetrate normal intact skin: the skin appendages (sweat glands and hair follicles), together comprising the shunt route, or the intact epidermis, as illustrated in Fig. 1.

Typically, one square centimeter of human skin yields 10 hair follicles, 15 sebaceous glands, and 100 sweat glands [52,53] that bypass the low diffusivity domain of the stratum corneum and which may function as diffusional shunts. However, the appendages provide a small fractional surface area, approximately 0.1% of the total skin area [54], and are widely believed to provide an insignificant pathway for most drug permeation, at least at pseudo-steady state [55–58]. More recent studies have questioned this concept, indicating that follicles may have more importance in percutaneous absorption than is generally assumed [59]. The appendageal route may be more significant for ions [60,61] and large polar molecules [62] which slowly permeate through intact stratum corneum.

The shunt route may provide the principal diffusion pathway immediately after drug application, as a prominent time delay prior to the establishment of steady state (the lag time) occurs for most molecules permeating across the bulk of the stratum corneum [54]. Shunt-route diffusion has been demonstrated within 5 min of drug application [63].

The major fraction of most diffusants permeates across the bulk of the intact horny layer. Two potential micropathways serve the stratum corneum, the transcellular and intercellular routes (Fig. 2). The principal pathway taken by a penetrant is decided mainly by the diffusant's partition coefficient [41]. Hydrophilic drugs should partition preferentially into the intracellular domains, whereas lipophilic penetrants (log P octanol–water typically >2) traverse the stratum corneum mainly via the intercellular route. (See the article Partition Coefficients in this volume.) Most diffusants permeate the stratum corneum by both routes; even highly oil-soluble drugs should partition to some minor extent into the corneocytes that contain some residual lipids. However, the tortuous intercellular pathway is widely considered to provide the principal route and the major barrier to the permeation of most drugs [34–36,42,46,58,64–66].

Transepidermal permeation is a complex process, with a variety of barriers to cross. Initially, a drug must first partition out of this vehicle into the stratum corneum before diffusing across the viable epidermis and dermis from where most permeants are cleared by the circulation [60]. The epidermis and dermis are essentially aqueous in nature and may thus provide a significant barrier to the further permeation of highly lipophilic drugs [67,68]. The skin is a metabolically active organ, and hence may transform drugs after topical application [69,70]. This biotransformation may very occasionally provide the rate-limiting step in the percutaneous absorption process [71,72].

The Permeation Process

Although the mechanisms for drug transport across the skin have yet to be fully elucidated, it is clear that the process is essentially one of passive diffusion. This is a phenomenon by which a diffusant moves down a concentration gradient (or more accurately, a chemical-potential gradient) by random molecular motion.

In the situation of a permeant entering the skin, diffusion is usually considered as unidirectional (i.e., the concentration gradient is directed only into the skin). This unidirectional diffusion in an isotropic medium may be expressed mathematically by Eq. (1), Fick's second law of diffusion.

$$\frac{\partial C}{\partial t} = D \frac{\partial^2 C}{\partial x^2} \tag{1}$$

where C is the concentration of the diffusing substance, x the space coordinate measured normal to the section, D the diffusion coefficient, and t the time. With skin permeation studies in vitro, investigators often use a membrane clamped between two compartments, one containing a drug formulation (the donor) and the other a receptor solution providing sink conditions (essentially zero concentration). After sufficient time, steady-state diffusion across the membrane prevails. Under these conditions Eq. (1) may be simplified to Eq. (2).

$$\frac{dm}{dt} = \frac{DC_0}{h} \tag{2}$$

where m is the cumulative mass of permeant that passes per unit area through the membrane in time t; C_0 is the concentration of diffusant in the first layer of the membrane at the skin surface contacting the source of the penetrant; and h is the membrane thickness.

In most diffusion experiments, it is difficult to measure C_0, but C'_0, the concentration of diffusant in the donor phase bathing the membrane, may be easily determined, because C_0 and C'_0 are related, as shown by Eq. (3).

$$C_0 = PC'_0 \tag{3}$$

where P is the partition coefficient of the diffusant between the membrane and the bathing solution. Substitution of Eq. (3) into Eq. (2) yields Eq. (4).

$$\frac{dm}{dt} = \frac{DC'_0P}{h} \tag{4}$$

This is the classic and most important equation used in skin permeation studies. A graph of m, the cumulative amount of drug crossing a unit area of skin, against time yields a profile of the drug penetrating the membrane (Fig. 3).

Extrapolation of the pseudo-steady-state portion of the graph to the intercept on the time axis provides the lag time (L). This is the period during which the rate of diffusion across the membrane is increasing. Steady-state conditions prevail after approximately 2.7 times the lag time [1]. The lag time is related to the diffusion coefficient by Eq. (5).

$$L = \frac{h^2}{6D} \tag{5}$$

Thus, in theory, D may be obtained by measuring L, provided the membrane thickness, h, is known. In practice, this method for evaluating D has several disadvantages as the exact thickness of the stratum corneum is difficult to measure and may vary with penetration enhancer treatment. The measured thickness of the membrane does not allow for a tortuous pathway for diffusion and, for stratum corneum, the value obtained for D is therefore an apparent one. Additionally, lag times obtained from permeation experiments with human skin tend to be very variable and include a component arising from penetrant-horny layer binding.

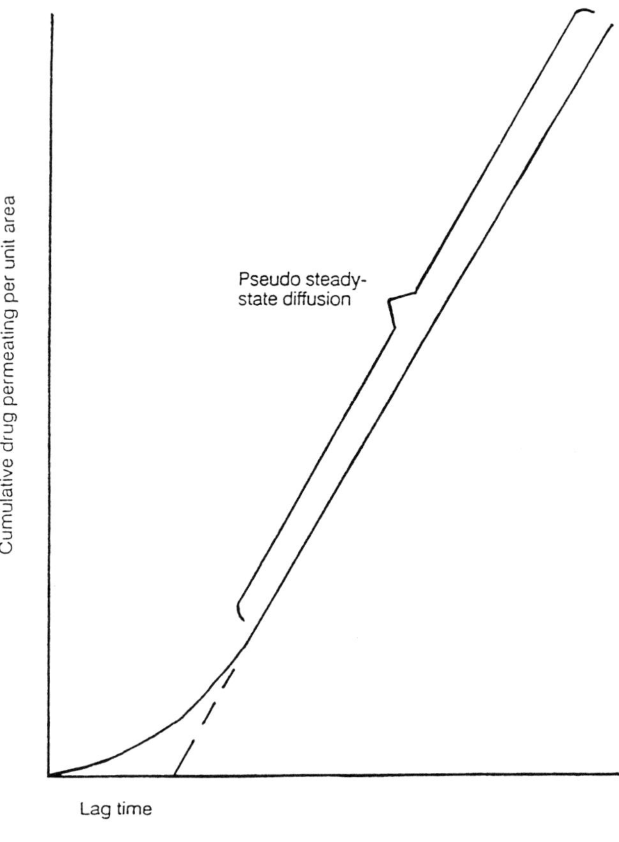

FIG. 3. A typical permeation profile for a molecule diffusing across human skin.

The permeability coefficient of a diffusant through a membrane, Kp, may be defined by Eq. (6),

$$Kp = \frac{PD}{h} \tag{6}$$

which may be substituted into Eq. (4) to give Eq. (7).

$$\frac{dm}{dt} = C_0'Kp \tag{7}$$

The expression dm/dt, the rate of change of cumulative mass of diffusant that passes per unit area through the membrane, is termed the flux of diffusant, J, and may be evaluated from the steady-state portion of a drug permeation profile. Hence, Eq. (8) holds.

$$J = C_0'Kp \tag{8}$$

Thus, if the donor concentration and the flux of permeant are known, the permeability coefficient may be determined. The permeability coefficient is widely used to characterize the percutaneous absorption of drugs as it represents the flux of drug per unit skin area per unit concentration.

It should be noted that the relationship quoted in Eq. (8) applies to a simple, inert membrane. When applied to human skin, several assumptions have to be made:

1. Transport across the skin is by passive diffusion only [60].
2. The horny layer provides the rate-determining barrier and the diffusants are rapidly cleared from the dermal side [58].
3. The stratum corneum is uniform in character, although it is not homogeneous [60].
4. The drug dissolves in the stratum corneum [73].

It should be noted that the relationships derived above apply only to pseudo-steady-state diffusion, that is, the linear portion of Fig. 3. Furthermore, Fickian diffusion theory is applicable to an isotropic medium. Skin is a multilayered heterogeneous membrane, and hence, apparent diffusion coefficients calculated from Eqs. (5) and (6) incorporate errors caused by drug–skin binding or deviations from ideal solution behavior. A surprising fact is how well these simple equations correlate with skin-permeation phenomena. More detailed accounts of relevant permeation theory and treatments of diffusional barriers in parallel and series are provided in the literature [1,74–76].

Experimental Techniques

This section reviews briefly some of the main procedures that have proved valuable in studying the effects and mechanisms of action of penetration enhancers.

Permeation Studies

Developmental studies for skin preparations seldom involve in vivo permeation studies because factors such as drug delivery and analysis, skin temperature, and experimental design may be more easily regulated in vitro. However, some in vivo protocols have been performed with penetration enhancers on guinea pigs [77] and rats [78,79]. Several techniques are used for in vitro penetration studies with penetration enhancers.

Diffusion Cells. Diffusion cells basically comprise two compartments with a membrane clamped between the donor and receptor sections (Fig. 4). Diffusion cells with a fixed volume of agitated donor and receptor solutions may be used to evaluate the steady-state flux of a drug or penetration enhancer. Cells for imitation of in vivo conditions often use a flow-through receptor fluid equating to the blood supply, with an unstirred donor phase equivalent to a drug formulation. By using diffusion cells, the conditions for drug delivery may be controlled; drug permeation may vary with, for example, the condition of the stratum corneum, skin temperature, donor or receptor pH, membrane hydration, and the thermodynamic activity of the donor formulation.

Membrane Selection. Most transdermal delivery studies are performed with a view to evaluating the in vivo human situation. Clearly, the most appropriate membrane for diffusion studies is the human skin. It provides considerable inter- and intrasample vari-

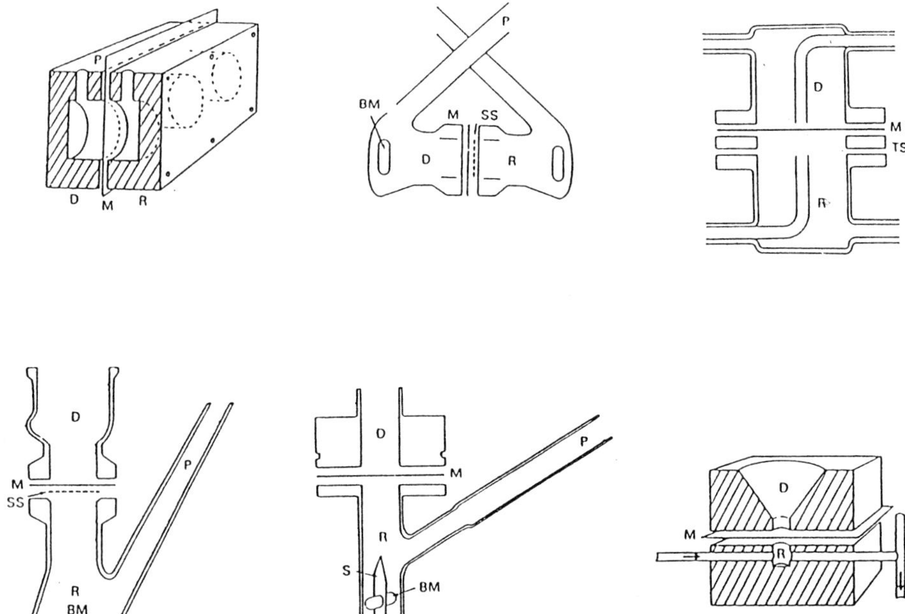

FIG. 4. Diffusion cells for the study of percutaneous absorption. Key: D, donor compartment; R, receptor compartment; M, membrane; P, sampling port; BM, bar magnet; SS, stainless steel support; TS, Teflon support; S, polyethylene sail.

ability [80,81], and drug diffusivity through the stratum corneum varies with body site [82,83]. However, the availability of human skin, or lack of it, has often dictated the choice of membrane in permeation studies.

Most in vitro permeation studies unfortunately use animal skin. The hairless mouse provides a widely used alternative to human tissue [84–88], whereas other workers prefer the rabbit [89], guinea pig [90–92], rat [93–97], or shed snake skin [89,98]. However, the limitations of animal models for predicting in vitro permeation through human skin have been well documented [99–105]. Whenever possible, human skin should be used in preference to an animal model!

Differential Scanning Calorimetry

Useful information regarding the modes of action of penetration enhancers may be gained by thermal analysis of the horny layer, notably differential scanning calorimetry (DSC). Thermal analysis has been used to investigate the uptake and binding of water in stratum corneum [106–109]. The molecular origins of thermal events arising from DSC of human stratum corneum were proposed by Van Duzee, whose work revealed four major endothermic transitions over the temperature range −50°C to +170°C [110]. Figure 5 illustrates a typical DSC thermal profile of hydrated stratum corneum. Van Duzee identified these transitions as: T_2 (75°C) lipid melting; T_3 (85°C) denaturation of α-keratin; and T_4 (107°C) denaturation of a nonfibrous protein. Subsequent studies have demonstrated that these temperatures of transitions vary considerably with the hydration level of human stratum corneum [111,113] and the animal species [114–118].

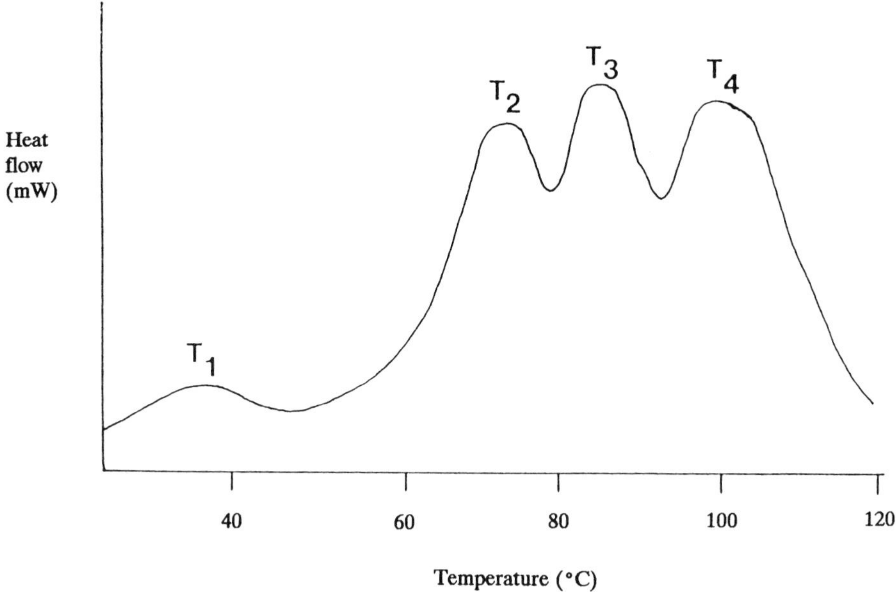

FIG. 5. Typical differential calorimetry (DSC) trace of hydrated human stratum corneum.

Interpretation of the endothermic transitions is becoming clearer, with T_1 widely accepted to arise from melting of sebaceous lipids and/or fat contamination of the samples. Alternatively, T_1 may develop from minor structural rearrangement within the lipid bilayers of the stratum corneum. However, this transition is not present in all samples and appears to depend to a large extent on sample preparation [112]. Thus, endotherm T_1 is not important when investigating the action mechanisms of penetration enhancers.

Endotherm T_2 is generally attributed to the melting of bilayer lipids. The peak is reversible on heating, cooling, and reheating and is removed from stratum corneum by known lipid solvents such as a chloroform–methanol system [110,114]. The endotherm T_4 is associated with protein denaturation, probably arising from an α-keratin conformational change of intracellular protein [111,113].

Interpretations of endotherm T_3 are varied, although there is general agreement that this transition does not arise from the denaturation of α-keratin as reported by Van Duzee [110]. Several workers have proposed that T_3 is due to a lipid–protein complex associated with the corneocyte cell membranes [112,119,120]. However, other investigators have produced evidence contrary to this interpretation of T_3. Using neonatal rat stratum corneum, Al-Saidan et al. showed a considerable rise in membrane permeability to alkanols when the tissue was preheated to 80°C (i.e., above T_3), yet no significant permeability increase was observed by preheating to 75°C (i.e., below T_3) [121]. If T_2 is due to the complete disruption of the barrier lipids, preheating to 75–80°C (both temperatures above T_2) would have an equal effect on membrane permeability, and both temperatures would greatly increase permeant diffusion. Clearly this is not the case, and the results of Al-Saidan et al. demonstrate that T_3 arises from the disruption of ''barrier'' lipids. Further evidence against the involvement of lipid–protein complex of the horny-cell membrane for endotherm T_3 was supplied by Swartzendruber et al. [122]. These authors report that exhaustive chloroform–methanol lipid extraction of the stratum corneum membrane does not remove lipids associated with the corneocyte membranes, yet thermal analysis of the horny layer following chloroform–methanol extraction shows no T_3 [110,112]. Thus, T_3 may not arise from the disruption of a lipid–protein complex of the horny-cell membrane.

Other evidence to suggest that T_3 is attributable to thermal events within the barrier (i.e., intercellular) lipids is provided by Goodman and Barry [111,113] who demonstrated that T_2 and T_3 are associated with the melting of bilayer lipids. The endotherm T_3 may be attributable to the melting (or disordering) of lipid bilayers as the polar head group packings of the molecules disrupt.

The literature contains only a few detailed accounts of DSC investigations of penetration-enhancer modifications of stratum corneum thermal events. Azone (1-dodecylazacycloheptan-2-one or laurocapram) was shown to shift the lipid-associated endotherms T_2 and T_3 to lower temperatures in human, hairless mouse, and porcine stratum corneum, results consistent with disordering of the intercellular lipids [111,113, 120,123–125]. Other enhancers studied by thermal analysis include dimethylsulfoxide [111,126], pyrrolidones [113,126], oleic acid [113,118,124], surfactants [127], octadecanoic acid [128], and terpenes [129–132]. All these chemicals alter the lipid endothermic transition temperatures, indicating that a potential mode of action for such accelerants is via disordering the intercellular bilayer structure, thus increasing drug diffusivity through the horny layer.

Infrared Spectroscopy

Early applications of infrared spectroscopy to human skin have been reviewed [46]. Fourier transform infrared (FTIR) spectroscopy is widely used for studies of penetration enhancer interactions with stratum corneum. Oertel used infrared spectroscopy to investigate protein conformational changes induced by organic sulfoxides in human stratum corneum [132]. Workers have examined stratum corneum water content in vivo by attenuated total reflectance (ATR) techniques [132,134]. Fourier transform infrared has been used to complement the DSC technique in order to investigate lipid thermotropic transitions in human, porcine, and hairless mouse stratum corneum [112,115–117]. A modern study investigated the content and organization of stratum corneum lipids by sequential stripping of layers from the ventral forearm of human volunteers [135]. The authors report that the horny-layer barrier varies across its thickness and that the intercellular lipid bilayers are more disordered nearer the skin surface than deeper in the tissue. A shift to a lower frequency was reported in lipid C-H antisymmetric stretching frequency with the sequential stripping, indicating that the barrier lipids were more highly ordered deeper in the tissue.

The literature yields few reports on the use of FTIR to investigate penetration enhancers with stratum corneum constituents. The effects of *n*-alkanols on hairless mouse skin have been investigated [136]. A later study reports that ethanol does not "fluidize" (or disorder) the stratum corneum lipids in the human ventral forearm skin [137]. The versatility of FTIR as a technique for probing enhancer actions, has been demonstrated. Thus, Mak et al. studied penetration enhancement in vivo using attenuated total reflectance (ATR)-FTIR [138]. By selecting a model permeant with a functional group foreign to human skin, the study was able to monitor drug permeation (4-cyanophenol, containing a —C≡N group) in the presence and absence of a penetration enhancer (oleic acid). The authors concluded that the oleic acid interacted with horny-layer lipids and disordered their structure, hence facilitating drug diffusion. This protocol also demonstrated some of the advantages of FTIR over other analytical methods (e.g., DSC); the technique is noninvasive, rapid, and may be used for in vivo experiments with human volunteers.

Vasoconstrictor Assay

A technique widely used to assess the activity and bioavailability of corticosteroid formulations and modified to assess penetration enhancer actions is the vasoconstrictor or blanching test. It relies on a drug eliciting a local vasoconstriction effect that can be assessed and thus quantified. For practical purposes, the test applies only to a limited number of drugs, principally corticosteroids.

Using an occluded vasoconstrictor assay, the bioavailability of mechlorisone dibutyrate from various polar solvents was shown to be under thermodynamic control [139]. Based on occluded and nonoccluded vasoconstrictor assays, various penetration enhancers (including Azone, oleic acid, and 2-pyrrolidone) were shown to increase the bioavailability of betamethasone-17-benzoate [25,140]. As with FTIR spectroscopy, the vasoconstrictor assay allows in vivo evaluations of enhancer effects in human volunteers.

X-Ray Diffractometry

X-ray diffractometry (XRD) has provided information on the molecular structure of the stratum corneum. Wide- or low-angle x-ray diffraction has been used to study several biological membranes [141]. Such reports have shown that mammalian epidermal keratin exists predominantly in the α form, with an α-to-β transformation occuring between 60 and 80°C [142–144]. Wide-angle x-ray diffraction has also been applied to the lipid domain of mammalian stratum corneum and the results have been reviewed by Potts [46] and Garson et al. [145]. Interestingly, Garson et al. concluded that intracellular keratin develops as β-sheets rather than the widely accepted concept of α-keratin [145]. More recently, small-angle X-ray scattering (SAXS) has probed the intercellular lipid matrix; results are given in Table 1. Studies by Bouwstra and co-workers showed that lipid lamellar spacings are independent of tissue water content, although treatments with penetration

TABLE 1 Small-Angle X-ray Scattering Data of Mammalian Stratum Corneum

Stratum Corneum and Treatment	Temperature (°C)	Repeat Distance (nm)	Reference
Human	Ambient	5.0–8.0	146
Human and skin softener	Ambient	3.0–4.5	
Mouse	25	13.1, 6.0	49
Mouse couplet	25	12.6, 6.3, 3.2, 2.3	
Mouse		None detected	
Mouse, preheated to 75°C	75 25	13.1, 6.0	
Human	Ambient	6.5	147
Human	Ambient	6.5, 13.4	148
Mouse	Ambient	13.1	149
Mouse, fatty acid deficient, hydrated	Ambient	13.19	
Mouse, fatty acid deficient, dry	Ambient	12.96	

enhancers do alter small-angle diffractograms [147,148]. The application of XRD to stratum corneum structural analysis is novel and promises to provide valuable information regarding the molecular structure of the tissue.

Electron Spin Resonance

Electron spin resonance (ESR) is a technique useful for studying a variety of biological membranes [150,151]. It has been used to probe the barrier nature of the stratum corneum and to investigate lipid-phase transitions in normal and x-linked ichthyotic human stratum corneum [152]. This technique offers three advantages over other physical-chemical techniques: it displays phase transitions within membrane microenvironments and indicates the polarity of the microenvironment. In addition, its sensitivity to molecular events is higher than that of techniques such as DSC. However, the methodology has several disadvantages, notably the potential for the spin probe itself to perturb the highly ordered lipid structure. Rehfeld and co-workers investigated thermal events in murine stratum corneum and isolated membrane complex [153], and ESR was utilized to probe the action mechanisms of skin penetration enhancers in human stratum corneum [154]. As with XRD, ESR promises to be a useful technique for studying molecular interactions within the horny layer.

Penetration Enhancers

To reduce the resistance of the stratum corneum and its biological variability, penetration enhancers (accelerants or absorption promoters) are incorporated into skin preparations. An ideal penetration enhancer can be defined as a chemical with the unique property in relation to skin that it reversibly reduces the barrier resistance of the horny layer without damaging any viable cells [1]. The attributes of the ideal enhancer may be listed as follows [155,156]:

- It should be pharmacologically inert, possessing no action of itself at receptor sites anywhere in the body.
- It should be nontoxic, nonirritating, and nonallergenic.
- Onset of action should be rapid, and duration of activity should be predictable and suitable for the drug used.
- Upon removal of the enhancer, the horny layer should immediately and fully recover its normal barrier property.
- The barrier function of the skin should reduce in one direction only. Endogenous materials should not be lost to the environment by diffusion out of the skin.
- The accelerant should be chemically and physically compatible with all drugs and adjuvants to be formulated in topical preparations and devices.
- If liquid and to be used at high volume fractions, it should be a suitable solvent for drugs.
- It should spread well on the skin, with a suitable skin ''feel.''

- It should readily formulate into dermatological preparations, transdermal devices, and skin adhesives.
- It should be inexpensive, odorless, tasteless, and colorless to be cosmetically acceptable.

To date, no material has been found to possess all the ideal properties of a penetration enhancer, but numerous chemicals have been studied that have some of the more desirable features.

Types of Penetration Enhancers

Sulfoxides and Similar Compounds

Dimethylsulfoxide (DMSO), the classic skin-penetration enhancer, is a powerful aprotic solvent which is colorless, nearly odorless, and hygroscopic. DMSO is a vehicle for idoxuridine in the treatment of severe herpetic infections of the skin and is particularly successful against *Herpes simplex.*

For 30 years, DMSO has been investigated as a skin penetration enhancer for a wide range of drugs, including antibiotics, steroids, narcotics, and salicylates. Barry [1] reviewed the literature up to 1983; more recent studies are detailed in Table 2. A simple numerical assessment of DMSO activity may be derived from the literature by defining an enhancement ratio (ER), calculated as the ratio of drug permeation after sulfoxide treatment to that before treatment.

Although DMSO is an excellent accelerant for a wide variety of drugs, it creates problems. The activity of the sulfoxide is highly concentration dependent [163], with 60% and above generally required to produce a significant effect. At such high concentrations, DMSO produces erythema and wheals [164], irreversible skin damage [165], and delamitation of the stratum corneum and denaturation of its proteins [162]. Another side effect is the production of dimethylsulfide, a DMSO metabolite which produces ha-

TABLE 2 Recent Studies of Dimethylsulfoxide (DMSO) as Skin-Penetration Enhancer

Drug	DMSO concentration (%)	Membrane	Temperature (°C)	ER[a]	Reference
Flufenamic acid	5[b]	Rabbits in vivo	Ambient	3	157
Acyclovir	100	Guinea pig in vitro	Ambient	3	158
Acyclovir	100	Guinea pig in vitro	Ambient	3	159
5-Ethyl-2′-deoxyuridine	95	Guinea pig in vitro	25	19	160
Naloxone	10[c]	Human in vitro	37	1	161
Methanol	100	Hairless mouse in vitro	37	20	162
Vidarabine	30	Hairless mouse in vitro	37	1	163
	50			14	
	75			23	
	100			32	
1-Hexanol	100	Rat in vitro	37	9	126

[a]ER = Enhancement ratio, calculated from the literature as drug permeations after DMSO treatment vs. control drug permeation

[b]In petroleum base.

[c]In propylene glycol.

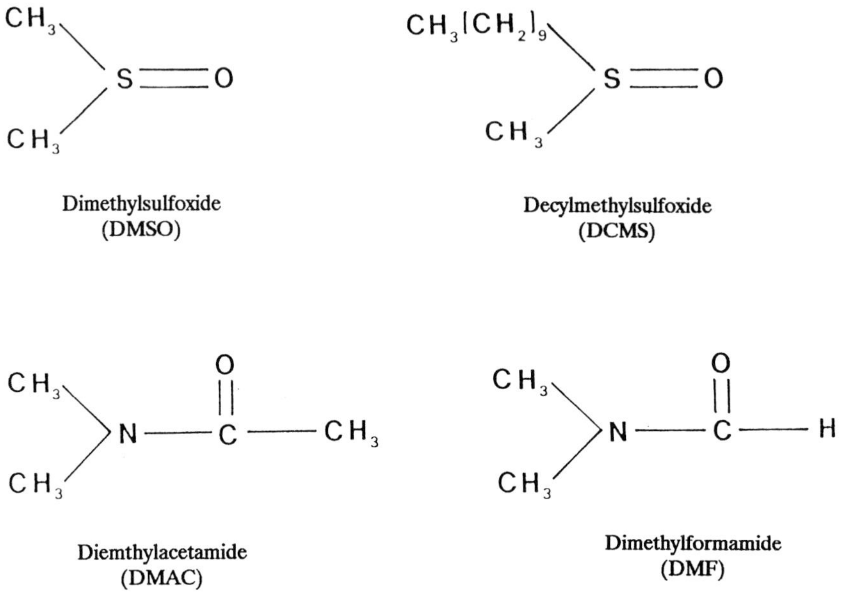

Dimethylsulfoxide
(DMSO)

Decylmethylsulfoxide
(DCMS)

Diemthylacetamide
(DMAC)

Dimethylformamide
(DMF)

FIG. 6. Structural formulas of some sulfoxides and chemically similar skin penetration enhancers.

litosis. Such repercussions have prevented widespread clinical use of DMSO and prompted a search for other, structurally related penetration enhancers (Fig. 6).

Dimethylacetamide (DMAC) and dimethylformamide (DMF) are powerful aprotic solvents with chemical structures similar to that of DMSO. Both promote in vitro permeation of griseofulvin and hydrocortisone but are less active than DMSO [166,167]. Local anesthesia with lidocaine was enhanced in the guinea pig by DMF and DMAC, and 75% DMAC in water provided a seven-fold increase in the blood concentration of the drug [168]. As a 10% solution in propylene glycol, DMAC yielded a 25% increase in naloxone flux across human skin in vitro [161].

Dimethylformamide was an effective enhancer for the model compound octanol, increasing the permeability coefficient through human skin in vitro threefold, and for caffeine, providing a 12-fold increase in drug permeation [169]. However, this study concluded that DMF induced irreversible membrane damage which accounted for the large increase in caffeine permeation. Extending this study, the enhancing effect of DMF in human volunteers in vivo was investigated using the vasoconstrictor assay [25,140]. DMF doubled the bioavailability of betamethasone-17-benzoate. It also produced a fourfold increase in aspirin flux across human skin in vitro [140]. *N*-Methylformamide (NMF) has also been utilized to promote the permeation of a variety of drugs in vitro. The amounts of mannitol, hydrocortisone, and progesterone permeating human skin were increased 191-, 82-, and 27-fold by NMF [171].

A homologous series of alkyl methylsulfoxides has been evaluated as potential accelerants [172]. In the series, ranging from DMSO to tetradecylmethylsulfoxide, the most active enhancer was decylmethylsulfoxide (DCMS), which promoted permeation of sodium nicotinate and thiourea across guinea pig skin. Recent studies with DCMS are shown in Table 3. The reversibility of DCMS action was demonstrated by Cooper [173], and a concentration-dependent effect was revealed by Touitou and Abed [84]. Literature

TABLE 3 Recent In Vitro Studies of Decylmethylsulfoxide (DCMS) as Skin-Penetration Enhancer

Drug	DCMS Concentration (%)[a]	Vehicle[b]	Membrane	Temperature (°C)	ER[c]	Reference
Urea	100		Human	22	110	173
Pentanol	100			22	1	
5-Fluorouracil	5	PG	Hairless mouse	22	2	84
	40	PG		22	70	
Naloxone	10	PG	Human	37	31	161
5-Fluorouracil	4	Water	Human	37	76	101
			Hairless mouse	37	102	
	15	PG	Human	37	4	
			Hairless mouse	37	9	
5-Fluorouracil	15	PG	Human	37	6	174
	4	Water		37	35[d],4[e]	
Estradiol	15	PG[f]		37	3.3[d]	
					1.1[e]	
	4	Water		37	3.6[d]	
Leuenkephalin	100mM	pH 7 buffer	Hairless mouse	37	5.4[f]	88
Oxymorphone	5		Human	37	1458[g]	102
HCl	1			37	299	
Base	1			37	0.2	

[a]Unless otherwise stated.
[b]PG = Propylene glycol.
[c]ER = Enhancement ratio, calculated from the literature as drug permeation after DCMS treatment vs. control drug permeation.
[d]Initial enhancement effect.
[e]Enhancement after 10 h.
[f]Aqueous donor and receptor solutions.
[g]Enhancement after 48 h.

results, including those given in Table 3, show DCMS to be an effective enhancer for hydrophilic molecules (including ionized molecules [173]) but not for more lipophilic compounds.

Pyrrolidones

Pyrrolidones and derivatives have been considered as potential accelerants for a variety of drugs (Fig. 7 and Table 4). These promoters apparently provide more activity toward hydrophilic drugs than toward lipophilic permeants.

N-Methyl-2-pyrrolidone (NMP) accelerates the permeation of the nonsteroidal anti-inflammatory drug mefanamic acid across rabbit skin in vivo [176]. Pyrrolidones also increase the bioavailability of the topical steroid betamethasone-17-benzoate in human volunteers as assessed by the vasoconstrictor assay [25,140]. 2-Pyrrolidone (2-P) and NMP create superior stratum corneum reservoirs of the drug compared with an inert vehicle. However, these papers drew attention to the fact that the pyrrolidones produced erythema in some volunteers, although the effect was short-lived.

Using a series of alkyl-substituted pyrrolidones, Sasaki et al. monitored transdermal permeation and skin accumulation of the accelerants and a model permeant, phenol red, for rat skin in vivo and in vitro [182]. In a further study, accumulation of the model permeant and the enhancers was found to be concentration dependent [183]. By combining

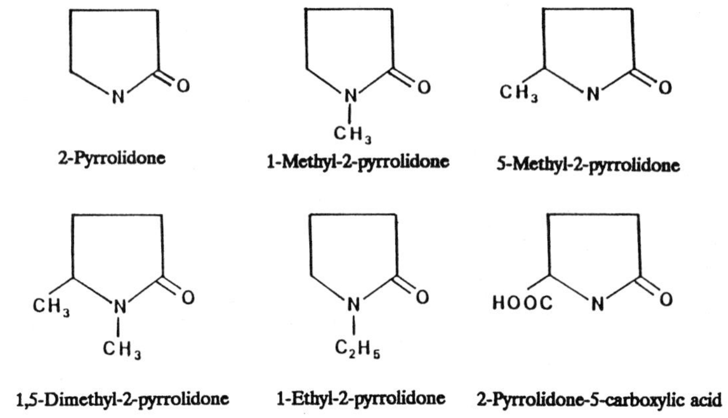

2-Pyrrolidone 1-Methyl-2-pyrrolidone 5-Methyl-2-pyrrolidone

1,5-Dimethyl-2-pyrrolidone 1-Ethyl-2-pyrrolidone 2-Pyrrolidone-5-carboxylic acid

FIG. 7. Structural formulas of pyrrolidone skin-penetration enhancers.

NMP with 1-lauryl-2-pyrrolidone as a vehicle for transdermal delivery, the permeation of phenol red and 5-fluorouracil was dramatically increased [179].

Unfortunately, despite the marked accelerant activity of the pyrrolidones for various drugs, the widespread use of these agents may be constrained because they damage skin, especially at high concentrations [156].

Fatty Acids

Percutaneous drug absorption has been increased by a wide variety of long-chain fatty acids, the most popular of which is oleic acid. Brief details of some of the uses of fatty acids as skin-penetration enhancers are provided in Tables 5 and 6.

A vasoconstrictor assay showed that oleic acid in propylene glycol increased the bioavailability of betamethasone-17-benzoate, whereas incorporation of the acid in an inert vehicle such as dimethylisosorbide provided no such improvement [140]. Other in vivo studies illustrated that oleic acid in propylene glycol is an effective accelerant for nicardipine and ketorolic acid in rhesus monkeys [189] and for azidothylmidine (AZT) in rats [96]. The interaction of oleic acid with horny-layer components has also been investigated in vivo using ATR-FTIR spectroscopy (see above) [113,137,138]. However, oleic acid can irritate the skin, producing erythema and edema in rabbits [185].

Various fatty acids were investigated as accelerants for the drug naloxone [161] in a protocol that illustrated the influence of chain length, branching, and bond saturation on enhancer activity. Lauric acid (C12) was the most effective straight-chain homolog, and cis double bonds in the alkyl chains increased fatty acid activity. Lauric acid is also an effective enhancer for indomethacin, testosterone, and 5-fluorouracil [187].

A "push-pull" mechanism has been proposed for the enhancement of theophylline and adenosine by alkanecarboxylic acids [190,191]. Excess free energy in the donor phase maintains maximum thermodynamic activity of theophylline (the "push" effect), and the accelerants increased drug solubility in the skin (the "pull" effect).

Alkyl esters of fatty acids also act as penetration enhancers. Methyl caprate raises the permeation of vitamin D_3, minoxidil, erythromycin, triamcinalone acetonide, hydrocortisone, and testosterone across hamster skin [192], whereas fatty acid esters enhance hydrocortisone butyrate propionate penetration in rats [193].

TABLE 4 Recent Studies of Pyrrolidones as Skin-Penetration Enhancers[a]

Drug	Pyrrolidone Concentration[b]	Membrane	Temperature (°C)	ER[c]	Reference
Methanol	80% 2-P in water	Human	30	2.3	169
Caffeine				0.83	
Mannitol	100% 2-P	Human	30	1.2	175
	100% NMP			1.6	
Caffeine	100% 2-P	Human	33	3.5[d]	170
Aspirin				7.2[d]	
Mefenamic acid	2% NMP	Rabbit in vivo	Ambient	1.5	176
Naloxone	10% in PG:	Human	37		161
	NMP			1.1	
	HEP			1.1	
	CHP			2.1	
	DAPP			2.4	
	CAP			34.5	
	TAP			24	
Mannitol	100% 2-P	Human	30	448	171
Hydrocortisone				95	
Progesterone				22.6	
Mannitol	100% NMP			256	
Hydrocortisone				8.7	
Progesterone				17.5	
Metronidazole	5% NMP in PG	Human	Ambient	0.95	177,178
	5% NMP in IPM			3.8	
	100% NMP			2.7	
5-Fluorouracil	2 mmol/mL NMP + LP in IPM	Rat	32	32.5	179
Indomethacin	2 mmol/mL in water:	Rat	32		180
	NMP			2.7[e]	
	HP			34.2[e]	
	LP			152[e]	
Sulfaguanidine	2 mmol/mL in water:	Rat	32		181
	NMP			23	
	HP			237	
	LP			275	
Aminopyrine	NMP			3.5	
	HP			23.5	
	LP			12.9	
1-Hexanol	100% 2-P	Rat	37	7	126

[a]In vitro unless otherwise stated.

[b]2-P = 2-pyrrolidone; NMP = 1-methyl-2-pyrrolidone; HEP = *N*-hydroxyethylpyrrolidone; CHP = *N*-cyclohexylpyrrolidone; DAPP = *N*-dimethylaminopropylpyrrolidone; CAP = *N*-cocoalkylpyrrolidone; TAP = *N*-tallowalkylpyrrolidone; LP = 1-lauryl-2-pyrrolidone; HP = 1-hexyl-2-pyrrolidone; PG = propylene glycol; IPM = isopropyl myristate.

[c]ER = Enhancement ratio, calculated from the literature as drug permeation after pyrrolidone treatment vs. control drug permeation.

[d]Calculated from maximum flux values.

[e]Calculated from flux values.

TABLE 5 Recent In Vitro Studies of Oleic Acid (OA) as Skin-Penetration Enhancer

Drug	OA Concentration (%)[a]	Vehicle[b]	Membrane	Temperature (°C)	ER[c]	Reference
Salicylic acid	0.1M	PG	Human	22	28	184
Metronidazole	1	PG	Human	Ambient	3	178
	5	PG			16	
	10	PG			15	
Naloxone	10	PG	Human	37	22	161
Mannitol	5	PG	Human	30	81	171
Hydrocortisone					60	
Progesterone					2.0	
5-Fluorouracil	5	PG	Human	32	20	101
			Hairless mouse		149	
5-Fluorouracil	5	PG	Human	32	17	174
Estradiol					3.5	
Naloxone	10	PG	Human	37	14	185
5-Fluorouracil	5	PG	Human	32	56	186
Estradiol					36	
5-Fluorouracil	5	PG	Human	32	31	104
			Hairless mouse		185	
			American black rat snake		2.3	
			Indian python dorsal		7.3	
			Indian python ventral		13.4	
Propranolol	3.3	PG–ethanol–water	Rabbit	Ambient	7.2	89
4-Cyanophenol	5	PG	Porcine	Ambient	35	138
Piroxicam	0.25	buffer	Hairless mouse	32	1.1	118
	0.25	buffer + 40% ethanol			200	

[a]Unless otherwise stated.
[b]PG = Propylene glycol.
[c]ER = Enhancement ratio, calculated from the literature as drug permeation after OA treatment vs. control drug permeation.

TABLE 6 Recent In Vitro Studies of Fatty Acids (FA) as Skin-Penetration Enhancers

Drug	FA Concentration[a]	Membrane	Temperature (°C)	ER[b]	Reference
Metronidazole	Linoleic acid in PG	Human	Ambient		178
	1%			10	
	5%			17	
	10%			26	
Naloxone	10% in PG	Human	37		161
	Heptanoic acid			29	
	Capric acid			117	
	Lauric acid			147	
	Stearic acid			14	
Indomethacin	10% capric acid in matrix	Hairless mouse	Ambient	8.8	188
Naloxone	10% in PG	Human	37		185
	Palmitoleic acid			38	
	Palmitelaidic acid			28	
Oxymorphone base	10% myristic acid in PG	Human	37	85	102
Oxymorphone HCl				6.7	
Naloxone	0.5 M capric acid in PG	Human	37	31	187
Testosterone				3.6	
Benzoic acid				1.5	
Indomethacin				47	
5-Fluorouracil				66	
Methotrexate				1.3	
Naloxone	0.5 M lauric acid in PG			38	
Testosterone				5.5	
Benzoic acid				1.3	
Indomethacin				102	
5-Fluorouracil				58	
Methotrexate				1.4	

[a]PG = Propylene glycol.
[b]ER = Enhancement ratio, calculated from the literature as drug permeation after fatty acid treatment vs. control drug permeation.

Azone

Azone was the first molecule specifically designed as a skin-penetration enhancer. Chemically it may be considered as a hybrid of a cyclic amide, as in the pyrrolidones, with an alkyl sulfoxide. It has low irritancy and is active at low concentrations (typically 0.1 to 5%). As with oleic acid and terpenes, the cosolvent is an important factor in Azone activity; the polar solvent propylene glycol often acts synergistically with Azone [194].

Azone enhances the skin transport of a wide variety of drugs including steroids, antibiotics, and hydrophilic and lipophilic permeants; its potency has been extensively reviewed [195]. Subsequent studies have shown Azone to be effective toward 5-fluorouracil [104,186], alkanols and steroids [125], and hydrocortisone [196]. The dose-dependent effects have been described [125,196].

A series of Azone derivatives have been synthesized [91,94], and members shown to be effective in promoting acyclovir permeation across hairless mouse and rat skin delivered from a variety of vehicles [197]. Diffusion of drugs with a range of lipophilicities was improved by combination with the Azone derivatives [92].

The absorption, metabolism, and excretion of Azone in humans have been investigated [198,199] as has its toxicity [200].

Surfactants

Surfactants are exclusively used in pharmaceutical, pesticide, and cosmetic formulations, and employed as skin-penetration enhancers for a range of drugs. Surfactants usually consist of a lipophilic alkyl or aryl chain with a hydrophilic head group. They may be classified according to the nature of the head group as anionic (sodium lauryl sulfate, SLS), cationic (cetyltrimethyl ammonium bromide), nonionic (the Synperonic NP series) or, if pH-dependent, zwitterionic (*N*-dodecyl-*N*,*N*-dimethylbetaine). Surfactants as accelerants have been reviewed in detail by Walters [201,202].

In studies that demonstrated that SLS is a powerful irritant, transepidermal water loss in volunteers in vivo was increased [203,204]. Indeed, anionic surfactants, such as SLS and cationic surfactants, strongly irritate skin, swell the stratum corneum, and interact with keratin [205]. The two commercial divalent anionic surfactants preparations, phenylsulfonate CA (70% w/v calcium dodecyl benzenesulfonate) and empicol ML26/F (26.5% w/v magnesium lauryl sulfate), damage human skin in vitro [206]. However, this can be prevented by using nonionic surfactants from the Synperonic NP and PE series in an equimolar mixture with the charged surfactant [206]; the nonionic surfactants themselves are harmless.

Tween 20 (a nonionic polysorbate surfactant) increased the flux of hydrocortisone and lidocaine across hairless-mouse skin [207,208], although other reports found no such evidence. This surfactant did not promote nicardipine or ketorolac permeation in vivo in monkeys [189] or 5-fluorouracil through human skin or snake skin in vitro [104,186]. This anomaly may be attributable to the selection of membranes for permeation studies, because 0.1% Tween 20 in normal saline improved 5-fluorouracil permeation sixfold across hairless mouse skin [104]. This membrane is particularly sensitive to disturbance, and it can be concluded that, in general, nonionic surfactants are, at most, only weak enhancers.

Many traditional dermatological formulations containing ionic surfactants, such as creams stabilized by mixed emulsifiers, probably depend at least in part for their therapeutic activity on the action of the surfactants as accelerants.

Urea

Urea is used as a hydrating agent in the treatment of scaling conditions, such as psoriasis, ichthyosis, and other hyperkeratotic skin conditions. It is mildly keratolytic and hence may affect skin keratin, particularly after prolonged contact.

Urea is available as a 10% cream and as such doubles the water-holding capacity of the horny layer but has little effect on the epidermal water barrier [209]. It increases the activity and bioavailability of the hydrocortisone in Alphaderm cream [210] and promotes the onset of erythema induced by hexyl nicotinate [155,211]. Percutaneous absorption of indomethacin across rabbit skin in vivo is improved by urea [212]. However, 10% urea in propylene glycol does not increase naloxone permeation through human skin in vitro [161], and as a 10% aqueous solution has no effect on the permeation of benzyl nicotinate in vivo [213].

Cyclic, unsaturated urea analogs were synthesized as a series of safe, biodegradable transdermal penetration enhancers [214]. Studies showed some of these analogs to be as effective as Azone in promoting indomethacin diffusion across shed snake and hairless mouse skin [215]. A series of C12 alkyl- and aryl-substituted urea analogs has been synthesized as penetration enhancers [216]. These analogs were moderately effective accelerants applied to human skin in vitro from propylene glycol, for the model hydrophilic drug 5-fluorouracil, whereas urea itself was ineffective.

Alcohols and Glycols

Of the various alcohols studied as skin penetration enhancers, ethanol is most widely used. As a solvent, it increases the flux of levonorgestrel sixfold, estradiol 40-fold, hydrocortisone 20-fold, and 5-fluorouracil fourfold through rat skin [217]. Permeation of estradiol through human skin in vivo can be improved by delivering the steroid from a saturated solution in 95% ethanol [218]. Ethanol is also used to promote estradiol permeation through hairless mouse skin [219,220]. However, the ethanol concentration can affect its activity. An ethanol–water system promotes salicylate ion diffusion across human stratum corneum at an ethanol volume fraction of 0.63 [221]. Higher ethanol volume fractions reduced permeation. Similar observations were made for nitroglycerine [222], where volume fractions of 0.7 or below improved drug flux across human skin but higher alcohol concentrations inhibited penetration. At high concentrations, ethanol and other lower alcohols can extract stratum corneum lipids and dehydrate stratum corneum membranes; these effects should be considered when examining the results of permeation experiments.

Other alkanols used as promoters include lauryl and linolenyl alcohol, which, as 10% solutions in propylene glycol, increased naloxone flux through human skin 29- and 73-fold, respectively [161]. 1-Octanol and 1-propanol increased the flux of salicylic acid across hairless mouse skin [223], and the former provided the optimum chain length to enhance nicotinamide permeation across hairless mouse skin in vitro [136]. Octanol has also been used successfully to promote indomethacin diffusion across hairless mouse skin [188]. The effects of alcohol alkyl-chain length and branching on levonorgestrel permeation through rat skin have been studied [224]; 1-butanol was the most effective enhancer with lower activity reported for branched alcohols.

Glycols are widely used in topical and cosmetic preparations, and several have been evaluated as potential enhancers. Propylene glycol shows mild accelerant activity toward 5-fluorouracil [104,186,216] and estradiol [186,225], whereas other glycols inhibit drug diffusion. Butane-1,2-diol reduces estradiol flux through human skin in vitro [225] and propane-1,3-diol did not promote nicardidpine or ketorolac penetration through monkey skin in vivo [189]. Polyethylene glycol (PEG) 400 reduced the permeability coefficient of estradiol through hairless mouse skin as the glycol concentration increased [226], with a similar trend reported for oxaprozin and guanabenz in human skin [227].

Other Materials

The safest and most widely used penetration enhancer is water [1]. The occlusive nature of many topical products, such as ointments and transdermal patches, increases the hydration of underlying stratum corneum. Generally, an increase in hydration diminishes the resistance of the skin to hydrophilic and lipophilic permeant diffusion [228–232].

Various amines and derivatives have been selected as accelerants. *N*,*N*-diethyl-*m*-toluamide is an insect repellent that enhances the permeation of a range of drugs, including ibuprofen and steroids, across hairless mouse skin [233]. Dodecylamine in propylene glycol improves the flux of testosterone, naloxone, 5-fluorouracil, and indomethacin through human skin in vitro [187), and an ethoxylated amine, *N,N*-bis(2-hydroxyethyl)oleylamine, has been used to augment salicylate anion and caffeine cation movement across human skin [234]. Dodecyl-*N,N*-dimethylamino acetate promotes indomethacin passage through snake skin [235,236]. However, some skin moisturizers, such as sodium pyroglutaminate and *N*-hydroxyethylacetamide, lower the bioavailability of benzyl nicotinate in human volunteers in vitro [213].

Other materials cited as penetration enhancers include *n*-alkanols [97], *n*-alkanes [237], and Orgelase, a leech enzyme that disaggregates the cells of human skin [238].

Essential Oils, Terpenes, and Terpenoids

Essential oils are the volatile, fragrant substances extracted from the flowers, fruit, leaves, and roots of many plants. Various essential oils have been utilized as flavorings, perfumes, and medicines for hundreds of years and their toxicities are well documented [239]. Chemical analysis of essential oils has revealed that they are a complex mixture of compounds including aromatic and nitrogen- and sulfur-containing moieties and terpenes.

The term "terpene" usually describes a compound which is a constituent of an essential oil and contains carbon, hydrogen, and possibly oxygen but is not aromatic. Terpenoid compounds are unified by their chemical structure, being based on isoprene (C_5H_8) units. The terpenes may thus be classified according to the number of isoprene units they contain; monoterpenes (C_{10}) have two isoprene units, sesquiterpenes (C_{15}) have three, and diterpenes (C_{20}) have four. Terpenes may also be subdivided into acyclic, monocyclic, bicyclic, and so forth. The structural formulas of some terpenes and terpenoids assessed as penetration enhancers are given in Fig. 8.

Terpenes have varied applications; for example, menthol is traditionally used in inhalation pharmaceuticals and has a mild antipruritic effect when incorporated into emollient preparations. It also is employed as a fragrance and to flavor toothpastes, peppermint sweets, and mentholated cigarettes. Details of terpenoid biosynthesis, chemistry, and reactions are outside the scope of this article but are well documented in the literature [240–242].

Despite the widespread medicinal usage of many terpenes, there are relatively few reports of their penetration-enhancing properties. 1,8-Cineole (eucalyptol) has been used to promote the percutaneous absorption of several lipophilic drugs through hairless mouse skin [243]. In addition, 1-carvone and eugenol have been patented as skin-penetration enhancers [244,245].

Camphor and eucalyptus oil, as a vehicle containing 50% ethanol, increase the total flux of nicotine permeating hairless mouse skin but have no effect on the kinetics of drug diffusion [246]. However, the authors make no comment on the effects of the ethanolic vehicle on the integrity of hairless mouse skin.

Several terpenoid cyclohexanone derivatives have been evaluated as accelerants for ketoprofen and indomethacin [247,248]. In vitro studies were performed on newborn pig skin, and in vivo experiments on shaved rats. The authors concluded that the promoting effects observed with "bulky" cyclohexanone derivatives were due to an action on the stratum corneum lipid structure, as no change in drug partitioning was detected. Compounds containing an azacyclo ring (similar to Azone) and acyclic terpene hydrocarbon

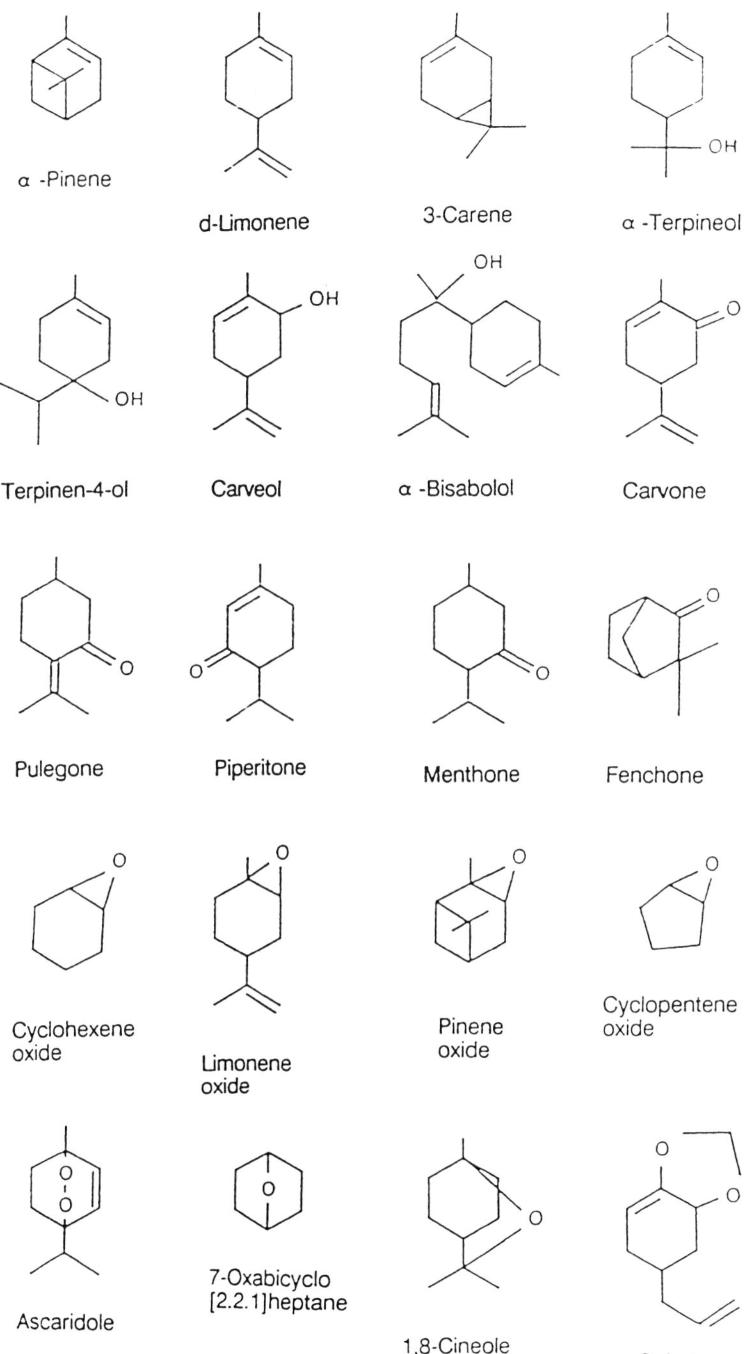

FIG. 8. Structural formulas of simple terpenes and terpenoids.

chains have been evaluated as accelerants for a variety of drugs [91–94,197]. These studies illustrated that azocyclo ring size has little effect on the potency of the accelerants, whereas the length of the hydrophobic terpene chain has a marked effect; a chain length of 12 carbon atoms provided optimal activity. It was concluded that the enhancers operated by increasing the partitioning of drugs into the stratum corneum but did not modify drug diffusivity through the membrane, although the results suggested that the accelerant effects may vary with the species of animal skin used (hairless mouse and rat skins yielded different results).

The essential oils of eucalyptus, chenopodium, and ylang-ylang have been used as penetration enhancers in excised human skin [249]. The most active oil, eucalyptus, increased the permeability coefficient of 5-fluorouracil 34-fold. As an extension of this study, 17 cyclic monoterpenes and terpenoids were evaluated for accelerant activity toward hydrophilic 5-fluorouracil in human skin [128–131,250–252] Hydrocarbon terpenes (e.g., d-limonene) were least active and cyclic ether terpenes (e.g., 1,8-cineole) were most active. Hydrocarbon and cyclic ether terpenes showed similar enhancement toward estradiol permeation through human skin, providing a four- to fivefold increase in membrane permeability coefficients [253].

Some monocyclic monoterpenes have been used as penetration enhancers for lipophilic indomethacin in rat skin [79,254]. Hydrocarbon terpenes were potent enhancers; notably, limonene proved to be as effective as Azone and was active at a concentration of 1% in a gel ointment. The authors concluded that the terpenes have no appreciable effect on drug partitioning and, hence, limonene alters the diffusional barrier function of the stratum corneum. The cyclic monoterpenes that increased permeation of indomethacin had a lipophilic index above zero, whereas oxygen-containing terpenes (e.g., carvone, 1,8-cineole) were ineffective. In a subsequent study, menthol and menthone increased diazepam absorption across rat skin, but less than hydrocarbon monoterpenes [97]. Transdermal permeation of prednisolone, a lipophilic anti-inflammatory steroid, has been improved by the acetone extract of cardamom seed [86]. The active constituents of the extract, the monoterpene terpineol and acetyl terpineol, were more effective than Azone in promoting drug diffusion, although the study used excised shaved mouse skin. Bisabolol, a monocyclic unsaturated sesquiterpene, is an inflammatory-inhibiting agent in skin care products. In propylene glycol, it increases the diffusivity of 5-fluorouracil (5-FU) and triamcinalone acetonide in human skin in vitro [255].

Recently, 12 sesquiterpenes were investigated as putative penetration enhancers for human skin [261]. Pretreatment of epidermal membranes with sesquiterpene oils, or using solid sesquiterpenes saturated in dimethyl isosorbide, increased the absorption rate of 5-FU. Enhancers with polar functional groups were generally more potent than pure hydrocarbons, and enhancers with the least "bunched" structures were the most active. The largest effect was observed following pretreatment with nerolidol, which increased 5-FU flux over 20-fold. Molecular modeling suggested that terpenes with structures suitable for alignment within lipid lamellae were the most potent enhancers. Sesquiterpene enhancers had long durations of action, implying that they did not wash out of the skin easily. Sesquiterpene effects were thus almost fully maintained for at least 4.5 days following pretreatment, which demonstrated poor reversibility.

Small-angle x-ray diffraction investigations of terpene enhancer actions on the lipid barrier in human skin showed that d-limonene and 1,8-cineole markedly reduce bilayer periodicity. Nerolidol, a long-chain sesquiterpene, actually reinforces lipid bilayer periodicity, possibly by orienting alongside stratum corneum lipids [262].

Currently, natural products receive considerable interest in the pharmaceutical industry and, as indicated in the above reviews, terpenes may provide relatively safe, clinically acceptable enhancers for lipophilic and hydrophilic drugs.

Penetration-Enhancer Action

Absorption enhancers may encourage drug permeation across the skin via several mechanisms, and much research is now devoted to elucidating the molecular basis for their actions. Some enhancers are reported to increase the vehicle solubility of a drug [218,222]. Permeation of vehicle components into the skin may then promote drug partitioning into the tissue, an effect responsible for "reservoir formation" following pyrrolidone use [205].

Long-term tissue hydration may form polar channels for drug diffusion [231]. However, this conclusion was drawn from a study using hairless mouse skin over 140 h of experimentation. The integrity of such a membrane after 50 h is questionable [101], and the results are not relevant to humans. High concentrations of ethanol (>50%) have been reported to form pores in the stratum corneum [220], although such an effect may be attributable to the lipid extraction properties of *n*-alkanols [136].

The transport mechanism for ionic drug diffusion into the stratum corneum can be improved by controlling the pH and hence drug ionization [234]. Thus, anions such as salicylate may be transported into the skin against their own concentration gradient.

The lipid-protein-partitioning (LPP) theory has been formulated to correlate literature reports and describe the potential action modes of penetration enhancers [50,51,186,256]. According to this scheme, accelerants may act by one or more of three main mechanisms:

1. Disruption of the highly ordered structure of stratum corneum lipids,
2. Interaction with intracellular protein, and
3. Improved partitioning of a drug, coenhancer, or cosolvent into the stratum corneum.

Studies by Aungst et al. broadly support this theory [187]. Skin-permeation enhancers were described according to their effects on drug solubilization in the vehicle, improvement in partitioning, effects on the barrier nature of the stratum corneum, and effects on solvent permeation.

Many examples of such interactions are cited in the literature [205,256]. Numerous accelerants, including fatty acids (especially cis-unsaturated such as oleic acid), Azone, and terpenes, reduce the order of intercellular lipid domains, an effect that has been well characterized by DSC [41]. Other enhancers, such as nonionic surfactants and keratolytic urea, interact with the corneocyte protein component of the horny layer. Increased partitioning of drugs into the stratum corneum has been reported following pyrrolidone treatments, and the synergism of action noted between propylene glycol and Azone is probably caused by the glycol facilitating Azone permeation into the tissue [195].

A chemical useful as a model enhancer, whose molecular basis of action is becoming clearer, is oleic acid. Infrared spectroscopic studies by Potts and co-workers have revealed that the acid acts by disruption of intercellular lipid domains [118,136–138]. More recent studies implied that oleic acid may coexist as pools in the ordered stratum

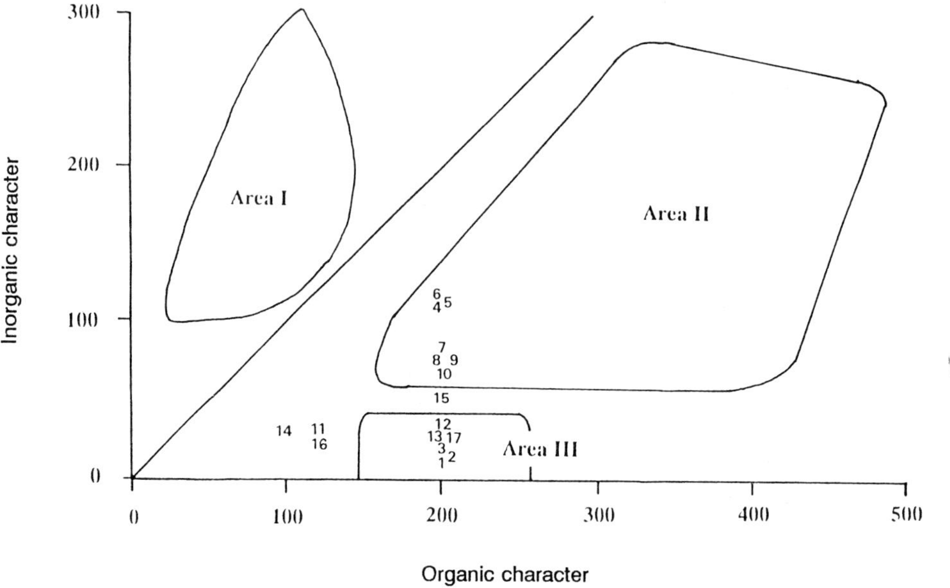

FIG. 9. A conceptual diagram for the classification of skin penetration enhancers. Key: 1, pinene; 2, limonene; 3, carene; 4, terpeneol; 5, terpinen-4-ol; 6, carveol; 7, carvone; 8, pulegone; 9, piperitone; 10, menthone; 11, cyclohexene oxide; 12, limonene oxide; 13, pinene oxide; 14, cyclopentene oxide; 15, ascaridole; 16, 7-oxabicyclo[2.2.2]heptane; 17, 1,8-cineole. (Modified from Hori et al. [259].)

corneum lipid bilayers [257]. Pooling may provide a pathway of diminished resistance for drug transport, with diffusion dependent on the permeant's nature. Such defects in the lipoidal barrier of the stratum corneum may explain the increased permeation of hydrophilic or even ionized molecules, but the authors intimate that oleic acid pools do not act as open pores in the lipid bilayers.

An alternative mechanism for penetration-enhancer action has been proposed, whereby an accelerant may alter the solvent nature of viable epidermal and dermal tissue and promote partitioning of a lipophilic drug from the horny layer into the lower layers of the skin [258]. Such a procedure would increase the clearance rate of the drug. However, for a practical in vivo situation, such alterations of the viable tissue probably would cause excessive skin irritation and damage, making the agent clinically unacceptable.

Based on a conceptual diagram (Fig. 9), accelerants have been classified according to their organic and inorganic character [259] into three areas: Area I in which enhancers are solvents, Area II contains accelerants for hydrophilic compounds, and Area III contains promoters for lipophilic compounds. The solvent area (Area I) contains DMSO and 2-pyrrolidone, compounds that probably exert their enhancing effects mainly by displacing water from around the lipid head groups to create a solvation shell [41,256], although partitioning effects also may be important. Area II includes molecules such as Azone and oleic acid, which probably insert between intercellular lipids, thereby disrupting the ordered bilayer structures [41].

From the present author's own data, terpene activities toward a model hydrophilic (5-fluorouracil) and a model lipophilic (estradiol) drug may be described by an enhancement ratio (ER) where

$$\text{ER} = \frac{\text{Drug permeability coefficent after terpene treatment}}{\text{Drug permeability coefficent before terpene treatment}}$$

These values are represented in Fig. 10 and clearly show that the terpenes have a range of activities toward both drugs.

The alcohol and ketone terpenes lie in Area II of the conceptual diagram, which suggests that the enhancers should increase hydrophilic drug permeation. The studies show that these terpenes are indeed effective enhancers for 5-fluorouracil (hydrophilic) but ineffective for estradiol (lipophilic). Of the other terpenes, the hydrocarbons fall in Area III of the diagram, indicating that they are effective promoters for lipophilic compounds, a prediction verified by the results. The oxide terpenes are scattered in Fig. 9. The terpene, 1,8-cineole is located in the area for enhancers of lipophilic compounds, and did promote estradiol permeation. However, it was also the most effective terpene for promoting 5-fluorouracil permeation, implying that it should be in Area II. Cyclopentene oxide and 7-oxabicyclo[2.2.1]heptane, both effective accelerants for 5-fluorouracil, are near the x-axis but are outside Area II, and ascaridole is situated between Areas II and III.

Thus the conceptual diagram may help to predict the activity of some terpenes (hydrocarbons, alcohols, and ketones) but may mislead if applied to other terpenes (e.g., oxides). The diagram also implies that a penetration enhancer may be effective for either hydrophilic or lipophilic compounds, suggesting that the two effects are mutually exclusive. This is clearly not always true as 1,8-cineole is effective in promoting both 5-fluorouracil and estradiol.

The results of this work indicate that the terpenes appear to be generally more effective accelerants for hydrophilic than for lipophilic compounds (Fig. 10). For example, 1,8-cineole produces an enhancement ratio of 94.5 for 5-fluorouracil and only 4.40 for

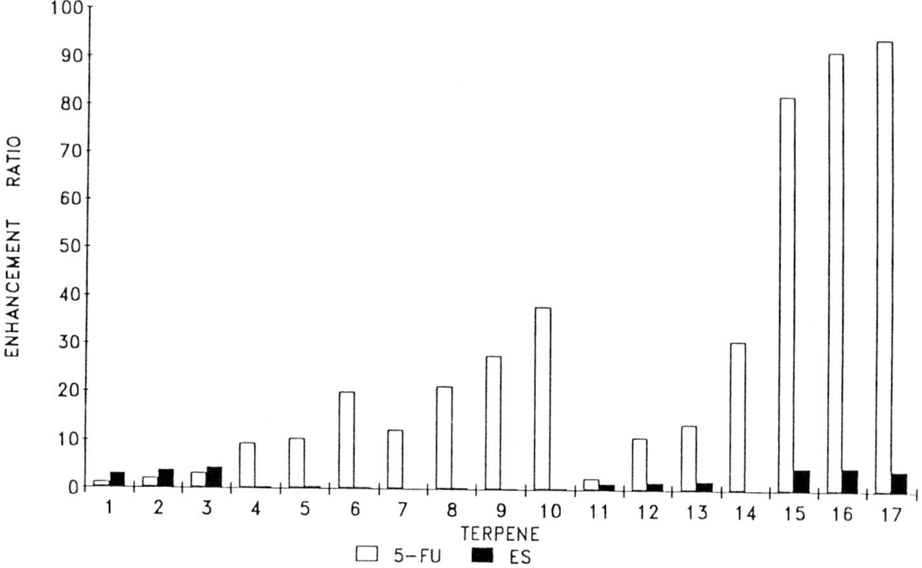

FIG. 10. The accelerant activities of some monoterpenes and terpenoids toward 5-fluorouracil (5-FU, □) and estradiol (ES, ■) in human skin in vitro expressed as enhancement ratios. (See Fig. 9 for key.)

estradiol. However, these small results may mislead as the scope for enhancement of these two drugs varies considerably. Hydrophilic drugs in general have greater potential for enhancement because their permeability coefficients are low, whereas lipophilic drugs have less capacity because their unmodified coefficients already approach a maximum value [260].

To deal with this complication and to describe the activities of penetration enhancers in a more informative way, an enhancement index (EI) has been proposed [253]. The enhancing abilities of chemicals may be more usefully quantified if viewed with respect to the maximum achievable drug permeation, that is, with the barrier layer of the skin removed. The maximum achievable enhancement depends, in part, on the partition coefficient of the permeant. The log *P* (octanol–water) is thus provided as a superscript to the EI, and the maximum ER, provided by stripping the stratum corneum from the skin, is given in a subscript. These two values provide information that places into context the accelerant effect. The EI is calculated as the percentage of the maximum achievable ER induced by enhancer treatment. However, the definition of the ER, which is the ratio of drug permeability coefficients determined after enhancer treatment to that before enhancer treatment, dictates that an ER of 1.0 indicates that an accelerant has no penetration-enhancing activity. To correct for this, the EI is defined as:

$$\mathrm{EI}_{\text{maximum ER}}^{\text{permeant log }P} = \frac{(\text{Enhancement ratio after accelerant treatment}) - 1}{(\text{Maximum enhancement ratio, stratum corneum removed}) - 1} \times 100$$

The EIs of the terpenes measured for 5-fluorouracil and estradiol are given in Fig. 11. These values, for example, show that although the enhancement ratio for 1,8-cineole toward 5-fluorouracil is high (94.5), in terms of the maximum achievable enhancement the terpene activity is low $\mathrm{EI}_{\mathrm{M8400}}^{\mathrm{P}-0.89} = 1.1\%$. On the other hand, for estradiol, although the enhancement ratio is apparently low (4.40), $\mathrm{EI}_{\mathrm{M42}}^{\mathrm{P2.29}} = 8.3\%$, that is, the terpene shows eight times more activity toward the lipophilic drug than toward the hydrophilic permeant, based on assessments of the maximum achievable effect.

Figure 11 indicates that the hydrocarbon and oxide terpenes are more active, in terms of the maximum possible enhancement, toward estradiol than toward 5-fluorouracil, whereas the alcohol and ketone terpenes are more effective with the hydrophilic drug. For estradiol, the hydrocarbon and cyclic ether terpenes (e.g., 1,8-cineole) produce between 5 and 10% of the maximum enhancement, that is, equivalent to up to 10% of the stratum corneum resistance being removed, a value at which the resistance of other skin layers or clearance into the receptor fluid may become significant. For 5-fluorouracil, the hydrocarbons remove less than 0.1% of the barrier resistance, and even the relatively effective cyclic ether terpenes remove only 1% of the stratum corneum resistance. ''Accelerants'' providing ERs of less than 1.0 actually inhibit drug permeation; such agents provide a negative EI. These results imply that, using the conceptual diagram of Hori et al. [259], the oxide terpenes should be located with the hydrocarbon terpenes in the area for enhancers of lipophilic drugs, Area III. Figure 9 shows that this is the case, despite the scatter of the terpenes on the diagram.

The literature provides a fuller consideration of the use of EIs [253]. This concept permits a simple, direct comparison of enhancer activities toward different permeants and informs investigators as to how close (or otherwise) they have approached the ideal situation of complete chemical removal of the horny-layer barrier.

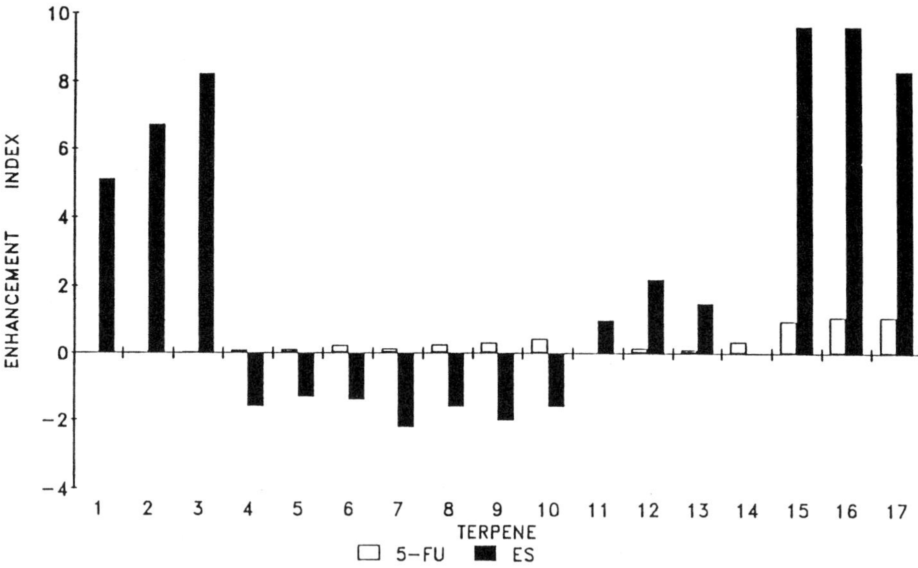

FIG. 11. The enhancing activities of some monoterpenes and terpenoids towards 5-fluorouracil (5-FU, □) and estradiol (ES, ■) in human skin in vitro, expressed as enhancement indices. (See Fig. 9 for key.)

Conclusions

The stratum corneum presents a formidable barrier to transdermal drug delivery, although penetration enhancers offer potential for reversibly reducing this barrier function. A wide variety of chemicals has been used as skin-penetration enhancers, but fundamental investigations of their modes of action are still in their infancy. By using modern analytical techniques such as DSC, FTIR spectroscopy, XRD and, in the future, FT Raman spectroscopy [263,264], the molecular basis of accelerant action may be soon assessed. Additionally, toxicological studies on many synthetic penetration enhancers are required before such agents are approved by the regulatory authorities for clinical use.

Meanwhile, the number of research papers devoted to the subject of skin penetration enhancers appears to grow exponentially year by year. Recent publications include further work on Azone and its derivatives [265–275], Transcutol [273], dodecyl-L-pyroglutamate [274], dodecyl *N,N*-dimethylamino acetate [275] and isopropionate [276] (both biodegradable), aminocaproic acid esters [277], nonane and nonanol [278,279], terpenes [280,281], and cationic [282] and nonionic [283] surfactants. The role that ethanol plays in transdermal delivery has been considered further [284–288], together with the effect of tricaprylin [289], Azone, isopropyl myristate, Sefsol-318, and menthol [290]. The enhancing effects of pyrrolidone derivatives [291–294], propylene glycol [295], propylene glycol with fatty acids [296], and *N,N*-diethyl-*m*-toluamide (DEET) [287] have been further investigated. Cyclodextrins are widely used in the pharmaceutical sciences and their possible effects in percutaneous absorption have now been considered by several authors [298–301]. Finally, lauroylsarcosine [302], bile acids [303], and sucrose laurate should be mentioned, the last for topical preparations of cyclosporin A [304].

Bibliography

Barry, B. W., *Dermatological Formulations: Percutaneous Absorption*, Marcel Dekker, Inc., New York and Basel, 1983.

Bronaugh, R. L., and Maibach, H. I., eds., *Percutaneous Absorption*, 2nd ed., Marcel Dekker, Inc., New York and Basel, 1989.

Bronaugh, R. L. and Maibach, H. I., eds., *In Vitro Percutaneous Absorption: Principles, Fundamentals and Applications*, CRC Press, Boca Raton, FL, 1991.

Gurner, R., and Teubner, A., eds., *Dermal and Transdermal Drug Delivery*, Wissenschaftliche Verlagsgesellschaft mbH, Stuttgart, 1993.

Walters, K. A., and Hadgraft, J., eds., *Pharmaceutical Skin Penetration Enhancement*, Marcel Dekker, Inc., New York, Basel and Hong Kong, 1993.

References

1. Barry, B. W., *Dermatological Formulations: Percutaneous Absorption*, Marcel Dekker, Inc., New York and Basel, 1983.
2. Guy, R. H., and Hadgraft, J., Transdermal drug delivery: The ground rules are emerging, *Pharm. Int.*, 6:112 (1985).
3. Powers, M. S., Schenkel, L., Darley, P. E., Good, W. R., Balestra, J. C., and Place, V. A., Pharmacokinetics and pharmacodynamics of transdermal dosage forms of 17β-estradiol: comparison with conventional oral estrogens used for hormone replacement, *Am. J. Obstet. Gynecol.*, 152:1099 (1985).
4. Chetkowski, R. J., Meldrum, D. R., Steingold, K. A., Randle, D., Luk, J. K., Eggena, P., Hershman, J. M., Alkjaersig, N. K., Fletcher, A. P., and Judd, H. L., Biologic effects of transdermal estradiol., *N. Engl. J. Med.*, 314:1615 (1986).
5. Chien, Y. W., Chien, T. Y., Bagdon, R. E., Huang, Y. C., and Bierman, R. H., Transdermal dual-controlled delivery of contraceptive drugs: formulation development, in vitro and in vivo evaluations, and clinical performance, *Pharm. Res.*, 6:1000 (1989).
6. Crust, M. P., Ganger, K. F., and Whitehead, M. I., Administration of steroids by skin patches, *Res. Reprod.*, 21:1 (1989).
7. Yum, S. I., Transdermal therapeutic systems and rate controlled drug delivery, *Med. Prog. Technol.*, 15:47 (1989).
8. Meyer, B. R., O'Mara, V., and Reidenberg, M. M., A controlled clinical trial of the addition of transdermal scopolamine to a standard metoclopramide and dexamethasone antiemetic regimen, *J. Clin. Oncol.*, 5:1994 (1987).
9. Langley, M. S., and Heel, R. C., Transdermal clonidine; a preliminary review of its pharmacodynamic properties and therapeutic efficacy, *Drugs*, 35:123 (1988).
10. Ornish, S. A., Zisook, S., and McAdams, L. A., Effects of transdermal clonidine treatment on withdrawal symptoms associated with smoking cessation; a randomized, controlled trial, *Arch. Intern. Med.*, 148:2027 (1988).
11. Green, J. J., and Cordes, D. H., Transdermal clonidine therapy and nicotine withdrawal, *West J. Med.*, 151:79 (1989).
12. Parra, R. O., and Gregory, J. G., Treatment of post-orchiectomy hot flashes with transdermal administration of clonidine, *J. Urol.*, 143:753 (1990).
13. Corbo, M., Liu, J. C., and Chien, Y. W., Transdermal controlled delivery of propranolol from a multilaminate adhesive device, *Pharm. Res.*, 6:753 (1989).
14. Corbo, M., Liu, J. C., and Chien, Y. W., Bioavailability of propranolol following oral and transdermal administration in rabbits, *J. Pharm. Sci.*, 79:584 (1990).

15. Gourlay, G. K., Kowalski, S. R., Plummer, J. L., Cherry, D. A., Gaukroger, P., and Cousins, M. J., The transdermal administration of fentanyl in the treatment of postoperative pain: pharmacokinetics and pharmacodynamic effects, *Pain*, 37:193 (1989).
16. Plezia, P. M., Kramer, T. H., Linford, J., and Hameroff, S. R., Transdermal fentanyl: pharmacokinetics and preliminary clinical evaluation, *Pharmacother.*, 9:2 (1989).
17. Gourlay, G. K., Kowalski, S. R., Plummer, J. L., Cherry, D. A., Szekely, S. M., Mather, L. E., Owen, H., and Cousins, M. J., The efficacy of transdermal fentanyl in the treatment of postoperative pain: a double blind comparison of fentanyl and placebo systems, *Pain*, 40:21 (1990).
18. Buchkremer, G., and Minneker, E., Efficiency of multimodel smoking cessation therapy combining transdermal nicotine substitution with behavioral therapy, *Meth. Find. Clin. Pharmacol.*, 11:215 (1989).
19. Dubois, J. P., Sioufi, A., Muller, P. H., Mauli, D., and Imhof, P. R., Pharmacokinetics and bioavailability of nictone in healthy volunteers following single and repeated administration of different doses of transdermal nicotine systems, *Meth. Find. Clin. Pharmacol.*, 11:187 (1989).
20. Carey, P. O., Howards, S. S., and Vance, M. L., Transdermal testosterone treatment of hypogonadal men, *J. Urol.*, 140:76 (1988).
21. Ahmed, S. R., Boucher, A. E., Manni, A., Santen, R. J., Bartholomew, M., and Demers, L. M., Transdermal testosterone therapy in the treatment of male hypogonadism, *J. Clin. Endocrinol. Metab.*, 66:546 (1988).
22. Cunningham, G. R., Cordero, E., and Thornby, J. I., Testosterone replacement with transdermal therapeutic systems; physiological serum testosterone and elevated dihydrotestosterone levels, *JAMA*, 261:2525 (1989).
23. Pikal, M. J., Transport mechanisms in iontophoresis. I. A theoretical model for the effect of electroosmotic flow on flux enhancement in transdermal iontophoresis, *Pharm. Res.*, 7:118 (1990).
24. Roberts, M. S., Singh, J., Yoshida, N., and Currie, K. I., Iontophoretic transport of selected solutes through human epidermis. In: *Prediction of Percutaneous Penetration: Methods, Measurements, Modelling* (R. C. Scott, R. H. Guy, and J. Hadgraft, eds.), IBC Technical Services Ltd., London, 1990, p. 231.
25. Barry, B. W., Southwell, D., and Woodford, R., Optimisation of bioavailability of topical steroids: penetration enhancers under occlusion, *J. Invest. Dermatol.*, 82:49 (1984).
26. Idson, B., Vehicle effects in percutaneous absorption, *Drug Metab. Rev.*, 14:207 (1983).
27. Kubota, K., Yamada, T., Ogura, A., and Ishizaki, T., A novel differential method of vehicle models for topically applied drugs: Application to a therapeutic timolol patch, *J. Pharm. Sci.*, 79:170 (1990).
28. Murphy, T. M., and Hadgraft, J., A physicochemical interpretation of phonophoresis in skin penetration enhancement. In: *Prediction of Percutaneous Penetration: Methods, Measurement, Modelling* (R. C. Scott, R. H. Guy, and J. Hadgraft, eds.), IBC Technical Services Ltd., London, 1990, p. 333.
29. Wilkes, G. L., Brown, I. A., and Widnauer, R. H., The biomechanical properties of skin, *CRC Crit. Rev. Bioeng.*, p. 453 (1973).
30. Millington, P. F., and Wilkinson, R., *Skin; Biological Structure and Function*, Vol. 9, Cambridge University Press, New York, 1983.
31. Wood, E. J., and Bladon, P. T. *The Human Skin; Studies in Biology Series*, No. 164, Edward Arnold, London 1985.
32. Marks, R. M., Barton, S. P., and Edwards, C., *The Physical Nature of the Skin*, MTP Press Ltd., Lancaster, 1988.
33. Lampe, M. A., Burligame, A. L., Whitney, J., Williams, M. L., Brown, B. E., Roitman, E., and Elias, P. M., Human stratum corneum lipids: characterization and regional variations, *J. Lipid Res.*, 24:120 (1983).

34. Elias, P. M., Goerke, J., and Friend, D. S., Mammalian epidermal barrier layer lipids: composition and influence on structure, *J. Invest. Dermatol.*, 69:535 (1977).
35. Elias, P. M., Epidermal lipids, membranes and keratinization, *Int. J. Dermatol.*, 20:1 (1981).
36. Elias, P. M., Epidermal lipids, barrier function, and desquamation, *J. Invest. Dermatol.*, 80:445 (1983).
37. Wertz, P. W., and Downing, D. T., Stratum corneum: biological and biochemical considerations. In: *Transdermal Drug Delivery; Developmental Issues and Research Initiatives* (J. Hadgraft, and R. H. Guy, eds.), Marcel Dekker, Inc., New York and Basel, 1989, Chap. 1.
38. Wertz, P. M., Madison, K. C., and Downing, D. T., Covalently bound lipids of human stratum corneum, *J. Invest. Dermatol.*, 92:109 (1989).
39. Michaels, A. S., Chanderasekaran, S. K., and Shaw, J. E., Drug permeation through human skin: theory and in vitro experimental measurement, *A. I. Ch. E. J.*, 21:985 (1975).
40. Chanderasekaran, S. K., and Shaw, J. E., Factors influencing the percutaneous absorption of drugs, *Curr. Probl. Dermatol.*, 7:142 (1978).
41. Barry, B. W., Mode of action of penetration enhancers in human skin, *J. Control. Rel.*, 6:85 (1987).
42. Elias, P. M., and Friend, D. S., The permeability barrier in mammalian epidermis, *J. Cell Biol.*, 65:180 (1975).
43. Grayson, S., and Elias, P. M., Isolation and lipid biochemical characterization of stratum corneum membrane complexes: implications for the cutaneous permeability barrier, *J. Invest. Dermatol.*, 78:128 (1982).
44. Williams, M. L., and Elias, P. M., The extracellular matrix of stratum corneum: role of lipids in normal and pathological function, *CRC Crit. Rev. Ther. Drug Carrier Syst.*, 3:95 (1987).
45. Knutson, K., Potts, R. O., Guzek, D. B., Golden, G. M., McKie, J. E., Lambert, W. J., and Higuchi, W. I., Macro- and molecular physical-chemical considerations in understanding drug transport in the stratum corneum. In: *Advances in Drug Delivery Systems* (J. M. Anderson, and S. W. Kim, eds.), Elsevier, Amsterdam, Vol. 1, 1986, p. 67.
46. Potts, R. O., Physical characterisation of the stratum corneum: the relationship of mechanical and barrier properties to lipid and protein structure. In: *Transdermal Drug Delivery; Developmental Issues and Research Initiatives* (J. Hadgraft, and R. H. Guy, eds.), Chap. 2, Marcel Dekker, Inc., New York and Basel, 1989.
47. Wertz, P. W., Madison, K. C., and Downing, D. T., Covalently bound lipids of human stratum corneum, *J. Invest. Dermatol.*, 92:109 (1989).
48. Wertz, P. W., Swartzendruber, D. C., Kitko, D. J., Madison, K. C., and Downing, D. T., The role of corneocyte lipid envelopes in cohesion of the stratum corneum, *J. Invest. Dermatol.*, 93:169 (1989).
49. White, S. H., Mirejovsky, D., and King, G. I., Structure of lamellar lipid domains and corneocyte envelopes of murine stratum corneum: an X-ray diffraction study, *Biochemistry*, 27:3725 (1988).
50. Barry, B. W., The LPP theory of skin penetration. In: *In vitro Percutaneous Absorption; Principles, Fundamentals and Applications* (R. L. Bronaugh, and H. I. Maibach, eds.), CRC Press, Boca Raton, FL, 1991, p. 165.
51. Barry, B. W., Lipid-protein-partitioning theory of skin penetration enhancement, *J. Control. Rel.*, 15:237 (1991).
52. Lubowe, I. I., *New Hope for Your Skin*, Dutton, New York, 1963.
53. Wells, F. W., and Lubowe, I. I., *Cosmetics and The Skin*, Von Nostrand, Reinhold, New York, 1964.
54. Scheuplein, R. I., Mechanisms of percutaneous absorption. II. Transient diffusion and the relative importance of various routes of skin penetration, *J. Invest. Dermatol.*, 48:79 (1967).

55. Blank, I. H., Penetration of low-molecular weight alcohols into skin. I. The effect of concentration of alcohol and type of vehicle, *J. Invest. Dermatol.*, 43:415 (1964).
56. Kligman, A. M. In: *The Epidermis* (M. Montagu, and W. C. Lobitz, eds.), Academic Press, new York, 1964, p. 387.
57. Malkinson, F. D. In: *The Epidermis* (M. Montagu, and W. C. Lobitz, eds.), Academic Press, New York, 1964, p. 435.
58. Scheuplein, E. J., and Blank, I. H., Permeability of the skin, *Physiol. Rev.*, 51:702 (1971).
59. Illel, B., Schaefer, H., Wepierre, J., and Doucet, O., Follicles play an important role in percutaneous absorption, *J. Pharm. Sci.*, 80:424 (1991).
60. Tregear, R. T., The permeability of mammalian skin to ions, *J. Invest. Dermatol.*, 46:16 (1966).
61. Scheuplein, R. J., Percutaneous absorption after twenty-five years: or "old wine in new wineskins," *J. Invest. Dermatol.*, 67:31 (1976).
62. Wahlberg, J. E., Effect of anionic, cationic and nonionic detergents on the percutaneous absorption of sodium chromate ^{51}Cr in the guinea pig, *Acta Dermato-Venereol.*, 48:549 (1968).
63. Shelley, W. B., and Melton, F. M., Factors accelerating the penetration of histamine through normal intact human skin, *J. Invest. Dermatol.*, 13:61 (1949).
64. Sweeney, T. M., and Downing, D. T., Role of lipids in epidermal barrier to water diffusion, *J. Invest. Dermatol.*, 55:135 (1970).
65. Curatolo, W., The lipoidal permeability barriers of the skin and alimentary tract, *Pharm. Res.*, 4:271 (1987).
66. Stoughton, R. B., Percutaneous absorption of drugs, *Annu. Rev. Pharmacol. Toxicol.*, 29:55 (1989).
67. Higuchi, T., Design of chemical structure for optimal dermal delivery, *Curr. Probl. Dermatol.*, 7:121 (1978).
68. Flynn, G. L., Mechanism of percutaneous absorption from physicochemical evidence. In: *Percutaneous Absorption* (R. L. Bronaugh and H. I. Maibach, eds.), Marcel Dekker, Inc., New York and Basel, 1985, p. 17.
69. Frienkel, R. K., Carbohydrate metabolism of epidermis. In: *Biochemistry and Physiology of the Skin* (L. A. Goldsmith, ed.), Vol. I., Oxford University Press, Oxford, 1983, p. 328.
70. Martin, R. J., Denyer, S. P., and Hadgraft, J., Skin metabolism of topically applied compounds, *Int. J. Pharm.*, 39:23 (1987).
71. Smith, L. H., and Holland, J. M., Interaction between benzo(a)pyrene and mouse skin in organ culture, *Toxicology*, 21:47 (1981).
72. Holland, J. M., Kao, J. Y., and Whitaker, M. J., A multisample apparatus for kinetic evaluation of skin penetration in vitro: the influence of viability and metabolic status of the skin, *Toxicol. Appl. Pharmacol.*, 72:272 (1984).
73. Scheuplein, R. J., Mechanism of percutaneous adsorption. I. Routes of penetration and the influence of solubility, *J. Invest. Dermatol.*, 45:334 (1965).
74. Flynn, G. L., Yalkowski, S. H., and Roseman, T. J., Mass transport phenomena and models: theoretical concepts, *J. Pharm. Sci.*, 63:479 (1974).
75. Crank, J., *The Mathematics of Diffusion*, 2nd ed., Oxford University Press (Clarendon), London, 1975.
76. Guy, R. H., and Hadgraft, J., Physicochemical aspects of percutaneous penetration and its enhancement, *Pharm. Res.*, 5:753 (1988).
77. Spruance, S. L., McKeough, M., Sugibayashi, K., Robertson, F., Gaede, P., and Clark, D. S., Effect of Azone and propylene glycol on penetration of trifluorothymidine through skin and efficacy of different topical formulations against cutaneous herpes simplex virus infections in guinea pigs, *Antimicrob. Agents Chemother.*, 26:819 (1984).
78. Ohshima, T., Yoshikawa, H., Takada, K., and Muranishi, S., Enhancing effect of absorption promoters on percutaneous absorption of a model dye (6-carboxyfluorescein) as a poorly ab-

sorbable drug. III. Histological study after addition of various absorption promoters in rats, *J. Pharmacobio-Dyn.*, 9:223 (1986).

79. Okabe, H., Takayama, K., Ogura, A., and Nagai, T., Effect of limonene and related compounds on the percutaneous absorption of indomethacin, *Drug Design Del.*, 4:313 (1989).
80. Maibach, H. I., In vivo percutaneous penetration of corticoids in man and unresolved problems in their efficacy, *Dermatologica*, 152 (Suppl.1):11 (1976).
81. Southwell, D., Barry, B. W., and Woodford, R., Variations in permeability of human skin within and between specimens, *Int. J. Pharm.*, 18 299 (1984).
82. Feldmann, R. J., and Maibach, H. I., Regional variation in percutaneous penetration of ^{14}C cortisol in man, *J. Invest. Dermatol.*, 48:181 (1967).
83. Bennett, S. L., and Barry, B. W., The use of human scalp and abdominal skin as in vitro models for percutaneous absorption. In: *Skin Models; Models to Study Function and Disease of Skin* (R. Marks and G. Plewig, eds.), Springer-Verlag, Berlin, 1987, p. 245.
84. Touitou, E., and Abed, L., Effect of propylene glycol, Azone and *n*-decylmethyl sulphoxide on skin permeation kinetics of 5-fluorouracil, *Int. J. Pharm.*, 27:89 (1985).
85. Huq, A. S., Ho, N. F. H., Husari, N., Flynn, G. L., Jetzer, W. E., and Condie, L., Permeation of water contaminative phenols through hairless mouse skin, *Arch. Environ. Contam. Toxicol.*, 15:557 (1986).
86. Yamahara, J., Kashiwa, H., Kishi, K., and Fujimura, H., Dermal penetration enhancement by crude drugs: in vitro skin permeation of prednisolone enhanced by active constituents in cardamon seed, *Chem. Pharm. Bull.*, 37:855 (1989).
87. Susten, A. S., Dames, B. L., and Niemeier, R. W., In vivo percutaneous absorption studies of volatile solvents in hairless mice. I. Description of a skin depot, *J. Appl. Toxicol.*, 6:43 (1986).
88. Choi, H. K., Flynn, G. L., and Amidon, G. L., Transdermal delivery of bioactive peptides: the effect of *n*-decylmethyl sulfoxide, pH and inhibitors on enkephalin metabolism and transport, *Pharm. Res.*, 7:1099 (1990).
89. Ogiso, T., and Shintani, M., Mechanism for the enhancement effect of fatty acids on the percutaneous absorption of propranolol, *J. Pharm. Sci.*, 79:1065 (1990).
90. Sheth, N. V., Freeman, D. J., Higuchi, W. I., and Spruance, S. L., The influence of Azone, propylene glycol and polyethylene glycol on in vitro skin penetration of trifluorothymidine, *Int. J. Pharm.*, 28:201 (1986).
91. Okamoto, H., Hashida, M., and Sezaki, H., Structure-activity relationship of 1-alkyl- or 1-alkenylazacycloalkanone derivatives as percutaneous penetration enhancers, *J. Pharm. Sci.*, 77:418 (1988).
92. Okamoto, H., Hashida, M., and Sezaki, H., Effect of 1-alkyl or 1-alkenylazacycloalkanone derivatives on the penetration of drugs with different lipophilicities through guinea pig skin, *J. Pharm. Sci.*, 80:39 (1991).
93. Okamoto, H., Ohyabu, M., Hashida, M., and Sezaki, H., Enhanced penetration of mitomycin C through hairless mouse and rat skin by enhancers with terpene moieties, *J. Pharm. Pharmacol.*, 39:531 (1987).
94. Okamoto, H., Tsukahara, H., Hashida, M., and Sezaki, H., Effect of 1-alkyl- or 1-alkenylazacycloalkanone derivatives on penetration of mitomycin C through rat skin, *Chem. Pharm. Bull.*, 35:4605 (1987).
95. Sasaki, H., Kojima, M., Mori, Y., Nakamura, J., and Shibasaki, J., Enhancing effect of pyrrolidone derivatives on transdermal drug delivery. I, *Int. J. Pharm.*, 44:15 (1988).
96. Seki, T., Kawaguchi, T., Sugibayashi, K., Juni, K., and Morimoto, Y., Percutaneous absorption of azidothymidine in rats, *Int. J. Pharm.*, 57:73 (1989).
97. Hori, M., Satoh, S., Maibach, H. I., and Guy, R. H., Enhancement of propranolol hydrochloride and diazepam skin absorption in vitro: effect of enhancer lipophilicity, *J. Pharm. Sci.*, 80:32 (1991).

98. Itoh, T., Magavi, R., Casady, R. L., Nishihata, T., and Rytting, J. H., A method to predict the percutaneous permeability of various compounds: shed snake skin as a model membrane, *Pharm. Res.*, 7:1302 (1990).
99. Bond, J. R., and Barry, B. W., Damaging effect of acetone on the permeability barrier of hairless mouse skin compared with that of human skin, *Int. J. Pharm.*, 41:91 (1988).
100. Bond, J. R., and Barry, B. W., Limitations of hairless mouse skin as a model for in vitro permeation studies through human skin: hydration damage, *J. Invest. Dermatol.*, 90:486 (1988).
101. Bond, J. R., and Barry, B. W., Hairless mouse skin is limited as a model for assessing the effects of penetration enhancers in human skin, *J. Invest. Dermatol.*, 90:810 (1988).
102. Aungst, B. J., Blake, J. A., Rogers, N. J., and Hussain, M. A., Transdermal oxymorphone formulation development and methods for evaluating flux and lag times for two skin permeation-enhancing vehicles, *J. Pharm. Sci.*, 79:1072 (1990).
103. Sherertz, E. F., Sloan, K. B., and McTiernan, R. G., Transdermal delivery of 5-fluorouracil through skin of hairless mice and humans in vitro: a comparison of the effect of formulations and a prodrug, *Arch. Dermatol. Res.*, 282:463 (1990).
104. Rigg, P. C., and Barry, B. W., Shed snake skin and hairless mouse skin as model membranes for human skin during permeation studies, *J. Invest. Dermatol.*, 94:235 (1990).
105. Sato, K., Sugibayashi, K., and Morimoto, Y., Species differences in percutaneous absorption of nicorandil, *J. Pharm. Sci.*, 80:104 (1991).
106. Bulgin, J. J., and Vinso, L. J., The use of differential thermal analysis to study the bound water in stratum corneum membranes, *Biochem. Biophys. Acta*, 136:551 (1967).
107. Walkley, K., Bound water in stratum corneum measured by differential scanning calorimetry, *J. Invest. Dermatol.*, 59:335 (1972).
108. Inove, T., Tsuji, K., Okamoto, K., and Toda, K., Differential scanning calorimetric studies on the melting behaviour of water in stratum corneum, *J. Invest. Dermatol.*, 86:689 (1986).
109. Takenouchi, M., Suzuki, H., and Tagami, H., Hydration characteristics of pathologic stratum corneum: evaluation of bound water, *J. Invest. Dermatol.*, 87:574 (1986).
110. Van Duzee, B. F., Thermal analysis of human stratum corneum, *J. Invest. Dermatol.*, 65:404 (1975).
111. Goodman, M., and Barry, B. W., Differential scanning calorimetry of human stratum corneum: effects of penetration enhancers Azone and dimethyl sulphoxide, *Anal. Proc.*, 23:397 (1986).
112. Golden, G. M., Guzek, D. B., Harris, R. R., McKie, J. E., and Potts, R. O., Lipid thermotropic transitions in human stratum corneum, *J. Invest. Dermatol.*, 86:255 (1986).
113. Goodman, M., and Barry, B. W., Action of penetration enhancers on human stratum corneum as assessed by differential scanning calorimetry. In: *Percutaneous Absorption*, 2nd ed., Chap. 33 (R. L. Bronaugh and H. I. Maibach, eds.), Marcel Dekker, Inc., New York and Basel, 1989.
114. Rehfeld, S. J., Lampe, M. A., and Elias, P. M., Do lipid phase transitions underline cohesion and dyshesion of stratum corneum? *J. Invest. Dermatol.*, 78:327 (1981).
115. Knutson, K., Potts, R. O., Guzek, D. B., Golden, G. M., McKie, J. E., Lambert, W. J., and Higuchi, W. I., Macro- and molecular-physical considerations in understanding drug transport in the stratum corneum, *J. Control. Rel.*, 2:67 (1985).
116. Golden, G. M., McKie, J. E., and Potts, R. O., The role of stratum corneum lipid fluidity in transdermal drug flux, *J. Pharm. Sci.*, 76:25 (1986).
117. Golden, G. M., Guzek, D. B., Kennedy, A. H., McKie, J. E., and Potts, R. O., Stratum corneum lipid phase transitions and water barrier properties, *Biochemistry*, 26:2382 (1986).
118. Francoeur, M. L., Golden, G. M., and Potts, R. O., Oleic acid: the effects on stratum corneum in relation to (trans)dermal drug delivery, *Pharm. Res.*, 7:621 (1990).
119. Knutson, K., Potts, R. O., Guzek, D. B., Golden, G. M., McKie, J. E., Lambert, W. J., and Higuchi, W. I., Macro- and molecular physical-chemical considerations in understudy-

ing drug transport in the stratum corneum. In: *Advances in Drug Delivery Systems* (J. M. Anderson and S. W. Kim, eds.), Elsevier, Amsterdam, 1986, p. 67.

120. Bouwstra, J. A., Peschier, L. J. C., Brussee, J., and Bodde, H. E., Effect of N-alkyl-azacycloheptan-2-one including Azone on the thermal behaviour of human stratum corneum, *Int. J. Pharm.*, 52:47 (1989).

121. Al-Saidan, S. M. H., Winfield, A. J., and Selkirk, A. B., Effect of preheating on the permeability of neonatal rat stratum corneum to alkanols, *J. Invest. Dermatol.*, 89:430 (1987).

122. Swartzendruber, D. C., Wertz, P. W., Madison, K. C., and Downing, D. T., Evidence that the corneocyte has a chemically bound lipid envelope, *J. Invest. Dermatol.*, 88:709 (1987).

123. Goodman, M., and Barry, B. W., Differential scanning calorimetry of human stratum corneum: effect of Azone, *J. Pharm. Pharmacol.*, 37 (Suppl.):80P (1985).

124. Goodman, M., and Barry, B. W., Action of skin penetration enhancers Azone, oleic acid and decylmethylsulphoxide: permeation and differential scanning calorimetry studies, *J. Pharm. Pharmacol.*, 38 (Suppl.):71P (1986).

125. Lambert, W. J., Higuchi, W. I., Knutson, K., and Krill, S. L., Dose-dependent enhancement effects of Azone on skin permeability, *Pharm. Res.*, 6:798 (1989).

126. Winfield, A. J., and Taylor, P. M., Thermal analysis as a screen for potential skin penetration enhancers. In: *Prediction of Percutaneous Penetration*; *Methods, Measurements, Modelling* (R. C. Scott, R. H. Guy, and J. Hadgraft, eds.), IBC Technical Services Ltd., London, 1990, p. 412.

127. French, E. J., Pouton, C. W., and Steele, G., Fluidization of lipid bilayers by non-ionic surfactants: structure-activity studies using a fluorescent probe. In: *Prediction of Percutaneous Penetration*; *Methods, Measurements, Modelling* (R. C. Scott, R. H. Guy, and J. Hadgraft, eds.), IBC Technical Services Ltd., London, 1990, p. 308.

128. Williams, A. C., and Barry, B. W., Permeation, FTIR and DSC investigations of terpene penetration enhancers in human skin, *J. Pharm. Pharmacol.*, 41 (Suppl.):12P (1989).

129. Williams, A. C., and Barry, B. W., Techniques for elucidating the modes of action of terpene penetration enhancers, *Proc. Int. Symposium on Present Developments and Future Challenges in Transdermal Drug Delivery*, II, Karger, Basel, 1989, p. 5.

130. Williams, A. C., and Barry, B. W., Correlation of differential scanning calorimetric parameters with skin penetration enhancing activity of terpenes, *Pharm. Res.*, 7 (Suppl.):112 (1990).

131. Williams, A. C., and Barry, B. W., Differential scanning calorimetry does not predict the activity of terpene penetration enhancers in human skin, *J. Pharm. Pharmacol.*, 42 (Suppl.):156P (1990).

132. Oertel, R. P., Protein conformational changes induced in human stratum corneum by organic sulfoxides: an infrared spectroscopic investigation, *Biopolymers*, 16:2329 (1977).

133. Potts, R. O., Guzek, D. B., Harris, R. R., and McKie, J. E., A non-invasive, in vivo technique to quantitatively measure water concentration of the stratum corneum using attenuated total-reflectance infrared spectroscopy, *Arch. Dermatol. Res.*, 277:489 (1985).

134. Mak, V. H. W., Potts, R. O., and Guy, R. H., Does hydration affect intercellular lipid organization in the stratum corneum?, *Pharm. Res.*, 8:1064 (1991).

135. Bommannan, D., Potts, R. O., and Guy, R. H., Examination of stratum corneum barrier function in vivo by infrared spectroscopy, *J. Invest. Dermatol.*, 95:403 (1990).

136. Kai, T., Mak, V. H. W., Potts, R. O., and Guy, R. H., Mechanism of skin penetration enhancement: effect of *n*-alkanols on the permeability barrier, *Proc. Int. Symp. Control. Rel. Bioactive. Mater.*, 15:211 (1988).

137. Guy, R. H., Mak, V. H. W., Kai, T., Bommannan, D., and Potts, R. O., Percutaneous penetration enhancers: mode of action. In: *Prediction of Percutaneous Penetration*; *Methods, Measurements, Modelling* (R. C. Scott, R. H. Guy, and J. Hadgraft, eds.), IBC Technical Services Ltd., London, 1990, p. 213.

138. Mak, V. H. W., Potts, R. O., and Guy, R. H., Percutaneous penetration enhancement in vivo measured by attenuated total reflectance spectroscopy, *Pharm. Res.*, 7:835 (1990).
139. Woodford, R., and Barry, B. W., Optimization and bioavailability of topical steroids: thermodynamic control, *J. Invest. Dermatol.*, 79:388 (1982).
140. Bennett, S. L., Barry, B. W., and Woodford, R., Optimization of bioavailability of topical steroids: non-occluded penetration enhancers under thermodynamic control, *J. Pharm. Pharmacol.*, 37:298 (1984).
141. Franks, N. P., and Levine, Y. K., Low-angle X-ray diffraction. In: *Membrane Spectroscopy* (E. Grell, ed.), Springer-Verlag, Berlin, 1981, p. 437.
142. Rudell, K. M., The protein of the mammalian epidermis, *Adv. Protein Chem.*, 7:253 (1952).
143. Baden, H. P., and Gifford, A. M., Isometric contraction of epidermis and stratum corneum with heating, *J. Invest. Dermatol.*, 54:298 (1970).
144. Baden, H. P., Goldsmith, L. A., and Bonar, L., Conformational changes in the α-fibrous proteins of epidermis, *J. Invest. Dermatol.*, 60:215 (1973).
145. Garson, J. C., Doucet, J., Leveque, J. L., and Tsoucaris, G., Oriented structure in human stratum corneum revealed by x-ray diffraction, *J. Invest. Dermatol.*, 96:43 (1991).
146. Fribert, S. E., Osborne, D. W., and Tombridge, T. L., X-ray diffraction study of human stratum corneum, *J. Soc. Cosmet. Chem.*, 36:349 (1985).
147. Bouwstra, J. A., de Vries, M. A., Gooris, G. S., Bras, W., Brussee, J., and Ponec, M., Thermodynamic and structural aspects of the skin barrier, *J. Control. Rel.*, 15:29 (1991).
148. Bouwstra, J. A., Bras, W., and Gooris, G. S., Structural aspects of stratum corneum, *Proc. Int. Conf. Prediction of Percutaneous Penetration*; *Methods, Measurements, Modelling*, Southampton, U.K., 1991.
149. Hou, S. Y. E., Mitra, A. K., White, S. H., Menon, G. K., Ghadially, R., and Elias, P. M., Membrane structures in normal and essential fatty acid-deficient stratum corneum: characterization by ruthenium tetroxide staining and x-ray diffraction, *J. Invest. Dermatol.*, 96:215 (1991).
150. Griffith, H. O., and Jost, P. C., Lipid spin labels in biological membranes. In: *Spin Labelling*; *Theory and Applications* (L. J. Berliner, ed.), Academic Press, New York, 1976, p. 453.
151. Schreier, S., Polnaszek, C. F., and Smith, I. C. P., Spin labels in membranes; problems in practice, *Biochim. Biophys. Acta*, 515:375 (1978).
152. Rehfeld, S. J., Plachy, W. Z., Williams, M. L., and Elias, P. M., Calorimetric and electron spin resonance examination of lipid phase transitions in human stratum corneum: molecular basis for normal cohesion and abnormal desquamation in recessive x-linked ichthyosis, *J. Invest. Dermatol.*, 91:499 (1988).
153. Rehfeld, S. J., Plachy, W. Z., Hou, S. Y. E., and Elias, P. M., Localization of lipid microdomains and thermal phenomena in murine stratum corneum and isolated membrane complexes: an electron spin resonance study, *J. Invest. Dermatol.*, 95:217 (1990).
154. Gay, C. L., Hadgraft, J., Kellaway, I. W., Evans, J. C., and Rowlands, C. C., The effects of skin penetration enhancers on human stratum corneum lipids; an electron spin resonance study. In: *Prediction of Percutaneous Penetration*; *Methods, Measurements, Modelling* (R. C. Scott, R. H. Guy, and J. Hadgraft, eds.), IBC Technical Services Ltd., London, 1990, p. 322.
155. Hadgraft, J., Penetration enhancers in percutaneous absorption, *Pharm. Int.*, 5:252 (1984).
156. Woodford, R., and Barry, B. W., Penetration enhancers and the percutaneous absorption of drugs: an update, *J. Toxicol. Cut. Occular Toxicol.*, 5:165 (1986).
157. Hwang, C. C., and Danti, A. G., Percutaneous absorption of flufenamic acid in rabbits: effect of dimethyl sulfoxide and various nonionic surface active agents, *J. Pharm. Sci.*, 72:857 (1983).

158. Spruance, S. L., McKeough, M. B., and Cardinal, J. R., Dimethylsulfoxide as a vehicle for topical antiviral chemotherapy, *Ann. N. Y. Acad. Sci.*, 411:28 (1983).
159. Spruance, S. L., McKeough, M. B., and Cardinal, J. R., Penetration of guinea pig skin by acyclovir in different vehicles and correlation with the efficacy of topical therapy of experimental cutaneous herpes simplex virus infection, *Antimicrob. Agents Chemother.*, 25:10 (1984).
160. Spruance, S. C., Freeman, D. J., and Sheth N. V., Comparison of topically applied 5-ethyl-2′-deoxyuridine and acyclovir in the treatment of cutaneous herpes simplex virus infection in guinea pigs, *Antimicrob. Agents Chemother.*, 28:203 (1985).
161. Aungst, B. J., Rogers, N. J., and Shefter, E., Enhancement of naloxone penetration through human skin in vitro using fatty acids, fatty alcohols, surfactants, sulfoxides and amides, *Int. J. Pharm.*, 33:225 (1986).
162. Kurihara-Bergstrom, T., Flynn, G. L., and Higuchi, W. I., Physicochemical study of percutaneous absorption enhancement by dimethylsulfoxide: kinetic and thermodynamic determinants of dimethyl sulfoxide mediated mass transfer of alkanols, *J. Pharm. Sci.*, 75:479 (1986).
163. Kurihara-Bergstrom, T., Flynn, G. L., and Higuchi, W. I., Physicochemical study of percutaneous absorption enhancement by dimethylsulfoxide: dimethylsulfoxide mediation of vidarabine (ara-A) permeation of hairless mouse skin, *J. Invest. Dermatol.*, 89:274 (1987).
164. Kligman, A. M., Topical pharmacology and toxicology of dimethylsulfoxide, *JAMA*, 193:796 (1965).
165. Al-Saidan, S. M. H., Selkirk, A. B., and Winfield, A. J., Effect of dimethylsulphoxide concentration on the permeability of neonatal rat stratum corneum to alkanols, *J. Invest. Deramtol.*, 89:426 (1987).
166. Munro, D. D., and Stoughton, R. B., Dimethylacetamide (DMAC) and dimethylformamide (DMFA) effect on percutaneous absorption, *Arch. Dermatol.*, 92:585 (1965).
167. Munro, D. D., The relationship between percutaneous absorption and stratum corneum retention, *Br. J. Dermatol.*, 81 (Suppl.):92 (1969).
168. Akerman, B., Haegerstam, G., Pring, B. G., and Sandberg, R., Penetration enhancers and other factors governing percutaneous local anaesthesia with lidocaine, *Acta Pharmacol. Toxicol.*, 45:58 (1979).
169. Southwell, D., and Barry, B. W., Penetration enhancers for human skin: mode of action of 2-pyrrolidone and dimethylformamide on partition and diffusion of model compounds water, *n*-alcohols and caffeine, *J. Invest. Dermatol.*, 80:507 (1983).
170. Southwell, D., and Barry, B. W., Penetration enhancement in human skin: effect of 2-pyrrolidone, dimethylformamide and increased hydration on finite dose permeation of aspirin and caffeine, *Int. J. Pharm.*, 22:291 (1984).
171. Barry, B. W., and Bennett, S. L., Effect of penetration enhancers on the permeation of mannitol, hydrocortisone and progesterone through human skin, *J. Pharm. Pharmacol.*, 39:535 (1987).
172. Sekura, D. L., and Scala, J., The percutaneous absorption of alkyl methyl sulfoxides, *Adv. Biol. Skin*, 12:257 (1972).
173. Cooper, E. R., Effect of decylmethyl sulfoxide on skin penetration. In: *Solution Behaviour of Surfactants: Theoretical and Applied Aspects* (K. L. Wittal and E. J. Fendler, eds.), Plenum Press, New York, 1982, p. 1505.
174. Goodman, M., and Barry, B. W., Action of penetration enhancers on human skin as assessed by the permeation of model drugs 5-fluorouracil and estradiol. I. Infinite dose technique, *J. Invest. Dermatol.*, 91:323 (1988).
175. Akhter, S. A., Bennett, S. L., Waller, I. L., and Barry, B. W., An automated diffusion apparatus for studying skin penetration, *Int. J. Pharm.*, 21:17 (1984).

176. Naito, S. I., Nakamori, S., Awataguchi, M., Nakajima, T., and Tominaga, H., Observations on and pharmacokinetic discussion of percutaneous absorption of mefenamic acid, *Int. J. Pharm.*, 24:127 (1985).
177. Mollgaard, B, Hoelgaard, A., and Baker, E., Vehicle effect on topical drug delivery—effect of *N*-methylpyrrolidone, polar lipids and Azone on percutaneous drug transport, *Proc. Intern. Symp. Control. Rel. Bioact. Mater.*, 15:209 (1988).
178. Hoelgaard, A., Mollgaard, B., and Baker, E., Vehicle effect on topical drug delivery. IV. Effect of *N*-methylpyrrolidone and polar lipids on percutaneous drug transport, *Int. J. Pharm.*, 43:233 (1988).
179. Sasaki, H., Kojima, M., Nakamura, J., and Shibasaki, J., Enhancing effect of combining two pyrrolidone vehicles on transdermal drug delivery, *J. Pharm. Pharmacol.*, 42:196 (1990).
180. Sasaki, H., Kojima, M., Nakamura, J., and Shibasaki, J., Enhancing effect of pyrrolidone derivatives on transdermal penetration of phenolsulfonphthalein and indomethacin from aqueous vehicle, *Chem. Pharm. Bull.*, 38:797 (1990).
181. Sasaki, H., Kojima, M., Nakamura, J., and Shibasaki, J., Enhancing effect of pyrrolidone derivatives on the transdermal penetration of sulfaguanidine, aminopyrine and sudan III, *J. Pharmacobio-Dyn.*, 13:200 (1990).
182. Sasaki, H., Kojima, M., Mori, Y., Nakamura, J., and Shibasaki, J., Enhancing effect of pyrrolidone derivatives on transdermal drug delivery. I., *Int. J. Pharm.*, 44:15 (1988).
183. Sasaki, H., Kojima, M., Mori, Y., Nakamura, J., and Shibasaki, J., Enhancing effect of pyrrolidone derivatives on transdermal drug delivery. II. Effect of application concentration and pretreatment of enhancer, *Int. J. Pharm.*, 60:177 (1990).
184. Cooper, E. R., Increased skin permeability for lipophilic molecules, *J. Pharm. Sci.*, 73:1153 (1984).
185. Aungst, B. J., Structure/effect studies of fatty acid isomers as skin penetration enhancers and skin irritants, *Pharm. Res.*, 6:244 (1989).
186. Goodman, M., and Barry, B. W., Lipid-protein-partitioning (LPP) theory of skin enhancer activity: finite dose technique, *Int. J. Pharm.*, 57:29 (1989).
187. Aungst, B. J., Blake, J. A., and Hussain, M. A., Contributions of drug solubilization, partitioning, barrier disruption and solvent permeation to the enhancement of skin permeation of various compounds with fatty acids and amines, *Pharm. Res.*, 7:712 (1990).
188. Chien, Y. W., Xu, H., Chiang, C. C., and Huang, Y. C., Transdermal controlled administration of vidomethacin. I. Enhancement of skin permeability, *Pharm. Res.*, 5:103 (1988).
189. Yu, D., Sanders, L. M., Davidson, G. W., Marvin, M. J., and Ling, T., Percutaneous absorption of nicardipine and ketorolac in rhesus monkeys, *Pharm. Res.*, 5:457 (1988).
190. Kadir, R., Stempler, D., Liron, Z., and Cohen, S., Delivery of theophylline into excised human skin from alkanoic acid solutions: A "push-pull" mechanism, *J. Pharm. Sci.*, 76:774 (1987).
191. Kadir, R., Stempler, D., Liron, Z., and Cohen, S., Penetration of adenosine into excised human skin: The enhancement factor, *J. Pharm. Sci.*, 77:409 (1988).
192. Chukwumerije, O., Nash, R. A., Matias, J. R., and Orentreich, N., Studies on the efficacy of methyl esters of *n*-alkyl fatty acids as penetration enhancers, *J. Invest. Dermatol.*, 93:349 (1989).
193. Ozawa, Y., Yamahira, T., Sunada, H., and Nadai, T., Influence of fatty acid-alcohol esters on percutaneous absorption of hydrocortisone buyrate propionate, *Chem. Pharm. Bull.*, 36:2145 (1988).
194. Wotton, P. K., Mollgaard, B., Hadgraft, J., and Hoelgaard, A., Vehicle effects on topical drug delivery. III. Effect of Azone on the cutaneous permeation of metronidazole and propylene glycol, *Int. J. Pharm.*, 24:19 (1985).
195. Wiechers, J. W., and de Zeeuw, R. A., Transdermal drug delivery: efficacy and potential applications of the penetration enhancer Azone, *Drug Design Del.*, 6:87 (1990).

196. Hou, S. Y. E., and Flynn, G. L., Enhancement of hydrocortisone permeation of human and hairless mouse skin by 1-dodecylazacycloheptan-2-one, *J. Invest. Dermatol.*, 93:774 (1989).
197. Okamoto, H., Muta, K., Hashida, M., and Sezaki, H., Percutaneous penetration of acyclovir through excised hairless mouse skin: effect of vehicle and percutaneous penetration enhancer, *Pharm. Res.*, 7:64 (1990).
198. Wiechers, J. W., Herder, R. E., Drenth, B. F. H., and de Zeeuw, R. A., Skin stripping as a potential method to determine in vivo cutaneous metabolism of topically applied drugs, *J. Soc. Cosmet. Chem.*, 40:367 (1989).
199. Wiechers, J. W., Drenth, B. F. H., Adolfsen, F. A. W., Prins, L., and de Zeeuw, R. A., Disposition and metabolic profiling of the penetration enhancer Azone. I. In vivo studies. Urinary profiles of hamster, rat, monkey and man, *Pharm. Res.*, 7:496 (1990).
200. Ponec, M., Haverkort, M., Soei, Y. L., Kempenaar, J., Brussee, J., and Bodde, H., Toxicity screening of *N*-alkylazacycloheptan-2-one derivatives in cultured human skin cells; structure–toxicity relationships, *J. Pharm. Sci.*, 78:738 (1989).
201. Walters, K. A., Penetration enhancers and their use in transdermal therapeutic systems. In: *Transdermal Drug Delivery: Developmental Issues and Research Initiatives* (J. Hadgraft and R. H. Guy, eds.), Chap. 10, Marcel Dekker, Inc., New York and Basel, 1989.
202. Walters, K. A., Surfactants and percutaneous absorption. In: *Prediction of Percutaneous Penetration; Methods, Measurements, Modelling* (R. C. Scott, R. H. Guy, and J. Hadgraft, eds.), IBC Technical Services Ltd., London, 1990, p. 148.
203. Tupker, R. A., Pinnagoda, J., and Nater, J. P., The transient and cumulative effect of sodium lauryl sulphate on the epidermal barrier assessed by transepidermal water loss: interindividual variation, *Acta Derm. Venereol. (Stockh.)*, 70:1 (1990).
204. Van Neste, D., In vivo prediction of sodium lauryl sulphate-induced skin damage. In: *Prediction of Percutaneous Penetration; Methods, Measurements, Modelling* (R. C. Scott, R. H. Guy, and J. Hadgraft, eds.), IBC Technical Services Ltd., London, 1990, p. 388.
205. Bodde, H. E., Verhoeven, J., and van Driel, L. M. J., The skin compliance of transdermal drug delivery systems, *Crit. Rev. Ther. Drug Carrier Syst.*, 6:87 (1989).
206. Eagle, S. C., Barry, B. W., and Scott, R. C., Inhibition of the damaging activity of divalent anionic surfactants on human skin. In: *Prediction of Percutaneous Penetration; Methods, Measurements, Modelling* (R. C. Scott, R. H. Guy, and J. Hadgraft, eds.), IBC Technical Services Ltd., London, 1990, p. 417.
207. Sarpotdar, P. P., and Zatz, J. L., Percutaneous absorption enhancement by nonionic surfactants, *Drug Dev. Ind. Pharm.*, 12:1625 (1986).
208. Sarpotdar, P. P., and Zatz, J. L., Evaluation of penetration enhancement of lidocaine by nonionic surfactants through hairless mouse skin in vitro, *J. Pharm. Sci.*, 75:176 (1986).
209. Grice, K., Sattar, H., and Baker, H., Urea and retinoic acid in ichthyosis and their effect on transepidermal water loss and water holding capacity of stratum corneum, *Acta Derm. (Stockh.)*, 53:114 (1973).
210. Woodford, R., and Barry, B. W., Alphaderm cream (1% hydrocortisone plus 10% urea): investigation of vasoconstrictor activity, bioavailability and application regimes in human volunteers, *Curr. Ther. Res.*, 35:759 (1984).
211. Beastall, J., Guy, R. H., Hadgraft, J., and Wilding, I., The influence of urea on percutaneous absorption, *Pharm. Res.*, 3:294 (1986).
212. Naito, S. I., and Tsai, Y. H., Percutaneous absorption of indomethacin from ointment bases in rabbits, *Int. J. Pharm.*, 8:263 (1981).
213. Lippold, B. C., and Hackemuller, D., The influence of skin moisturizers on drug penetration in vivo, *Int. J. Pharm.*, 61:205 (1990).
214. Wong, O., Huntington, J., Konishi, R., Rytting, J. H., and Higuchi, T., Unsaturated cyclic ureas as new non-toxic biodegradable transdermal penetration enhancers, I. Synthesis, *J. Pharm. Sci.*, 77:967 (1988).

215. Wong, O., Tsuzuki, N., Nghiem, B., Kuehnhoff, J., Itoh, T., Masaki, K., Huntingdon, J., Konishi, R., Ryttig, J. H., and Higuchi, T., Unsaturated cyclic ureas as new non-toxic biodegradable transdermal penetration enhancers, II. Evaluation study, *Int. J. Pharm.*, 52:191 (1989).
216. Williams, A. C., and Barry, B. W., Urea analogues in propylene glycol as penetration enhancers in human skin, *Int. J. Pharm.*, 56:43 (1989).
217. Friend, D. R., Catz, P., and Heller, J., Transdermal permeation enhancers for drugs, *Proc. Intern. Symp. Control. Rel. Bioact. Mater.*, 15:152 (1988).
218. Pershing, L. K., Lambert, L. D., and Knutson, K., Mechanism of ethanol-enhanced estradiol permeation across human skin in vivo, *Pharm. Res.*, 7:170 (1990).
219. Higuchi, W. I., Rohr, U. D., Burton, S. A., Liu, P., Fox, J. L., Ghanem, A. H., Mahmoud, H., Borsadia, S., and Good, W. R., Effect of ethanol on the transport of β-estradiol in hairless mouse skin. In: *Controlled Release Technology; Pharmaceutical Applications* (P. I. Lee and W. R. Good, eds.), ACS Symposium Series 348, Chap. 17, American Chemical Society, Washington, 1987.
220. Ghanem, A. H., Mahmoud, H., Higuchi, W. I., Rohr, U. D., Borsadia, S., Liu, P., Fox, J. L., and Good, W. R., The effects of ethanol on the transport of β-estradiol and other permeants in hairless mouse skin. II. A new quantitative approach, *J. Control. Rel.*, 6:75 (1987).
221. Kurihara-Bergstrom, T., Knutson, K., De Noble, L. J., and Goates, C. Y., Percutaneous absorption enhancement of an ionic molecule by ethanol-water systems in human skin, *Pharm. Res.*, 7:762 (1990).
222. Berner, B., Mazzenga, G. C., Otte, J. H., Steffens, R. J., Juang, R. H., and Ebert, C. D., Ethanol:water mutually enhanced transdermal therapeutic system II: Skin permeation of ethanol and nitroglycerin, *J. Pharm. Sci.*, 78:402 (1989).
223. Soan, K. B., Siver, K. G., and Koch, A. M., The effect of vehicle on the diffusion of salicyclic acid through hairless mouse skin, *J. Pharm. Sci.*, 75:744 (1986).
224. Friend, D., Catz, P., Heller, J., Reid, J., and Baker, R., Transdermal delivery of levonorgestrel I. Alkanols as permeation enhancers in vitro, *J. Control. Rel.*, 7:243 (1988).
225. Mollgaard, B., and Hoelgaard A., Permeation of estradiol through skin, effect of vehicles, *Int. J. Pharm.*, 15:185 (1983).
226. Valia, K. H., and Chien, Y. W., Long-term skin permeation kinetics of estradiol (I): Effect of drug solubilizer—polyethylene glycol 400, *Drug Devel. Ind. Pharm.*, 10:951 (1984).
227. Sarpotdar, P. P., Gaskill, J. L., and Giannini, R. P., Effect of polyethylene glycol 400 on the penetration of drugs through human cadaver skin in vitro, *J. Pharm. Sci.*, 75:26 (1986).
228. Wurster, D. E., and Kramer, S. F., Investigation of some factors influencing percutaneous absorption, *J. Pharm. Sci.*, 50:288 (1961).
229. McKenzie, A. W., and Stoughton, R. B., Method for comparing percutaneous absorption of steroids, *Arch. Dermatol.*, 86:608 (1962).
230. Behl, C. R., Flynn, G. L., Kurihara, T., Harper, N., Smith, W., Higuchi, W. I., Ho, N. F. H., and Pearson, C. L., Hydration and percutaneous absorption. I. Influence of hydration on alkanol permeation through hairless mouse skin, *J. Invest. Dermatol.*, 75:346 (1980).
231. Walters, K. A., Walker, M., and Olejnik, O., Hydration and surfactant effects on methyl nicotinate penetration through hairless mouse skin, *J. Pharm. Pharmacol.*, 37 (Suppl.):81P (1985).
232. Lambert, W. J., Higuchi, W. I., Knutson, K., and Krill, S. L., Effects of long-term hydration leading to the development of polar channels in hairless mouse stratum corneum, *J. Pharm. Sci.*, 78:925 (1989).
233. Windheuser, J. J., Haslam, J. L., Caldwell, L., and Shaffer, R. D., The use of *N,N*-diethyl-*m*-toluamide to enhance dermal and transdermal delivery of drugs, *J. Pharm. Sci.*, 81:1211 (1982).

234. Hadgraft, J., Walters, K. A., and Wotton, P. K., Facilitated percutaneous absorption: a comparison and evaluation of two in vitro models, *Int. J. Pharm.*, 32:257 (1986).
235. Fleeker, C., Wong, O., and Rytting, J. H., Facilitated transport of basic and acidic drugs in solutions through snake skin by a new enhancer—dodecyl *N,N*-dimethylamino acetate, *Pharm. Res.*, 6:443 (1989).
236. Wong, O., Huntington, J., Nishihata, T., and Rytting, J. H., New alkyl *N,N*-dialkyl-subsituted amino acetates as transdermal penetration enhancers, *Pharm. Res.*, 6:286 (1989).
237. Mollgaard, B., and Hoelgaard, A., Vehicle effects on topical drug delivery. II. Concurrent skin transport of drugs and vehicle components, *Acta Pharm. Suec.*, 20:443 (1983).
238. Williams, D. G., and Hadgraft, J., Medicinal leech hyaluronidase as a potential skin penetration enhancer: in-vitro permeation studies, *J. Pharm. Pharmacol.*, 42 (Suppl.):85P (1990).
239. Opdyke, D. L. J., Monographs on fragrance raw materials, *Food Cosmet. Toxicol.*, 11-17 (Suppl.): (1973–1979).
240. Simonsen, J. L., *The Terpenes*, Cambridge University Press, New York, 1953.
241. Pinder, A. R., *The Chemistry of the Terpenes*, Chapman and Hall Ltd., London, 1960.
242. Newman, A. A., *Chemistry of Terpenes and Terpenoids*, Academic Press, London and New York, 1972.
243. Zupan, J. A., Use of eucalyptol for enhancing skin permeation of bio-affecting agents, *Eur. Pat.* 0069385, 1982.
244. Leonard, T. W., Mikula, K. K., and Schlesinger, M. S., Carvone enhancement of transdermal drug delivery, *U.S. Pat.* 4,888,360 (1989).
245. Leonard, T. W., Mikula, K. K., and Schlesinger, M. S., Eugenol enhancement of transdermal drug delivery, *U.S. Pat.* 4,888,362 (1989).
246. Nuwayser, E. S., Gay, M. H., De Roo, D. J., and Blaskovich, P. D., Transdermal nicotine—an aid to smoking cessation, *Proc. Intern. Symp. Control. Rel. Bioact. Mater.*, 15:213 (1988).
247. Nagai, T., Yi, Q. D., Higuchi, R. I., Akitoshi, Y., and Takayama, K., Effect of cyclohexanone derivatives on percutaneous absorption of ketoprofen and indomethacin, *Proc. Intern. Symp. Control. Rel. Bioact. Mater.*, 15:154 (1988).
248. Danyi, Q., Takayama, K., and Nagai, T., Effect of cyclohexanone derivatives on in vitro percutaneous absorption of indomethacin, *Drug Design Del.*, 4:323 (1989).
249. Williams, A. C., and Barry, B. W., Essentials oils as novel human skin penetration enhancers, *Int. J. Pharm.*, 57:R7 (1989).
250. Williams, A. C., and Barry, B. W., The use of terpenes as skin penetration enhancers. In: *Prediction of Percutaneous Penetration*; *Methods*, *Measurements*, *Modelling* (R. C. Scott, R. H. Guy, and J. Hadgraft, eds.), IBC Technical Services, Ltd., London 1990, p. 224.
251. Williams, A. C., and Barry, B. W., Terpenes and the lipid-protein-partitioning theory of skin penetration enhancers, *Pharm. Res.*, 8:17 (1991).
252. Barry, B. W., and Williams, A. C., Terpenes as skin penetration enhancers. In: *Pharmaceutical Skin Penetration Enhancement* (K. A. Walters and J. Hadgraft, eds.), Marcel Dekker, Inc., New York and Basel, 1993, p. 95.
253. Williams, A. C., and Barry, B. W., The enhancement index concept applied to terpene penetration enhancers for human skin and model lipophilic (oestradiol) and hydrophilic (5-fluorouracil) drugs, *Int. J. Pharm.*, 74:157 (1991).
254. Nagai, T., Okabe, H., Ogura, A., and Takayama, K., Effect of limonene and related compounds on the percutaneous absorption of indomethacin, *Proc. Intern. Symp. Control. Rel. Bioact. Mater.*, 16:181 (1989).
255. Kadir, R., and Barry, B. W., α-Bisabolol, a possible safe penetration enhancer for dermal and transdermal therapeutics, *Int. J. Pharm.*, 70:87 (1991).

256. Barry, B. W., Action of skin penetration enhancers—the lipid-protein-partitioning theory, *Int. J. Cosmet. Sci.*, 10:281 (1988).
257. Ongpipattanakul, B., Burnette, R. R., Potts, R. O., and Francoeur, M. L., Evidence that oleic acid exists in a separate phase within stratum corneum lipids, *Pharm. Res.*, 8:350 (1991).
258. Guy, R. H., and Hadgraft, J., Selection of drug candidates for transdermal drug delivery. In: *Transdermal Drug Delivery; Developmental Issues and Research Initiatives* (J. Hadgraft and R. H. Guy, eds.), Marcel Dekker, Inc., New York and Basel, 1989, p. 59.
259. Hori, M., Satoh, S., and Maibach, H. I., Classification of percutaneous penetration enhancers: A conceptual diagram. In: *Percutaneous Absorption; Mechanisms, Methodology, Drug Delivery* (R. L. Bronaugh and H. I. Maibach, eds.), 2nd ed., Marcel Dekker, Inc., New York and Basel, 1989, p. 197.
260. Flynn, G. L., and Stewart, B., Percutaneous drug penetration: Choosing candidates for transdermal development, *Drug Develop. Res.*, 13:169 (1988).
261. Cornwell, P. A., and Barry, B. W., *J. Pharm. Pharmacol.*, in press (1994).
262. Cornwell, P. A., Barry, B. W., Bouwstra, J. A., and Gooris, G. S., Small-angle x-ray diffraction investigations of terpene enhancer actions on the lipid barrier in human skin, *3rd International Conference on Prediction of Percutaneous Penetration: Methods, Measurements, Modelling*, Montpellier, France, 1993.
263. Anigbogu, A. N. C., Williams, A. C., Barry, B. W., and Edwards, H. G. M., *J. Pharm. Pharmacol.*, 45 (Suppl.):53P (1993).
264. Anigbogu, A. N. C., Williams, A. C., Barry, B. W., and Edwards, H. G. M., Fourier transform Raman spectroscopy in the study of interactions between terpene penetration enhancers and human skin, *3rd International Conference on Prediction of Percutaneous Penetration: Methods, Measurements, Modelling*, Montpellier, France, 1993.
265. Engblom, J., and Engström, S., Azone and the formation of reversed mono- and bicontinuous lipid-water phases, *Int. J. Pharm.*, 98:173 (1993).
266. Michniak, B. B., Player, M. R., Chapman, J. M., Jr., and Sowell, J. W., Sr., In vitro evaluation of a series of Azone analogs as dermal penetration enhancers. I, *Int. J. Pharm.*, 91:85 (1993).
267. Michniak, B. B., Player, M. R., Fuhrman, L. C., Christensen, C. A., Chapman, J. M., Jr., and Sowell, J. W., Sr., In vitro evaluation of a series of Azone analogs as dermal penetration enhancers. II. (Thio) amides, *Int. J. Pharm.*, 94:203 (1993).
268. Brain, K. R., Hadgraft, J., Lewis, D., and Allan, G., The influence of Azone on the percutaneous absorption of methotrexate, *Int. J. Pharm.*, 71:R9 (1991).
269. Hoogstraate, A. J., Verhoef, J., Brussee, J., Ijzermann, A. P., Spies, F., and Boddé, H. E., Kinetics, ultrastructural aspects and molecular modelling of transdermal peptide flux enhancement by *N*-alkylazacycloheptanones, *Int. J. Pharm.*, 76:37 (1991).
270. Ogiso, T., Iwaki, M., Bechako, K., and Tsutsumi, Y., Enhancement of percutaneous absorption by laurocapram, *J. Pharm. Sci.*, 81:762 (1992).
271. Okamoto, H., Hashida, M., and Sezaki, H., Effect of 1-alkyl- or 1-alkenylazacycloalkanone derivatives on the penetration of drugs with different lipophilicities through guinea pig skin, *J. Pharm. Sci.*, 80:39 (1991).
272. Schückler, F., and Lee, G., Measuring the uptake of Azone into excised human stratum corneum from thin polymer films, *J. Pharm. Pharmacol.*, 45:162 (1993).
273. Watkinson, A. C., Hadgraft, J., and Bye, A., Aspects of the transdermal delivery of prostaglandins, *Int. J. Pharm.*, 74:229 (1991).
274. Schückler, F., and Lee, G., Relating the concentration-dependent action of Azone and dodecyl-L-pyroglutamate on the structure of excised human stratum corneum to changes in drug diffusivity, partition coefficient and flux, *Int. J. Pharm.*, 80:81 (1992).
275. Hirvonen, J., Rytting, J. H., Paronen, P., and Urtti, A., Dodecyl *N,N*-dimethylamino acetate and Azone enhance drug penetration across human, snake, and rabbit skin, *Pharm. Res.*, 8:933 (1991).

276. Turunen, T. M., Buyuktimkin, S., Buyuktimkin, N., Urtti, A., Paronen, P., and Rytting, J. H., Enhanced delivery of 5-fluorouracil through shed snake skin by two new transdermal penetration enhancers, *Int. J. Pharm.*, 92:89 (1993).
277. Dolezal, P., Hrabálek, A., and Semecký, V., ϵ-Aminocaproic acid esters as transdermal penetration enhancing agents, *Pharm. Res.*, 10:1015 (1993).
278. Melendres, J. L., Nangia, A., Sedik, L., Hori, M., and Maibach, H. I., Nonane enhances propranolol hydrochloride penetration in human skin, *Int. J. Pharm.*, 92:243 (1993).
279. Hori, M., Satoh, S., Maibach, H. I., and Guy, R. H., Enhancement of propranolol hydrochloride and diazepam skin absorption in vitro: Effect of enhancer lipophilicity, *J. Pharm. Sci.*, 80:32 (1991).
280. Cornwell, P. A., and Barry, B. W., The routes of penetration of ions and 5-fluorouracil across human skin and the mechanisms of action of terpene skin penetration enhancers, *Int. J. Pharm.*, 94:189 (1993).
281. Yano, T., Kanetake, T., Saita, M., and Noda, K., Effects of l-menthol and dl-camphor on the penetration and hydrolysis of methyl salicylate in hairless mouse skin, *J. Pharmacobio-Dyn.*, 14:663 (1991).
282. Kushla, G. P., and Zatz, J. L., Correlation of water and lidocaine flux enhancement by cationic surfactants in vitro, *J. Pharm. Sci.*, 80:1079 (1991).
283. Bialik, W., Walters, K. A., Brain, K. R., and Hadgraft, J., Some factors affecting the in vitro penetration of ibuprofen through human skin, *Int. J. Pharm.*, 92:219 (1993).
284. Friend, D. R., and Smedley, S. I., Solvent drag in ethanol/ethyl acetate enhanced skin permeation of d-norgestrel, *Int. J. Pharm.*, 97:39 (1993).
285. Obata, Y., Takayama, K., Maitani, Y., Machida, Y., and Nagai, T., Effect of ethanol on skin permeation of nonionized ionized diclofenac, *Int. J. Pharm.*, 89:191 (1993).
286. Hatanaka, T., Shimoyama, M., Sugibayashi, K., and Morimoto, Y., Effect of vehicle on the skin permeability of drugs: polyethylene glycol 400-water and ethanol–water binary solvents, *J. Control. Rel.*, 23:247 (1993).
287. Liu, P., Higuchi, W. I., Song, W., Kurihara-Bergstrom, T., and Good, W. R., Quantitative evaluation of ethanol effects on diffusion and metabolism of β-estradiol in hairless mouse skin, *Pharm. Res.*, 8:865 (1991).
288. Liu, P., Kurihara-Bergstrom, T., and Good, W. R., Cotransport of estradiol and ethanol through human skin in vitro: understanding the permeant/enhancer flux relationship, *Pharm. Res.*, 8:938 (1991).
289. Uchida, T., Lee, C. K., Sekiya, N., and Goto, S., Enhancement effect of an ethanol/Panasate 800 binary vehicle on anti-inflammatory drug permeation across excised hairless mouse skin, *Biol. Pharm. Bull.*, 16:168 (1993).
290. Morimoto, Y., Sugibayashi, K., Kobayashi, D., Shoji, H., Yamazaki, J., and Kimura, M., A new enhancer-coenhancer system to increase skin permeation of morphine hydrochloride in vitro, *Int. J. Pharm.*, 91:9 (1993).
291. Lambert, W. J., Kudla, R. J., Holland, J. M., and Curry, J. T., A Biodegradeable transdermal penetration enhancer based on *N*-(2-hydroxyethyl)-2-pyrrolidone I. Synthesis and characterization, *Int. J. Pharm.*, 95:181 (1993).
292. Kim, C.-K., Hong, M.-S., Kim, Y.-B., and Han, S.-K., Effect of penetration enhancers (pyrrolidone derivatives) on multilamellar liposomes of stratum corneum lipid: a study by UV spectroscopy and differential scanning calorimetry, *Int. J. Pharm.*, 95:43 (1993).
293. Sasaki, H., Kojima, M., Mori, Y., Nakamura, J., and Shibasaki, J., Enhancing effect of pyrrolidone derivatives on transdermal penetration of 5-fluorouracil, triamcinolone acetonide, indomethacin, and flurbiprofen, *J. Pharm. Sci.*, 80:533 (1991).
294. Seki, T., Kawaguchi, T., Juni, K., Sugibayashi, K., and Morimoto, Y., Sustained transdermal delivery of zidovudine via controlled release of penetration enhancer, *J. Control. Rel.*, 17:41 (1991).

295. Kasting, G. B., Francis, W. R., and Roberts, G. E., Skin penetration enhancement of triprolidine base by propylene glycol, *J. Pharm. Sci.*, 82:551 (1993).
296. Komata, Y., Inaoka, M., Kaneko, A., and Fujie, T., In vitro percutaneous absorption of thiamine disulfide from a mixture of propylene glycol and fatty acid, *J. Pharm. Sci.*, 81:744 (1992).
297. Moody, R. P., Wester, R. C., Melendres, J. L., and Maibach, H. I., Dermal absorption of the phenoxy herbicide 2,4-D dimethylamine in humans: effect of DEET and anatomic site, *J. Toxicol. Environ. Health.*, 36:241 (1992).
298. Vollmer, U., Müller, B. W., Mesens, J., Wilffert, B., and Peters, T., In vivo skin pharmacokinetics of liarozole: percutaneous absorption studies with different formulations of cyclodextrin derivatives in rats, *Int. J. Pharm.*, 99:51 (1993).
299. Loftsson, T., and Bodor, N., Effects of 2-hydroxypropyl-β-cyclodextrin on the aqueous solubility of drugs and transdermal delivery of 17β-estradiol, *Acta Pharm. Nord.*, 1:185 (1989).
300. Loftsson, T., Brewster, M. E., Derendorf, H., and Bodor, N., 2-Hydroxypropyl-β-cyclodextrin: properties and usage in pharmaceutical formulations, *Pharm, Ztg. Wiss.*, 136:5 (1991).
301. Loftsson, T., Ólafsdóttir, B. J., and Bodor, N., The effects of cyclodextrins on transdermal delivery of drugs, *Eur. J. Pharm. Biopharm.*, 37:30 (1991).
302. Aioi, A., Kuriyama, K., Shimizu, T., Yoshioka, M., and Uenoyama, S., Effects of vitamin E and squalene on skin irritation of a transdermal absorption enhancer, lauroylsarcosine, *Int. J. Pharm.*, 93:1 (1993).
303. Carelli, V., Di Colo, G., Nannipieri, E., and Serafini, M. F., Bile acids as enhancers of steroid penetration through excised hairless mouse skin, *Int. J. Pharm.*, 89:81 (1993).
304. Lerk, P. C., and Sucker, H., Application of sucrose laurate in topical preparations of cyclosporin A, *Int. J. Pharm.*, 92:203 (1993).

BRIAN W. BARRY
ADRIAN C. WILLIAMS

INDEX TO VOLUME 11